Dermato-toxicology

Dermato-toxicology

second edition

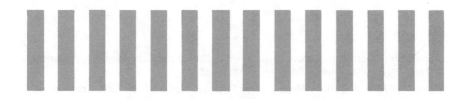

edited by

Francis N. Marzulli
National Academy of Sciences

Howard I. Maibach
University of California
San Francisco Medical Center

HEMISPHERE PUBLISHING CORPORATION
Washington   New York   London

DISTRIBUTION OUTSIDE THE UNITED STATES
McGRAW–HILL INTERNATIONAL BOOK COMPANY
Auckland   Bogotá   Guatemala   Hamburg   Johannesburg   Lisbon
London   Madrid   Mexico   Montreal   New Delhi   Panama   Paris
San Juan   São Paulo   Singapore   Sydney   Tokyo   Toronto

Chapter 23 was adapted from material published in *Clinical and Experimental Dermatology* and is reprinted with permission from the editor.

Chapter 26, "Drug- and Heavy Metal-Induced Hyperpigmentation" by R. D. Granstein and A. J. Sober, was reprinted with permission from the *Journal of the American Academy of Dermatology*, 5:1–18, 1981.

DERMATOTOXICOLOGY, Second Edition

1 2 3 4 5 6 7 8 9 0   B C B C   8 9 8 7 6 5 4 3 2

This book was set in Press Roman by Hemisphere Publishing Corporation. The editors were Anne Shipman and Mary Dorfman; the designers were Lilia N. Guerrero and Sharon Martin DePass; the production supervisor was Miriam Gonzalez; and the typesetter was Sandra F. Watts.
BookCrafters, Inc., was printer and binder.

Library of Congress Cataloging in Publication Data
Main entry under title:

Dermatotoxicology.

    Rev. ed. of: Dermatotoxicology and pharmacology.
c1977.
    Bibliography: p.
    Includes index.
    1. Skin–Diseases. 2. Toxicology. 3. Contact dermatitis. 4. Dermatopharmacology. I. Marzulli, Francis Nicholas, date. II. Maibach, Howard I. [DNLM: 1. Skin diseases–Etiology. WR 140 D43518]
RL72.D47   1983   616.5   82-9234
ISBN 0-89116-250-X   AACR2

contents

contributors

Robert B. Armstrong, M.D.
Department of Dermatology, Columbia University, College of Physicians and Surgeons, 630 West 168th Street, New York, New York 10032

Monica C. Bischoff
Associate, Institute of Neurotoxicity, Albert Einstein College of Medicine, 1300 Morris Park Avenue, Bronx, New York 10461

Fred G. Bock, Ph.D.
Roswell Park Memorial Institute, New York State Department of Health, 666 Elm Street, Buffalo, New York 14263

Robert L. Bronaugh, Ph.D.
Dermal and Ocular Toxicology Branch, Food and Drug Administration, 200 C Street, S.W., Washington, D.C. 20204

K. D. Crow, M.D.
Wiltshire Area Health Authority, Swindon Health District, Princess Margaret Hospital, Okus Road, Swindon SN1 4JU, England

Paul H. Dugard, Ph.D.
Central Toxicology Laboratory, Imperial Chemical Industries Limited, Alderly Park, Cheshire, England

Henry F. Edelhauser, Ph.D.
Department of Ophthalmology, Medical College of Wisconsin, Milwaukee, Wisconsin 53201

John H. Epstein, M.D.
Department of Dermatology, University of California, San Francisco Medical Center, 3rd Avenue and Parnassus, San Francisco, California 94143

William L. Epstein, M.D.
Department of Dermatology, University of California, San Francisco Medical Center, 3rd Avenue and Parnassus, San Francisco, California 94143

Gerald A. Gellin, M.D.
Department of Dermatology, University of California, San Francisco Medical Center, 3rd Avenue and Parnassus, San Francisco, California 94143

Albert Giles, Jr., B.S.
Division of Toxicology, Food and Drug Administration, 200 C Street, S.W., Washington, D.C. 20204

Richard D. Granstein, M.D.
Department of Dermatology,
Massachusetts General Hospital, Boston,
Massachusetts 02114

Leonard C. Harber, M.D.
Department of Dermatology, Columbia
University, College of Physicians and
Surgeons, 630 West 168th Street,
New York, New York 10032

Niels Hjorth, M.D.
Department of Dermatology, Gentofte
Hospital, DK-2900 Hellerup, Copenhagen,
Denmark

Kays Kaidbey, M.D.
Department of Dermatology, University of
Pennsylvania, School of Medicine, 34th
at Spruce, Philadelphia, Pennsylvania 19104

Georg Klecak, M.D.
Department of Biological and Pharma-
ceutical Research, F. Hoffman-La Roche
& Company, Ltd., Basle, Switzerland

Albert M. Kligman, M.D.
Department of Dermatology, University of
Pennsylvania, School of Medicine, 34th
at Spruce, Philadelphia, Pennsylvania 19104

Andrija Kornhauser, Ph.D.
Division of Toxicology, Food and Drug
Administration, 200 C Street, S.W.,
Washington, D.C. 20204

Arthur H. McCreesh, Ph.D.
U.S. Army Environmental Hygiene Agency,
Toxicology Division, Aberdeen Proving
Ground, Maryland 21010

T. O. McDonald, Ph.D.
Alcon Laboratories, Fort Worth, Texas
76101

Bertil Magnusson, M.D.
Department of Dermatology, University
of Lund, Malmo, Sweden

H. C. Maguire, Jr., M.D.
Dermatology Department, Hahnemann
Medical College, 230 North Broad,
Philadelphia, Pennsylvania 19102

Howard I. Maibach, Ph.D.
Department of Dermatology, University of
California, San Francisco Medical Center,
3rd Avenue and Parnassus, San Francisco,
California 94143

Francis N. Marzulli, Ph.D.
National Academy of Sciences, 2101
Constitution Avenue, N.W., Washington,
D.C. 20037

C. G. Toby Mathias, M.D.
Department of Dermatology, University of
California, San Francisco Medical Center,
3rd Avenue and Parnassus, San Francisco,
California 94143

Torkil Menné, M.D.
Department of Dermatology, Gentofte
Hospital, DK-2900 Hellerup, Copenhagen,
Denmark

John E. Milner, M.D.
Department of Environmental Health,
SC-34, School of Public Health and
Community Medicine and Department of
Dermatology, School of Medicine, University
of Washington, 1959 N.E. Pacific, Seattle,
Washington 98195

Patrick K. Noonan, Ph.D.
Departments of Pharmaceutical Chemistry
and Dermatology, University of California,
San Francisco Medical Center, 3rd Avenue
and Parnassus, San Francisco, California
94143

John R. T. Reeves, Ph.D.
University of California, San Francisco
Medical Center, 3rd Avenue and Parnassus,
San Francisco, California 94143

Edward L. Rongone, M.D.
Department of Biochemistry, Creighton
University School of Medicine, 24th and
California, Omaha, Nebraska 68131

Van Seabaugh, M.A.
Consumer Product Safety Commission,
200 C Street, S.W., 5th Floor, Washington,
D.C. 20204

John A. Shadduck, Ph.D.
*Department of Pathology, University
of Texas, Southwestern Medical School,
Dallas, Texas 75235*

Alan R. Shalita, M.D.
*Division of Dermatology, State University
of New York, Downstate Medical School,
New York, New York 11203*

Arthur J. Sober, M.D.
*Department of Dermatology, Massachusetts
General Hospital, Boston, Massachusetts
02114*

Peter S. Spencer, Ph.D.
*Institute of Neurotoxicology, Albert Einstein
College of Medicine, 1300 Morris Park
Avenue, Bronx, New York 10461*

Marshall Steinberg, Ph.D.
*Hazleton Laboratories America, Inc., 9200
Leesburg Pike, Vienna, Virginia 22180*

Frederick Urbach, M.D.
*Center for Photobiology, Temple University
School of Medicine, 3401 North Broad,
Philadelphia, Pennsylvania 19140*

Geo von Krogh, M.D.
*Department of Dermatology, University of
California, San Francisco Medical Center,
3rd Avenue and Parnassus, San Francisco,
California 94143*

Jan E. Wahlberg, M.D.
*Department of Occupational Dermatology,
National Board of Occupation Safety and
Health and Karolinska Sjukhuset, Stock-
holm, Sweden*

Wayne Wamer, B.S.
*Division of Toxicology, Food and Drug
Administration, 200 C Street, S.W.,
Washington, D.C. 20204*

Ronald C. Wester, Ph.D.
*Department of Dermatology, University of
California, San Francisco Medical Center,
3rd Avenue and Parnassus, San Francisco,
California 94143*

preface

This edition updates many chapters of the first edition and eliminates certain topics found only in that edition (sweat and sebaceous gland toxicology, histologic and immunologic aspects of contact dermatitis, effects of drugs on cutaneous microbial flora, and cutaneous manifestations of food intolerance). The intent is to limit the size of this edition while increasing the scope of certain subjects.

We revised the order of presentation beginning with a brief description of the skin itself, its structure, function, and biochemistry. From this background information we proceed to a discussion of the barrier functions of skin and factors involved in dermal penetration with the thought that a topically applied substance must first penetrate the skin if it is to sensitize, irritate, or result in systemic effects. We present a more comprehensive treatment of this important subject with greater attention to practical and *in vitro* studies as well as theoretical considerations.

We follow this with an expanded section on skin sensitization, including a comparison of animal and human findings. Information on skin irritation has been up-dated.

We expanded our coverage of photobiology because of increasing recent interest and concerns in this area.

Finally, we introduce varied subjects of more than peripheral interest to many dermatotoxicologists, such as skin carcinogenesis, chloracne, pigmentation, eczema, urticaria, granulomas, hair, and sebaceous gland toxicology. Neurotoxic substances and toxicity from heavy metals are also discussed. Eye irritation is placed near the end of the book not because of a lack of importance but simply because the eye, though it shares many anatomic similarities to skin, is a separate and distinctly unique organ.

Test methods suggested by the Interagency Regulatory Liaison Group (IRLG) and Organization for Economic Cooperation and Development (OECD) are provided as appendixes for those toxicologists interested in regulatory agency guidelines. The IRLG is no longer a functioning group, however, and their guidelines are included for interest only.

Recent activities by animal welfare groups have resulted in a reappraisal of animal test methods with interest in using tissues or cell cultures in place of animals. The development of the Ames test for predicting carcinogenic potential was a leading stimulus to this type of effort. However, the Ames test has its limitations and toxicologists have been concerned for years about the applicability of animal tests to humans. But there is an even greater divergence between *in vitro* systems and humans. Tests involving complicated mechanisms, such as those that occur in immunology, require intact animals and become exceedingly difficult to replace by *in vitro* methods. The rabbit eye test for eye irritation has received wide adverse publicity by animal welfare groups. Yet, even with its limitations, the rabbit eye has an important capacity not shared by tissue cultures—it offers a time-frame for recovery when injured. Also, it possesses anatomical structures such as the cornea, iris, and conjunctiva that are not unlike those of humans. If investigators treat the rabbit eye with the care used in human ocular experimentation this should substantially alleviate public concern for this issue.

In the future we may see a proliferation of *in vitro* test methods as pressures to replace animal testing develop. Only time will tell how useful they are.

Francis N. Marzulli
Howard I. Maibach

preface
to the first edition

Dermatotoxicology, a relatively new discipline, is defined as a science that deals with adverse skin effects and the substances that produce them. This volume represents a first attempt at consolidating recent developments in various aspects of skin research of interest and concern to researchers in dermatotoxicology.

Three key subdisciplines are skin irritation, skin sensitization, and skin penetration. Skin metabolism and skin carcinogenesis are related important subdisciplines. Pharmacologic aspects of skin are for the most part concerned with skin appendages such as the eccrine glands and the pilosebaceous apparatus.

A section on immunology is included as the basis of understanding allergic contact dermatitis. The science of immunology has undergone an explosion of new developments, some of which provide a better understanding of the complicated mechanisms that may be involved in skin sensitization. Eye irritation is included in this volume primarily because of a traditional linkage of eye and skin irritation.

Different in scope from those texts that deal with clinical dermatology or cosmetic science, this volume attempts to provide useful background, reference, and up-to-date state of the art information in areas such as skin irritation, skin sensitization, and skin penetration. The contents should be of special interest to those engaged in evaluating toxicologic safety; much of the impetus to the development of dermatotoxicology as a separate discipline derives from government regulations suggesting and sometimes demanding that certain products applied to the skin should be evaluated for toxic hazard prior to reaching the market place. This volume provides background information rather than specific test methodologies.

Because recent developments in some of these areas have been rapid and because of the time involved in the preparation of any such volume, some parts may be outdated by publication date. Certain chapters that were expected to have involved more extensive coverage were reduced in scope and others were eliminated in order to meet deadlines. We believe nevertheless that this represents a satisfactory beginning in this relatively new discipline and that it fulfills a need and provides a groundwork on which future authors can build.

We want to acknowledge the assistance in the review of manuscripts by Carl Bruch, John Lucas, Helen Reynolds, Joseph McLoughlin, Max Samter, Andrew Ulsamer, Robert Hehir, Van Seabaugh, Anne Wolven, Paige Yoder, William Markland, Leon Sanders, and Elizabeth Weisburger. We thank Mary Phillips, our editor at Hemisphere, for her valuable assistance in transforming our manuscript into a book.

Francis N. Marzulli
Howard I. Maibach

Dermato-
toxicology

1

skin structure, function, and biochemistry

■ Edward L. Rongone ■

INTRODUCTION

The normal sequence of metabolic transformations in an individual is the governing factor in determining one's state of health. The great majority of these processes occur in tissues and organs that are well protected from the environment. However, the skin, which has many important physiological functions in humans, is exposed to all elements of the environment. The outward appearance of skin is dependent not only on its environment but also on complex metabolic pathways within the skin and other organs of the body. The complex biotransformations that occur in the skin are often referred to as "cutaneous metabolism."

Skin, one of the largest organs of the body, constitutes approximately 10% of the normal body weight. Several important functions have been attributed to skin, such as regulation of the body temperature, protection from the environment, and partial regulation of water loss and retention. A newer function attributed to skin is its role as a temporary storage site for glucose when blood glucose is elevated (Johnson and Fusaro, 1972.)

Several other important biochemical properties are associated with the skin, such as melanin formation regulated by the melanocyte-stimulating hormone (Lerner and McGuire, 1961), epinephrine stimulation of the sweat glands (Wada, 1950), protein synthesis (Freedberg, 1972), androgen regulation of sebum production by the sebaceous glands (Strauss and Pochi, 1963), insulin regulation of carbohydrate and lipid metabolism (Kahlenberg and Kalant, 1966; Hsia et al., 1966a, 1966b), and complete regeneration of viable

1

epidermal cells. More specific examples of biotransformations occurring within the skin will be discussed in the appropriate sections of this chapter. Only a brief description of skin will be given here, since this topic is covered extremely well in many books related to dermatology and histology (Rothman, 1954; Montagna, 1962; Pillsbury, 1971).

PROPERTIES OF SKIN

Structure

The skin is an organ consisting of two different layers that are derived from different germ layers. These layers are known as epidermis and dermis, and their characteristics are different. The thinner, outer layer (epidermis) is epithelial tissue derived from ectoderm. The thicker, relatively inert inner layer (dermis) consists mainly of connective tissue and has a mesodermal origin. The dermis constitutes approximately 90-95% of the mass of human skin, whereas the smaller epidermal layer accounts for the major portion of the biochemical transformations that occur in skin. However, the skin appendages that extend down into the dermal layer, such as sweat glands, hair follicles, and sebaceous glands, are also metabolically important. These appendages are formed during embryonic development from developing epidermal cells that invade the developing dermal layer.

Skin thickness varies with location in humans. The epidermis is approximately 0.1 mm and the dermis 2-4 mm thick. The skin on the palms and soles has a much thicker epidermis than that in other areas. The skin at these locations has a thick layer of keratin, whereas the skin at other locations has a relatively thin layer. The dermoepidermal interface is characterized by dermoepidermal ridges and interpapillary pegs. Dermoepidermal ridges provide maximum interface area between the epidermis and dermis. This dermoepidermal relationship is of great importance when one considers that the nutrients for the epidermis must come from the dermis, since there is no blood supply in the epidermis.

Epidermal Characteristics

The epidermis is a thin layer of cells overlying the dermis. It consists of several types of cells. The innermost type is known as the stratum germinativum (basal cell layer), and is followed by the stratum spinosum (prickle cell layer), stratum granulosum, stratum lucidum, and (the outermost layer) stratum corneum. The combined stratum spinosum and stratum germinativum are often referred to as the Malpighian layer. The basal cell layer consists of one layer of columnar epithelial cells which, upon division, are pushed up into the prickle cell layer. In humans, the prickle cell layer consists of several layers, believed to be held together by tiny intercellular fibrils known as tonofibrils (Odland, 1960) that pass from one cell to another.

As the prickle cells approach the surface of the skin they become larger and form the stratum granulosum, which is two to four cells thick. The keratohyalin granules are formed in this layer. In the stratum granulosum the nuclei are either broken up or dissolved, resulting in the death of the epidermal cell, and the number of cytoplasmic granules increased.

The next layer, stratum lucidum, is ill defined except in areas of thick skin. This layer is said to consist of eleidin, which is presumed to be a transformation product of the keratohyalin present in the stratum granulosum. In the outermost layer, the stratum corneum, the eleidin has been converted into keratin, which represents the ultimate fate of the epidermal cell. Keratin, continuously sloughed off or worn away, must continuously be replaced by the cells beneath it. This sequential transformation and migration of the living basal cells to the dead epithelial cells of the stratum corneum (horny scales) represents a protective action of the skin against foreign objects that penetrate the outer skin barriers. The time required for a basal cell to migrate from the stratum germinativum to the outer part of the stratum corneum has been estimated to be 26–28 days. The extremely metabolically active basal cells lie adjacent to the dermis, which has the only blood supply to the skin and a higher oxygen tension than the other layers of the epidermis.

Dermal Characteristics

The dermis is a thick fibrous network of collagen and elastin, which serves as a supporting unit for the epidermis. It is composed of two layers. The outer, thinner one is called the papillary layer because of its prominent papillae, and it merges with the thicker reticular layer. The papillary layer has a finer structure than the reticular layer because its collagen fibers are not as coarse as those in the reticular layer. The papillae are well nourished by the capillaries that are prominent in them, and the biologically active epidermis is supplied with its essential nutrients by these capillaries. Exchange of nutrients and waste products between the blood and epidermis occurs by diffusion through the dermis, which is thought to serve as a large reservoir of nutrients for the metabolically active epidermis (Johnson and Fusaro, 1972). The blood supply to the skin appears to exceed the nutritional needs of the epidermis; Champion (1970) reported that blood flow rates vary from slightly more than 0 to approximately 2.5 ml/min/100 g tissue, which is adequate to meet nutritional needs. High blood flow rates (100 ml/100 g tissue), which may occur at times in the extremities, are considered to be for the dissipation of body heat. Burton (1961) reported that a blood flow rate of 0.1 ml/min/ 100 g tissue would supply adequate oxygen for the metabolic needs of the skin.

The dermis contains several types of cells, namely fibroblasts, fat cells, macrophages, histiocytes, mast cells, and cells associated with the blood vessels and nerves of the skin. The predominant cell is the fibroblast, which is associated with biosynthesis of the fibrous proteins and ground substances.

Hyaluronic acid, chondroitin sulfates, and mucopolysaccharides are a few of the macromolecular ground substances.

Several investigators (Van Scott and Reinertson, 1961; Billingham and Silver, 1967) have reported that in transplant experiments the differentiation and type (pathological or normal) of epidermal tissue is usually controlled by the dermis. The dermis has an abundance of water, which is available to the body during periods of water deprivation (Eisele and Eichelberger, 1945; Flemister, 1941–1942). Excellent reviews related to skin and its water-binding relationships have been written by Carruthers (1962) and Bentley (1970).

Cutaneous Appendages

The appendages of skin are hair follicles, sebaceous glands, eccrine and apocrine sweat glands, hair, nails, and arrectores pilorum muscle.

In the second month of fetal development, small epidermal growths invade the underlying dermis. These growths are first observed in regions of the eyebrows, chin, and upper lips. General development occurs at about the fourth month over the major portion of the body. These invaginations eventually become hair follicles, which give rise to hair growth. Hair follicles develop at fixed distances, and as the surface area increases they become more widely separated; however, no new follicles are developed after birth. The wide variance in follicle densities at different locations in the adult is accounted for by the highly variable increase of surface area between various body sites (Szabo et al., 1958). Hair follicles extend from the dermis through the epidermal layer at a slight angle. The deeper portion of a hair follicle has a bulblike structure, which extends into the deeper layers of dermis. At the lower edge of this bulblike structure is the dermal papilla (germinal matrix of cells), which is bathed in a highly vascularized connective tissue. This tissue of the hair follicle papilla is one of the most metabolically active in the body.

The epidermal invagination between the germinal matrix and the skin surface becomes canalized and is known as the external root sheath of the hair follicle. Near the surface of the skin the external root sheath exhibits layers somewhat similar to those in the epidermis, but as it extends downward toward the germinal papilla it tends to lose some of the more outward layers.

As the cells of the germinal matrix proliferate, the uppermost ones are forced up into the external root sheath. As they move farther up the sheath the transition into keratin occurs, and growing hair eventually protrudes from the epidermis. The sebaceous glands are usually formed in the upper third of the hair follicle as it develops and they grow out into the surrounding dermis. The ducts of the sebaceous glands empty into the follicles at the site where they were formed. Sebaceous glands are distributed over most of the body; exceptions are the palms, soles, and lower lip. They vary in size and number depending on the area of skin. Areas of greatest concentration occur on the scalp, nose, forehead, face, and axillary regions.

The sebaceous glands synthesize and secrete their characteristic lipids into the pilary canal and subsequently to the surface of the skin. The glands are holocrine and their secretions (sebum) are related directly to the size and turnover rate of the glands. Areas of the body that tend to become oily generally have the greatest density of hair follicles and sebaceous glands.

The size and cellular turnover rates of the sebaceous glands are under hormonal control, with particular sensitivity to the androgens. Epstein and Epstein (1966) employed autoradiographic techniques in the elucidation of cell renewal and differentiation in the human sebaceous gland. Using [³H] thymidine, they demonstrated that radioactivity was present in the outer layers of the sebaceous gland in the germinative layer 40 min after injection of the isotope. The labeled cells were pushed to the center of the gland within 7-9 days and began to differentiate at approximately 14 days. The ultrastructural events in the sebaceous gland's life cycle were reviewed by Zelickson (1967), who divided the cells into three different types: (1) peripheral cells, which are located next to the basement membrane and are rich in ribosomes; (2) partially differentiated cells, which are active in the synthesis and storage of sebum droplets; and (3) fully differentiated cells, which contain vacuoles that will be released when the cells rupture.

Normal sebum secretion by the sebaceous gland is a result of several processes: (1) proliferation of the basal cells of the gland, (2) forcing of basal cells toward the cavity of the gland as cell multiplication continues, (3) accumulation of lipids in the cells as they migrate toward the center of the gland, and (4) necrosis of the cells, which results in expulsion of the cellular debris as sebum.

Expulsion of the sebum into the pilary canal and eventually the hair follicle can be caused by contraction of the minute arrector pili muscle. Contraction of this muscle also causes the hair to become erect. At times this occurs during fear, which has led to the old saying about "hair standing on end."

The activity of hair follicles changes in a cyclic fashion, resulting in three stages of hair growth: (1) growing phase (anagen), (2) transitional phase (catagen), and (3) resting phase (telogen). The reader is referred to an excellent book edited by Montagna and Ellis (1958) for more details on hair growth.

Sweat glands are simple tubular glands, which number approximately 3 million over the entire body. There are 3,000 per square inch in the palm. Each gland consists of two parts, the secretory part and the excretory duct. The secretory part, which is located immediately below the dermis in the subcutaneous tissue, is coiled and twisted on itself and engulfed in blood vessels. After extensive coiling it changes into an excretory duct, which extends toward the surface. The ducts follow a spiral pathway through the dermis and epidermis and open in the surfaces of the ridges of the skin.

Sweat glands are divided into two classes, the eccrines and the apocrines. Eccrine sweat glands are distributed over the entire body, and their main function is secreting water to cool the skin's surface and subsequently to dissipate excess body heat. These glands are sensitive to environmental and pyrogenic changes in temperature and to certain types of nervous stimuli. They may be inhibited by anticholinergics and stimulated by sympathomimetic drugs.

Apocrine sweat glands, more localized than the eccrines, are found in the axillary areas, genitalia, and nipples. They are larger than the eccrine glands, are coiled and tubular, and do not open onto the skin's surface. Like sebaceous glands, they empty their secretions directly into the pilary canal. These secretions then reach the outer surface of the epidermis with the sebum of the sebaceous gland. Human apocrine glands are poorly innervated compared to eccrine glands. The amount of apocrine sweat is small compared to eccrine sweat; its chemical composition is difficult to ascertain since it is expelled in conjunction with sebum. Apocrine secretion is odorless, and characteristic odors attributed to it arise from the decomposition products of bacterial action on the constituents of the secretion at the skin's surface. Controlling these odors is a primary concern of the cosmetic industry.

Fingernails and toenails develop from the epidermis during the end of the third month of embryonic life. The rate of nail growth differs at different ages and may be affected by hormonal deficiencies, certain diseases, and, at times, by psychological disturbances (Ham and Leeson, 1961).

CARBOHYDRATE METABOLISM IN THE SKIN

Enzymes

In many instances, metabolic pathways can be more reliably identified through the enzymes related to them than through the metabolic products. An excellent example is the relationship between the citric acid cycle and amino acid metabolism. Oxalacetic acid and α-ketoglutaric acid are intermediates in the citric acid cycle, but they may also be produced by deamination of their respective amino acids, aspartic and glutaric acids. Other intermediates of the citric acid cycle may be related to lipid metabolism.

Histochemical and biochemical techniques have been used in identifying enzymes in skin, and for general purposes it may be said that skin possesses most of the major metabolic pathways. The metabolic pathways in skin have been investigated by general procedures involving, for example, tissue slices of whole skin, epidermis and dermis homogenates, and differential centrifugation. A technique for the perfusion of isolated dog skin, reported by Kjaersgaard (1954), was used by Halprin and Chow (1961) when they observed the incorporation of $[^{14}C]$ acetate into citric acid cycle intermediates by dog skin. Their preparations were enzymatically active up to 48 h if heparinized and kept in a deep-freeze.

Enzymes associated with aerobic and anaerobic glycolysis in skin have been demonstrated in several species as well as man (Cruickshank et al., 1957, 1958; Zelickson, 1960; Griesemer and Gould, 1954; Rippa and Vignali, 1965; Halprin and Ohkawara, 1966a, 1966b; Mier and Cotton, 1970; Kondo and Gerna-Torsellini, 1974).

Enzyme activities are higher in the epidermis than in the dermis (Weber, 1964).

Oxygen uptake by skin was demonstrated by several investigators, suggesting the presence of the citric acid cycle in skin (e.g., Halprin and Chow, 1961).

The hexose monophosphate shunt has been demonstrated in skin in humans and other species (Freinkel, 1960; Pomerantz and Asbornsin, 1961). The detection of glucose-6-phosphogluconic dehydrogenase was reported by Rippa and Vignali (1965), Halprin and Ohkawara (1966a, 1966b), Freinkel (1960), and Jacobson and Davidson (1962).

Since the skin uses glycogen as well as glucose as a source of energy, the identification of enzymes for its synthesis and breakdown has been undertaken by many investigators. Braun-Falco (1954) showed by histochemical methods that fetal human epidermis contained large amounts of glycogen up to 6 months of age, whereas glycogen could only be found in the stratum spinosum and keratohyalin-containing cells of the adult. These experiments are of interest since glycogen may be detected in the basal cells of the epidermis under inflammatory stimuli and traumatic conditions (Lobitz et al., 1962). Glycogen was detected in the basal cells 4 hr after trauma reached a maximum and approximately 8–16 hr later, and then decreased. Adachi (1962) has shown that in dogs glycogen synthesis first decreases after X-ray irradiation and then increases and reaches a maximum rate in 24 hr. A simultaneous decrease in phosphorylase activity and an increase in UDPG synthetase occurred.

Halprin and Ohkawara (1966a) demonstrated the presence in human epidermis of the glycogen synthesizing enzymes UDPG pyrophosphorylase and glycogen synthetase, as well as hexokinase, phosphoglucomutase, glucose-6-phosphate dehydrogenase, phosphorylase, and UDPG dehydrogenase. Adachi (1961) showed the presence of glycogen synthetase in dog skin and demonstrated that perfusion of $[^{14}C]$glucose through living dog skin resulted in the recovery of radioactive glycogen, and that glycogen synthesis was in a dynamic equilibrium with its degradation.

Glycogen degradation may follow two different metabolic processes in human epidermis. Weber (1964) and Johnson and Fusaro (1972) cite several references related to the identification of an α-amylase in skin. The action and purpose of the α-amylase needs clarification.

Enzymes related to glycogen breakdown in skin by the phosphorylase system have been described by Adachi (1961), Mier and Cotton (1967), Leathwood and Ryman (1971), and Ellis and Montagna (1958). Sato and Dobson (1970) demonstrated Mg-K-Na-activated ATPase enzyme systems in the palmar sweat glands of the rhesus monkey.

DeBersaques (1977) determined the activities of eight enzymes related to carbohydrate metabolism in human epidermal tumors. He observed that the activities were increased in basal cell epithelioma, variable in squamous cell epithelioma and verruca seborrheica, and lowered in keratoacanthoma. The results of DeBersaques are shown in Table 1.

Cutaneous Glucose

Several excellent reviews have been published on carbohydrates in skin (Pillsbury, 1931; Rothman, 1954; Johnson and Fusaro, 1972). Carbohydrates in skin became of interest to investigators after the report of Urbach and Fantl (1928) describing the glucose content of human skin. Investigations have indicated that the glucose content of skin never exceeds that of blood and that there is a direct correlation of skin glucose to blood glucose (Schragger, 1962; Urbach and Lentz, 1945). Values of skin glucose are estimated to be approximately 40–75% of blood glucose values. Urbach and Lentz (1945) investigated cutaneous glucose tolerance curves in humans and observed that cutaneous glucose levels increased similarly to blood glucose levels; however, they decreased at a slower rate. Later, using more refined techniques, Johnson and Fusaro (1972) and Peterka and Fusaro (1965) did similar experiments and observed similar results. Their investigations of fasting skin glucose levels indicated that (1) fasting levels varied widely within experimental groups (31–63 mg/100 g), (2) average glucose concentration was constant over a period of months and, (3) average glucose content of the backs of different groups were constant (46–48 mg/100 g).

Glucose Metabolism

Under normal conditions, glucose enters cells. Upon entering, it becomes phosphorylated to form glucose 6-phosphate, which may then be utilized for anabolic pathways such as the biosynthesis of glycogen or the macromucopolysaccharides. UDP-glucose is essential for these biosynthetic pathways. UDP-glucose, the glucose donor in the biosyntheses of glycogen and

TABLE 1   Average Enzyme Activities in Tumor Tissue
Compared to Those in Epidermis, Taken as 100^a

Tumor	Citr Syn	Citr Ly	ICDH-NAD	Fu	ME	Glu DH	Gly3 PDH	GSS Red
Basal cell epithelioma	129	147	216	115	132	134	157	134
Squamous cell epithelioma	140	82	124	104	120	106	90	90
Verruca seborrheica	126	102	139	97	103	159	111	142
Keratoacanthoma	72	90	122	82	70	116	57	81

^{a}Abbreviations: Citr Syn, Citrate synthetase; Citr Ly, ATP citrate lyase; ICDH-NAD, Isocitrate dehydrogenase; Fu, Fumarase; ME, Malic enzyme; Glu DH, Glutamate dehydrogenase; Gly3 PDH, Glycerol-3-phosphate dehydrogenase; and GSS Red, Glutathione reductase.

mucopolysaccharides, is an activated form of glucose, just as ATP and acetyl CoA are activated forms of orthophosphate and acetate, respectively. The glucose 6-phosphate may also enter the catabolic pathways, namely the glycolytic pathway which eventually leads to the production of pyruvate. Pyruvate may then be further metabolized to lactate, the major pathway in the epidermis, or it may be decarboxylated and converted to acetyl CoA. The acetyl CoA then enters into other anabolic pathways, such as fatty acid and sterol biosynthesis, or condenses with oxalacetate and enters the tricarboxylic acid cycle for the formation of additional energy. Glucose 6-phosphate may also be metabolized through the hexose monophosphate shunt, where it is utilized for the production of reduced NADP ($NADP + H \rightarrow NADPH$), or it may be converted into pentoses, which may be used in nucleic acid synthesis. The degree of glucose utilization in skin through these alternate pathways differs quantitatively from that in liver or muscle. The major product of glucose metabolism in skin is lactic acid, produced through the Embden-Meyerhof pathway, whereas in the liver the pyruvic acid formed is converted mainly to acetyl CoA. Investigations also strongly suggest that quantitatively more glucose is metabolized through the hexose monophosphate shunt than the tricarboxylic acid cycle (Freinkel, 1960). Since Pillsbury (1931) reported the presence of lactate in skin, several other investigators have demonstrated that the epidermis converts most of its glucose to lactic acid (Gilbert, 1964; Cruickshank et al., 1957; Halprin and Ohkawara, 1966c). Johnson and Fusaro (1972) calculated that the epidermis of a 70-kg man produces approximately 17 g of lactate per day and that the skin contains a lactate pool four times that of blood. Their analysis of whole human skin for lactate resulted in an average of 33 mg/100 g tissue. They suggested that this large lactate pool is mainly a result of its production by the epidermis. Lactate was also found in sweat and its concentration appeared to be associated with the sweating rate (Johnson and Fusaro, 1972; Rothman, 1954). Lactate concentration was inversely proportional to the sweating rate, whereas the total amount excreted paralleled the sweating rate.

Freinkel (1960) reported data suggesting that lactate is the major metabolite of [U-^{14}C]glucose, [6-^{14}C]glucose and [1-^{14}C]glucose. Her quantitative data indicated that less than 2% of the glucose entered the tricarboxylic acid cycle, whereas approximately 70% was converted into lactate. More CO_2 was produced by the hexose monophosphate shunt than in the Krebs cycle.

Adachi and Uno (1969) demonstrated the production of lactate by resting and growing human hair follicles. More than 90% of the glucose utilized went into lactate formation, and the growing hair follicle utilized twice the amount of [^{14}C]glucose indicated by [^{14}C]carbon dioxide and [^{14}C]lactic acid determinations. Their experiment demonstrated the presence of the tricarboxylic acid cycle and hexose monophosphate shunt in anagen and telogen hair follicles. They concluded that the Embden-Meyerhof pathway is the major one for glucose utilization and ATP production in the hair follicle, with a much smaller sector being metabolized through the tri-carboxylic acid cycle. The activity of the hexose-monophosphate shunt, which provides pentose and NADPH for the synthesis of fatty acids, nucleic acids, and so forth, was increased fourfold in the growing hair follicles. Adachi and Uno (1969) demonstrated that it is essential to identify the location and the period of growth of the hair follicles because enzymatic activity differs not only in different structures of the hair follicles but also at different stages of the hair growth.

Weiner and Van Heyningen (1952) demonstrated that sweat lactic acid is independent of serum lactate concentration and suggested that the conversion of carbohydrate to lactate could theoretically supply sufficient energy for the formation of sweat. In attempts to determine the source of sweat lactate, Gordon et al. (1971) injected [^{14}C] glucose and lactate intravenously in humans and demonstrated that sweat lactate is a metabolite of blood glucose.

Prolonged fasting in humans diminishes glucose consumption, with preferential metabolism of the ketone bodies (β-hydroxybutyrate and aceto-acetate) or free fatty acids in brain, cardiac, and striated muscle (Owen et al., 1967, 1969; Owen and Reichard, 1971; Shipp et al., 1961). Since Gordon et al. (1971) showed that blood glucose is the major source of sweat lactate in the nonfasted state, Benson et al. (1974) attempted to determine whether the sweat gland continues to depend on carbohydrate in the fasted state. The sweat gland utilized [^{14}C] glucose at approximately the same rate in both the fasted and the nonfasted state, is in contrast to the diminished glucose consumption by the brain and muscle during fasting conditions. Sweat lactate concentrations decreased only 19% and reached a new steady state. They demonstrated a significant sweat gland glycogen loss during sweating in fasted subjects, followed by an almost complete replenishment of the glycogen content 6 h after the conclusion of sweating, whereas no glycogen loss occurred in acclimatized subjects on an *ad libitum* diet after 2 h of sweating.

The effects of several pharmacological drugs on the sweat glands has been investigated (Gordon et al., 1968; Weiner and Van Heyningen, 1952; Ohara, 1951; Wolfe et al., 1970). Wolfe et al. (1970) incubated dissected human eccrine sweat glands with glucose in the presence and absence of epinephrine or methacholine and showed that the large amount of lactate present in sweat could be accounted for by its production in the sweat gland. The lactate produced was approximately 1.5 nmol per gland per hour in the absence of glucose and 2.7 nmol in the presence of physiologic concentrations of glucose. Both of the drugs enhanced lactate formation. Their experiments also demonstrated a depletion of sweat gland glycogen during the incubations indicating that both glycogen and glucose can be used as substrates for lactate production. Sato and Dobson (1971) investigated the effect of Mecholyl (acetyl methylcholine), epinephrine, and ouabain on glucose metabolism of freshly dissected human and monkey paw eccrine sweat glands. Both species exhibited glycolytic activity, which was enhanced by mecholyl and epinephrine. Ouabain inhibited $^{14}CO_2$ production in both unstimulated and stimulated glands. All concentrations of mecholyl stimulated ATP production. Mecholyl was a better stimulator than epinephrine, and epinephrine was biphasic, with the higher concentrations inhibiting and the lower concentrations enhancing ATP production.

Gluconeogenesis requires the bypass of three irreversible reactions catalyzed by glucose-6-phosphatase, phosphofructokinase, and pyruvate kinase. A glyconeogenic pathway would require only the last two enzymatic pathways to be bypassed. These two reverse reactions are controlled by the enzymes fructose-1,6-diphosphatase and pyruvate carboxylase plus phosphoenolpyruvate carboxykinase. Although the existence of a glyconeogenic pathway was dismissed as unlikely for many years, Peters and White (1976) demonstrated the presence of a glycogenic pathway in rat skin. They demonstrated the presence of the three key enzymes fructose-1,6-diphosphatase, pyruvate carboxylase, and phosphoenolpyruvate carboxykinase and the incorporation of pyruvate and alanine into skin glycogen.

Hansen et al. (1980) studied the biosynthesis of proteoglycans in skin and aorta of rats by using subcutaneous sponge implants. Their experiments demonstrated that rat aorta contained a predominance of sulfated glycosaminoglycans, in particular heparan sulfate, whereas skin had a predominance of hyaluronic acid and dermatan sulfate. The rate of biosynthesis of the proteoglycans was higher in skin than in aorta. A sequential change was observed in the granulation tissue, with an initial high content of hyaluronic acid followed by increasing amounts of chondroitin sulfate and dermatan sulfate in older granulation tissue.

The enzyme activities of collagen galactosyltransferase and collagen glycosyltransferase in human skin vary with age (Anttinen, 1977). The activities are greatest in fetal skin and are higher in children's skin than that of adults. Galactosyltransferase and glucosyltransferase activities in fetal skin were approximately 4 and 6 times those of adult skin, respectively.

Incubation of D-[^{3}H] glucosamine with slices of pig ear skin resulted in the biosynthesis of labeled epidermal glycosaminoglycan. When the epidermis was separated from the dermis before the incubation, no labeled epidermal glycosaminoglycan was synthesized. Although King and Tabiowa (1980) showed that the dermis appeared to be essential for the synthesis of the epidermal glycosaminoglycans, they postulate that synthesis does not occur in the dermis.

Sears et al. (1977) demonstrated the incorporation of L-[1-^{3}H] fucose into glycoproteins by confluent human skin fibroblasts in a linear manner up to 48 h and their release into the fibroblast culture media.

Secretion of acid mucopolysaccharides was inhibited by clobetasone butyrate, clobetasol propionate, betamethasone valerate, and cortisol (Priestly, 1978).

Energy Source of Epidermis

The epidermis is in a constant state of regeneration and requires a constant supply of energy to maintain its 3–4 wk turnover rate. It may obtain its energy needs in terms of ATP by several mechanisms, among which glycolysis and respiration appear to be extremely important. Although glycolysis is an important catabolic process in skin, it is a poor source of ATP. In glycolysis, the maximal rate of ATP production in the epidermis is approximately 0.1 μmol/hr/mg fresh tissue in the presence of physiologic blood concentrations of glucose (Decker, 1971). Most glucose is metabolized to lactate and only a very small amount is converted to CO_2 by way of the tricarboxylic acid cycle; therefore other energy sources appear to be necessary. Other possible sources of energy to the epidermis are the lipids and fatty acids. Cellular phospholipids are considered to be major endogenous nutrients for epidermal energy. Johnson and Fusaro (1972) suggest that the acetoacetate produced in the liver and shunted to the peripheral tissue may be a major source of energy for the skin, since the acetoacetate can be converted to acetoacetyl CoA in the peripheral tissue. The acetoacetyl CoA is then readily cleaved by thiolase to acetyl CoA, which may enter the Krebs cycle by combining with oxaloacetate and eventually be oxidized to CO_2 with the resultant production of ATP.

Decker (1971) states that respiration generates most of the energy for the epidermis (0.5 μmol ATP/hr/mg tissue) and that the main respiratory *in vitro* pathways of the epidermis are the tricarboxylic acid cycle and β-oxidations of lipids. In discussing energy production and requirements for the metabolic reactions occurring in the skin, one must consider all phases of metabolism, which is beyond the scope of this chapter. The reader is referred to two excellent review articles (Johnson and Fusaro, 1972; Decker, 1971).

Glycogen Storage Diseases

Skin glycogen is in a dynamic state. Glycogen synthesis in skin is assumed to be similar to that in liver and muscle since several of the enzymes associated with these processes have been identified in skin. By using the vacuum blistering technique, Leathwood and Ryman (1971) demonstrated the presence of glycogen phosphorylase, amylo-1,6-glucosidase, and acid α-glucosidase in human skin epidermis.

Leathwood and Ryman used modified procedures involving epidermis obtained from patients with type II and type V glycogen storage diseases. In type II, Pompe's disease, there is a generalized lack of lysosomal α-glucosidase, whereas type V, McArdle's disease, appears to be related to a lack of muscle phosphorylase activity. Their experiments demonstrated an absence of acid α-glucosidase in the epidermis of two patients with type II disease, whereas the epidermis of a patient with type V disease had normal levels of phosphorylase activity. Leathwood and Ryman suggested that the vacuum blistering technique may be a useful tool for the diagnosis of type II glycogen storage disease since they obtained negative results for acid α-glucosidase activity.

Hug et al. (1969) showed the presence of membrane-bound vacuoles in fibroblasts from type II glycogen storage disease patients and suggested that cultured fibroblasts may be used to study disease mechanisms and screen therapeutic agents without hazard to the patients.

A deficiency of the enzyme glucosylceramide: β-glucosidase results in glucosylceramidosis, better known as Gaucher's disease. This enzyme is a lysosomal enzyme related to the degradation of mammalian glycosphingolipid metabolism. Mueller and Rosenberg (1977, 1979) demonstrated the presence of this enzyme in human fibroblast.

DeBruyn et al. (1977) investigated the possibility of using hair roots for the detection of galactosemia. They demonstrated the presence of galactokinase and galactose-1-phosphate in roots of human hair and developed a radiochemical microassay for detecting both enzymes in hair roots.

Effects of Insulin on Carbohydrates

Kahlenberg and Kalant (1966) investigated glucose uptake with thigh skin obtained postmortem from diabetics of the maturity-onset type and from subjects who had no history of diabetes. They observed glucose uptake rates of approximately 3.89 and 2.60 mg/hr/g skin for the nondiabetics and diabetics, respectively. On addition of insulin (0.1 unit/ml) uptake by the skin in the diabetic group increased 27%, whereas the nondiabetic group showed very little increase. Hsia and co-workers reported an increase of glucose uptake in the presence of insulin, which resulted in increased lipogenesis and CO_2 formation from radioactive glucose (see section on lipogenesis).

Germinario and Oliveiara (1974) demonstrated that insulin stimulated the stereospecific carrier-mediated hexose transport in cultured skin fibroblasts.

Increased degradation of ^{125}I-labeled low-density lipoprotein (LDL) by cultured human skin fibroblasts occurred when the cells were preincubated with insulin (Chart et al., 1978). This effect of insulin appeared to be mediated by the stimulation of LDL binding to its receptor site. The degradation was independent of glucose concentration in the incubation medium (Chart et al., 1979). The data suggest that insulin enhances LDL receptor activity by increasing the number of LDL receptors rather than by affecting binding affinity.

Psoriasis

Herdenstam (1962) reported that oxygen uptake and CO_2 production were greater in diseased and noninvolved psoriatic skin than in normal skin. Rippa and Vignali (1965) analyzed human epidermis for several enzymes associated with carbohydrate metabolism. Epidermal specimens were obtained from normal male subjects and subjects with localized psoriasis. Skin specimens were removed with a Gosset Dermotome. They demonstrated a significant rise in glucose-6-phosphate dehydrogenase and 6-phosphogluconate in psoriatic skin, with no significant changes in the level of phosphohexose isomerase and aldolase. Their work suggests that the rapidly regenerating psoriatic epidermis has a higher requirement for NADPH, resulting in an increase of the enzymes associated with NADPH production. The increased flow of glucose through the hexose monophosphate shunt is also necessary for the synthesis of pentoses needed in the increased nucleic acid formation. Halprin and Ohkawara (1966b) reported that the activities of several glycolytic enzymes were all higher in psoriatic epidermis than in adjacent normal-appearing epidermis, but they could not detect quantitative enzyme differences between the epidermis of normal subjects and normal-appearing epidermis of individuals with psoriasis. However, other investigators have reported enzymatic differences between the epidermis of normal subjects and normal-appearing epidermis of psoriatic subjects (Hammar, 1971; Serri et al., 1971).

Phosphofructokinase is considered one of the major regulatory enzymes in the glycolytic pathway in many tissues, such as brain, liver, heart, skeletal muscle, and diaphragm. Kondo and Adachi (1971, 1972) demonstrated that phosphofructokinase is also a regulatory enzyme of glycolysis in normal epidermis and its appendages. To determine whether phosphofructokinase is a major regulatory enzyme of glycolysis in psoriatic epidermis, Kondo and Gerna-Torsellini (1974) measured changes of ATP, glucose 6-phosphate, fructose 6-phosphate, fructose 1,6-diphosphate, and lactate after periods of ischemia. Their experiments demonstrated decreased levels of ATP, glucose, glucose 6-phosphate, and fructose 6-phosphate and increased levels of fructose 1,6-diphosphate and lactate. The depletion of the glycolytic intermediates before fructose 1,6-diphosphate and the accumulation of lactate suggest that phosphofructokinase is partially activated in psoriatic epidermis.

Mycophenolic acid, an inhibitor of guanosine-5-monophosphate synthesis, has been effective in treating severe psoriasis and experimental tumors in animals. Mycophenolic acid is conjugated immediately on absorption and circulates mainly as a glucuronide conjugate. Gomez et al. (1977) demonstrated that mouse skin homogenates were capable of hydrolyzing mycophenolic acid-β-D-glucuronide. They reported that mouse skin preparations possessed a higher β-glucuronide activity per milligram of protein than mouse liver, kidney, spleen, lung, heart, and small intestine.

Panconesi and Cappugi (1979) demonstrated a statistically significant reduction in the ability of psoriatic skin to synthesize PGE_2.

King et al. (1979) reported that the incorporation of [^{3}H]glucosamine into membrane-bound glycoproteins of involved psoriatic epidermal cells was also less than that in normal epidermal cells.

Saihan et al. (1980) observed that the level of the cyclic nucleotide cyclic GMP in untreated psoriatic plaques was increased dramatically over that in noninvolved skin. No significant changes were observed in cyclic AMP.

Freinkel and Traczyk (1980) demonstrated the presence of an acid and alkaline phospholipase in fetal rat epidermis and suggested that these enzymes play an important role in the degradative events in keratinization.

Cyclic AMP

Marks and Grimm (1972) reported a diurnal variation in mouse epidermal cyclic AMP that was inversely correlated with mitotic activity. Diurnal variations in cyclic AMP, cyclic GMP, and cyclic GMP/cyclic AMP ratios were determined in mouse epidermis by Garte and Belman (1980). Diurnal variations (60%) were observed in the cyclic AMP and cyclic GMP/cyclic AMP ratios, whereas cyclic GMP levels had a much greater variation (250%). Maximum peaks occurred between 10 a.m. and 2 p.m. for all three parameters.

Yoshikawa et al. (1975a) described a method for the microanalysis (less than 100 μg tissue) of cAMP in human epidermis, dermis, and hair follicles. Levels of cAMP in dermis, epidermis, and hair follicles (bulbs) were approximately 1, 2, and 5 pmol/μg dry weight of tissue, respectively. Yoshikawa et al. (1975b) also demonstrated that the rise in cAMP content of skin rapidly increases after removal from the body. It reaches it maximum level after 2 min (four times the initial level) and remains at this level for approximately 3 min, after which it decreases slowly. This observation is somewhat similar to that of Lowry et al. (1964) and Kondo and Adachi (1971), who reported that the levels of metabolic intermediates and related nucleotides of the glycolytic pathway change rapidly after removal of the brain and skin from the intact experimental animal.

Adachi et al. (1975) investigated the relationship of prostaglandins and cAMP in pigs and human epidermis. They demonstrated that prostaglandins E_1 and E_2 increased the concentration of cAMP in pig epidermis and in human epidermis from psoriatic subjects, whereas prostaglandins A, A_2, and $F_{2\alpha}$ were relatively ineffective. The observation that stimulation was not inhibited by propanolol (β-blocker) and that stimulations by PGE_2 and epinephrine were additive suggests that each drug acts independently on the epidermal adenyl cyclase system. Stimulations by PGE_1 and PGE_2 are not additive.

Mui et al. (1975) incubated skin with [^{3}H]adenine to label cAMP. The accumulation of [^{3}H]cAMP was then used as an index of adenyl cyclase activity. Their results demonstrate that the incorporation of tritium into cAMP was significantly lower in psoriatic plaques than in uninvolved skin of psoriatic patients or in skin of normal control subjects. The stimulation of adenyl cyclase by adrenaline in psoriatic plaques was approximately fivefold, whereas in uninvolved skin there was a 12- to 32-fold increase. Adenyl cyclase activity in uninvolved skin of psoriatic patients appeared normal, and the response of psoriatic plaques and normal skin to PGE_2 stimulation was similar.

The adenyl cyclase system and its regulatory actions extend into many phases of biochemical transformations. In skin, it is thought that the adenyl cyclase system is activated by independent receptors sensitive to the catecholamines, prostaglandins, histamine, and adenosine. Increased levels of cyclic AMP also may occur in skin when treated with short-chain alcohols. Iizuka et al. (1981) reported that trypsin increases cyclic AMP levels in pig skin.

Peters and White (1978) investigated the relation between cyclic AMP and biochemical changes in rat skin after epidermal hyperplasia induced by hexadecane. Immediately after topical application they observed a fall of cyclic AMP, which subsequently rose above the initial values. DNA synthesis increased by 6 h and reached a maximum concentration after 1 d. They illustrated that the induced hyperplasia caused changes in DNA synthesis and glycogen metabolism that were linked to the initial decrease of cyclic AMP concentrations.

Addition of adenosine to epidermis from humans or mice resulted in significantly increased levels of cyclic AMP. This adenosine-induced increase in cyclic AMP in epidermis was decreased by the addition of theophylline (Duell, 1980).

DiGiovanna et al. (1981) reported that lithium carbonate decreases the responsiveness of adenyl cyclase to the stimulants histamine, adenosine monophosphate, and epinephrine.

Aoyagi et al. (1980), in investigations of the effects of epidermal growth factor on pig epidermis, observed that an increase in intracellular cyclic GMP occurred when pig skin slices were incubated with epidermal growth factor. Since this stimulation requires several hours, they postulated that the effect on cyclic GMP is probably a consequence of the action of epidermal growth factor.

Green and Lewis (1979) reported the partial purification and characterization of deoxyguanosine kinase from pig skin.

LIPID METABOLISM

Surface Lipids of Human Skin

Natural surface lipids are derived from two major sources: the sebaceous glands and epidermis. In normal adults, sebum contributes most of the surface lipids because of the active sebaceous glands. The contribution of the sebaceous glands differs at various body sites. Sebaceous gland secretions in descending order are: face, back, chest, abdomen, arms, and legs. Many of the earlier discrepancies in the quantitation of skin lipids were due to methods of collection and location of samples (Cunliffe et al., 1971a; Cotterill et al., 1972). As procedures became more standardized, remarkable agreement was achieved between different laboratories. Nonpolar solvents such as hexane extract only surface lipids, whereas more polar solvents such as chloroform:methanol and methylene dichloride:methanol extract lipids from the epidermis as well (Nicolaides, 1963). Isolation, separation, and quantitation of surface lipids have been accomplished by column, thin-layer, and gas chromatography. The various classes of compounds identified include fatty acids, triglycerides, squalene, wax esters, sterol esters, sterols, and saturated hydrocarbons. Table 2 shows data (Lewis and Hayward, 1971; Felger, 1969) illustrating the relative concentrations of the constituents of surface lipids from sebum-rich areas of humans.

Lipids were extracted from isolated sebaceous glands of the scalp by Kellum (1967), and the major constituents identified were squalene, wax esters, and triglycerides. No free fatty acids were detected, which suggests that many if not all of the free fatty acids in surface lipids are bacterial hydrolytic products of sebum.

By using gas-liquid chromatography, James and Wheatley (1956) demonstrated the presence of free fatty acids containing 7-18 carbon atoms in

TABLE 2   Surface Lipids of Humans

Lipid class	Percentage of total sebum		
	Back[a]	Scalp[a]	Face[b]
Total lipid	100	100	100
Free fatty acid	16.0	29.6	24
Paraffins	1.3	0.8	1.3
Squalene	11.4	12.8	10.2
Wax	21.5	20.2	20.0
Sterol ester	2.9	2.6	2.2
Triglycerides	46.4	31.7	31.3
Free sterol	1.8	1.5	0.6
"Polar material"	–	–	8.1

[a]Lewis and Hayward, 1971.
[b]Felger, 1969.

skin lipids of the forearm. They detected unsaturated fatty acids with both odd and even numbers of carbon atoms as well as branched-chain fatty acids. Other investigators have obtained similar fatty acid patterns in their investigations of surface lipids from the backs of humans and from vernix caseosa (Haahti, 1961; Haahti et al., 1960). Downing (1963) demonstrated by gas-liquid chromatography that the vernix caseosa contained a higher proportion of saturated branched-chain fatty acids (78%) than the adult surface lipids (12%), which suggests that the branched acids are not bacterial metabolites but products of the sebaceous gland. They also detected branched unsaturated fatty acids. The vernix caseosa also contained 2-hydroxy fatty acids, which were predominantly branched and saturated. Karkkainen et al. (1965) and Nicolaides et al. (1972) analyzed the lipids of the vernix caseosa and substantiated the work of Downing. Sebaceous glands are probably the source of the branched acids (Downing and Strauss, 1974).

Nikkari (1969), Nicolaides et al. (1970), and Downing and Sharaf (1976) have shown that skin surface lipids of several mammals contain compounds that migrate like aliphatic diesters on thin-layer chromatograms. In the cow, rabbit, and domestic cat, these compounds were represented by 2-hydroxy acids esterified with long-chain fatty acids and alcohols. In the rat, mouse, and guinea pig, the diesters had lower mobility on thin-layer plates and were composed of long-chain 1,2-diols esterified with two equivalents of long-chain fatty acids. Surface lipids of dogs contained diols with intermediate mobilities. Sharaf et al. (1977) thoroughly investigated the skin surface lipids of dogs and reported that they consisted of sterol esters (42%), wax diesters (32%), free sterols (9%), polar lipids (7%), and unidentified components (10%). The diols were esterified with one long-chain fatty acid and one isovaleric acid moiety. The diols were mainly branched-chain C_{21} and C_{22} compounds with C_{20} and C_{21} branched fatty acids forming the esters. The sterols formed esters mainly with saturated C_{21} to C_{23} fatty acids. The esterified sterols contained 96% cholesterol and 4% lathosterol. Young et al. (1981) investigated the composition of the skin surface lipids of the gerbil. They contained sterol esters (10%), wax diesters (36%), triacylglycerol (26%), free fatty alcohols (8.8%), free fatty acids (5.4%), cholesterol (8.4%), and polar lipids (5%). The wax esters were comprised of saturated 1,2-diols with an odd carbon number esterified with two saturated fatty acids with even carbon numbers. The triacylglycerols and free fatty acid fractions had both saturated and unsaturated components. Cholesterol was the only esterified and free sterol identified. The sterol esters contained monoenoic and dienoic fatty acids. The fatty alcohols were all straight chain and most contained an even number of carbon atoms.

Several investigators reported on the changes in the composition of skin surface lipids during starvation and malnourishment (Pochi et al., 1970; Downing et al., 1972; Dogliotti et al., 1977; Straus et al., 1978). Strauss et al. (1978) reported that the squalene/wax ester ratio is increased in starved adults, whereas the opposite was observed in children with protein-caloric malnutrition. This difference may be due to different sources of surface lipids in adults and children. In adults, over 95% of the surface lipids are of sebaceous origin, whereas in children they are of epidermal origin. Since squalene and wax esters come from sebaceous glands, their percentage in surface lipids of children is low. Cholesterol, primarily of epidermal origin, was elevated in children. Triglycerides, which are derived from both epidermis and sebaceous gland, were unchanged in children, compared to adults. Straus et al. (1978) suggest that analysis of skin surface lipids may be used in determining the nutritional status of individuals since the squalene content and squalene/wax ester ratio of skin surface lipids can be correlated with other biochemical changes in protein-caloric malnutrition states.

Pochi et al. (1977) investigated the relation of skin surface lipid composition to acne, pubertal development, and steroid excretion in children. They observed a positive correlation between surface lipids and age. The lipid analyses indicated that the relative proportion of sebaceous lipids to epidermal lipids was higher in individuals with acne in all age groups studied. No significant correlation with the fatty acids was observed. A significant positive correlation was observed between the amount of sebaceous lipids and the urinary excretion of androsterone, etiocholanolone and 17-ketosteroids in boys and girls and of testosterone and dehydroepiandrosterone in boys. They suggested that surface lipid composition may be a potential indicator of very early onset of puberty.

Nazzaro-Porro et al. (1979) investigated the effect of aging on fatty acids in skin surface lipids. They observed, as others have, that composition, concentration, and structure vary according to age and sex and that the surface lipids of prepubertal children are similar to those of elderly individuals. The variations observed were mainly in the monoenes with less than 16 carbon atoms. The double bond was always observed to be a 6-7 ene in these compounds, whereas fatty acids with longer carbon chains had different positional isomers. The 9-10 monenes of the fatty acids in triglycerides, wax esters, and sterol esters were always higher in girls and women than in boys and men.

Sphingomyelinase, which hydrolyzes sphingomyelin to ceramide and phosphorylcholine, was identified in subcellular fractions of pig and human epidermis (Bowser and Gray, 1978). The optimum pH was 4.5 to 5 and enzymes from both sources exhibited Michaelis-Menten kinetics. Gatt and Bierman (1980) cultured human skin fibroblasts with liposomes containing sphingomyelin. The sphingomyelin was incorporated and metabolized by the fibroblasts and produced a reduction in LDL binding and degradation as well as an increase of acetate incorporation into sterols. Gatt and Bierman (1980) suggested that sphingomyelin can influence the regulation of cell surface LDL receptor and intracellular cholesterol balance.

Essential Fatty Acids

Essential fatty acid (EFA) deficiency develops in experimental animals reared on diets lacking essential fatty acids. In rats, this deficiency is characterized by scaliness of the tail and feet. The epidermis is hyperplastic and the stratum corneum dense. Transepidermal water loss is increased due to impaired barrier function of the skin. Tissue phospholipids have decreased amounts of linoleic and arachidonic acid and ω-9-eicosatrienoic acid is increased. Addition of essential fatty acids to the diet reverses these abnormalities. Prottey (1977) demonstrated that topical application of linoleic acid to rats restored the impaired barrier function to normal within 5 d, increased the linoleic acid content in skin lecithin, and had no effect on arachidonic acid in lecithin or on skin scaliness. Hartop et al. (1977) investigated the increased rates of transepidermal water loss in plaques of human psoriasis and in skin of EFA-deficient rats. Daily topical application for 2 wk of sunflower seed oil to the EFA-deficient rats resulted in a return to normal rates of transepidermal water loss, healing of the scaly skin condition, and increased incorporation of linoleic acid into epidermal phospholipid. Topical application of sunflower seed oil to psoriatic skin increased the linoleic acid content of epidermal phospholipid but had no effect on the rate of transepidermal water loss. Hartop et al. concluded that the impaired barrier function in psoriasis is not due to EFA deficiency. Elias et al. (1980) confirmed the reports of Prottey (1977) and Hartop et al. (1977). Takehisa and Kimura (1977) reported that branched fatty acids synthesized from leucine and valine increased in skin surface lipids in rats with an EFA deficiency. Lowe et al. (1979) investigated the effect of EFA deficiencies on epidermal DNA synthesis, epidermal thickness, and cyclic nucleotide levels in hairless mouse skin. They observed an increase in *in vitro* epidermal DNA synthesis and epidermal thickness. Cyclic AMP levels were significantly reduced, whereas changes in cyclic GMP were not significant; however, changes in cyclic AMP/cyclic GMP ratios were significantly decreased in EFA-deficient skin. Lowe et al. (1978) also reported that prostaglandin E and prostaglandin F levels, measured by radioimmunoassay, were lower in EFA-deficient mouse skin.

By using mass spectrometry and thin-layer chromatography, Hammarstrom et al. (1979) demonstrated that arachidonic acid is converted mainly to 12L-hydroxy-5,8,10,14-eicosatetraenoic acid (12-HETE) and prostaglandin E_2 by human epidermis and mouse dermis. Mouse epidermis formed HETE, PGD_2, and PGE_2. Thrombroxane B_2 and 6-keto-$PGF_{1\alpha}$ were not formed in appreciable amounts under the conditions used.

Wound Healing

Lord et al. (1980) reported that topically applied $PGF_{2\alpha}$ enhanced hexosamine formation in wounded guinea pig skin. This strongly suggests that $PGF_{2\alpha}$ may function during wound healing by accelerating the process of granulation.

Wound healing is adversely affected by hypoxia, and it has been suggested that healing may be enhanced by increasing inspired oxygen tension (Underfriend, 1966; Niinikoski, 1969; Stephens and Hunt, 1971). Kirk and Irvin (1977) investigated the effect of oxygen therapy on the healing of skin wounds and colonic anastomoses in rats. Sutured skin incisions and normal and ischemic colonic anastomoses were investigated in control animals breathing air and in test animals breathing 50% oxygen. Wound healing was followed by measurements of wound breaking strength, colonic bursting wall tension, and wound collagen after treatment with oxygen for 7 d. They observed no significant difference in skin wound healing or colonic anastomoses between control and experimental animals.

The effect of petrolatum on microsomal lipoxygenase activity in petrolatum-treated wound skin and normal skin was investigated by Penneys et al. (1980). They observed that microsomal preparations from petrolatum-treated wounded skin, with arachidonic acid as the substrate, had depressed lipoxygenase activity compared to those from untreated wounded skin. There was no difference between treated and untreated normal pig skin. They suggested that petrolatum may contain a constituent that interferes with proinflammatory processes.

Maines and Cohn (1977) reported the presence of heme oxygenase activity in intact skin and suggested that its elevation in skin is a response to specific stimuli and not a manifestation of nonspecific injury.

Although glycogen exists in very low concentration in adult epidermis, it accumulates for short periods of time in adult epidermis following injury as by ultraviolet light (Ohkawara et al., 1972) and irradiation (Adachi, 1941). Hoopes (1973) demonstrated that the maximal increase in glycogen content occurred 3 d after injury.

Lipid biosynthesis from glucose is increased in severe acne in both dermis and epidermis (Shuster et al., 1980).

Sebum

Investigations have shown that the composition of sebum is species-specific (Wheatley, 1956). Excellent reviews on the comparative chemistry of sebum and the control and measurement of sebum secretion were written by Nikkari (1974) and Shuster and Thody (1974), respectively. Numerous investigations have established the androgen-sebaceous gland relationship. Castrated males produce considerably less sebum than normal men. It has also been shown that administration of testosterone to castrated males (Pochi et al., 1962) or postmenopausal women (Strauss et al., 1962; Smith and Brunot, 1961) results in an increase in sebaceous gland activity. The observations that exogenous testosterone does not increase sebum production in normal males (Strauss et al., 1962) and that administration of human chorionic gonadotropin to adult males results in no change in sebum secretion (Pochi and Strauss, 1974) suggest that maximal stimulation of the sebaceous gland occurs with endogenous testosterone. However, pharmacologic doses of methyl testosterone or testosterone propionate do cause a detectable increase in sebum production (Pochi and Strauss, 1974). Other workers have reported that testosterone resulted in an increase of skin surface lipids (Jarrett, 1959).

Dehydroepiandrosterone (DHH) or DHA sulfate augments sebum secretion (Wilson and Gloyan, 1970; Drucker et al., 1972). Subcutaneous administration of progesterone to adult male rats resulted in decreased sebum secretion, whereas in adult female rats a slight increase was observed (Thody and Shuster, 1978). In castrated adult rats, progesterone caused an increase in sebum production in both sexes. Simpson et al. (1979) reported that progesterone applied topically to males had no effect on sebum production, whereas in females a significant reduction of sebum excretion was observed, the maximal effect occurring at the end of 2 mo.

Sebaceous gland activity may be influenced by caloric intake. Sebum production was measured in fasting subjects (Pochi et al., 1970), and diminished secretions occurred 2-4 wk after the onset of fasting. The composition of surface lipids was also altered. Lower caloric intake resulted in a reduction of the triglycerides, fatty acids, wax esters, cholesterol, and cholesterol esters. However, no significant change in squalene occurred. The decreased sebum production may in part be explained by decreased androgen production in individuals on prolonged total caloric intakes (Schultz et al., 1964; Hendrikx et al., 1968). In a similar study Downing et al. (1972) demonstrated a change in the sebaceous gland lipids of the forehead in humans after 5 days without food. Decreased synthesis of all lipids occurred except for squalene, and this change was reversed by returning to a normal diet.

Surface Lipids in Acne

Krakow et al. (1973) reported that the fatty acid octadeca-5,8-dienoic acid is present in higher concentration in the sebum of acne patients.

Several investigators have reported little difference in the composition of skin surface lipids of patients with acne and controls. However, Powell and Beveridge (1970) demonstrated an increase in the esters and a decrease in the triglyceride content of forehead sebum from acne subjects. Cunliffe et al. (1971b), in a study with 410 subjects, observed an increase in the wax esters in males and females with acne as well as a significant decrease of free fatty acids in males with severe acne.

Puhvel et al. (1975) investigated the effect of microorganisms on the lipid content of isolated human sebaceous glands. They dissected, pooled, homogenized, and sterilized human sebaceous glands and, using a peptone-yeast extract as a growth medium, cultured *Propionibacterium acnes, P. granulosum,* and *Staphylococcus epidermidis* subgroup II. They analyzed the sebaceous lipids by means of thin-layer chromatophy before and after bacterial growth. The most striking effect of the bacteria was their hydrolysis of the sebaceous triglycerides followed by their esterification of sebaceous cholesterol to cholesteryl esters. The work of Puhvel et al. emphasized the importance of considering skin bacteria modifications of substrates when investigating metabolic processes in the skin or other tissues. Pablo and Fulton (1975) investigated the effect of several antibiotics on the ratio of free fatty acids to fatty esters in sebum by using a Wilks Skin Analyzer in conjunction with infrared spectroscopy and observed a significant depression of the ratio after treatment for 1 wk. The antibiotic clindamycin caused the most dramatic reduction of the FFA/FE ratio.

Synthesis of Lipids

Nicolaides et al. (1955) demonstrated that human skin is active in lipogenesis when they incubated human scalp skin with [^{14}C]acetate and detected ^{14}C uptake in fatty acids, squalene, and sterols. Subsequently, Nicolaides and Rothman (1955) proposed that sterol synthesis occurred in the epidermis and squalene synthesis occurred in the sebaceous gland. Later, Vroman et al. (1969) investigated lipogenesis in preputial skin of the newborn and in adult abdominal skin by *in vitro* studies with [1-^{14}C]acetate. The formed metabolites were separated on unisil and florisil columns and subsequently identified by gas-liquid chromatography. They identified ^{14}C-labeled fatty acids that contained 14-26 carbon atoms.

Palmitic acid and stearic acid were the major ^{14}C-labeled fatty acids identified, with lesser amounts of: 14:0, 15:0, 16:1, 18:1, 18:2, 20:0, 20:1, 22:0, 24:0, 24:1, and 26:0 ^{14}C-labeled acids.

The data of Vroman et al. demonstrated that the labeled carbon was most actively incorporated in the polar lipid fraction (28-36%), followed by the free sterol fraction (22-26%) and then the triglycerides (13-16%). Less label was detected in the hydrocarbon fraction (6-14%), wax and sterol esters (2-3%), diglycerides (1-4%), monoglycerides (5%), and fatty acids (5-12%). Skin from the two locations appeared to synthesize the different lipid classes in similar proportions; however, the abdominal skin appeared to be less active.

Although arachidonic acid (20:4) comprises approximately 9% of the fatty acids in skin, no radioactive 20:4 acid was identified in these experiments.

Wilkinson (1970b, 1972) carried out *in vitro* experiments with [1-^{14}C]acetate using isolated epidermal cells, human preputial skin, mouse skin, and isolated labeled linoleic acid. The data indicated that labeling occurred almost entirely by acetate exchange, since oxidative fission resulted in a monocarboxylic fragment with essentially no label.

The biosynthetic pathway for branched fatty acids has not been elucidated. Experiments of Wheatley et al. (1961, 1967), in which they perfused the leg skin of dogs with labeled isoleucine, valine, and leucine and found that they were incorporated into fatty acids, suggest that the anteiso and iso acids may be derived from these compounds.

Several free unsaturated fatty acids were isolated and identified in human hair lipids (Weitkamp et al., 1947). The chain lengths of the unsaturated fatty acids varied from 11–20 carbon atoms. In the fatty acids with 16 carbon atoms or more, the most characteristic double bond was between C-6 and C-7 (Δ^6). However, several different unsaturated C_{17} and C_{18} fatty acids were tentatively identified, which had the following structures: $C_{17-1}\Delta^6$; $C_{17-1}\Delta^8$; $C_{17-2}\Delta^{6,8}$; $C_{18-1}\Delta^6$; $C_{18-1}\Delta^9$; $C_{18-3}\Delta^{6,8,9}$. The unsaturated fatty acids with 11, 12, 13, 14, 15, and 16 carbon atoms had double bonds located at Δ^2, Δ^3, Δ^4, Δ^5, and Δ^6, respectively. Nicolaides et al. (1964) also demonstrated that the Δ^6 double bond was predominant and that unsaturation in other monoenoic (over C_{16}) acids was displaced by one or more two-carbon units. Oleic acid, $C_{18-1}\Delta^9$, again was the exception. Unsaturated C_{16} and C_{18} fatty acids were reported to be components of wax-sterol esters and triglycerides (Felger, 1969). Fatty acids containing up to 30 carbon atoms were isolated from vernix caseosa, and both Δ^6 and Δ^9 unsaturation were present (Downing and Greene, 1968). In the longer-chain fatty acids unsaturation occurred two carbon units removed from the Δ^6 and Δ^9 positions, Δ^9 being the more prevalent in fatty acids containing more than 17 carbon atoms.

Wheatley et al. (1973) demonstrated the incorporation of acetate, pyruvate, and L-lactate into lipids in the absence of glucose by guinea pig ear skin. Their data indicated that acetate incorporation was lowest, and lactate incorporation not only was highest but was also concentration-dependent. These investigators suggest that the HMP shunt may not function as a regulatory mechanism in cutaneous lipogenesis.

Wheatley (1974) investigated the incorporation rates of several representative compounds as precursors for lipogenesis by guinea pig ear skin slices. The classes of compound tested were: short-chain fatty acids, glucose, glycolysis products, Kreb's cycle acids, and selected amino acids. Incorporation rates were expressed as nanomoles of precursor incorporated into nonsaponifiable material and fatty acids; [1,2-^{14}C]acetate (64 nmol/g/hr); [1-^{14}C]propionate (50 nmol/g/hr), and [1-^{14}C]butyrate (147 nmol/g/hr) were actively incorporated into fatty acids. [U-^{14}C]D-glucose (54 nmol/g/hr);

[2-^{14}C]pyruvate (104 nmol/g/hr); [2-^{14}C]D,L-lactate (55 nmol/g/hr; [1,5-^{14}C]citrate (4.6 nmol/g/hr), and [2,3-^{14}C]succinate (7.0 nmol/g/hr) were also actively incorporated into fatty acids. Of the amino acids tested, [U-^{14}C]L-alanine (91 nmol/g/hr); [U-^{14}C]L-leucine (70 nmol/g/hr), and [U-^{14}C]L-isoleucine (35 nmol/g/hr) had the highest rates of incorporation into fatty acids, whereas [1,2-^{14}C]glycine (1 nmol/g/hr); [U-^{14}C]L-lysine (2 nmol/g/hr), and [Me-^{14}C]L-methionine (1.5 nmol/g/hr) had the lowest rates of incorporation into fatty acids. [U-^{14}C]L-aspartate and [U-^{14}C]L-glutamate had intermediate rates of incorporation. The rates of incorporation of these compounds into the nonsaponifiable fraction were similar except at a lower level.

Lipogenesis was compared in human epidermal and dermal preparations (Hsia et al., 1970) by using *in vitro* techniques. The epidermal preparation was obtained by the suction blistering technique and 2 *M* NaI soaking procedure (Hambrick and Blank, 1954). Underlying dermal tissue was obtained by normal skin biopsy procedures. The tissues were incubated with [1-^{14}C]acetate and the uptake of ^{14}C was compared in eight classes of lipids (hydrocarbons, sterol esters, waxes, triglycerides, sterols, diglycerides, monoglycerides, and fatty acids). Although both tissues incorporated labeled carbon in all eight classes of compounds, the epidermis was quantiatively more active than the dermis in the synthesis of neutral lipids and sterols. The data of Hsia et al. also suggest that squalene and triglycerides are produced by sebaceous glands. This work was in agreement with investigations carried out by other researchers (Nicolaides and Wells, 1957; Nicolaides and Rothman, 1955).

Lipogenesis was investigated in epidermis obtained by the suction blistering technique from male subjects (ages 25–49) before and after ingestion of 100 g glucose by Hsia et al. (1970). They observed an increase of [^{14}C]acetate uptake into lipids by the epidermis after the glucose loading. These results reinforce their earlier observation (Hsia et al., 1966b) that skin specimens obtained from diabetic patients incorporated less ^{14}C from [1-^{14}C]acetate into lipids than specimens from normal subjects. Experiments by Ziboh and Hsia (1969) demonstrated that the skin obtained from diabetic rats (alloxan-treated) also had faulty lipogenic activity, which was corrected by insulin treatment. They observed that lipogenic activity fluctuated with L-glycerol-3-phosphate levels and that the addition of L-glycerol-3-phosphate to incubation media enhanced lipogenesis. These results seem to indicate that there is an endogenous metabolic regulation of lipid synthesis in the epidermis.

Hydroxy acids have been isolated from skin by several investigators (Downing, 1963; Ansari et al., 1970). These acids exist in trace amounts and are reported to be completely saturated and branched and apparently of epidermal origin.

Fatty Alcohols

Fatty alcohols in human surface lipids include alcohols with both odd and even numbers of carbon atoms (Brown et al., 1954; Hougen, 1955).

Unsaturated alcohols also exist in both branched and straight-chain carbon compounds. The chain length of the alcohols ranges from C_{12} to C_{27} and the unsaturated alcohols exist mainly as C_{20}, C_{22}, and C_{24} compounds (Haahti and Horning, 1963; Boughton and Wheatley, 1959; Downing, 1965; Nicolaides, 1967). Free fatty alcohols have not been detected as such in human surface lipids; they exist as esters of fatty acids or as diesters with 2-hydroxyacids which occur in vernix caseosa (Downing, 1963; Ansari et al., 1970). The major saturated alcohol constituents are formed from even-numbered straight-chain fatty acids containing 14–24 carbon atoms. The major monoene alcohol contains 20 carbon atoms, and there are lesser amounts of C_{24} and C_{27} alcohols. The positions of the double bonds appear to be similar to those of the fatty acids found in human surface lipids. The biosynthesis from fatty acids is unresolved, although mechanisms have been proposed (Sand et al., 1969).

Prostaglandins

Prostaglandins (PG) are a relatively new class of important biologically active compounds, which have widespread biological actions. They are present in a wide variety of mammalian tissues and appear to be modulators of intracellular metabolism (Horton, 1969). Prostaglandins are 20-carbon fatty acids that contain a five-carbon ring (C-8 to C-12). The major classes are designated PGA, PGB, PGE, and PGF, followed by a subscript that denotes the number of double bonds. Prostaglandins differ from one another in the number and positions of the double bonds and hydroxyl groups. The biochemical precursors of prostaglandins *in vivo* are C_{20} polyunsaturated fatty acids, which are required in the diets of mammals. The essential fatty acid precursor of PGE and PGE_2 is 5,8,11,14-eicosatetraenoic (arachidonic) acid. The relationship of prostaglandins to cutaneous metabolism is indirectly implied by the adverse skin reactions that occur in mammals with essential fatty acid deficiencies. Burr and Burr (1929, 1930) were the first to describe the symptoms of an essential fatty acid deficiency in rats. The typical skin lesions observed in these rats were excessive scaliness of tails and feet. The symptoms were accompanied by decreased fertility, urine excretion, and growth.

Ziboh and Hsia (1972) analyzed the scaly lesions of rats on an essential fatty acid diet. These lesions showed marked increases of monoenoic acids (16:1 and 18:1) and eicosatrienoic acid (20:3) with concurrent decreases of dienoic acid (18:2) and tetraenoic acid (20:4). Intraperitoneal injections of PGE_2 had no effect on the lesions of these rats, whereas topical application of PGE_2 to the lesions cleared them but did not alter the fatty acid composition of the skin. Failure of the intraperitoneal route of application may be explained by the rapid *in vivo* inactivation of the prostaglandins. Incubation of ^{14}C-labeled glucose with skin specimens from fatty acid-deficient rats resulted in a fourfold increase in the incorporation of radioactive carbon into lipid fractions and a three- to fourfold enhancement of the monohexosphosphate shunt pathway. Ziboh and Hsia suggest that the beneficial effects of PGE_2 on the scaly lesions may be due to its inhibitory effect on abnormal sterol esterification in the skin of these essential fatty acid-deficient rats.

Prostaglandins have been isolated and identified from rat and human skin by Jouvenaz et al. (1970) and Mathur and Gandhi (1972). PGE_2 and PGF_2 have also been isolated from the affected skin of patients with Kaposi's sarcoma (Bhana et al., 1971). Jouvenaz et al. (1970) and van Dorp (1971), using gas chromatography reported that the major portion of prostaglandin activity resides in the epidermis of rat skin. Mathur and Gandhi (1972) reported concentrations of 760-2,140 ng PG (expressed in terms of PGE_1) per gram of wet skin in biopsy specimens of human thighs. The values reported for the albino rat skin, epidermis, and dermis were approximately 732, 1,539, and 592 ng/g wet tissue, respectively. Mathur and Gandhi also demonstrated that erythemal doses (2-8 MED) of UV radiation to albino rats caused an increase of both epidermal and dermal prostaglandins. Arturson et al. (1973) recovered prostaglandins from human burn blister fluid and demonstrated that the contraction of smooth muscle was due to PGE_2 and PGF_2 present in the fluid.

Bergstrom et al. (1965) reported that intravenous injection of PGE_1 in humans caused inflammation and a pronounced edema at the site of injection. Horton (1969) demonstrated increased permeability of pig cutaneous vessels after the injection of PGE_1. Soloman et al. (1968) also reported an erythematous reaction that lasted 2-10 hr in patients after injecting PGE_1 intradermally. Juhlin and Michaelsson (1969) administered PGE_1, PGE_2, PGF_1, and PGF_2 intradermally to subjects and observed that PGE_1 and PGE_2 were the most effective vasodilators. The mode of action of the prostaglandins in vasodilation is somewhat obscure, but Kumar and Soloman (1972) suggest that the early part of what becomes a prolonged vasodilatory response initiated by PGE_1 is mediated by histamine release. Crunkhorn and Willis (1971) also suggest that cutaneous vascular permeability may be mediated by prostaglandin-induced histamine response. Prostaglandins have been associated with the lyosomal enzymes associated with inflammation (Brocklehurst, 1971). DiRosa and Willoughby (1971) reported that the effects of prostaglandins in inflammation were correlated with the migration of leukocytes to traumatic area. Therefore, it is possible that the presence of prostaglandins at inflammatory sites may be due to release from the invading cells or biosynthesis within the skin itself. Kischer (1969) reported that PGE_1 and PGB_1 enhanced the growth and maturation of chick embryo skin in tissue culture by stimulating epidermal proliferation and keratinization.

Ziboh and Hsia (1971) demonstrated the biosynthesis of prostaglandins from arachidonic acid in rat skin. They incubated $[1\text{-}^{14}C]$ arachidonic acid with rat skin homogenates and isolated and identified PGE_2 as the major metabolic product as well as two minor metabolites. They demonstrated that PGE_2 enhanced the production of CO_2 and lipids from differentially labeled glucose by rat and human skin. Using $[1\text{-}^{14}C]$ glucose and $[6\text{-}^{14}C]$ glucose, they demonstrated that PGE_2 acted similarly to insulin in stimulating both the hexose monophosphate shunt and the glycolytic pathways of glucose in skin; however, the degree of stimulation was less than that of insulin. Jonsson and Anggard (1972) demonstrated the biosynthesis and metabolism of PGE_2 and $PGF_{2\alpha}$, using tritiated arachidonic acid. Ziboh (1973) reported that the microsomal fraction of human epidermal cell synthesized prostaglandins, demonstrating that the prostaglandin synthesis system was membrane-bound.

Aso et al. (1975) analyzed extracts of guinea pig and human epidermis for prostaglandins PGE_1, PGE_2, and $PGF_{2\alpha}$ by radioimmunoassay procedures and found that the three existed in approximately equal concentrations. The total concentrations were 62.0 and 148 ng/g wet weight for the guinea pig and human epidermis, respectively. They also demonstrated the conversion of labeled arachidonic acid to PGE_2 and PGF_2 by guinea pig epidermal homogenates; the rates of formation of PGE_2 and PGF_2 were 10 and 2.5 pmol/mg protein/30 min. Homogenates from psoriatic epidermis produced less PGE_2 from arachidonic acid than homogenates from nonpsoriatic epidermis. Aso et al. also demonstrated six- to ninefold increase in cAMP when guinea pig epidermal slices were incubated with PGE_1 ($3-6 \times 10^{-6}$ M) and theophylline (2×10^{-3} M). The synthesis of PGE_2, a potent proinflammatory agent, and its conversion into the potent anti-inflammatory agent $PGF_{2\alpha}$ by the NADPH-dependent enzyme PGE_2-9-ketoreductase has been demonstrated (Lesie, 1973; Lee, 1975; Stone, 1975). Ziboh et al. (1977) reported that skin preparations from psoriatic plaques and EFA-deficient rats showed increase conversion of PGE_2 to $PGF_{2\alpha}$. Hensby et al. (1976) reported the biosynthesis of PGD_2 by rat skin.

Camp and Greaves (1980) compared the activities of NAD^+-dependent 15-hydroxyprostaglandin dehydrogenases obtained from rat skin and lung tissues. There was a 5-fold greater dehydrogenase activity in the lung tissue than the skin tissue. However, the total weight of the skin was approximately 23 times that of the lung. The experiments indicate that cutaneous prostaglandin catabolism may be of great importance since the entire skin contained approximately $4\frac{1}{2}$ times as much 15-hydroxyprostaglandin dehydrogenase activity.

The physiological role of phospholipases in skin has been investigated (Long, 1970; Poulos, 1973; Vonkeman et al., 1968; Gryglewski et al., 1976; Nijkamp, 1976; Hong and Levine, 1975; Ziboh and Lord, 1979). Hydrolysis of phospholipids in cutaneous tissue with resultant release of arachidonic acid and ultimate production of the prostaglandins appears to be important in cutaneous inflammation. Experimental data indicate that anti-inflammatory steroids inhibit the release of arachidonic acid from phosphatidylcholine in blood vessel membranes, lungs, and tissue cultures. Ziboh and Lord (1979) reported that phosphatidylcholine hydrolysis by skin phospholipase A2 was inhibited by the anti-inflammatory steroids, cortisol, and triamcinolone acetonide, and was enhanced by histamine, bradykinin, retinoic acid, and cholera enterotoxin. The hydrolysis of phosphatidylcholine was enhanced by low concentrations of PGE_2

and $PGF_{2\alpha}$, suggesting a feedback mechanism for the release of arachidonic acid from phosphatidylcholine with concurrent synthesis of prostaglandins.

Hulan and Kramer (1977) investigated the effect of long-chain monoenes on PGE_2 synthesis by rat skin. They reported that the highest level of synthesis occurred in rats fed diets containing corn oil. This is not surprising, since corn oil has a higher concentration of 18:2N-6, the precursor of arachidonic acid required for PGE_2 synthesis. They confirmed the observation of Ziboh et al. (1978) that 18:1N-9 was an inhibitor of PGE_2 synthesis. Hulan and Kramer (1977) reported that skin from rats with the most severe dermal lesions and alopecia had the lowest capacity for PGE_2 synthesis.

An increase of arachidonic acid, PGE_2, and $PGF_{2\alpha}$-like material resulted when human abdominal skin was irradiated with ultraviolet light (290–320 nm). These compounds reached maximum concentrations at the end of 24 h and returned to normal at 48 h, although the erythema was still maximal (Hensby et al., 1980).

Gorman et al. (1979) found that human foreskin fibroblasts synthesize PGI_2 and that adenylate cyclase of these cells is more sensitive to PGI_2 than PGE_2.

Investigations by Voorhees and Duell (1971) and Hsia et al. (1972) suggest that control of cAMP and cGMP levels may be important in regulation of the growth and function of skin. Cyclic nucleotide phosphodiesterase, the hydrolytic enzyme that cleaves cAMP, has been detected in epidermal tissue and studied by several investigators (Mier and Urselmann, 1972; Marks and Raab, 1974; King et al., 1974, 1975). Many other articles have been published on cAMP and prostaglandins; the reader is referred to reviews by Kuehl (1974) and Goldyne (1975).

Kuehl (1972) and Lord and Ziboh (1978) demonstrated the presence of prostaglandin receptors in rat and human skin. Lord (1978) reported that the receptor sites are associated mainly with the smooth and endoplasmic reticulum in rat skin. Human skin membranes have a high degree of specificity and affinity for binding PGE_2. Protein components appear to be important constituents of these receptor sites since trypsin and heat inhibit this binding. Membrane exposure to ultraviolet light prevented membrane binding for PGE_2. This inhibitory effect of ultraviolet light irradiation could be prevented by the oxidizing agents 5,5'-dithiobis-2-nitrobenzoic acid and α-tocopherol.

Lipid Synthesis and Insulin

Skin actively participates in the biosynthesis of lipids (Vroman et al., 1969; Ziboh et al., 1970; Hsia et al., 1970). Hsia et al. (1966b) showed that the depressed lipogenesis that occurs in human skin during conditions of diabetic acidosis is corrected with insulin administration and that insulin stimulated *in vitro* lipogenesis in human skin. Later, Ziboh and Hsia (1969) demonstrated an impairment of lipogenesis in the skin of alloxan-treated rats, which could be corrected by insulin administration. Ziboh et al. (1971) showed that insulin enhanced glucose uptake by skin 24–108% (depending on the experimental conditions). Epinephrine (1 $\mu g/ml$) had no effect on glucose uptake, whereas in conjunction with insulin it had a synergistic effect. Using [U-^{14}C] glucose, [1-^{14}C] glucose, and [6-^{14}C] glucose, they demonstrated that glucose is an effective precursor for lipogenesis in rat skin. In *in vitro* experiments 1 g of skin converted 300–400 nmol of glucose carbon into lipids and 400–600 nmol of CO_2 from glucose per hour.

Bacteria

Antibacterial and antifungal properties have been attributed to fatty acids and their esters in skin surface lipids. The extent of their contribution is in doubt. Their antibacterial and antifungal properties are becoming important because of their extensive use in cosmetics and pharmaceuticals. Kabara (1975) reported the effect of nine straight-chain fatty acids (C_6–C_{18}) on 12 gram-positive organisms and observed that capric, lauric, myristic, myristoleic, palmitic, palmitoleic, linoleic, and linolenic acids possessed different degrees of antibacterial activity. Lauric acid had the greatest activity. These fatty acids had no antibacterial activity against gram-negative organisms.

Cove et al. (1980) analyzed the sebum excretion rate, bacterial population, and production rate of free fatty acids on human skin of girls 18–21 yr of age. Their results support previous reports that free fatty acids are produced as a result of Micrococcaceae and skin Propionibacteriaceae action and that the size of the bacterial colony is not dependent on the excretion rate of sebum. Weissmann and Noble (1980) observed that exposure to long-wave ultraviolet irradiation increased the excretion of skin lipids, decreased the density of propionibacteria, and caused a transient rise of aerobic cocci on the arm.

METABOLISM OF PROTEINS

Deoxyribonucleic acid (DNA) is known to play a key role in genetic coding and ribonucleic acid (RNA) in the biosynthesis of proteins. Investigators have repeatedly demonstrated the presence of DNA in the nucleus and RNA in the cytosol of cells. Mammalian epidermal cells are no exception. The complex process of protein synthesis is attributed to several constituents, such as ribosomal RNA; messenger RNA; the pool of amino acids, energy sources, and cytoplasmic enzymes known as aminoacyl-t-RNA synthetase; and a carrier of activated amino acids known as transfer RNA. When the genetic code was broken, it was demonstrated that the specificity of the protein-synthesizing mechanism was related to the sequence of triplet nucleotide codons in mRNA, which in turn was determined by a series of triplet nucleotides in DNA. The three different RNA species (rRNA, mRNA, and tRNA) are synthesized on the DNA template. Ribosomal RNA and ribosomal proteins unite and form the ribosomal subunits on which protein synthesis occurs. Messenger RNA accounts for the amino acid specificity of the synthesized proteins and tRNA functions as a carrier for specific amino acids, which are activated by aminoacyl-tRNA synthetase. Extensive details of protein synthesis and the genetic code are reviewed by Crick (1966), Bernstein et al. (1970), and Freedberg (1972).

Early investigations related to protein synthesis in the epidermis were accomplished by administration of ^{14}C- or ^{3}H-labeled thymidine followed by detection of the radioactivity in different parts of the epidermis. Schultze and Oehlert (1960) reported that $1\frac{1}{2}$ hr after administration of [^{3}H]thymidine to young adult rats and mice, radioactive nuclei were found only in the basal layer of the epidermis and esophageal epithelium. Later, Fukuyama and Bernstein (1961) administered [^{3}H]thymidine to newborn rats by intraperitoneal injections and analyzed skin for radioactivity at various time intervals up to 4 days. They observed that the nuclei of the basal layer contained radioactivity within 15 min, and after 12 hr most of the label was restricted to the basal layer. They reported the presence of label in the spinous layer 12 hr after administration and in the granular layer after 2 days. By the third day labeled cells were decreasing in the basal layer, and by the fourth and fifth days labeled cells had decreased in the spinous and granular layers, respectively. These data suggest that DNA synthesis occurs in the basal layer and the rate of cellular movement in newborn rat epidermis is 4 days on the average.

RNA synthesis in newborn rat epidermis was investigated by Fukuyama and Bernstein (1963) in experiments similar to their previous ones with [^{3}H]thymidine. The labeled precursor in this case was [^{3}H]cytidine. They reported RNA synthesis in all layers of the epidermis except the stratum corneum. They also reported that there appear to be different locations of protein synthesis in the epidermis. Around the same time, Freedberg and Baden (1964), using *in vitro* methods with guinea pig epidermal slices, concluded that most protein synthesis occurs in the basal layer of cells. Later, Fukuyama et al. (1965) and Fukuyama and Epstein (1968) demonstrated differential incorporation of labeled amino acids into the epidermis of newborn rats. Leucine, glycine, and alanine were taken up primarily in the basal cell layer, whereas arginine, histidine, and methionine were taken up mainly into the granular layer. Their results also suggested that two different classes of proteins may be synthesized in these layers.

Freedberg and Matsui (1968) noted that the concentration of the synthetase enzymes in newborn guinea pig epidermis is greater than in adult epidermis and also that the specific activity in newborn skin is three times that in adult skin. Freedberg (1972) compared the incorporation of amino acids into peptides by three different systems, namely liver, hair root cells, and epidermis. His data indicated that leucine, alanine, proline, threonine, and serine were most actively incorporated, whereas methionine and histidine were incorporated at a much lower level. Citrulline and ornithine were essentially not incorporated. In the epidermal preparation, leucine and valine were the most actively incorporated amino acids, followed by glutamic acid and serine. Cysteine had a relatively low rate of incorporation. In the hair root preparation, cysteine was by far the most actively incorporated amino acid. Arginine, serine, and proline were relatively high. Surprisingly, glycine had a rather low incorporation.

Penneys and Muench (1971) showed that human epidermis is an extremely rich source of aminoacyl-tRNA synthetases. Several investigators demonstrated that hair follicles are extremely active in protein synthesis (Clarke and Rogers, 1970; Steinert and Rogers, 1971a, 1971b).

Churchill and Speakman (1970) and Clarke and Rogers (1970) suggested that large polyribosomes may be involved in the synthesis of epidermal fibrous proteins. Freedberg (1972) suggested that epidermal keratin molecules may be synthesized on large membrane-bound polyribosomal complexes and polymerization may occur before their release from the complexes.

Flaxman and Harper (1975) maintained organ cultures of adult human skin in a chemically defined medium without serum for 7 days. They observed that the stratum corneum was orthokeratotic and that a significant increase of DNA synthesis occurred during the first 5 days.

Prottey and Ferguson (1974) reported that cultured epidermal cells from the dorsal skin of albino guinea pigs exhibit enhanced cellular metabolism, especially dehydrogenase activity, DNA synthesis, and phospholipid turnover, for the first 6 days.

Investigations related to protein synthesis in psoriatic epithelium have lagged behind those in normal epithelial tissue. Amino acid uptake and glycine transport are more rapid in psoriatic tissue than in normal epithelium. Freedberg (1967) reported that psoriatic epithelium synthesized more protein per unit time than normal epithelium *in vitro*. However, he postulated that it may be an abnormal synthesis of protein (Freedberg, 1972).

Im and Hoopes (1974) investigated the concentrations of glucose, glycogen, and ATP in the peripheral and central layers of sebaceous glands and in the epidermis. They found a decreasing concentration gradient of both carbohydrates from the periphery to the center of the glands, whereas the ATP concentrations were rather constant throughout the gland. Their data indicated that 78% of the detected NADP existed as NADPH. They reported a thorough analysis of 29 enzymes in sebaceous glands and epidermis. Relatively high aminotransferase activities suggested that amino acid metabolism may contribute significantly to the overall metabolism of the sebaceous glands.

Many hormones have been implicated in the regulation of collagenase production (Gross, 1976). In estrogen-treated animals, collagen catabolism is inhibited to a greater extent than its overall resorption, and it was suggested that this effect is due to decreased amounts of collagenase produced by the uterus (Ryan and Woessner, 1971, 1972). In human skin explants in culture Koob et al. (1980) demonstrated that collagenase synthesis is prevented by 10^{-8} M dexamethasone, 5×10^{-4} M dibutyryl cyclic AMP, or 2.5×10^{-3} M theophylline. Progesterone, which inhibits collagenase production in rat uterine cultures, exhibited no inhibition in human skin cultures.

Cortisol inhibition of collagen synthesis and degradation was reported by several investigators (Berliner and Nabors, 1967). Pratt and Aronow (1966) reported that cortisol decreased the rate of thymidine and uridine incorporation into DNA and RNA was depressed with a resultant decrease in the rate of growth of mouse fibroblast. Synthesis of DNA was depressed earlier and to a greater degree than RNA. Saarni et al. (1978) reported that in short-term experiments cortisol did not alter the synthesis of DNA, sulfated glycosamino-glycans, or collagen in human fetal skin fibroblast; however, the synthesis of hyaluronic acid was decreased.

Several enzymes with ribonuclease activity have been isolated and partially purified from adult guinea pig epidermis (Melbye and Freedberg, 1977). Polyamines, especially spermidine, enhance the activity of ribonuclease of both microbial and mammalian origin. Melbye and Freedberg (1977) reported that the effect of spermidine on ribonuclease activity appears not to be general, because the activity of only three of the isolated ribonucleases was increased; the remaining six ribonucleases were inhibited by all polyamine concentrations tested.

Ornithine decarboxylase is a rate-limiting enzyme in the biosynthetic pathway that converts ornithine into the polyamine putrescine before cutaneous spermidine and spermine biosynthesis. The polyamines function in cutaneous DNA, RNA, and protein synthesis during cutaneous cell proliferation. Bolton et al. (1981) observed that ornithine decarboxylase activity increased in guinea pig ear after mild wounds.

Ornithine decarboxylase and S-adenosylmethionine decarboxylase activities were increased after a single topical application of tetradecanoylphorbol acetate to mice (Boutwell et al., 1978). The ornithine decarboxylase activity increased 250-fold at 4.5 h and returned to baseline levels at 12 h, whereas S-adenosylmethionine decarboxylase reached its maximum activity after 12 h but did not return to baseline levels for several days.

Buehler et al. (1977) investigated the activities of ornithine decarboxylase and S-adenosylmethionine decarboxylase in skin fibroblast during cell growth in normal and cystic fibrosis patients during the synthesis of polyamines. They observed a linear relation between increased S-adenosylmethionine activity and putrescine concentration. S-Adenosylmethionine decarboxylase activity increased as the cells reached confluence, whereas ornithine decarboxylase activity increased during early exponential growth and decreased as the cells reached confluence. Growth-promoting stimuli such as hair plucking (Morrison and Goldsmith, 1978) and wounding (Clark-Lewis and Murray, 1978) caused increases of ornithine decarboxylase in skin. Geronemus et al. (1979) reported that topical application of nitrofurazone (Furacin) resulted in a decrease in the rate of wound healing in pig skin. Lesiewicz and Goldsmith (1980) demonstrated that nitrofurazone inhibits ornithine decarboxylase induction for approximately 48 h and suggested that the induction of ornithine decarboxylase may be a necessary preliminary event in wound healing.

Topical application of 12-O-tetradecanoylphorbol-13-acetate (TPA) to mouse skin resulted in the induction of epidermal ornithine decarboxylase activity (Verma et al., 1980). The induction was inhibited by prior treatment of the skin with inhibitors of prostaglandin synthesis, in the following sequence: indomethacin $>$ naproxen $>$ flufenamic acid $>$ acetylsalicylic acid. The inhibitory effect of indomethacin appeared to be specific; however, the inhibition by the prostaglandin synthesis inhibitors was overcome by simultaneous application of PGE_1, PGE_2, PGD_2, or the 6,9-thio analog of PGI_2 with TPA.

Transglutaminases have been demonstrated in human epidermis (Ogawa and Goldsmith, 1976; Goldsmith and Martin, 1975) as well as the hair follicles of several species. The primary substrate for hair follicle transglutaminase is a citrilline-rich protein that is present in the medulla and internal root sheath of the hair; the primary substrate for the epidermal transglutaminase is still undetermined.

Tyrosine aminotransferase activity has been demonstrated in the skin of mice (Pomerantz and Li, 1978), humans, and rats (Thorpe and Goldsmith, 1980).

Age-dependent changes in propyl and lysyl hydroxylase activity of human skin have been reported (Anttinen et al., 1978; Tuderman and Kivirikko, 1977). Both enzyme activities were higher in fetal skin than adult skin. Murad et al. (1980) observed this age-related phenomenon when human skin fibroblasts from different age levels were investigated.

Guinea pig and human skin contain enzymes associated with the inactivation of histamine. Francis et al. (1977) and Yamamoto et al. (1977) demonstrated that this degradation may be due to N-methyltransferase activity, which results in the production of methyl histamine.

Rats subjected to acute or chronic protein deprivation show significant suppression of the mechanisms related to protein catabolism, resulting in a rapid decrease of urinary nitrogen, hydroxyproline, and creatinine. Dawson and Milne (1977) found that protein deprivation caused changes in the solubility of skin collagen, suggesting an increase in its rate of maturation. They suggested that the effects of protein deficiency on skin collagen in rats depend on the previous dietary history of the animals.

Werenne and Revel (1978) investigated the effect of DNA and interferon on protein phosphorylation in human foreskin fibroblasts. They observed that DNA induced phosphorylation if the cells were treated long enough for the induction of interferon. Thymidine incorporation into epidermal growth factor was inhibited by human interferon; maximum inhibition occurred after treatment of cells with interferon before the onset of DNA synthesis. Lin et al. (1980) reported that pretreatment of human fibroblasts with interferon inhibited the effect of epidermal growth factor without affecting its receptor binding.

STEROLS AND STEROIDS

Steroid-Sebum Relationship

The relationship of sebum production to hormones has been investigated by several research groups (Ebling, 1948, 1957a, 1957b; Lasher et al., 1954,

1955; Lorincz and Lancaster, 1957; Woodbury et al., 1965; Thody and Shuster, 1970, 1971, 1972, 1973; Goolamali et al., 1974). It is well known that thyroxine, androgens (testicular as well as adrenal), and the pituitary gland play a role in sebum secretion. Testosterone stimulates sebum production in both normal and castrated rats. However, the pituitary gland is necessary for a maximum response in the rat (Ebling et al., 1969). The colchicine method of Ebling (1974, 1957a, 1957b) shows that increased mitosis is one factor associated with sebaceous gland stimulation by androgens. Sebaceous glands of castrated rats become larger after testosterone administration (Ebling, 1948, 1957a), whereas the response to testosterone in hypophysectomized-castrated rats is insignificant (Lasher et al., 1954, 1955; Ebling, 1957b). Thody and Shuster (1970, 1971) demonstrated that the surface fat of hypophysectomized-castrated rats was significantly less than that of castrated rats. Later, investigators reported the presence of a previously unrecognized pituitary sebotropic hormone in rats and humans (Thody and Shuster, 1972; Shuster and Thody, 1974; Burton et al., 1972; Goolamali et al., 1974) and suggested that it is a melanocyte-stimulating hormone. Recently, Ebling et al. (1975), using matched littermates, demonstrated that the response of sebaceous glands to testosterone is practically eliminated by hypophysectomy and that it may be completely restored by subcutaneous injections of pure bovine growth hormone. It has long been established that antiandrogenic steroids, nonsteroidal antiandrogens, and estrogens inhibited sebum production.

Lutsky et al. (1975) studied the effect of the powerful nonsteroidal antiandrogen flutamide (α,α,α-trifluoro-2-methyl-4'-nitro-m-propionoltuidide) on the sebaceous gland activity of rats when administered orally for 24 days at 20 mg/day. This compound reduced the number, size, and sebum production in ovariectomized, testosterone-stimulated rats. When applied topically to the flank organs (androgen-sensitive cutaneous sebaceous struc-tures) of testosterone-propionate treated female hamsters for 14 days, *in vitro* inhibition of ^{14}C uptake from sodium [1-^{14}C]acetate into lipids occurred. However, when applied to the flank organs of intact male hamsters it had no effect on the pattern of endogenous lipids of the sebaceous gland, even though there was a marked reduction in the size of the flank organ.

The hormonal control of sebaceous glands in rats is thought to act on at least two levels, mitosis and intracellular synthesis. The androgens are considered to act at both levels and the decrease of sebum production by antiandrogen is thought to take place at the same sites. Estrogens are considered to have no effect on mitosis and exhibit their biological effect at the level of intracellular synthesis (Ebling, 1974).

Sterols

Sterols in skin have been the subject of much controversy since the work of Roffo, who implicated cholesterol in the genesis of skin cancer by reasoning that exposure to sunlight caused most skin tumors and also enhanced the cholesterol content of skin. It was further postulated that UV irradiation altered the cholesterol and that the alteration products possessed carcinogenic properties. Subsequently it was suggested that steroid peroxides were the active substances, forming peroxido free radicals that enhanced oxidation of cell nutrients and consequently increased cell metabolism and growth. Lo and Black (1972) investigated the effect of mercury arc lamp irradiation on [^{14}C]cholesterol. They tentatively identified by chromatography the following oxidative products: cholestan-3β,5α,6β-triol; 7α- and 7β-hydroxycholesterol, 7-ketocholesterol-α-oxide. Formation of these products was approximately proportional to exposure time to the mercury arc lamp. It was of interest that 7-ketocholesterol was identified, since this compound has been reported to have carcinogenic properties when administered to experimental animals. The relationship of cholesterol to skin carcinogenesis remains obscure.

Srere et al. (1950) demonstrated that [^{14}C]acetate is converted by rat skin into labeled cholesterol. Subsequently, by use of *in vitro* techniques with human scalp preparations, it was demonstrated that the greater portion of [^{14}C]acetate was incorporated into the squalene fraction, and a much smaller amount was incorporated into cholesterol.

Squalene exists in relatively high concentrations in human sebum, whereas it is virtually absent in sebum from other mammals (Nikkari, 1974). Squalene is synthesized by the sebaceous gland of human skin, while the keratinizing epidermis is responsible for sterol synthesis. The high concentration of squalene in the sebaceous gland is apparently due to a lack of enzymes necessary for its conversion to sterols or the presence of an inhibitor for the conversion.

Wilson (1963) demonstrated two different pathways for the biosyntheses of cholesterol from lanosterol by rat skin and the preputial gland. The Kandutsch-Russel or "saturated side chain" pathway appeared to be by far the predominant one in whole rat skin whereas the Bloch or "unsaturated" pathway plays a minor role. The difference between the two pathways is in the intermediary steps between lanosterol and cholesterol. In the Kandutsch-Russel pathway, reduction of the lanosterol side chain to form dihydro-lanosterol takes place before any modification of the steroid nucleus occurs. 7-Dehydrocholesterol is formed in this pathway and eventually may be converted to vitamin D in the presence of sunlight. In the Bloch pathway, modifications of the steroid nucleus occur first to form desmosterol, after which the side-chain double bond is reduced to form cholesterol. Gaylor (1963) reported that rat skin synthesizes lanosterol from squalene and that this conversion occurs faster in epidermis than in dermis.

Steroids in Human Skin Surface Lipids

The presence of steroid hormones or their metabolites in human skin surface lipids was first reported by Dubovie (1954) and was confirmed by

Carrie and Ruhrmann (1955). Dubovie reported that 17-ketosteroids were present in small amounts, since a fraction obtained from the skin surface lipids by Girard separation gave a positive Zimmerman reaction. Dubovie (1960) expanded his work and presented values for 17-ketosteroids, 3-hydroxysteroids, and 17-hydroxysteroids in human hair fat. Cook and Lorincz (1963) confirmed the work of Dubovie by using enzymatic steroid assay procedures. They used the steroid-specific dehydrogenase enzymes 3α-hydroxysteroid dehydrogenase and 3β,17β-hydroxysteroid dehydrogenase, derived from *Pseudomonas testosterone*. They demonstrated the presence of 3α-hydroxysteroids and 3β,17β-hydroxysteroids in skin surface lipids, with the 3α-hydroxysteroids being present in greater concentrations, and concluded that the concentrations in normal and acned subjects do not differ.

Oertel and Treiber (1969), using spectrophotometric methods, reported microgram amounts of steroids in sebum collected from the scalp and thigh of humans. In an attempt to confirm this, Karunkaran et al. (1973) used labeled steroids as monitors for recoveries and gas chromatographic analysis for the identification and quantitation of steroids in the sebum obtained from face, thigh, and scalp of men. The amounts detected were much lower than those reported by other investigators (Oertel and Treiber, 1969; Dubovie, 1967). They reported evidence for the presence of androstanedione, androstenedione, dihydrotestosterone, androsterone, and dehydroepiandrosterone. Testosterone and etiocholanolone were not detected.

Histochemical Investigations

The presence of hydroxysteroid dehydrogenases in human sebaceous glands appears to be associated with the location of the glands (Baillie et al., 1965). Baillie et al. used the formation of monoformazan or diformazan granules as an indicator system. They reported that human sebaceous glands from the upper part of the back contained seven hydroxysteroid dehydrogenases: 2α, 3β, 16β, and 17β, whereas the forearm was devoid of them. The 3β- and 16β-hydroxysteroid dehydrogenases were very active in areas that are prone to acne vulgaris, whereas the 3α-, 11β-, and 17β-hydroxysteroid dehydrogenases were moderately active, and the 6β- and 20β-hydroxysteroid dehydrogenases were the least active. The same general pattern was observed in acned subjects, except that 3β- and 16β-hydroxysteroid dehydrogenase activity was lower. Later, histochemical studies by Baillie et al. (1966) demonstrated changes in hydroxysteroid dehydrogenase activity relative to age and sex. Histochemical investigations by Julesz et al. (1966a, 1966b) demonstrated a preferential accumulation of 17-ketosteroids in skin obtained from areas of maximum hair growth.

In Vitro Biotransformation of Androgens in Human Skin

Numerous investigators have reported that skin is capable of activation or inactivation of several steroidal hormones. In many instances, these transformations are very similar to those in endocrine organs. These alterations

include activation of the weak androgen dehydroepiandrosterone to testosterone, followed by further activation of testosterone to 5α-dihydrotesto-
sterone and eventually inactivation of 5α-dihydrotestosterone.

Wotiz et al. (1956) reported that human skin was capable of metabolizing
testosterone. By using paper chromatography and IR spectophotometry, they
detected eight radioactive Zimmermann positive spots. They demonstrated that
skin metabolized testosterone at a greater rate than several other normal and
malignant tissues, except for breast cancer tissue, which metabolized testosterone approximately three times as rapidly as skin.

Subsequently, testosterone was incubated with human male mammary
skin obtained from a patient with Kleinfelter's syndrome (Rongone, 1966). By
use of column chromatography in conjunction with gas-liquid chromatography, 5α-androstane-3,17-dione; 3α-hydroxy-5α-androstane-17-one; 5α-
androstane-3,17-dione; androst-4-ene-3,17-dione and 3α-hydroxy-5β-androstane-
17-one were identified as metabolites. It is the consensus that reduction of the
Δ^4 bond in steroids proceeds by the 5α route in skin.

Cameron et al. (1966) reported *in vitro* formation of testosterone and
androst-4-ene-3,17-dione from dehydroepiandrosterone (DHA). This was the
first report indicating that human skin could convert the Δ^5-3β hydroxyl group
to the Δ^4-3 keto group. It suggested that skin cholesterol could be converted to
a biologically active steroid in skin. The conversion of cholesterol to pregnenolone has not been demonstrated to occur in skin. It has been suggested that
one of the main pathways of DHA metabolism to androsterone in skin is
through androstene-3,17-dione and testosterone.

It appears that one characteristic difference between cutaneous steroid
metabolism and systemic metabolism is the stereospecific reduction at C-5.
Approximately equivalent amounts of the 5α and 5β isomers are formed in
the systemic pathways. Mauvais-Jarvis et al. (1969) reported that the 5α/5β
ratio of urinary C_{19} steroids is three times greater when testosterone is applied
topically than when it is administered intravenously and six times greater than
when it is given orally. This investigation indicates that topically applied
steroids are indeed absorbed through the skin and enter the systemic
metabolic pool. Cutaneous absorption of steroids has been observed several
times, and the effects of topically applied estrogens on males, resulting in
secondary female characteristics, are well known.

Faredin et al. (1967) incubated [4-C^{14}]dehydroepiandrosterone with
male pubic skin and reported the isolation and identification of 3α-hydroxy-5α-
androstane-17-one; 5α-androstane-3,17-dione; androst-4-ene-3,17-dione; androst-
5-ene-3β,17β-diol; 17β-hydroxy-androst-5-ene-3-one; 7α-hydroxydehydroepian-
drosterone; 7-ketodehydroepiandrosterone; epiandrosterone; testosterone; 16α-
hydroxydehydroepiandrosterone and 5β-androstane-3,17-dione.

Faredin et al. (1969) extended their investigations on [4-^{14}C]dehydro-
epiandrosterone and reported identification of the metabolite 17β-hydroxy-
DHA, previously unreported in humans. However, the main 7-hydroxy
metabolite was the 7α isomer. The mechanism of the 7β-hydroxyl metabolite

is unresolved; that is, reduction of 7-keto-KHA or direct 7β-hydroxylation of DHA.

A third possible pathway for DHA metabolism in skin was reported by Gallegos and Berliner (1967) and Faredin et al. (1969) when they demonstrated the conversion of DHA to androst-4-ene-3,17-diol with human male skin in organ cultures and skin, respectively. Gallegos and Berliner also reported the formation of androst-4-ene-3,17-dione; testosterone; and DHA sulfate. The ability of the skin to form water-soluble steroids was later confirmed by Berliner et al. (1968) in male and female skin.

Gomez and Hsia (1968) incubated [4-^{14}C] testosterone and [4-^{14}C] androst-4-ene-3,17-dione with adult skin obtained at autopsy and with neonatal abdominal and foreskin, and demonstrated the formation of 5α-dihydrotestosterone, 5α-androstanedione; androsterone; and epiandrosterone. These data were confirmed by Wilson and Walker (1969). Wilson and Walker also reported a difference in the 5α-reductase activity of skin from different anatomical sites. Activities were high in labia majora, scrotum, prepuce, and clitoris, and low in the mons, trunk, and limb areas. They also reported that 5α-steroid hydrogenase activity increases in the prepuce for the first 3 months after birth and then falls until adult levels are attained.

Oertel and Treiber (1967) administered [7α-^{3}H] dehydroepiandrosterone [^{35}S] sulfate intravenously to normal male subjects and isolated several labeled metabolites in skin and sweat extracts. They reported that up to 95% of the steroids present in the skin extracts were sulfoconjugates, whereas 90% of the steroids in the sweat extracts were in the free steroid fraction. They concluded that endogenous sulfoconjugated DHA is metabolized in human skin and that the sulfoconjugated metabolites undergo hydrolysis prior to excretion in sweat. It has been reported that adult human skin contains both hydrolytic enzymes β-glucuronidase and steroid sulfatase (Mesirow and Stoughton, 1954; Kim and Herrmann, 1968).

Shoulder skin from male subjects with and without acne was incubated in Krebs improved Ringer I solution with the labeled steroid substrates [7α-^{3}H] dehydroepiandrosterone, [7α-^{3}H] androstenedione, and [7α-^{3}H] testosterone (Hay and Hodgins, 1974). No marked metabolic changes were observed between the acned and control subjects. The acne tissue formed greater amounts of 5α-dihydrostestosterone from testosterone than the control. Cooper et al. (1978) reported that the activities of the enzymes 5α-reductase and 17β-hydroxysteroid dehydrogenase do not automatically increase with increased sebaceous gland activity.

A combination of estrogens and glucocorticoid treatment daily suppressed sebum production in women with severe acne (Saihan and Burton, 1980).

Androgen Metabolism in Experimental Animals

Several of the appendages of the skin are androgen-responsive tissues. This makes steroid metabolic investigations in skin somewhat more difficult than similar studies in other responsive tissues. To elucidate the effects of the different skin appendages, Hay and Hodgins (1977) investigated steroid-related enzymes in epidermis, sweat glands, sebaceous glands, hair follicles, and dermis isolated from human forehead and axillary skin. All the appendages investigated contained $17\beta,3\beta$ and 3α-hydroxysteroid dehydrogenase activity, 3β-hydroxysteroid dehydrogenase-Δ^4-Δ^5-isomerase activity, and 5α-reductase activity. Ninety percent of the Δ^5-3β-hydroxysteroid dehydrogenase activity of the forehead skin was localized in the sebaceous glands. Approximately 50% of the 5α-reductase of forehead skin was found in the sebaceous glands; the sweat glands of the axillary skin contained a slightly greater amount.

The biological action of testosterone is considered to be dependent on its conversion to 5α-dihydrotestosterone by the enzyme 5α-reductase. 5α-Dihydrotestosterone then binds to specific cytosol receptors and is transported into the nuclei, where the androgen-receptor complex binds to an acceptor that is mainly chromatin. Eventually, there is an increase in RNA synthesis.

Localization of 5α-reductase in the nucleus is considered the characteristic feature of target organs (Frederiksen and Wilson, 1971 and Nozu and Tamaoki, 1974); in nontarget organs it is located in the cytosol (Wilson and Gloyna, 1970).

Bazzano and Reisner (1974) administered [^{3}H]testosterone intravenously to 4-month-old castrated rats and determined the comparative rate of *in vivo* uptake of testosterone and metabolites by skin and accessory sex organs at different time intervals. They observed peak uptake of [^{3}H]testosterone in the prostate and skin within 45 min, whereas radioactivity was still increasing in the preputial gland and seminal vesicles 90 min after injection. However, the major metabolite was 5α-dihydrotestosterone in all of the tissues. Comparative quantitative results of androgen uptake in skin, expressed as counts per minute per total amount of tissue $\times 10^{-5}$, were: testosterone, 114; dihydrotestosterone, 19; androstenedione, 9; androstanedione, 9; and androstandiol, 6.

Several investigators have studied the metabolism of testosterone by the rat preputial gland (Bardin et al., 1970; Bullock et al., 1970; Richardson and Axelrod, 1971). Richardson and Axelrod (1971) incubated [7α-^{3}H]testosterone with preputial gland nuclei and isolated 5α-dihydrotestosterone, 5α-androstane-$3\beta,17\beta$-diol, and 3-epiandrosterone. In their investigations with minced rat preputial glands they observed that dihydrotestosterone represented approximately 70% of the metabolites formed. Their investigations support the work of Fang et al. (1969) and Bruchovsky and Wilson (1968) who showed that androgen target tissues retain 5α-dihydrotestosterone. Recently, Adachi (1974) has reported the presence of androgen receptor proteins in the hamster sebaceous gland.

Dehydroepiandrosterone metabolism by the rat preputial gland has been investigated, and androstenedione was identified as a metabolite (Bazzano and Reisner, 1974).

Testosterone Metabolism and Hair Growth

Schweikert and Wilson (1974) investigated the relationship of testosterone and hair growth in resting (telogen) and growing (anagen) hair roots from different anatomical sites of men and women. The major metabolites of [1,2-^{3}H] testosterone in all cases were 5α reduced and 17-keto products. The formation of 17-ketosteroid metabolites was decreased in resting hairs from all anatomical sites, whereas dihydrotestosterone formation was decreased only in resting hair roots from the scalp. A higher metabolic rate was observed at all locations of the scalp of bald men compared to corresponding sites of women and nonbald men, and a significantly higher metabolic rate was observed in the frontal area of bald men.

Adachi and Kano (1970) reported that particulate fractions obtained from human scalp hair follicles contained adenyl cyclase activity, which was inhibited by 5α-androstan-17β-ol-3-one (dihydrotestosterone) but not by testosterone, and that it was activated by estrone.

Unbound testosterone, the substrate for the 5α-reductase in skin, may originate from circulating testosterone or from the transformation of C_{19} steroids such as androstenedione within the target cells (Ito and Horton, 1971).

The 5α-reductase distribution in skin varies in the appendages of skin. The 5α-reductase activity in axillary skin of both men and women was highest in the sweat glands, followed by the sebaceous glands. Hair follicles were significantly lower than sebaceous glands (Takayasu et al., 1980).

Isolated hair follicles metabolize testosterone by reduction of the 4-5 double bond to form 5α-dihydrotestosterone and 17β-hydroxysteroid dehydrogenation (Fayekas and Dandor, 1972; Schweikert and Wilson, 1974). Anagen hair follicles demonstrated a greater 5α-reductase activity than resting hair follicles.

A statistically significant increase of 5α-reductase activity was observed in resting hair follicles in patients with polycystic ovaries compared to normal individuals (Miyazaki et al., 1978). This phenomenon was not observed in growing hair follicles.

The conversion of [^{3}H] testosterone to 5α-androstane-3α,17β-diol and 5α-androstane-3β,17β-diol in skin from women with hirsutism was significantly greater than in skin homogenates from normal women (Kuttenn et al., 1977) but the same as the value for normal men. Patients with idiopathic hirsutism had the highest conversion values. Androstenedione was the principal androgen secreted in hirsutism. Svensson et al. (1979) demonstrated differences in 5α-reductase activity between scrotal skin of hypospadic and normal men.

Five metabolites were isolated when dehydroepiandrosterone was incubated with human scalp hair follicles. Androstenedione, androstenediol, and 7α-hydroxydehydroepiandrosterone were identified. Androstenediol and 7α-hydroxydehydroepiandrosterone were the major metabolites. The 7α-hydroxylation, cytochrome P-450 system was inhibited by metyrapone and a carbon monoxide atmosphere. The formation of androstenediol was not inhibited by either metyrapone or CO. The enzyme system responsible for the hydroxylation was associated with the subcellular particulate fraction (Vermorken et al., 1979).

Wright and Giacomini (1980) studied the metabolism of ^{3}H-labeled 17β-hydroxy-5α-androstane-3-one in subcellular fractions of human female pubic skin. They observed that both cytosol and microsomal fractions converted dihydrotestosterone to mainly 5α-androstane-3α,17β-diol and 5α-androstane-3α,17β-diol. In the cytosol incubations, the rate of 3α-diol formation was greater than that of 3β-diol when NADPH was the cofactor, whereas 3β-diol was the major metabolite when NADH was used. 5α-Androstane-3β,17β-diol was the main product formed in the microsomal incubations whether NADH or NADPH was used.

The pattern of C_{19} steroid metabolism appears to change somewhat under different physiological conditions. Moretti et al. (1978) reported that testosterone metabolism in basal cell epitheliomas differs from that of normal surrounding skin. They reported a significant decrease in 5α-reductase activity in basal cell epitheliomas with a resultant decrease in dihydrotestosterone and androstanediol production; no significant change occurred in 17β-hydroxysteroid activity.

In rats fed a magnesium-deficient diet, the mast cell population decreased in the skin (Belanger, 1977). Administration of large doses of testosterone to males and estradiol to females moderated the loss of mast cells in skin and depressed the mast cell population increase in bone marrow.

Dehydroepiandrosterone inhibited thymidine incorporation into normal human skin fibroblasts (Saenger and New, 1977), which resulted in decreased cellular proliferation.

Biotransformations of C_{21} Steroids

Although Malkinson et al. (1959) observed the conversion of cortisol to cortisone, the relationship of skin and C_{21} steroids has not been investigated to the same extent as that of androgen and skin. This may be explained largely by the fact that the sebaceous gland appears to be a target organ for the androgens.

Several years later Hsia et al. (1964) demonstrated that [4-^{14}C]hydrocortisone was converted to several unidentified metabolites by human skin. The following year these investigators reported that human skin lost its ability to metabolize cortisol a few hours after death; however, the activity was restored by adding TPNH generating systems. Both dermis and epidermis were capable of metabolizing cortisol, and this property is not related to sebaceous glands and hair follicles because skin from the sole, which has neither sebaceous glands nor hair follicles, metabolized cortisol (Hsia et al., 1965). Later Hsia and Hao (1966) demonstrated the conversion of [4-^{14}C]cortisol to several metabolites by slices of human skin. The metabolites isolated by paper chromatography and isotopic dilution procedures were: cortison, 4-pregnene-

11β,17α,20β,21-tetraol-3-one (Reichstein's substance E); 4-pregnene-11β,17α,-20α,21-tetraol-3-one; 4-pregnene-17α,20β,21-triol-3,11-dione (U); 4-pregnene-17α,2α,21-triol-3,11-dione; allodihydrocortisol; and allotetrahydrocortisol. The latter two metabolites were detected only from incubation mixtures with foreskin and not from incubations with skin from other anatomical sites.

Progesterone was actively metabolized by human skin and vaginal mucosa to the 5α isomers (Frost et al., 1969). The metabolites identified were: 5α-pregnane-3,20-dione; 5α-pregnane-3α-ol-20-one; 5α-pregnane-3β-ol-20-one; 5α-pregnane-3β,20α-diol; 4-pregnene-20α-ol-3-one; and 5α-pregnane-3α,20α-diol. The major pathway of metabolism in both tissues followed the 5α-pregnane route. Relatively less 5α-pregnane metabolites were formed in abdominal skin (17%) than in foreskin (52%) or vaginal mucosa (63%), except for 5α-pregnane-3α,20α-diol. Garzan and Berliner (1970) demonstrated the conversion of progesterone to 6β-hydroxyprogesterone by human skin and skin fibroblasts obtained from the same skin specimen and grown in cell cultures.

Recently, Gomez et al. (1975) reported on the metabolism of [4-^{14}C]-progesterone by subcellular fractions of human skin. They reported the presence of a membrane-bound 5α-reductase and a soluble 20α-hydroxysteroid dehydrogenase, both of which utilize TPNH as a cofactor.

Primate skin (squirrel monkey) is capable of converting pregnenodone to progresterone (Rongone, 1969).

There is no known effect of the progesterone metabolites in skin, and the effects of progesterone are highly questionable. Hsia (1971) reported that progesterone inhibits the production of 5α-dihydrotestosterone by microsomes of human skin. He also reported data pertaining to the relationship between the structure of steroids and their inhibitory effect on the 5α reduction of testosterone by microsomes of human skin. Steroids that are strong inhibitors are: progesterone (93%), deoxycorticosterone acetate (86%), deoxycorticosterone (85%), and androstenedione (76%), 19-nontestosterone (55%), and 17α-hydroxyprogesterone (54%). Steroids with mild or weak inhibitory effects are: corticosterone (24%), epitosterone (24%), 4-androstene-11β-ol-3,17-dione (23%), 4-androstene-3,11,17-trione (8%), estrone (8%), and cortisone (5%).

Progesterone and 5α-pregnane-3,20-dione inhibit the conversion of [1,2-^{3}H]dihydrotestosterone to 5α-androstane-3α,17β-diol and 5α-androstane-3β,17α-diol by the cytosolic and microsomal cellular subfractions of pubic skin. The 5α-pregnane-3,20-dione acted as a competitive inhibitor for both 3α- and 3β-hydroxysteroid dehydrogenases (Giacomini and Wright, 1979).

Systemic corticosteroid therapy frequently results in hirsutism, purpeva, stria, skin atrophy, and other Cushing-like syndromes. Systemic administration of corticosteroids may also result in skin lesions characterized by hemorrhagic longitudinal linear tearing (Gottlieb et al., 1980).

Betamethasone applied topically to the skin of normal individuals increased cutaneous blood flow (Kjeldstrup et al., 1978). [^{3}H]Betamethasone-

17-valerate was converted to [³H]betamethasone by human whole skin, epidermis, and dermis. After 6 h of incubation with these preparations, [³H]betamethasone-17-valerate appeared to be resistant to metabolism through oxidation but was susceptible to hydrolysis in skin (Rawlins et al., 1979).

Protein synthesis in skin was decreased following glucocorticoid treatment (Newman and Cutroneo, 1978; Cutroneo and Counts, 1975; Uitto et al., 1972). Cutroneo and Clarke (1979) demonstrated that glucocorticoids have not only an antianabolic effect but also an anticatabolic effect on proteins in skin.

The addition of cortisol, free L-amino acids, or a combination of both resulted in increased protection of skin at subzero temperatures. The most protective agent for protein synthesizing activity and the membrane integrity of the cutaneous cells was ATP added to the various storage media (DeLoecker et al., 1980).

Long-term treatment of rabbits with prednisolone resulted in increased degradation of newly synthesized collagen as well as cell biosynthesis in damaged skin (Manthorpe et al., 1980). Prednisolone also inhibited the biosynthesis of glycosaminoglycans and decreased the total amount of glycosaminoglycans and nucleic acids in skin.

Priestly (1978) demonstrated that both clobetasol propionate and betamethansone valerate inhibited the synthesis of collagen and other proteins by fibroblasts. Collagen synthesis was inhibited to a greater degree than synthesis of the other proteins.

Using baby foreskin fibroblasts, Ponec et al. (1979) demonstrated that cortisol-17-butyrate and clobetasol-17-propionate caused a specific decrease in the synthesis of collagen. However, no decrease in cellular prolyl hydroxylase activity occurred.

Estrogen

Frost et al. (1966) demonstrated the interconversion of estrone and 17β-estradiol by the foreskin of the newborn. The equilibrium appeared to be toward the conversion of 17β-estradiol to estrone. Experiments with fresh surgical abdominal skin specimens also showed conversion of 17β-estradiol to estrone. Bazzano and Reisner (1974) reported that rat preputial gland and human sebaceous glands microdissected from $CaCl_2$-treated whole skin also convert 17β-estradiol to estrone.

Subcutaneous and topical administration of estradiol to young mice at different ages resulted in an increase of hyaluronic acid and water content in mouse skin (Uzuka et al., 1979). The increase appeared to be dependent on dose, number of estradiol injections, and age. This increase of hyaluronic acid was blocked by simultaneous administration of estradiol and an antiestrogen.

Receptors

Investigations during the 1960s suggested that the skin is a target organ for several steroid hormones. The past 10 yr have proved that this is true and that there are steroid receptors in mammalian skin. An accepted theory of steroid action is that steroids affect target cells by complexing to special proteins called receptors, which are present only in target cells. The complex migrates into the nucleus and binds to the chromatin, which causes an alteration of gene expression. Receptors have been demonstrated in mammalian skin for the estrogens, androgens, glucocorticoids, and progesterone (Bakert et al., 1977; Eppenburger and Hsia, 1972; Uzuka et al., 1978; Giannopoulos et al., 1974). Although androgen receptors have been reported and identified in genital and interscapular skin of humans (Kaufman et al., 1976; Evan et al., 1977; Bonne et al., 1977) and human skin fibroblast (Kennan et al., 1975; Griffen et al., 1976), no evidence of estrogen receptors was reported in human skin until recently.

A low-capacity, high-affinity estradiol-binding protein in the cytosol of human face skin was found by Hasselquist et al. (1980).

A method for the assay of androgen receptors in human skin cytosol was devised by Mowszowicz et al. (1981). These investigators measured the androgen-binding capacity of human skin cytosol by using 5α-[^{3}H] dihydrotesto-sterone. They observed that the androgen receptor binding capacity was a function of age, sex, and anatomic site in normal and pathological conditions. Androgen receptors have been detected in duck preen glands, the counterpart of human sebaceous glands, by using dextran-coated charcoal absorption (Daniel et al., 1977).

Androgen Metabolism by Chicken Uropygial Gland

The uropygial gland is the unique cutaneous gland of birds and it is the homologue of the sebaceous glands of mammals. The lipids of the uropygial gland have been analyzed by several investigators (Haahti et al., 1964; Odham, 1967; Nicolaides et al., 1968; Jacob and Zeman, 1972) and in general resemble the lipids of mammalian sebum. The major lipids of waterfowl are predominantly branched-chain, saturated monoester waxes (Haahti et al., 1964; Odham, 1967).

Rongone and co-workers (1967, 1968) investigated the metabolism of androgens by chicken uropygial glands. Uropygial gland metabolizes [4-^{14}C]-testosterone and [4-^{14}C] androstene-3,17-dione similarly to skin. Testosterone metabolites identified by gas chromatography, column chromatography, and crystallization to constant specific activity were 3α-hydroxy-5α-androstane-17-one; 5α-androstane-3,17-dione; and 5α-androstane-3α,17β-diol. Incubation of androstenedione with uropygial homogenates resulted in identification of the metabolites 3α-hydroxy-5α-androstane-17-one and 5α-androstane-3α,17β-diol.

Bile Acids

The pruritus of cholestasis is caused by retention of bile acids with their accumulation in the skin. Ghent et al. (1977) cast doubt on this belief when they demonstrated (1) that there was no consistent relation between pruritus and concentrations of either total or individual bile acids in serum, and (2) that concentrations of bile acids on the skin surface were not correlated with pruritus. They suggested that bile acid metabolites in skin may lead to the production and accumulation of pruritogenic substances, variable responses in itch threshold, or an intermediate mediator of itch sensation to bile acids.

Fibroblast cultures have become a common tool in many different investigations, such as diagnosis of genetic disorders, viral transformations, properties of plasma membranes, metabolic transformations, and so on. The origin of the fibroblastic cells is of great importance. It was demonstrated by Conrad et al. (1977) that the fibroblastlike cells from cornea, heart, and skin of embryonic chicks show characteristic differences when grown *in vitro*. Schneider et al. (1977) showed significant differences between fibroblasts obtained from skin and lung of human fetuses, although they have morphological similarities. Lemonnier et al. (1980) demonstrated that skin fibroblasts had faster growth, smaller cell volume, and lower glucose consumption than to aponeurosis fibroblasts.

Human fibroblasts cultured from foreskin and abdominal skin converted androstenedione to estrone (Schweikert et al., 1976; Schweikert, 1977). Mowszowicz et al. (1980) demonstrated that 5α-reductase activity increased in cultured skin fibroblasts with successive subcultures.

Several investigators, using cultured fibroblasts from genital skin, reported that an inherited deficiency of 5α-reductase, which converts testosterone to dihydrotestosterone in androgen target tissue, may result in a specific form of male pseudohermaphroditism (Moore et al., 1975; Griffin et al., 1976; Peterson et al., 1977; Sanger et al., 1978; Kuttenn et al., 1979; Savage et al., 1980).

Kishore and Boutwell (1980) demonstrated that mouse epidermis contains a cytosolic oxidase and reductase capable of oxidizing and reducing retinal. The oxidase has an optimum pH of 8.5 and its activity is enhanced slightly by the addition of either FAD or NAD. The reductase's optimum pH is 6.0 and its activity was enhanced 5- to 7-fold by the addition of reduced NAD or NADPH.

Photochemical conversion of 7-dehydrocholesterol to previtamin D_3 in skin by sunlight is well established (Holick et al., 1977, 1979, 1980). Holick et al. (1981) proposed a new mechanism controlling cutaneous photosynthesis of previtamin D_3. When skin is initially exposed to ultraviolet radiation, the 7-dehydrocholesterol is converted to previtamin D_3, which can undergo isomerization to D_3 or photoisomerization to lumisterol$_3$ and tachysterol$_3$. After prolonged exposure to sun, pre-D_3 synthesis reaches a level at about 10–15% of the original 7-dehydrocholesterol. Since vitamin-D-binding protein has no affinity or minimum affinity for the inert products lumisterol$_3$ and tachysterol$_3$, very small amounts of these photoisomers go into the circulation; they are probably sloughed off in the normal turnover of skin. The investigators reported that the photoproduction of lumisterol$_3$ is significantly greater in hypopigmented skin than in heavily pigmented skin.

Kuttan (1980) demonstrated that prolyl hydroxylase activity was lower in the skin of scorbutic guinea pigs. This low prolylhydroxylase could be enhanced by adding ascorbate, ferrous ions, and α-ketoglutarate before the assay.

Fung and Khachadurian (1980) showed that polyoxyethylated cholesterol depresses cholesterol synthesis by inhibiting β-hydroxy-β-methylglutarylCoA (HMG-CoA) reductase and decreases cholesteryl ester formation by inhibiting acyl-CoA:cholesterol acyltransferase in cultured skin fibroblasts.

Bickers (1978) demonstrated that the activity of aryl hydrocarbon hydroxylase, a cytochrome P-450 dependent enzyme, is increased in skin after topical application of coal to humans. Studies with animals demonstrated that topical application of coal tar also caused an increased in liver aryl hydrocarbon hydroxylase after percutaneous absorption.

REFERENCES

Abe, T., Ohkido, M., and Yamamoto, K. 1978. Studies on skin surface barrier functions: Skin surface lipids and transepidermal water loss in atopic skin during childhood. *J. Dermatol.* 5:223–229.

Adachi, K. 1961. Metabolism of glycogen in the skin and the effect of x-rays. *J. Invest. Dermatol.* 37:381–395.

Adachi, K. 1962. Metabolism of glycogen in the skin and the effect of x-rays. *J. Invest. Dermatol.* 37:381–393.

Adachi, K. 1974. Receptor proteins for androgen in hamster sebaceous glands. *J. Invest. Dermatol.* 62:217–223.

Adachi, K. and Kano, M. 1970. Adenyl cyclase in human hair follicles; its inhibition by dihydrotestosterone. *Biochem. Biophy. Res. Commun.* 41:884–890.

Adachi, K. and Uno, H. 1969. Glucose metabolism of growing and resting human hair follicles. *Am. J. Physiol.* 215:1234–1239.

Adachi, K., Yoshikawa, K., Halprin, K. and Levine, V. 1975. Prostaglandin and cyclic AMP in epidermis: Evidence for the independent action of prostaglandins and adrenaline on the adenyl cyclase system in pig and human epidermis, normal and psoriatic. *Br. J. Dermatol.* 92:381–388.

Ansari, N. M. A., Fu, H. C. and Nicolaides, N. 1970. Fatty acids of the alkane diol esters of vernix caseosa. *Lipids* 5:279–282.

Anttinen, H., Orva, S., Ryhanen, L. and Kivirikko, K. I. 1973. Assay of protocollagen lysyl hydroxylase activity in the skin of human subjects and changes in the activity with age. *Clin. Chim. Acta* 47:289–292.

Anttinen, H., Oikarinen, A. and Kivirikko, K. I. 1977. Age-related changes in human skin collagen galactosyltransferase and collagen glucosyltransferase activities. *Clin. Chim. Acta* 76:95–101.

Aoyasi, T., Adachi, K., Halprin, K. M. and Levine, V. 1980. The effects of epidermal growth factor on the cyclic nucleotide system in pig epidermis. *J. Invest. Dermatol.* 74:238–241.

Arturson, G., Hamberg, M. and Jonsson, C. E. 1973. Prostaglandins in human burn blister fluid. *Acta Physiol. Scand.* 87:270–276.

Arumugham, R. and Bose, S. M. 1979. Effect of protein deficiency on the metabolism of glycoproteins and glycosaminoglycans in albino rat skin. *Acta Biochim. Pol.* 26:295–301.

Aso, K., Deneau, D. G., Krulig, L., Wilinson, D. I. and Farber, E. M. 1975. Epidermal synthesis of prostaglandins and their effect on levels of cyclic adenosine 3′,5′-monophosphate. *J. Invest. Dermatol.* 64:326–331.

Baillie, A. H., Calman, K. C. and Milne, J. A. 1965. Histochemical distribution of hydroxysteroid dehydrogenases in human skin. *Br. J. Dermatol.* 77:610–616.

Baillie, A. H., Thompson, J. and Milne, J. A. 1966. The distribution of hydroxysteroid dehydrogenase in human sebaceous glands. *Br. J. Dermatol.* 78:451–457.

Baker, J. F., Christian, R. A., Simpson, P. and White, A. M. 1977. The binding of topically applied glucocorticoids to rat skin. *Br. J. Dermatol.* 96:171–178.

Bardin, C. W., Bullock, L., Schneider, G., Allison, J. E. and Stanley, A. J. 1970. Pseudohermaphrodite rat; end organ insensitivity to testosterone. *Science* 167:1136–1137.

Baynes, J. and Levine, M. 1977. The role of histidine in human epidermis. *Br. J. Dermatol.* 97:387–394.

Bazzano, G. S. and Reisner, R. M. 1974. Steroid pathways in sebaceous glands. *J. Invest. Dermatol.* 62:211–216.

Belanger, L. F. 1977. Variations in the mast cell population of skin and bone marrow in magnesium-deprived rats. The influence of sex hormones. *J. Nutr.* 107:2164–2170.

Benson, J. W., Buja, M. L., Thompson, R. H. and Gordon, R. S. 1974. Glucose utilization by sweat glands during fasting in man. *J. Invest. Dermatol.* 63:287–291.

Bentley, J. P. 1970. The biological role of the ground substance mucopoly-saccharides. In *Advances in biology of skin*, vol. 10, pp. 103–121. eds. W. Montagna, J. B. Bently, R. L. Dobson. New York: Meredith.

Bergstrom, S., Carlson, L. A. and Ekelund, L. G. 1965. Cardiovascular and metabolic response to infusions of prostaglandin E_1 and to simultaneous infusions of noradrenaline and prostaglandin E_1 in man. *Acta Physiol. Scand.* 64:332–339.

Berliner, D. L. and Nabors, C. J. 1967. Effects of corticosteroids on fibroblast functions. *J. Reticuloendothel. Soc.* 4:284–313.

Berliner, D. L., Pasqualine, J. R. and Gallegos, A. J. 1968. The formation of water soluble steroids by human skin. *J. Invest. Dermatol.* 50:220–224.

Bernstein, I. A., Chakrabarti, S. G., Kumaroo, K. K. and Sibrack, L. A. 1970. Synthesis of protein in mammalian epidermis. *J. Invest. Dermatol.* 55:291–302.

Bhattacharyya, A. K. and Connor, W. E. 1979. Effect of different dietary fats on daily loss of sterols from the skin of man. *Nutr. Metab.* 23:384–390.

Bickers, D. R. and Kappas, A. 1978. Human skin aryl hydrocarbon hydroxylase. Induction by coal tar. *J. Clin. Invest.* 62:1061–1068.

Billingham, R. E. and Silver, W. K. 1967. Studies on the conservation of epidermal specifices of skin and certain mucosas in adult mammals. *J. Exp. Med.* 125:429–446.

Bolton, L. L., Constantine, B. E. and Rovee, D. T. 1981. The kinetics of ornithine decarboxylase activity as a function of wounding in guinea pig ear epidermis. *J. Clin. Invest. Dermatol.* 76:480–483.

Bonne, C., Saurat, H.-H., Chivot, M., Lehuschet, D. and Raynaud, J. 1977. Androgen receptor in human skin. *Br. J. Dermatol.* 97:501–504.

Booth, B. A., Polak, K. L. and Uitto, J. 1980. Collagen biosynthesis by human skin fibroblasts. I. Optimization of the culture conditions for synthesis of type I and type III procollagens. *Biochim. Biophys. Acta* 607:145–160.

Boughton, B. and Wheatley, V. R. 1959. Studies of sebum. 9. Further studies of the unsaponifiable matter of human forearm "sebum." *Biochem. J.* 73:144–149.

Boutwell, R. K., O'Brien, T. G., Verma, A. K., Weekes, R. G., DeYoung, L. M.,

Ashendel, C. L. and Astrup, E. G. 1978. The induction of ornithine-decarboxylase activity and its control in mouse skin epidermis. *Adv. Enzyme Regul.* 17:89–112.

Bowser, P. A. and Gray, G. M. 1978. Sphingomyelinase in pig and human epidermis. *J. Invest. Dermatol.* 70:331–335.

Braun-Falco, O. 1954. Histochemisohe and morphologische studien an nor-maler and pathologisch. Veranderter haut. *Arch. Dermatol. Syphilol.* 198:111–198.

Brocklehurst, W. E. 1971. Role of kinins and prostaglandins in inflammation. *Proc. R. Soc. Med.* 64:4–6.

Brown, R. A., Young, W. S. and Nicolaides, N. 1954. Analysis of high molecular weight alcohols by the mass spectrometer. The wax alcohols of human hair fat. *Anal. Chem.* 26:1653–1654.

Bruchovsky, N. and Wilson, J. D. 1968. The conversion of testosterone to 5α-androstane-17β-ol-3-one by rat prostate *in vivo* and *in vitro*. *J. Biol. Chem.* 243:2012–2021.

Buehler, B., Wright, R., Schott, S., Darby, B. and Rennert, O. M. 1977. Ornithine decarboxylase and *S*-adenosyl methionine decarboxylase in skin fibroblasts of normal and cystic fibrosis patients. *Pediatr. Res.* 11:186–190.

Bullock, L., Schneider, G. and Bardin, C. W. 1970. Steroid reductase activity in tissues from rats with end organ insensitivity to testosterone. *Life Sci.* 9:701–705.

Burr, G. O. and Burr, M. M. 1929. A new deficiency disease produced by a rigid exclusion of fat from the diet. *J. Biol. Chem.* 82:345–367.

Burr, G. O. and Burr, M. M. 1930. On the nature and role of the fatty acids essential in nutrition. *J. Biol. Chem.* 86:587–621.

Burton, A. C. 1961. Special features of the circulation of the skin. *Adv. Biol. Skin* 2:117–122.

Burton, J. L., Libman, L. J., Cunliffe, W. J., Wilkinson, R., Hall, R. and Shuster, S. 1972. Sebum excretion in acromegaly. *Br. Med. J.* 1:406–408.

Cameron, E. H. D., Baillie, A. H., Grant, J. K., Milne, J. A. and Thomson, J. 1966. Transformation *in vitro* of [7α-^{3}H]-dehydroepiandrosterone to [^{3}H]-testosterone by skin from men. *J. Endocrinol.* 35:XIX (abstract).

Camp, R. and Greaves, M. W. 1980. The catabolism of prostaglandins by rat skin. *Biochem. J.* 186:153–160.

Carrie, C. and Ruhrmann, H. 1955. Uber den Gehalt der Hau-toberflachenlipoide on 17-ketosteroiden. *Hautarzt* 6:9.

Carruthers, C. 1962. *Biochemistry of skin in health and disease*, p. 153. Springfield, Ill.: Thomas.

Chait, A., Bierman, E. L. and Albers, J. J. 1978. Regulatory role of insulin in the degradation of low density lipoprotein by cultured human skin fibroblasts. *Biochim. Biophys. Acta* 529:292–229.

Chait, A., Bierman, E. L. and Albers, J. J. 1979. Low-density lipoprotein receptor activity in cultured human skin fibroblasts. Mechanism of insulin-induced stimulation. *J. Clin. Invest.* 64:1309–1319.

Champion, R. H. 1970. In *An introduction to the biology of the skin*, pp. 114–123. Oxford: Blackwell.

Churchill, L. and Speakman, P. T. 1970. Protein synthesis in mammalian epidermis: Are polyribosomes involved in fibrous protein biosynthesis? *Biochem. J.* 117:67P–68P.

Clarke, D. M. and Rogers, G. E. 1970. Protein synthesis in the hair follicle. II. Polysomes and amino acid incorporation. *J. Invest. Dermatol.* 55:425–432.

Clark-Lewis, I. and Murray, A. W. 1978. Tumor promotion and the induction of epidermal ornithine decarboxylase activity in mechanically stimulated mouse skin. *Cancer Res.* 38:494–497.

Conrad, G. W., Hart, G. W. and Chen, Y. 1977. Differences *in vitro* between fibroblast-like cells from cornea, heart and skin of embryonic chicks. *J. Cell Sci.* 26:119–138.

Cook, T. J. and Lorincz, A. L. 1963. Enzyme determination of hydroxy steroids in human skin surface lipids. *J. Invest. Dermatol.* 41:265–268.

Cook, T. J. and Spector, A. R. 1964. Excretion of intravenously administered radioactive hydrocortisone in skin surface lipids. *J. Invest. Dermatol.* 43:413–414.

Coombes, E. J., Shakespeare, P. G. and Batstone, G. F. 1980. Lipoprotein changes after burn injury in man. *J. Trauma* 11:971–975.

Cooper, M. J., Hay, J. B., McGibbon, D. and Shuster, S. 1978. Correlations between androgen metabolism and sebaceous-gland activity. *Biochem. Soc. Trans.* 6:970–972.

Cotterill, J. A., Cunliffe, W. J. and Williamson, B. 1971. Severity of acne and sebum excretion rate. *Br. J. Dermatol.* 85:93–94.

Cotterill, J. A., Cunliffe, W. J. and Williamson, B. 1972. Variations in skin surface lipid composition and sebum excretion rate with different sampling techniques. II. *Br. J. Dermatol.* 86:356–360.

Cove, J. H., Holland, K. T. and Cunliffe, W. J. 1980. An analysis of sebum excretion rate, bacterial population and the production rate of free fatty acids on human skin. *Br. J. Dermatol.* 103:383–386.

Crick, F. H. C. 1966. The genetic code—Yesterday, today and tomorrow. *Cold Spring Harbor Symp. Quant. Biol.* 31.

Cruickshank, C. N. D., Trotter, M. D. and Cooper, J. R. 1957. Studies on the carbohydrate metabolism of skin. *Biochem. J.* 66:285–289.

Cruickshank, C. N. D., Hershey, F. B. and Lewis, C. 1958. Isocitric dehydrogenase activity of human epidermis. *J. Invest. Dermatol.* 30:33–37.

Crunkhorn, P. and Willis, A. L. 1971. Interaction between prostaglandins E and F given intradermally in the rat. *Br. J. Pharmacol.* 41:507–512.

Cunliffe, W. J. and Shuster, S. 1969. The rate of sebum excretion in man. *Br. J. Dermatol.* 81:697–704.

Cunliffe, W. J., Cotterill, J. A. and Williamson, B. 1971a. Variations in skin surface lipid composition with different sampling techniques. I. *Br. J. Dermatol.* 85:40–45.

Cunliffe, W. J., Cotterill, J. A. and Williamson, B. 1971b. Skin surface lipids in acne. *Br. J. Dermatol.* 85:496.

Cutroneo, K. R. and Clarke, D. H. 1979. Decreased protein degradation in the skin of glucocorticoid-treated newborn rats. *Biochem. Pharmacol.* 28:3229–3231.

Cutroneo, K. R. and Counts, D. F. 1975. Anti-inflammatory steroids and collagen metabolism: Glucocorticoid-mediated alterations of prolyl hydroxylase activity and collagen synthesis. *Mol. Pharmacol.* 11:632–639.

Daerr, W. H., Gianturco, S. H., Patsch, J. R., Smith, L. C. and Gotto, A. M., Jr. 1980. Stimulation and suppression of 3-hydroxy-3-methylglutaryl coenzyme A reductase in normal human fibroblasts by high density lipoprotein subclasses. *Biochim. Biophys. Acta* 619:287–301.

Daniel, J. Y., Vignon, F., Assenmacher, I. and Rochefort, H. 1977. Evidence of androgen and estrogen receptors in the preen gland of male ducks. *Steroids* 30:703–709.

Dawson, R. and Milne, G. 1978. The effects of dietary nitrogen level on the collagen of rat skin. *Br. J. Nutr.* 39:181-192.

DeBersaques, J. 1977. Enzymes of carbohydrate metabolism in human epidermal tumors. *J. Cutan. Pathol.* 4:32-37.

DeBersaques, J. 1979. Enzymes of carbohydrate metabolism in lesions of the palms and soles. *Arch. Dermatol. Res.* 265:343-345.

deBruyn, C. H., Raymakers, C., Wensing, A., Dei, T. L. and H'osli, P. 1977. Enzymes of galactose metabolism in human hair roots. *Br. J. Dermatol.* 97:487-495.

Decker, R. H. 1971. Nature and regulation of energy metabolism in the epidermis. *J. Invest. Dermatol.* 57:351-363.

DeLoecker, W., DeWever, F. and Pennickx, F. 1980. Metabolic changes in human skin preserved at −3 and at −196 degrees C. *Cryobiology* 17:46-53.

DeWind, L. T. 1980. Corticosteroids and skin tearing. *J. Am. Med. Assoc.* 244:1674-1675 (letter).

DiGiovanna, J. J., Aoyagi, T., Taylor, R. and Halprin, K. M. 1981. Inhibition of epidermal adenyl cyclase by lithium carbonate. *J. Invest. Dermatol.* 76:259-263.

DiRosa, M. and Willoughby, D. A. 1971. Screens for anti-inflammatory drugs. *J. Pharm. Pharmacol.* 23:297-298.

Dogliotti, M., Liebowitz, D. T., Downing, D. T. and Strauss, J. S. 1977. Nutritional influences of pellagra on sebum composition. *Br. J. Dermatol.* 97:25-28.

Downing, D. T. 1963. Fatty acid composition of vernix caseosa. *Aust. J. Chem.* 16:679-682.

Downing, D. T. 1965. Composition of the unsaponifiable matter of vernix caseosa. *Aust. J. Chem.* 18:1287-1291.

Downing, D. T. and Greene, R. S. 1968. Double bond positions in the unsaturated fatty acids of vernix caseosa. *J. Invest. Dermatol.* 50:380-386.

Downing, D. T. and Sharaf, D. M. 1976. Skin surface lipids of the guinea pig. *Biochim. Biophys. Acta* 431:378-389.

Downing, D. T. and Strauss, J. S. 1974. Synthesis and composition of surface lipids of human skin. *J. Invest. Dermatol.* 62:228-244.

Downing, D. T., Strauss, J. S. and Pochi, P. E. 1972. Changes in skin surface lipid composition induced by severe caloric restriction in man. *Am. J. Clin. Nutr.* 25:365-367.

Drevon, C. A., Attie, A. D., Pansburn, S. H. and Steinberg, D. 1981. Metabolism of homologous and heterologous lipoproteins by cultured rat and human skin fibroblasts. *J. Lipid Res.* 22:37-46.

Drucker, W. D., Blumberg, J. M., Gandy, H. M., David, R. R. and Verde, A. L. 1972. Biologic activity of dehydroepiandrosterone sulfate in man. *J. Clin. Endocrinol. Metab.* 35:48-54.

Dubovie, M. I. 1954. The secretion of sex steroids in some skin diseases. *Ukr. Biokhim. Zh.* 26:3.

Dubovie, M. I. 1960. Content of steroid hormones in the skin fat. *Vestn. Dermatol. Venerol.* 34:10.

Dubovie, M. I. 1967. Androgenic steroids in sebum. *Vestn. Dermatol. Venerol.* 41:14-21.

Duell, E. A. 1980. Adenosine-induced alterations in the adenosine $3',5'$-monophosphate levels in mammalian epidermis. *Mol. Pharmacol.* 18:49-52.

Ebling, F. J. 1948. Sebaceous glands. I. The effect of sex hormones on the sebaceous glands of the female albino rat. *J. Endocrinol.* 5:297–302.

Ebling, F. J. 1957a. The action of testosterone and oestradiol on the sebaceous glands and epidermis of the rat. *J. Embryol. Exp. Morphol.* 5:74–79.

Ebling, F. J. 1957b. The action of testosterone on the sebaceous glands and epidermis in castrated and hypophysectomized male rats. *J. Endocrinol.* 15:297–306.

Ebling, F. J. 1974. Hormonal control and methods of measuring sebaceous gland activity. *J. Invest. Dermatol.* 62:161–171.

Ebling, F. J., Ebling, E. and Skinner, J. 1969. The influence of pituitary hormones on the response of the sebaceous glands of the rat to testosterone. *J. Endocrinol.* 45:245–256.

Ebling, F. J., Ebling, E., Randall, V. and Skinner, J. 1975. The sebotrophic action of growth hormone (BGH) in the rat. *Br. J. Dermatol.* 92:325–332.

Eisele, C. W. and Eichelberger, L. 1945. Water, electrolyte and nitrogen content of human skin. *Proc. Soc. Exp. Biol. Med.* 58:97–100.

Elias, P. M., Brown, B. E. and Ziboh, V. A. 1980. The permeability barrier in essential fatty acid deficiency: Evidence for a direct role for linoleic acid in barrier function. *J. Invest. Dermatol.* 74:230–233.

Ellis, R. E. and Montagna, W. 1958. Histology and cytochemistry of human skin. *J. Histochem. Cytochem.* 6:201–207.

Eppenburger, U. and Hsia, S. L. 1972. Binding of steroid hormones by the 105,000 X g supernatant fraction from homogenates of rat skin and variations during the hair cycle. *J. Biol. Chem.* 247:5453–5469.

Epstein, E. H., Jr., and Epstein, W. L. 1966. New cell formation in human sebaceous glands. *J. Invest. Dermatol.* 46:453–458.

Essman, W. B. 1977. Serotonin and monoamine oxidase in mouse skin: Effects of cigarette smoke exposure. *J. Med.* 8:95–101.

Esvelt, R. P., DeLuca, H. F., Wichmann, J. K., Yoshizawa, S., Zurcher, J., Sar, M. and Stumpf, W. E. 1980. 1,25-Dihydroxyvitamin D_3 stimulated increase of 7,8-dehydrocholesterol levels in rat skin. *Biochemistry* 19:6158–6161.

Evan, D., Savage, M. O. and Binet, E. 1977. A specific and rapid determination of human skin dihydrotestosterone cytosol receptor. *Clin. Endocrinol. Metab.* 45:363–367.

Fang, S., Anderson, K. M. and Liao, S. 1969. Receptor proteins for androgens. *J. Biol. Chem.* 244:6584–6595.

Faredin, I., Fazekas, A. G., Kokai, K., Toth, I. and Julesz, M. 1967. The *in vitro* metabolism of $4\text{-}C^{14}$-dehydroepiandrosterone by human male pubic skin. *Eur. J. Steroids* 2:223–242.

Faredin, I., Toth, I., Fazekas, A. G., Kokai, K. and Julesz, M. 1968. Conjugation *in vitro* of $[4\text{-}^{14}C]$dehydroepiandrosterone sulfate by normal human female skin slices. *J. Endocrinol.* 41:295–296.

Faredin, I., Fazekas, A. G., Toth, I., Kokai, K. and Julesz, M. 1969. Transformation *in vitro* of $[4\text{-}^{14}C]$dehydroepiandrosterone into 7-oxygenated derivatives by normal human male and female skin tissue. *J. Invest. Dermatol.* 52:357–361.

Fazekas, A. G. and Sandor, T. 1972. Metabolism of androgens by isolated human hair follicles. *J. Steroid Biochem.* 3:485–492.

Felger, C. B. 1969. The etiology of acne. I. Composition of sebum before and after puberty. *J. Soc. Cosmet. Chem.* 20:565–575.

Ferrari, R. A., Chakrabarty, K., Beyler, A. L. and Wiland, J. 1978. Suppression of sebaceous gland development in laboratory animals by 17alpha-propyltestosterone. *J. Invest. Dermatol.* 71:320–323.

Flaxman, B. A. and Harper, R. A. 1975. Organ culture of human skin in chemically defined media. *J. Invest. Dermatol.* 64:96–99.

Flemister, L. J. 1941–42. Distribution of available water in animal tissue. *Am. J. Phsyiol.* 135:430–438.

Francis, D., Greaves, M. W. and Yamamoto, S. 1977. Enzymatic histamine degradation by human skin. *Br. J. Pharmacol.* 60:583–587.

Frederiksen, D. A. and Wilson, J. D. 1971. Partial characterization of the nuclear nicotinamide adenine dinucleotide phosphate: Δ^4-3-Ketosteroid 5α-oxidoreductase of rat prostate. *J. Biol. Chem.* 246:2584–2593.

Freedberg, I. M. 1967; Rashes and ribosomes. *N. Engl. J. Med.* 276:1135–1143.

Freedberg, I. M. 1972. Pathways and controls of epithelial protein synthesis. *J. Invest. Dermatol.* 59:56–65.

Freedberg, I. M. and Baden, H. P. 1964. Studies on epidermal protein metabolism: Incorporation of amino acids and nucleotides *in vitro. Clin. Res.* 10:266.

Freedberg, I. M. and Matsui, K. 1968. Factors controlling the early steps of epidermal protein synthesis. *J. Clin. Invest.* 47:36a.

Freinkel, R. K. 1960. Metabolism of glucose-C^{14} by human skin *in vitro. J. Invest. Dermatol.* 34:37–42.

Freinkel, R. K. and Traczyk, T. N. 1980. The phospholipases A of epidermis. *J. Invest. Dermatol.* 74:169–173.

Frost, P., Weinstein, G. D. and Hsia, S. L. 1966. Metabolism of estradiol-17β-ol and estrone in human skin. *J. Invest. Dermatol.* 46:584–585.

Frost, P., Gomez, E. C., Weinstein, G. D., Lamas, W. J. and Hsia, S. L. 1969. Metabolism of progesterone-4-^{14}C *in vitro* in human skin and vaginal mucosa. *Biochemistry* 8:948–952.

Fukuyama, K. and Bernstein, I. A. 1961. Autoradiographic studies of the incorporation of thymidine-^{3}H into deoxyribonucleic acid in the skin of young rats. *J. Invest. Dermatol.* 36:321–326.

Fukuyama, K. and Bernstein, I. A. 1963. Site of synthesis of ribonucleic acid in mammalian epidermis. *J. Invest. Dermatol.* 41:47–52.

Fukuyama, K. and Epstein, W. L. 1968. Protein synthesis studies of different species. *Am. J. Anat.* 122:269–273.

Fukuyama, K., Nakamura, T. and Bernstein, I. A. 1965. Differentially localized incorporation of amino acids in relation to epidermal keratinization in the newborn rat. *Anat. Rec.* 152:525–529.

Fung, C. H. and Khachadurian, A. K. 1980. Suppression of synthesis and esterification of cholesterol and stimulation of low density lipoprotein receptor activity by polyoxyethylated cholesterol in cultured human fibroblasts. *J. Biol. Chem.* 255:676–680.

Fung, C. H., Khachadurian, A. K., Wang, C. H. and Durr, I. F. 1977. Regulation of lipid synthesis by low density lipoproteins in cultured skin fibroblasts in homozygous familial hypercholesterolemia. *Biochim. Biophys. Acta* 487:445–457.

Gallegos, A. J. and Berliner, D. L. 1967. Transformation and conjugation of DHA by human skin. *J. Clin. Endocrinol.* 27:1214–1218.

Garzan, P. and Berliner, D. L. 1970. Adaptive enzymatic expression in the metabolism of progesterone during the life fibroblast cycle. *VIth Int. Meet. Reticuloendothel. Soc., Freiburg, Germany,* p. 48.

Garte, S. J. and Belman, S. 1980. Diurnal variation in cyclic nucleotide levels in normal and phorbol myristate acetate treated mouse epidermis. *J. Invest. Dermatol.* 74:224–225.

Gatt, S. and Bierman, E. L. 1980. Sphingomyelin suppresses the binding and utilization of low density lipoproteins by skin fibroblasts. *J. Biol. Chem.* 255:3371–3376.

Gaylor, J. L. 1963. Biosynthesis of skin sterols. III. Conversion of squalene to sterols by rat skin. *J. Biol. Chem.* 238:1643–1648.

Germinario, R. J. and Oliveira, M. 1979. Stimulation of hexose transport in cultured human skin fibroblasts by insulin. *J. Cell. Physiol.* 99:313–318.

Geronemus, R. G. and Mertz, P. M. 1979. Wound healing: The effects of topical antimicrobial agents. *Arch. Dermatol.* 115:1311–1314.

Ghent, C. N., Bloomer, J. R. and Klatskin, G. 1977. Elevations in skin tissue levels of bile acids in human cholestasis: Relation to serum levels and to pruritus. *Gastroenterology* 73:1125–1130.

Giacomini, M. and Wright, F. 1980. The effects of progesterone and pregnanedione on the reductive metabolism of dihydrotestosterone in human skin. *J. Steroid Biochem.* 13:645–651.

Giannopoulos, G., Hassan, Z. and Solomon, S. 1974. Glucocorticoid receptors in fetal and adult rabbit tissues. *J. Biol. Chem.* 249:2424–2427.

Gilbert, D. 1964. Demonstration of a respiratory control mechanism in human skin *in vitro*. *J. Int. Coll. Surg.* 42:45–49.

Gloor, M., Willebrandt, U., Thomer, G. and Kupferschmid, W. 1980. Water content of the horny layer and skin surface lipids. *Arch. Dermatol. Res.* 268:221–223.

Goldsmith, L. A. and Martin, C. M. 1975. Human epidermal transamidase. *J. Invest. Dermatol.* 64:316–321.

Goldyne, M. E. 1975. Prostaglandins and cutaneous inflammation. *J. Invest. Dermatol.* 64:377–385.

Gomez, E. C. and Hsia, S. L. 1968. *In vitro* metabolism of testosterone-4-^{14}C and Δ^4-androsterone-3,17-dione-4-^{14}C in human skin. *Biochemistry* 7:24–32.

Gomez, E. C., Frost, P. and Hsia, S. L. 1975. Transformations of progesterone by subcellular fractions of human skin. *J. Invest. Dermatol.* 64:240–244.

Gomez, E. C., Michaelover, J. and Frost, P. 1977. Cutaneous betaglucuronidase: Cleavage of mycophenolic acid by preparations of mouse skin. *Br. J. Dermatol.* 97:303–336.

Goolamali, S. K., Plummer, N., Burton, J. L., Shuster, S. and Thody, A. J. 1974. Sebum excretion and melanocyte-stimulating hormone in hypoadrenalism. *J. Invest. Dermatol.* 63:253–255.

Gordon, R. S., Wolfe, S. M., Cage, G. W. and Thompson, R. H. 1968. *In vitro* studies of human eccrine gland. *Fed. Proc.* 27:2983.

Gordon, R. S., Thompson, R. H., Muenzer, J. and Thrasher, D. 1971. Sweat lactate in man is derived from blood glucose. *J. Appl. Physiol.* 31:713–716.

Gorman, R. R., Hamilton, R. D. and Hopkins, N. K. 1979. Stimulation of human foreskin fibroblast adenosine 3':5'-cyclic monophosphate levels by prostacyclin (prostaglandin I2). *J. Biol. Chem.* 254:1671–1676.

Gottlieb, N. L. and Penneys, N. S. 1980. Spontaneous skin tearing during systemic corticosteroid treatment. *J. Am. Med. Assoc.* 243:1260–1261.

Greaves, M. W., Kingston, W. P. and Pretty, K. 1975. Action of a series of non-steroid and steroid anti-inflammatory drugs on prostaglandin biosynthesis by the microsomal fraction of rat skin. *Br. J. Pharmacol.* 53:470P.

Green, J. F. and Lewis, R. A. 1979. Partial purification and characterization of deoxyguanosine kinase from pig skin. *Biochem. J.* 183:547–553.

Griesemer, R. D. and Gould, E. 1954. A method for the study of intermediary carbohydrate metabolism of epidermis. I. Oxidation of acids of the citric acid cycle. *J. Invest. Dermatol.* 22:299–315.

Griffen, J. E., Punyashthiti, K. and Wilson, J. D. 1976. Dihydrotestosterone binding by cultured human fibroblasts. Comparison of cells from control subjects and from patients with hereditary male pseudohermaphroditism due to androgen resistance. *J. Clin. Invest.* 57:1342–1351.

Groshong, R., Gibson, D. A. and Baldessarini, R. J. 1977. Monoamine oxidase activity in cultured human skin fibroblasts. *Clin. Chim. Acta.* 80:113–120.

Gross, J. 1976. In *Biochemistry of Collagen,* eds. G. N. Ramachandran and A. H. Reddi, pp. 275–317. New York: Plenum.

Gryglewski, R. J., Panczenko, B., Korbut, R., Gradzinska, L. and Ocetkiewicz, A. 1975. Corticosteroids inhibit prostaglandin release from perfused mesenteric blood vessels of rabbit and from perfused lungs of sensitized guinea pig. *Prostaglandins* 10:343–355.

Haahti, E. 1961. Major lipid constituents of human skin surface with special reference to gas chromatographic methods. *Scand. J. Clin. Lab. Invest.* 13(Suppl. 59):1–108.

Haahti, E. and Horning, E. C. 1963. Isolation and characterization of saturated and unsaturated fatty acids and alcohols of human skin surface lipids. *Scand. J. Clin. Lab. Invest.* 15:73–78.

Haahti, E., Nikkari, T., Salmi, A. M. and Laaksonen, A. L. 1960. Fatty acids of vernix caseosa. *Scand. J. Clin. Lab. Invest.* 13:70–73.

Haahti, E., Langerspetz, K., Nikkari, T. and Fales, H. M. 1964. Lipids of the uropygial gland of birds. *Comp. Biochem. Physiol.* 12:435–437.

Halprin, K. M. and Chow, D. C. 1961. Metabolic pathways in perfused dog skin. *J. Invest. Dermatol.* 36:431–439.

Halprin, K. M. and Ohkawara, A. 1966a. Glucose and glycogen metabolism in the human epidermis. *J. Invest. Dermatol.* 46:43–50.

Halprin, K. M. and Ohkawara, A. 1966b. Carbohydrate metabolism in psoriasis: An enzymatic study. *J. Invest. Dermatol.* 46:51–69.

Halprin, K. M. and Ohkawara, A. 1966c. Lactate production and lactate dehydrogenase in the human epidermis. *J. Inverst. Dermatol.* 47:222–226.

Ham, W. A. and Leeson, T. S. 1961. The integumentary system (the skin and its appendages). In *Histology,* 4th ed., pp. 546–579. Philadelphia: Lippincott.

Hambrick, G. W. and Blank, H. J. 1954. Whole mounts for the study of skin and its appendages. *J. Invest. Dermatol.* 23:437–453.

Hammar, H. 1971. Hydroxylacyl-CoA dehydrogenase and glucose-6-phosphate dehydrogenase in normal human skin and in some papulosquamous diseases of the skin. *Acta Dermatol. Venereol. (Stockh.)* 51:93–97.

Hammarström, S., Lindgren, J. A., Marcelo, C., Duell, E. A., Anderson, T. F. and Voorhees, J. J. 1979. Arachidonic acid transformations in normal and psoriatic skin. *J. Invest. Dermatol.* 73:180–183.

Hammersen, G., Mandell, R. and Levy, H. L. 1975. Galactose-1-phosphate uridyl transferase in fibroblasts: Isozymes in normal and variant states. *Ann. Hum. Genet.* 39:147–151.

Hanigan, J. and Goldsmith, L. A. 1978. Endogenous substrates for epidermal transglutaminase. *Biochim. Biophys. Acta* 522:589–601.

Hansen, T. M., Garbarsch, C., Helin, G., Helin, P., Hølund, B., Kofod, B. and Lorenzen, I. 1980. Proteoglycans, DNA, and RNA in rat granulation tissue, skin, and aorta. Biochemical and histological studies. *Acta Pathol. Microbiol. Scand.* 88A:143–150.

Hartman, A. D. 1977. Lipoprotein lipase distribution in rat adipose tissues: Effect on chylomicron uptake. *Am. J. Physiol.* 232:E316–E323.

Hartop, P. J., Allenby, C. F. and Prottey, C. 1978. Comparison of barrier function and lipids in psoriasis and essential fatty acid-deficient rats. *Clin. Exp. Dermatol.* 3:259–267.

Hasselquist, M. B., Goldberg, N., Schroeter, A. and Spelsberg, T. C. 1980. Isolation and characterization of the estrogen receptor in human skin. *J. Clin. Endocrinol. Metab.* 50:76–82.

Hay, J. B. and Hodgins, M. B. 1974. Metabolism of androgens by human skin in acne. *Br. J. Dermatol.* 91:123–133.

Hay, J. B. and Hodgins, M. B. 1978. Distribution of androgen metabolizing enzymes in isolated tissues of human forehead and axillary skin. *J. Endocrinol.* 79:29–39.

Hendrikx, A., Heyns, W. and De Moor, P. 1968. Influence of a low-calorie diet and fasting on the metabolism of dehydroepiandrosterone sulfate in adult obese subjects. *J. Clin. Endocrinol.* 28:1525–1533.

Hensby, C. N., Kingston, W. P. and Greaves, M. W. 1976. Prostaglandins and skin. *Clin. Exp. Dermatol.* 1:385.

Hensby, C. N., Plummer, N. A., Black, A. K., Fincham, N. and Greaves, M. W. 1980. Time-course of arachidonic acid, prostaglandins E2 and F2 alpha production in human abdominal skin, following irradiation with ultraviolet wavelengths (290–320 nm). *Adv. Prostagland. Thromboxane Res.* 7:857–860.

Herdenstam, G. G. 1962. On the *in vitro* metabolism of labeled glucose in normal and psoriatic skin. *Acta Dermatol. Venereol. (Stockh.)* 42(Suppl. 47):1–62.

Holick, M. F., Frommer, J. E., McNeill, S. C., Richtand, N. M., Henley, J. W. and Potts, J. T., Jr. 1977. Photometabolism of 7-dehydrocholesterol to previtamin D_3 in skin. *Biochem. Biophys. Res. Commun.* 76:107–114.

Holick, M. F., Richtand, N. M., McNeill, S. C., Holick, S. A., Frommer, J. E., Henley, J. W. and Potts, J. T., Jr. 1979. Effect of NADP$^+$ and its analogs on the rose bengal-sensitized photoinactivation of d-erythrulose reductase from beef liver. *Biochemistry* 18:1003.

Holick, M. F., MacLaughlin, J. A., Clark, M. B., Potts, J. T., Jr., Anderson, R. R., Blank, I. H., Jr., Parrish, A. and Elias, P. 1980. Photosynthesis of previtamin D_3 in human skin and the physiologic consequences. *Science* 210:203–205.

Holick, M. F., MacLaughlin, J. A. and Doppelt, S. H. 1981. Regulation of cutaneous previtamin D_3 photosynthesis in man: Skin pigment is not an essential regulator. *Science* 211:590–593.

Holman, R. T. 1977. Essential fatty acids in human nutrition. *Adv. Exp. Med. Biol.* 83:515–534.

Hong, S. L. and Levine, L. 1976. Inhibition of arachidonic acid release from cells as the biochemical action of anti-inflammatory corticosteroids. *Proc. Natl. Acad. Sci. U.S.A.* 73:1730–1734.

Hoopes, J. E. and Im, M. J. 1973. Glycogen in regenerating epithelium during wound healing. *Surg. Forum* 24:523–525.

Horton, E. W. 1963. Action of prostaglandin E_1 on tissues which respond to bradykinin. *Nature (Lond.)* 200:892–893.

Horton, E. W. 1969. Hypotheses on physiological roles of prostaglandins. *Physiol. Rev.* 49:122–131.

Hougen, F. W. 1955. The constitution of the aliphatic alcohols in human sebum. *Biochem. J.* 59:302–309.

Hsia, S. L. 1971. Potentials in exploring biochemistry in human skin. *Essays Biochem.* 7:1–38.

Hsia, S. L. and Hao, Y. L. 1966. Metabolic transformation of cortisol-4-C^{14} in human skin. *Biochemistry* 5:1469–1474.

Hsia, S. L. and Hao, Y. L. 1967. Transformation of cortisone to cortisol in human skin. *Steroids* 10:489–500.

Hsia, S. L., Witten, V. H. and Hao, Y. L. 1964. *In vitro* metabolic studies of hydrocortisone-4-C^{14} in human skin. *J. Invest. Dermatol.* 43:407–411.

Hsia, S. L., Mussallem, A. J. and Witten, V. H. 1965. Further metabolic studies of hydrocortisone-4-^{14}C in human skin. Requirement for pyridine nucleotides and site of metabolism. *J. Invest. Dermatol.* 45:384–390.

Hsia, S. L., Sofer, G. and Lane, B. 1966a. Lipid metabolism in human skin. I. Lipogenesis from acetate-1-^{14}C. *J. Invest. Dermatol.* 47:437–442.

Hsia, S. L., Dreize, M. A. and Marquez, M. C. 1966b. Lipid metabolism in human skin. II. A study of lipogenesis in skin of diabetic patients. *J. Invest. Dermatol.* 47:443–448.

Hsia, S. L., Fulton, J. E., Jr., Fulghum, D. and Buch, M. N. 1970. Lipid synthesis from acetate-1-^{14}C by suction blister epidermis and other skin components. *Proc. Soc. Exp. Biol. Med.* 135:285–291.

Hsia, S. L., Wright, R., Mandy, S. H. and Halprin, K. 1972. Adenyl cyclase in normal and psoriatic skin. *J. Invest. Dermatol.* 59:109–113.

Hug, G., Schubert, W. K. and Soukup, S. 1969. Ultrastructure and enzymatic deficiency of fibrocyte cultures in type II glycogenosis. *J. Clin. Invest.* 48:40a.

Hulan, H. W. and Kramer, J. K. 1977. The effects of long-chain monoenes on prostaglandin E2 synthesis by rat skin. *Lipids* 12:604–609.

Iizuka, H., Kamigaki, K., Nemoto, O., Aoyagi, T. and Miura, Y. 1980. Effects of hydrocortisone on the adrenaline-adenylate cyclase system of the skin. *Br. J. Dermatol.* 102:703–710.

Iizuka, H., Aoyagi, T., Kamigaki, K., Kato, N., Nemoto, O. and Miura, V. 1981. Effects of trypsin on the cyclic AMP system of the pig skin. *J. Invest. Dermatol.* 76:511–513.

Im, M. J. and Hoopes, J. E. 1974. Enzymes of carbohydrate metabolism in normal human sebaceous glands. *J. Invest. Dermatol.* 62:153–160.

Ito, T. and Horton, R. 1971. The source of plasma dihydrotestosterone in man. *J. Clin. Invest.* 50:1621–1627.

Jablonska, S., Groniowski, M. and Dabrowski, J. 1979. Comparative evaluation of skin atrophy in man induced by topical corticoids. *Br. J. Dermatol.* 100:193–206.

Jacob, J. and Zeman, A. 1972. Das burzeldrusensekret der ringeltaube (Columba palumbus). *Hoppe Seylers Z. Physiol. Chem.* 353:492–494.

Jacobson, B. and Davidson, E. 1962. Biosynthesis of uronic acid by skin enzymes. *J. Biol. Chem.* 237:635–637.

James, A. T. and Wheatley, V. R. 1956. Studies of sebum. 6. The determination of the component fatty acids of human forearm sebum by gas-liquid chromatography. *Biochem. J.* 63:269–273.

Jarrett, A. 1959. The effects of progesterone and testosterone on surface sebum and acne vulgaris. *Br. J. Dermatol.* 71:102–116.

Johnson, J. A. and Fusaro, R. M. 1972. Role of skin in carbohydrate metabolism. *Adv. Metab. Disord.* 6:1–55.

Jonsson, C. E. and Anggard 1972. Biosynthesis and metabolism of prostaglandin E_2 in human skin. *Scand. J. Clin. Lab. Invest.* 29:289–297.

Jouvenaz, G. H., Nugteren, D. H., Beerthius, R. K. and van Dorp, D. A. 1970. A sensitive method for the determination of prostglandins by gas chromatography with electron-capture detection. *Biochim. Biophys. Acta* 202:231–234.

Juhlin, L. and Michaelsson, G. 1969. Cutaneous vascular reactions to prostaglandins in healthy subjects and in patients with urticaria and atopic dermatitis. *Acta Dermatol. Venereol. (Stockh.)* 49:251–261.

Julesz, M., Faredin, I. and Toth, I. 1966a. Steroids in human skin and hairs. I. Zimmerman chromogens in the skin of normal and hirsute women. IV. Neutral. 17-ketosteroids in human hairs. *Acta Med. Acad. Sci. Hung.* 22:25–52.

Julesz, M., Faredin, I. and Toth, I. 1966b. Steroids in human skin and hair. *2nd Int. Congr. Horm. Steroids* 3:327.

Kabara, J. J. 1975. Lipids as safe and effective antimicrobial agents for cosmetics and pharmaceuticals. *Cosmet. Perfum.* 90:21–25.

Kahlenberg, A. and Kalant, N. 1966. The effect of insulin and diabetes on glucose metabolism in human skin. *Can. J. Biochem.* 44:801–808.

Karkkainen, J., Nikkari, T., Ruponen, S. and Haahti, E. 1965. Lipids of vernix caseosa. *J. Invest. Dermatol.* 44:333–338.

Karunkaran, M. E., Pochi, P. E., Strauss, J. S., Valerio, E. A., Wotiz, H. H. and Clark, S. J. 1973. Androgen in skin surface lipids. *J. Invest. Dermatol.* 60:121–125.

Kassis, V., Weismann, K., Heiligstädt, H. and Sondergaard, J. 1977. Synthesis of prostaglandins by psoriatic skin. *Arch. Dermatol. Res.* 259:207–212.

Kaufman, M., Straisfeld, C. and Pinski, L. 1976. Specific 5α-dihydrotestosterone binding in labial skin fibroblasts cultured from patients with male pseudohermaphroditism. *Clin. Genet.* 9:457.

Kellum, R. E. 1967. Human sebaceous gland lipids. *Arch. Dermatol.* 59:218–220.

Kennan, B. S., Meyer, W. J., Hadjan, A. and Migeon, C. J. 1975. Androgen receptor in human skin fibroblasts: Characterization of a specific 17β-hydroxy-5α-androstan 3-one-protein complex in cell sonicates and nuclei. *Steroids* 25:535–552.

Kim, M. H. and Herrmann, W. L. 1968. *In vitro* metabolism of dehydroepiandrosterone sulfate in foreskin, abdominal skin and vaginal mucosa. *J. Clin. Endocrinol.* 28:187–191.

King, I. A. and Tabiowo, A. 1980. The dermis is required for the synthesis of extracellular glycosaminoglycans in cultured pig epidermis. *Biochim. Biophys. Acta* 632:234–243.

King, L. E., Jr., Florendo, N. T., Solomon, S. S. and Hashimoto, K. 1974. Cyclic 3',5'-nucleotide phosphodiesterase. I. Histochemical localization in rat skin. *J. Invest. Dermatol.* 62:485–492.

King, L. E., Jr., Solomon, S. S. and Hashimoto, I. 1975. Cyclic 3',5'-nucleotide phosphodiesterase in rat skin. *J. Invest. Dermatol.* 64:390–396.

Kirk, D. and Irvin, T. T. 1977. The role of oxygen therapy in the healing of experimental skin wounds and colonic anastomosis. *Br. J. Surg.* 64:100–103.

Kischer, C. W. 1969. Accelerated maturation of chick embryo skin treated with prostaglandin B_1; an electron microscopic study. *Am. J. Anat.* 124:491–512.

Kishore, G. S. and Boutwell, R. K. 1980. Enzymatic oxidation and reduction of retinal by mouse epidermis. *Biochem. Biophys. Res. Commun.* 94:1381-1386.

Kjaersgaard, A. R. 1954. Perfusion of isolated dog skin. *J. Invest. Dermatol.* 22:135-141.

Kondo, S. and Adachi, K. 1971. Phosphofructokinase regulation of glycolysis in skin. *J. Invest. Dermatol.* 57:175-179.

Kondo, S. and Adachi, K. 1972. The nature of the inhibition and activation of epidermal phosphofructokinase: An allosteric enzyme. *J. Invest. Dermatol.* 59:397-401.

Kondo, S. and Gerna-Torsellini, M. 1974. Phosphofructokinase (PFK) regulation of glycolysis in skin. *J. Invest. Dermatol.* 62:503-506.

Koob, T. J. and Jeffrey, J. J. 1974. Regulation of human skin collagenase activity of hydrocortisone and dexamethasone in organ culture. *Biochem. Biophys. Res. Commun.* 61:1083-1088.

Koob, T. J., Jeffrey, J. J., Eisen, A. Z. and Bauer, E. A. 1980. Hormonal interactions in mammalian collagenase regulation. Comparative studies in human skin and rat uterus. *Biochim. Biophys. Acta* 629:13-23.

Krajewska, E., DeClercq, E. and Shugar, D. 1978. Nucleoside-catabolizing enzyme activities in primary rabbit kidney cells and human skin fibroblasts. *Biochem. Pharmacol.* 27:1421-1426.

Krakow, R., Downing, D. T., Strauss, J. S. and Pochi, P. E. 1973. Identification of a fatty acid in human skin surface lipids apparently associated with acne vulgaris. *J. Invest. Dermatol.* 61:286-289.

Kristensen, J. K., Wadskov, S. and Henriksen, O. 1978. Dose-dependent effect of topical corticosteroids on blood flow in human cutaneous tissue. *Acta Derm.-Venereol.* 58:145-148.

Kucan, J. O. and Robson, M. C. 1978. Influence of topical steroids on bacterial proliferation in the burn wound. *J. Surg. Res.* 24:79-82.

Kuehl, F. A., Jr. 1974. Prostaglandins, cyclic nucleotides and cell function. *Prostaglandins* 5:325-340.

Kuehl, F. A., Jr. and Humes, J. L. 1972. Direct evidence for a prostaglandin receptor and its application to prostaglandin measurements. *Proc. Natl. Acad. Sci. U.S.A.* 69:480-484.

Kumar, R. and Soloman, L. W. 1972. Prostaglandins in cutaneous biology. *Arch. Dermatol.* 106:101-107.

Kunze, H. and Vog, W. 1971. Significance of phospholipase A for prostaglandin formation. *Ann. N.Y. Acad. Sci.* 180:123-125.

Kuttan, R. 1980. Activation of prolyl hydroxylase in tissue homogenates of scorbutic guinea pigs. *J. Nutr.* 110:1525-1532.

Kuttenn, F., Mowszowicz, I., Schaison, G. and Mauvais-Jarvis, P. 1977. Androgen production and skin metabolism in hirsutism. *J. Endocrinol.* 75:83-91.

Kuttenn, F., Mowszowicz, I., Wright, F., Baudot, N., Jaffiol, C., Robin, M. and Mauvais-Jarvis, P. 1979. Male pseudohermaphroditism: A comparative study of one patient with 5-alpha-reductase deficiency and three patients with the complete form of testicular feminization. *J. Clin. Endocrinol. Metab.* 49:861-865.

Lasher, N., Lorincz, A. L. and Rothman, S. 1954. Hormonal effects on sebaceous glands in the white rat. II. The effect of the pituitary adrenal axis. *J. Invest. Dermatol.* 22:25-31.

Lasher, N., Lorincz, A. L. and Rothman, S. 1955. Hormonal effects on sebaceous glands in the white rat. III. Evidence for the presence of a pituitary sebaceous gland tropic factor. *J. Invest. Dermatol.* 24:499–505.

Lau, Y. T., Lang, M. A. and Essig, A. 1979. Evaluation of the rate of basal oxygen consumption in the isolated frog skin and toad bladder. *Biochim. Biophys. Acta* 545:215–222.

Leathwood, P. D. and Ryman, B. E. 1971. Enzymes of glycogen metabolism in human skin with particular reference to differential diagnosis of the glycogen storage diseases. *Clin. Sci.* 40:261–269.

Leigh, I. M. and Sanderson, K. V. 1979. Cutaneous changes produced by prolonged systemic steroid therapy. *Br. J. Dermatol.* 101(Suppl. 17):71–73.

Lemonnier, F., Gautier, M., Wolfrom, C. and Lemonnier, A. 1980. Some metabolic differences between human skin and aponeurosis fibroblasts in culture. *J. Cell Physiol.* 104:415–423.

Lerner, A. B. and McGuire, J. S. 1961. Effect of alpha and beta melanocyte stimulating hormones on skin color of man. *Nature (Lond.)* 189:176–179.

Lesiewicz, J. and Goldsmith, L. A. 1980. Ornithine decarboxylase in skin. *J. Invest. Dermatol.* 75:207–210.

Lesiewicz, J. and Goldsmith, L. A. 1980. Inhibition of rat skin ornithine decarboxylase by nitrofurazone. *Arch. Dermatol.* 116:1225–1226 (letter).

Lewis, C. A. and Hayward, B. 1971. Human skin surface lipids. In *Modern trends in dermatology*, ed. P. Borrie, vol. 4, pp. 89–121. London: Butterworths.

Lin, S. L., Ts'o, P. O. and Hollenberg, M. D. 1980. The effects of interferon on epidermal growth factor action. *Biochem. Biophys. Res. Commun.* 96:168–174.

Lo, W. B. and Black, H. S. 1972. Formation of cholesterol derived photoproducts in human skin. *J. Invest. Dermatol.* 58:278–283.

Lobitz, W. C., Jr., Brophy, D., Larner, A. E. and Daniels, F., Jr. 1962. Glycogen response in human epidermal base cell. *Arch. Dermatol.* 86:207–211.

Long, V. J. W. 1970. Variations in lipid composition at different depths in the cow snout epidermis. *J. Invest. Dermatol.* 55:269–273.

Lord, J. T., Ziboh, V. A. and Warren, S. K. 1978. Specific binding of prostaglandin E_2 and $F_{2\alpha}$ by membrane preparations from rat skin. *Endocrinology* 102:1300–1309.

Lord, J. T. and Ziboh, V. A. 1979. Specific binding of prostaglandin E2 to membrane preparations from human skin: Receptor modulation by UVB-irradiation and chemical agents. *J. Invest. Dermatol.* 73:373–377.

Lord, J. T., Ziboh, V. A., Cagle, W. D., Kursunoglu, S. and Redmond, G. 1980. Prostaglandins in wound healing: Possible regulation of granulation. *Adv. Prostagland. Thromboxane Res.* 7:865–869.

Lorincz, A. L. and Lancaster, G. 1957. Anterior pituitary preparation with tropic activity for sebaceous, preputial and harderian glands. *Science* 126:124–125.

Lowe, N. J. and DeQuoy, P. R. 1978. Linoleic acid effects on epidermal DNA synthesis and cutaneous prostaglandin levels in essential fatty acid deficiency. *J. Invest. Dermatol.* 70:200–203.

Lowe, N. J. 1980. Epidermal ornithine decarboxylase, polyamines, cell proliferation, and tumor promotion. *Arch. Dermatol.* 116:822–825.

Lowry, O. H., Passonneau, J. V., Hasselberger, F. Y. and Schulz, D. W. 1964. Effect of ischemia on known substrates and cofactors of the glycolytic pathway in brain. *J. Biol. Chem.* 239:18–30.

Lutsky, B. N., Budak, B., Koziol, P., Monohan, M. and Neri, R. O. 1975. The effects of a nonsteroid antiandrogen, flutamide, on sebaceous gland activity. *J. Invest. Dermatol.* 64:412–417.

Maines, M. D. and Cohn, J. 1977. Bile pigment formation by skin heme oxygenase: Studies on the response of the enzyme to heme compounds and tissue injury. *J. Exp. Med.* 145:1054–1059.

Malkinson, F. D., Lee, M. W. and Cutukovic, I. 1959. *In vitro* studies of adrenal steroid metabolism in the skin. *J. Invest. Dermatol.* 32:101–108.

Mann, P. R., Williams, R. H. and Gray, G. M. 1980. Distribution of glycoproteins containing fucose in normal and psoriatic keratinocytes. *Br. J. Dermatol.* 102:649–657.

Manthorpe, R., Garbarsch, C. and Lorenzen, I. 1980. Long-term effect of glucocorticoid on connective tissue of aorta and skin. Morphological and biochemical studies of tissues from rabbits with intact and injured aortas. *Acta Endocrinol.* 95:271–281.

Marks, F. and Grimm, W. 1972. Diurnal fluctuation and β-adrenergic elevation of cyclic AMP in mouse epidermis *in vivo*. *Nature (Lond.)* 240:178–179.

Marks, F. and Raab, I. 1974. The second messenger system of mouse epidermis. IV. Cyclic AMP and cyclic GMP phosphodiesterase. *Biochim. Biophys. Acta* 334:368–377.

Mathur, G. P. and Gandhi, V. M. 1972. Prostaglandin in human and rat skin. *J. Invest. Dermatol.* 58:291–295.

Mauvais-Jarvis, P., Bercovici, J. P. and Gauthier, F. 1969. *In vitro* studies on testosterone metabolism by skin of normal males and patients with the syndrome of testicular feminization syndrome. *J. Clin. Endocrinol.* 29:417–421.

Melbye, S. W. and Freedberg, I. M. 1977. Epidermal nucleases. II. The multiplicity of ribonucleases in guinea-pig epidermis. *J. Invest. Dermatol.* 68:285–292.

Mesirow, S. L. and Stoughton, R. B. 1954. Demonstration of β-glucuronidase in human skin. *J. Invest. Dermatol.* 23:315–316.

Mier, P. D. and Cotton, D. W. K. 1967. Enzymes of the glycolytic pathway in skin. III. Phosphorylase. *Br. J. Dermatol.* 79:164–169.

Mier, P. D. and Cotton, W. K. 1970. Enzymes of the glycolytic pathway in skin. X. Enolase. *Br. J. Dermatol.* 82:27–31.

Mier, P. D. and Urselmann, E. 1972. Adenosine 3',5'-cyclic nucleotide monophosphate phosphodiesterase in skin. I. Measurement and properties. *Br. J. Dermatol.* 86:141–147.

Miyazaki, M., Takayasu, S., Karakawa, T., Aono, T., Kurachi, K. and Mutsumoto, K. 1978. Activity of testosterone 5-alpha-reductase in the hair follicles of women with polycystic ovaries. *J. Endocrinol.* 78:445–446.

Montagna, W. 1962. *The structure and function of skin,* 2nd ed. New York: Academic Press.

Montagna, W. and Ellis, R. A., eds. 1958. *The biology of hair growth.* New York: Acadmic Press.

Moretti, G., Cardo, P., Rampini, E. and Pellerano, S. 1978. Testosterone metabolism in basal cell epitheliomas. *J. Invest. Dermatol.* 71:361–362.

Morrison, D. M. and Goldsmith, L. A. 1978. Ornithine decarboxylase in rat skin. *J. Invest. Dermatol.* 38:300–313.

Mowszowicz, I., Riahi, M., Wright, F., Bouchard, P., Kuttenn, F. and Mauvais-Jarvis, P. 1981. Androgen receptor in human skin cytosol. *J. Clin. Endocrinol. Metab.* 52:338–344.

Mowszowicz, I., Kirchhoffer, M. O., Kuttenn, F. and Mauvais-Jarvis, P. 1980.

Testosterone 5-alpha-reductase activity of skin fibroblasts. Increase with serial subcultures. *Mol. Cell Endocrinol.* 17:41–50.

Mueller, O. T. and Rosenberg, A. 1977. Beta-glucoside hydrolase activity of normal and glucosylceramidotic cultured human skin fibroblasts. *J. Biol. Chem.* 252:825–829.

Mueller, O. T. and Rosenberg, A. 1979. Activation of membrane-bound glucosylceramide:beta-glucosidase in fibroblasts cultured from normal and glucosylceramidotic human skin. *J. Biol. Chem.* 254:3521–3525.

Mueller, O. T. and Rosenberg, A. 1977. β-Glucoside hydrolase activity of normal and glucosylceramidotic cultured human skin fibroblasts. *J. Biol. Chem.* 252:825–829.

Mui, M. M., Hsia, S. L. and Halprin, K. M. 1975. Further studies on adenyl cyclase in psoriasis. *Br. J. Dermatol.* 92:255–262.

Murad, S., Sivarajah, A. and Pinnell, S. R. 1980. Prolyl and lysyl hydroxylase activities of human skin fibroblasts: Effect of donor age and ascorbate. *J. Invest. Dermatol.* 75:404–407.

Murray, A. W., Solanki, V. and Verma, A. K. 1977. Accumulation of cyclic adenosine 3',5'-monophosphate in adult and newborn mouse skin: Responses to ischemia and isoproterenol. *J. Invest. Dermatol.* 68:125–127.

Nazzaro-Porro, M., Passi, S., Boniforti, L. and Belsito, F. 1979. Effects of aging on fatty acids in skin surface lipids. *J. Invest. Dermatol.* 73:112–117.

Newman, R. A. and Cutroneo, K. R. 1978. Glucocorticoids selectively decrease the synthesis of hydroxylated collagen peptides. *Mol. Pharmacol.* 14:185–198.

Nicolaides, N. 1963. Human skin surface lipids—Origins, composition and possible function. In *Advances in biology of skin*, vol. 4, *The Sebaceous Glands*, eds. W. Montagna, R. A. Ellis, A. F. Silver, pp. 167–187. Oxford: Pergamon.

Nicolaides, N. 1967. The monoene and other wax alcohols of human skin surface lipid and their relation to the fatty acids of this lipid. *Lipids* 2:266–275.

Nicolaides, N. and Rothman, S. 1955. The site of sterol and squalene synthesis in the human skin. *J. Invest. Dermatol.* 24:125–129.

Nicolaides, N. and Wells, G. C. 1957. On the biogenesis of the free fatty acids in human skin surface fat. *J. Invest. Dermatol.* 29:423–433.

Nicolaides, N., Reiss, O. K. and Langdon, R. G. 1955. Studies on the *in vitro* lipid metabolism of the human skin. *J. Am. Chem. Soc.* 77:1535–1538.

Nicolaides, N., Kellum, R. E. and Wooley, P. V. 1964. The structure of the free unsaturated fatty acids of human skin surface fat. *Arch. Biochem. Biophys.* 105:634–639.

Nicolaides, N., Fu, H. C. and Rice, G. R. 1968. The skin surface lipids of man compared with those of eighteen species of animals. *J. Invest. Dermatol.* 51:83–89.

Nicolaides, N., Fu, H. C., Ansari, M. N. A. and Rice, B. R. 1972. The fatty acids of wax esters and sterol esters from vernix caseosa and from skin surface lipids. *Lipids* 7:506–517.

Niinikoski, J. 1969. Effect of oxygen supply on the tensile strengths of a healing skin wound and experimental granulation tissue. *Acta Physiol. Scand. Suppl.* 334:28–33.

Nijkamp, F. P., Flower, R. J., Moncada, S. and Vane, J. R. 1976. Partial purification of rabbit aorta contracting substance-releasing factor and inhibition of its activity by anti-inflammatory steroids. *Nature (Lond.)* 263:479–482.

Nikkari, T. 1969. The occurrence of diester waxes in human vernix caseosa and in hair lipids of common laboratory animals. *Comp. Biochem. Physiol.* 129:795-803.

Nikkari, T. 1974. Comparative chemistry of sebum. *J. Invest. Dermatol.* 64:257-267.

Nitowsky, H. M. and Grunfeld, A. 1967. Lysosomal α-glucosidase in type II glycogenosis; activity of leucocytes and cell cultures in relationship to genotype. *J. Lab. Clin. Med.* 69:472-484.

Nozu, K. and Tamaoki, B. 1974. Intranuclear and intermicrosomal distributions of 3-oxo-5α-steroid:NADP⁺ Δ⁴-oxidoreductase in rat ventral prostate. *Biochim. Biophys. Acta* 348:321-333.

Obinata, A. and Endo, H. 1977. Induction of epidermal transglutaminase by hydrocortisone in chick embryonic skin. *Nature (Lond.)* 270:440-441.

Odham, J. 1967. Studies on feather waxes of waterfowl. *Ark. Kemi* 27:295-307.

Odland, G. F. 1960. A submicroscopic granular component in human epidermis. *J. Invest. Dermatol.* 34:11-15.

Oertel, G. W. and Treiber, L. 1969. Metabolism and excretion of C_{19}-C_{18}-steroids by human skin. *Eur. J. Biochem.* 7:234-238.

Ogawa, H. and Goldsmith, L. A. 1976. Human epidermal transglutaminase. *J. Biol. Chem.* 251:7281-7288.

Ogawa, H. and Goldsmith, L. A. 1977. Human epidermal transglutaminase. *J. Invest. Dermatol.* 68:32-35.

Ohara, K. 1951. Studies on oxygen consumption of human skin tissues with special reference to that of sweat glands. *Jap. J. Physiol.* 2:1-8.

Ohkawara, A. 1976. Glycogen metabolism and cyclic AMP in the hair follicle. In *Biology and Diseases of the Hair*, pp. 247-255. Baltimore: University Park.

Oikarinen, A. and Hannuksela, M. 1980. Effect of hydrocortisone-17-butyrate, hydrocortisone, and clobetasol-17-propionate on prolyl hydroxylase activity in human skin. *Arch. Dermatol. Res.* 267:79-82.

Oram, J. F., Shafrir, E. and Bierman, E. L. 1980. Triacylglycerol metabolism and triacylglycerol lipase activities of cultured human skin fibroblasts. *Biochim. Biophys. Acta* 619:214-227.

Owen, O. E. and Reichard, G. A. 1971. Human forearm metabolism during progressive starvation. *J. Clin. Invest.* 50:1536-1545.

Owen, O. E., Morgan, A. P., Kemp, H. G., Sullivan, J. M., Herrera, M. G. and Cahill, G. F. 1967. Brain metabolism during fasting. *J. Clin. Invest.* 46:1589-1595.

Owen, O. E., Felig, P., Morgan, A. P., Wahren, J. and Cahill, G. F. 1969. Liver and kidney metabolism during prolonged starvation. *J. Clin. Invest.* 48:574-583.

Oxlund, H. 1980. Changes in the biomechanical properties of skin and aorta induced by corticotrophin treatment. *Acta Endocrinol.* 94:132-137.

Oxlund, H., Fogdestam, I. and Viidik, A. 1979. The influence of cortisol on wound healing of the skin and distant connective tissue response. *Surg. Gynecol. Obstet.* 148:876-880.

Pablo, C. M. and Fulton, J. E. 1975. Sebum: Analysis by infared spectroscopy. *Arch. Dermatol.* 111:734-735.

Panconesi, E. and Cappugi, P. 1979. The biosynthesis of prostaglandins in psoriatic skin. *Acta Derm.-Venereol. (Suppl.)* 87:45-47.

Penneys, N. S. and Muench, K. H. 1971. Tryptophanyl-tRNA synthetase of human skin. *J. Invest. Dermatol.* 56:248.

Penneys, N. S., Eaglstein, W. and Ziboh, V. 1980. Petrolatum: Interference with the oxidation of arachidonic acid. *Br. J. Dermatol.* 103:257–262.

Peterka, E. S. and Fusaro, R. M. 1965. Cutaneous carbohydrate studies. II. The constancy of the glucose content of the skin on the back of normal persons. *J. Invest. Dermatol.* 45:177–178.

Peters, R. F. and White, A. M. 1976. The existence of a glyconeogenic pathway in rat skin. *Biochem. J.* 156:465–468.

Peters, R. F. and White, A. M. 1978. The relationship between cyclic adenosine 3',5'-monophosphate and biochemical events in rat skin after the induction of epidermal hyperplasia using hexadecane. *Br. J. Dermatol.* 98:301–314.

Pillsbury, D. M. 1931. The intrinsic carbohydrate metabolism of the skin. *J. Am. Med. Assoc.* 96:426.

Pillsbury, D. M. 1971. *A manual of dermatology.* Philadelphia: Saunders.

Plewig, G. 1974. Acne vulgaris; proliferative cells in sebaceous glands. *Br. J. Dermatol.* 90:623–630.

Pochi, P. E. and Strauss, J. S. 1966. Effect of cyclic administration of conjugated equine estrogens on sebum production in women. *J. Invest. Dermatol.* 47:582–585.

Pochi, P. E. and Strauss, J. S. 1974. Endocrinologic control of the development and activity of the human sebaceous gland. *J. Invest. Dermatol.* 62:191–201.

Pochi, P. E., Strauss, J. S. and Mescon, H. 1962. Sebum secretion and urinary fractional 17-ketosteroid and total 17-hydroxycorticoid excretion in male castrates. *J. Invest. Dermatol.* 39:475–483.

Pochi, P. E., Downing, D. T. and Strauss, J. S. 1970. Sebaceous gland response in man to prolonged total caloric deprivation. *J. Invest. Dermatol.* 55:303–309.

Pochi, P. E., Strauss, J. S. and Downing, D. T. 1977. Skin surface lipid composition, acne, pubertal development, and urinary excretion of testosterone and 17-ketosteroids in children. *J. Invest. Dermatol.* 69:485–489.

Pomerantz, S. H. and Asbornsen, M. T. 1961. Glucose metabolism in young rat skin. *Arch. Biochem. Biophys.* 93:147–152.

Pomerantz, S. H. and Li, J. P. 1978. Tyrosine aminotransferase in AKR/J albino and C57BL/6J black mouse skin. *J. Invest. Dermatol.* 70:240–245.

Ponec, M., de Haas, C., Kempenaar, J. A. and Bachra, B. N. 1979. Effects of glucocorticoids on cultured human skin fibroblasts. V. Influence of anabolic steroids on the inhibitory effects of clobetasol-17-propionate on cell proliferation and collagen synthesis. *Arch Dermatol. Res.* 266:75–82.

Ponec, M., Kempenaar, J. A., Van Der Meulen-Van-Harskamp, G. A. and Bachra, B. N. 1979. Effects of glucocorticosteroids on cultured human skin fibroblasts. IV. Specific decrease in the synthesis of collagen but no effect on its hydroxylation. *Biochem. Pharmacol.* 28:2777–2783.

Poulos, A., Voglmayr, J. K. and White, I. G. 1973. Phospholipid changes in spermatozoa during passage through the genital tract of the bull. *Biochim. Biophys. Acta* 306:194–202.

Powell, E. W. and Beveridge, G. W. 1970. Sebum excretion and sebum composition in adolescent men with and without acne vulgaris. *Br. J. Dermatol.* 82:243–249.

Pratt, W. B. and Aronow, L. 1966. The effect of glucocorticoids on protein and nucleic acid synthesis in mouse fibroblasts growing *in vitro. J. Biol. Chem.* 241:5244–5250.

Priestly, G. C. 1978. Effects of corticosteroids on the growth and metabolism of fibroblasts cultured from human skin. *Br. J. Dermatol.* 99:253–261.

Prottey, C. 1977. Investigation of functions of essential fatty acids in the skin. *Br. J. Dermatol.* 97:29–38.

Prottey, C. and Ferguson, T. F. M. 1974. The metabolic activity of primary cultures of guinea pig dorsal skin cells. *Br. J. Dermatol.* 91:681–686.

Puhvel, S. M., Reisnes, R. M. and Sakamoto, M. 1975. Analysis of lipid composition of isolated human sebaceous gland homogenates after incubation with cutaneous bacteria. Thin layer chromatography. *J. Invest. Dermatol.* 64:406–411.

Punnonen, R., Lövgren, T. and Kouvonen, I. 1980. Demonstration of estrogen receptors in the skin. *J. Endocrinol. Invest.* 3:217–221.

Rawlins, M. D., Shaw, V. and Shuster, S. 1979. The in vitro metabolism of betamethasone-17-valerate by human skin. *Br. J. Pharmacol.* 66:441P.

Richardson, G. S. and Axelrod, L. R. 1971. Metabolism of labeled testosterone by minces and nuclei of preputial glands of male rats. *Endocrinology* 88:890–894.

Rippa, M. and Vignali, C. 1965. The level of enzymes of the oxidative shunt and glycolysis in psoriatic skin. *J. Invest. Dermatol.* 45:78–80.

Rongone, E. L. 1966. Testosterone metabolism by human male mammary skin. *Steroids* 7:489–503.

Rongone, E. L. 1969. Conversion of pregnenolone to progesterone by primate skin. *Proc. Soc. Exp. Biol. Med.* 130:253–256.

Rongone, E. L. and Ferraro, F. M. 1968. Androst-4-ene-3,17-dione-4-^{14}C metabolism by homogenates of the chicken uropygial gland. I. Antibiotic concentrations necessary for inhibition of bacterial growth. *J. Pharm. Sci.* 57:1962–1965.

Rongone, E. L., Hill, M. and Burns, R. 1967. Testosterone metabolism by the chicken uropygial gland. *Steroids* 9:425–439.

Rosenthal, M. D. 1980. Selectivity in incorporation, utilization and retention of oleic and linoleic acids by human skin fibroblasts. *Lipids* 15:838–848.

Rothman, S. 1954. *Physiology and biochemistry of the skin,* pp. 210 and 472. Chicago: Univ. of Chicago Press.

Ryan, J. N. and Woessner, J. F. 1971. Mammalian collagenase: Direct demonstration in Homogenates of involuting rat uterus. *Biochem. Biophys. Res. Commun.* 44:144–149.

Ryan, J. N. and Woessner, J. F. 1972. Oestradiol inhibits collagen breakdown in the involuting rat uterus. *Biochem. J.* 127:705–713.

Saarni, H., Tammi, M. and Doharty, N. S. 1978. Decreased hyaluronic acid synthesis, a sensitive indicator of cortisol action on fibroblast. *J. Pharm. Pharmacol.* 30:200–201.

Sabeh, G., Alley, R. A., Robbins, T. J., Narduzzi, J. V., Kenny, F. M. and Danowski, T. S. 1969. Adrenalcortical indices during fasting obesity. *J. Clin. Endocrinol.* 29:373–376.

Saenger, P. and New, M. 1977. Inhibitory action of dehydroepiandrosterone (DHEA) on fibroblast growth. *Experientia* 33:966–967.

Saenger, P., Goldman, A. S., Levine, L. S., Korth-Schutz, S., Muecke, E. C., Katsumata, M., Doberne, Y. and New, M. I. 1978. Prepubertal diagnosis of steroid 5-alpha-reductase deficiency. *J. Clin. Endocrinol. Metab.* 46:627–634.

Saihan, E. M., Albano, J. and Burton, J. L. 1980. The effect of steroid dithranol therapy on cyclic nucleotides in psoriatic epidermis. *Br. J. Dermatol.* 102:565–569.

Saihan, E. M. and Burton, J. L. 1980. Sebaceous gland suppression in female acne patients by combined glucocorticoid-oestrogen therapy. *Br. J. Dermatol.* 103:139–142.

Sand, A. H., Hehl, J. L. and Schlenk, H. 1969. Biosynthesis of wax esters in fish. Reduction of fatty acids and oxidation of alcohols. *Biochemistry* 8:4851–4854.

Sansone, G., Davidson, W., Cummings, B. and Reisner, R. M. 1971. Sebaceous gland lipogenesis induced by testosterone: Early metabolic events. *J. Invest. Dermatol.* 57:144–148.

Sato, K. 1977. The physiology, pharmacology, and biochemistry of the eccrine sweat gland. *Rev. Physiol. Biochem. Pharmacol.* 79:51–131.

Sato, K. and Dobson, R. L. 1970. Enzymatic basis for the active transport of sodium in the duct and secretory portion of the eccrine sweat gland. *J. Invest. Dermatol.* 55:53–56.

Sato, K. and Dobson, R. L. 1971. Glucose metabolism of the isolated eccrine sweat gland. I. The effects of mecholyl, epinephrine and ouabain. *J. Invest. Dermatol.* 56:272–280.

Savage, M. O., Preece, M. A., Jeffcoate, S. L., Ransley, P. G., Rumsby, G., Mansfield, M. D. and Williams, D. I. 1980. Familial male pseudohermaphroditism due to deficiency of 5-alpha-reductase. *Clin. Endocrinol.* 12:397–406.

Schalla, W., Zesch, A. and Schaffer, H. 1974. The estimation of enzyme activity in living epidermal cells. *Br. J. Dermatol.* 91:489–501.

Schell, H., Hornstein, O. P. and Schwarz, W. 1980. Human epidermal cell proliferation with regard to circadian variation of plasma cortisol. *Dermatologica* 161:12–21.

Schneider, E. L., Mitsul, Y., Au, K. S. and Shorr, S. S. 1977. Tissue specific differences in cultured human diploid fibroblasts. *Exp. Cell Res.* 108:1–6.

Schragger, A. H. 1962. Ultramicro determination of epidermal glucose. *J. Invest. Dermatol.* 39:417–418.

Schultz, A. L., Kerlow, A. and Ulstrom, R. A. 1964. Effect of starvation on adrenal cortical function in obese subjects. *J. Clin. Endocrinol.* 24:1253–1257.

Schultze, B. and Oehlert, W. 1960. Autoradiographic investigations of incorporation of ^{3}H-thymidine into cells of the rat and mouse. *Science* 31:737–738.

Schweikert, H. U. 1979. Conversion of androstenedione to estrone in human fibroblasts cultured from prostate, genital and nongenital skin. *Horm. Metab. Res.* 11:635–640.

Schweikert, H. U. and Wilson, J. 1974. Regulation of human hair growth by steroid hormones. I. Testosterone metabolism in isolated hairs. *J. Clin. Endocrinol. Metab.* 38:811–819.

Schweikert, H. U., Milewich, I. and Wilson, J. D. 1976. Aromatization of androstenedione by cultured human fibroblasts. *J. Clin. Endocrinol. Metab.* 43:785–795.

Sear, C. H., Grant, M. E. and Jackson, D. S. 1977. Biosynthesis and release of glycoproteins by human skin fibroblasts in culture. *Biochem. J.* 168:91–103.

Seiter, C. W. and Summer, G. K. 1975. Glycogen metabolism in human skin fibroblasts. Influence of maltose on the activity of acid alpha-1,4-glucosidase. *Proc. Soc. Exp. Biol. Med.* 149:945–949.

Serri, F., Cerimele, D. and Torsellini, M. 1971. *Quantitative histochemical study of metabolic enzymes in diseased and symptom-free skin in psoriasis*, eds. E. M. Farber and A. J. Cox, pp. 255–261. Stanford, Calif.: Stanford Univ. Press.

Sharaf, D. M., Clark, S. J. and Downing, D. T. 1977. Skin surface lipids of the dog. *Lipids* 12:786.

Shipp, J. C., Opie, L. H. and Challoner, D. 1961. Fatty acid and glucose metabolism in the perfused heart. *Nature (Lond.)* 189:1018–1019.

Shuster, S. and Thody, A. J. 1974. The control and measurement of sebum production. *J. Invest. Dermatol.* 62:172–190.

Shuster, S., Cooper, M. F., McGibbon, D. and Wilson, P. D. 1980. Epidermal lipid biosynthesis in acne. *Br. J. Dermatol.* 103:127–130.

Simpson, N. B., Bowden, P. E., Forster, R. A. and Cunliffe, W. J. 1979. The effect of topically applied progesterone on sebum excretion rate. *Br. J. Dermatol.* 100:687–692.

Smith, J. G., Jr. and Brunot, F. R. 1961. Hormonal effects on aged human sebaceous glands. *Acta Dermatol. Venereol. (Stockh.)* 41:61–65.

Soloman, L. M., Juhlin, L. and Kirschenbaum, M. G. 1968. Prostaglandin on cutaneous vasculature. *J. Invest. Dermatol.* 51:280–282.

Spector, A. A., Denning, G. M. and Stoll, L. L. 1980. Retention of human skin fibroblast fatty acid modifications during maintenance culture. *In Vitro* 16:932–940.

Srere, P. A., Chaikoff, I. L., Tretimann, S. S. and Burstein, L. L. 1950. The extra-hepatic synthesis of cholesterol. *J. Biol. Chem.* 182:629–634.

Steinberg, D., Nestel, P. J., Weinstein, D. B., Remaut-Desmeth, M. and Chang, C. M. 1978. Interactions of native and modified human low density lipoproteins with human skin fibroblasts. *Biochim. Biophys. Acta* 528:199–212.

Steinert, P. M. and Rogers, G. E. 1971a. Protein biosynthesis in cell-free systems prepared from hair follicle tissue of guinea pigs. *Biochim. Biophys. Acta* 232:556–572.

Steinert, P. M. and Rogers, G. E. 1971b. The synthesis of hair keratin proteins *in vitro*. *Biochim. Biophys. Acta* 238:150–156.

Stephens, F. O. and Hunt, T. K. 1971. Effect of changes in inspired oxygen and oxygen and carbon dioxide tensions in wound tensile strength: An experimental study. *Ann. Surg.* 173:515–519.

Stewart, M. E. and Pochi, P. E. 1978. Antiandrogens and the skin. *Int. J. Dermatol.* 17:167–179.

Strauss, J. S. and Pochi, P. E. 1961. The quantitative gravimetric determination of sebum production. *J. Invest. Dermatol.* 36:292–298.

Strauss, J. S. and Pochi, P. E. 1963. The human sebaceous gland: Its regulation by steroid hormones and its use as an end-organ for assaying androgenicity *in vitro*. *Rec. Prog. Horm. Res.* 19:385–444.

Strauss, J. S., Kligman, A. M. and Pochi, P. E. 1962. The effect of androgens and estrogens on human sebaceous glands. *J. Invest. Dermatol.* 39:139–155.

Strauss, J. S., Vitale, J. J., Downing, D. T. and Franco, D. 1978. Surface lipid composition in children with protein-calorie malnutrition. *Am. J. Clin. Nutr.* 31:327–340.

Sutherland, B. M., Harber, L. C. and Kochevar, I. E. 1980. Pyrimidine dimer formation and repair in human skin. *Cancer Res.* 40:3181–3185.

Svensson, J., Eneroth, P., Gustafsson, J. A., Ritzén, M. and Stenberg, A. 1979. Reduction of androstenedione by skin *in vitro* and serum levels of gonadotrophins and androgens in men with hypospadias. *J. Endocrinol.* 82:395–401.

Szabo, G. 1958. The regional frequency and distribution of hair follicles in human skin. In *Biology of hair growth*, eds. W. Montagna and R. A. Ellis, pp. 33–38. New York: Academic Press.

Takayasu, S. 1979. Metabolism and action of androgen in the skin. *Int. J. Dermatol.* 18:681–692.

Takehisa, F. and Kimura, S. 1977. Effect of essential fatty acid deficiency on lipid of skin surface of rat. *J. Nutr. Sci. Vitaminol.* 23:431–437.

Thody, A. J. and Shuster, S. 1970. The effects of hypophysectomy and testosterone on the activity of sebaceous glands of castrated rats. *J. Endocrinol.* 47:219–224.

Thody, A. J. and Shuster, S. 1971. The effect of hypophysectomy on the response of the sebaceous gland to testosterone propionate. *J. Endocrinol.* 49:329–333.

Thody, A. J. and Shuster, S. 1972. Control of sebum secretion by posterior pituitary. *Nature (Lond.)* 237:346–347.

Thody, A. J. and Shuster, S. 1973. Possible role of MSH in the mammal. *Nature (Lond.)* 245:207–209.

Thody, A. J. and Shuster, S. 1978. Effect of progesterone on the sebaceous glands. *Postgrad. Med. J.* 54:88–90.

Thomas, G. 1980. Characteristics of prostaglandin E1 potentiation of inflammatory activity of some agents. *Prostaglandins* 19:39–50.

Thorpe, J. M. and Goldsmith, L. A. 1980. Tyrosine aminotransferase activity in skin. *J. Invest. Dermatol.* 75:371–372.

Tuderman, L. and Kivirikko, K. I. 1977. Immunoreactive prolyl hydroxylase in human skin, serum and synovial fluid: Changes in the content and components with age. *Eur. J. Clin. Invest.* 7:295–300.

Udenfriend, S. 1966. Formation of hydroxyproline in collagen. *Science* 152:1335–1340.

Urbach, E. and Fantl, P. 1928. Methoden zur quantitativchemichen analyse der haut. II. Zuckergehalt der normalen haut. *Biochem. Z.* 196:474–477.

Urbach, E. and Lentz, J. W. 1945. Carbohydrate metabolism and the skin. *Arch. Dermatol. Syphilol.* 52:301–306.

Uzuka, M., Nakajima, M. and Mori, Y. 1978. Estrogen receptor in the mouse skin. *Biochim. Biophys. Acta* 544:329–337.

van Dorp, D. 1971. Recent developments in the biosynthesis and the analysis of prostaglandins. *Ann. N.Y. Acad. Sci.* 180:181–195.

Van Scott, E. J. and Reinertson, R. P. 1961. The modulating influence of stromal environment on epithelial cells studied in human autotransplants. *J. Invest. Dermatol.* 36:109–131.

Verma, A. K. and Murray, A. W. 1974. The effect of benzo(a)pyrene on the basal and isoproterenol-stimulated levels of cyclic adenosine-3′,5′-monophosphate in mouse epidermis. *Cancer Res.* 34:3408–3413.

Verma, A. K., Ashendel, C. L. and Boutwell, R. K. 1980. Inhibition by prostaglandin synthesis inhibitors of the induction of epidermal ornithine decarboxylase activity, the accumulation of prostaglandins, and tumor promotion caused by 12-O-tetradecanoylphorbol-13-acetate. *Cancer Res.* 40:308–315.

Vermorken, A. J., Goos, C. M., Henderson, P. T. and Bloemendal, H. 1979. Hydroxylation of dehydroepiandrosterone in human scalp hair follicles. *Br. J. Dermatol.* 100:693–698.

Vonkeman, H. and Van Dorp, D. A. 1968. The action of prostaglandin synthetase on 2-arachidonyl-lecithin. *Biochim. Biophys. Acta* 164:430–433.

Voorhees, J. J. and Duell, E. A. 1971. Psoriasis as a possible defect of the adenyl cyclase-cyclic AMP cascade. *Arch. Dermatol.* 104:352–358.

Voorhees, J. J., Stawiski, M., Duell, E., Haddox, M. and Goldberg, N. 1973. Increased cyclic GMP and decreased cyclic AMP levels in the hyperplastic, abnormally differentiated epidermis of psoriasis. *Life Sci.* [I] 13:639–653.

Vroman, H. E., Nemecek, R. A. and Hsia, S. L. 1969. Synthesis of lipids from acetate by human preputial and abdominal skin *in vitro. J. Lipid Res.* 10:507–514.

Wada, M. 1950. Sudorific action of adrenalin on the human sweat glands and determination of their excitability. *Science* 111:376–377.

Wallace, S. M., Falkenberg, H. M., Runikis, J. O. and Stewart, W. D. 1979. Skin levels and vasoconstrictor assay of topically applied hydrocortisone. *Arch. Dermatol.* 115:440–441.

Weber, C. 1964. Some aspects of the carbohydrate metabolism of enzymes in the human epidermis under normal and pathological conditions. In *The epidermis*, eds. W. Montagna and W. S. Lobitz, pp. 453–470. New York: Academic Press.

Weiner, J. S. and Van Heyningen, R. E. 1952. Observations on lactate content of sweat. *J. Appl. Physiol.* 4:734–744.

Weinstein, G. D., Frost, P. and Hsia, S. L. 1968. *In vitro* interconversion of estrone and 17β-estradiol in human skin and vaginal mucosa. *J. Invest. Dermatol.* 51:4–10.

Weissmann, A. and Noble, W. C. 1980. Photochemotherapy of psoriasis: Effects on bacteria and surface lipids in uninvolved skin. *Br. J. Dermatol.* 102:185–193.

Weitkamp, A. W., Smilhanic, A. M. and Rothman, S. 1947. The free fatty acids of human hair fat. *J. Am. Chem. Soc.* 69:1936–1939.

Wérenne, J. and Revel, M. 1978. Triggering of protein phosphorylation in human cell system by interferon and double-stranded RNA. *Arch. Int. Physiol. Biochim.* 86:471–473.

Weitkamp, A. W., Smilhanic, A. M. and Rothman, S. 1947. The free fatty acids of human hair fat. *J. Am. Chem. Soc.* 69:1936–1939.

Wheatley, V. R. 1956. Sebum: Its chemistry and biochemistry. *Am. Perfum.* 68:37–47.

Wheatley, V. R. 1974. Cutaneous lipogenesis. Major pathways of carbon flow and possible interrelationships between the epidermis and sebaceous glands. *J. Invest. Dermatol.* 62:245–256.

Wheatley, V. R., Chow, D. C. and Keenan, F. D. 1961. Studies of the lipids of dog skin. II. Observations on the lipid metabolism of perfused surviving dog skin. *J. Invest. Dermatol.* 36:237–239.

Wheatley, V. R., Lipkin, G. and Woo, T. H. 1967. Lipogenesis from amino acids in perfused isolated dog skin. *J. Lipid Res.* 8:81–89.

Wheatley, V. R., Kumarisiri, M. and Brind, J. L. 1973. Cutaneous lipogenesis. IV. Role of the pentose phosphate pathway during lipogenesis in guinea pig ear skin. *J. Invest. Dermatol.* 61:357–365.

Wilkinson, D. I. 1970a. Positional isomers of monoene and diene fatty acids of human epidermal cells. *Arch. Biochem. Biophys.* 136:368–371.

Wilkinson, D. I. 1970b. Incorporation of acetate-1-C^{14} into fatty acids of isolated epidermal cells. *J. Invest. Dermatol.* 54:132–138.

Wilkinson, D. I. 1972. Polyunsaturated fatty acids of skin: Identification of ^{14}C-acetate incorporation. *Lipids* 7:544–547.

Wilson, J. D. 1963. Studies on the regulation of cholesterol synthesis in the skin and preputial gland of the rat. In *Advances in biology of skin*, vol. 4, *The sebaceous glands*, eds. W. Montagna, R. A. Ellis, A. F. Silver, pp. 148–166. Oxford: Pergamon.

Wilson, J. D. and Gloyna, R. W. 1970. The intranuclear metabolism of testosterone in the accessory organs of reproduction. *Rec. Prog. Horm. Res.* 26:309–336.

Wilson, J. D. and Walker, J. D. 1969. The conversion of testosterone to 5α-androstane-17β-ol-3-one (dihydrotestosterone) by skin slices of man. *J. Clin. Invest.* 48:371–379.

Wolfe, S., Cage, G., Ticke, L., Miller, H. and Gordon, R. S. 1970. Metabolic studies of isolated human eccrine sweat glands. *J. Clin. Invest.* 49:1880–1884.

Woodbury, L. P., Lorincz, A. L. and Ortega, P. 1965. Studies on pituitary sebotropic activity. I. A new sensitive assay method for sebotropic activity based on beta-glucuronidase content of preputial glands. *J. Invest. Dermatol.* 45:362–363.

Wotiz, H. H., Mescon, H., Doppel, H. and Leman, H. M. 1956. The *in vitro* metabolism of testosterone by human skin. *J. Invest. Dermatol.* 26:113–120.

Wright, F. and Giacomini, M. 1980. Reduction of dihydroestosterone to androstanediols by human female skin *in vitro*. *J. Steroid Biochem.* 13:639–643.

Wu, J. D. and Bailey, J. M. 1980. Lipid metabolism in cultured cells: Studies on lipoprotein-catalyzed reverse cholesterol transport in normal and homozygous familial hypercholesterolemic skin fibroblasts. *Arch. Biochem. Biophys.* 202:467–473.

Yamamoto, S., Francis, D. and Greaves, M. W. 1977. Enzymic histamine catabolism in skin and its possible clinical significance. *Clin. Exp. Dermatol.* 2:389–393.

Yeuns, D., Nacht, S. and Cover, R. E. 1981. The composition of the skin surface lipids of the gerbil. *Biochim. Biophys. Acta* 663:524–535.

Yoshikawa, K., Adachi, K., Halprin, K. M. and Levine, V. 1975b. Cyclic AMP in skin: Effects of acute ischaemia. *Br. J. Dermatol.* 92:249–254.

Yoshikawa, K., Adachi, K., Levine, V. and Halprin, K. M. 1975a. Microdetermination of cyclic AMP levels in human epidermis, dermis and hair follicles. *Br. J. Dermatol.* 92:241–249.

Yoshizato, K., Kikuyama, S. and Shioya, N. 1980. Stimulation of glucose utilization and lactate production in cultured human fibroblasts by thyroid hormone. *Biochim. Biophys. Acta* 627:23–29.

Zabel, J. 1979. Uptake of ^{3}H-testosterone in the skin of healthy women and in the skin of patients with acne vulgaris. *Acta Histochem.* 64:243–248.

Zelickson, A. S. 1960. Histochemical localization of mitochondria in human skin. *J. Invest. Dermatol.* 35:265–268.

Zelickson, A. S. 1967. In *Ultrastructure of normal and abnormal skin*, ed. A. S. Zelickson, pp. 144–153. Philadelphia: Lea and Febiger.

Ziboh, V. A. 1973. Biosynthesis of prostaglandin E_2 in human skin: Subcellular localization and inhibition by unsaturated fatty acids and anti-inflammatory drugs. *J. Lipid Res.* 14:377–384.

Ziboh, V. A. and Hsia, S. L. 1969. Lipogenesis in rat skin: A possible regulatory role of glycerol-3-phosphate. *Arch. Biochem. Biophys.* 131:131–162.

Ziboh, V. A. and Hsia, S. L. 1971. Prostaglandin E_2 biosynthesis and effects on glucose and lipid metabolism in rat skin. *Arch. Biochem. Biophys.* 146:100–109.

Ziboh, V. A. and Hsia, S. L. 1972. Effects of prostaglandin E_2 on rat skin: Inhibition of sterol ester biosynthesis and clearing of scaly lesions in essential fatty acid deficiency. *J. Lipid Res.* 13:458–467.

Ziboh, V. A. and Lord, J. T. 1979. Phospholipase A activity in the skin. Modulators of arachidonic acid release from phosphatidylcholine. *Biochem. J.* 184:383–390.

Ziboh, V. A., Dreize, M. A. and Hsia, S. L. 1970. Inhibition of lipid synthesis and glucose-6-phosphate dehydrogenase in rat skin by dehydroepiandrosterone. *J. Lipid Res.* 11:346–354.

Ziboh, V. A., Wright, R. and Hsia, S. L. 1971. Effects of insulin on the uptake and metabolism of glucose. *Arch. Biochem. Biophys.* 146:93–99.

Ziboh, V. A., Vanderhock, J. Y. and Lands, W. E. M. 1974. Inhibition of sheep vesicular gland oxygenase by unsaturated fatty acids from skin of essential fatty acid deficient rats. *Prostaglandins* 5:233–240.

Ziboh, V. A., Lord, J. T. and Penneys, N. S. 1977. Alterations of prostaglandin E2-9-ketoreductase activity in proliferating skin. *J. Lipid. Res.* 18:37–43.

2

cutaneous biotransformations and some pharmacological and toxicological implications

Patrick K. Noonan ■ Ronald C. Wester

INTRODUCTION

The skin is viewed as a passive membrane with a primary function of restricting the diffusion of substances into and out of the body. In its most simple form the skin can be described in terms of three basic layers: epidermis, dermis, and subcutaneous fat. The outermost layer of the epidermis is the stratum corneum, the major barrier to percutaneous absorption. Below the stratum corneum is the viable epidermal layer, the most metabolically active layer in skin (Laerum, 1969). This is a unique biological situation because any substance that penetrates the stratum corneum is then subjected to the drug-metabolizing properties of the viable epidermis. Lack of metabolism allows free passage of the unchanged chemical into the systemic circulation. Metabolism of the chemical results in obvious modification of the molecule. The result may be reduced pharmacological and/or toxicological activity. However, the reverse can also occur. Skin metabolizing enzymes can be induced, and they can convert nonactive chemical moieties into active pharmacological and toxicological agents.

This chapter reviews the chemical metabolizing potential of skin, relates this potential to enzyme induction and first-pass metabolism, and discusses some of the potential toxicological implications.

STEROID METABOLISM

Topical administration of steroids (e.g., hydrocortisone) is commonly utilized for some dermatologic disorders. The skin plays an important role in

71

the formation and catabolism of endogenous steroids and thus may play a role in the regulation of these endogenous hormones (Hsia, 1971). The following is a discussion of the various enzymatic reactions of steroid metabolism.

Alcohol Oxidation

There are several examples of the cutaneous metabolism of alicyclic alcohol groups present in many steroids. Hsia et al. (1965) observed that hydrocortisone (Fig. 1) can be metabolized by human skin to cortisone. Wotiz et al. (1956) found that testosterone was metabolized to at least seven metabolites in human skin. The major metabolite was Δ^4-androstene-3,17-dione (structure B in Fig. 2). Another example of alicyclic alcohol oxidation involves the estrogen estradiol. Skin contains the metabolic enzymes necessary for the oxidation of estradiol to estrone (Weinstein et al., 1968). The reaction is shown in Fig. 1. All of these oxidations were catalyzed in skin by the enzyme 17β-hydroxysteroid dehydrogenase.

Alicyclic Carbon Hydroxylation

Faredin et al. (1969) incubated dehydroepiandrosterone (DHA, structure C in Fig. 2) with slices of human abdominal skin and isolated several metabolites. The major metabolite (60%) was 7α-hydroxydehydroepiandro-

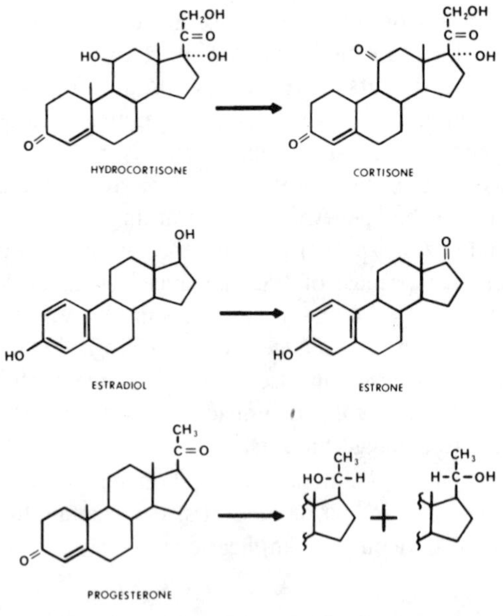

FIGURE 1 Cutaneous metabolism of several steroids. (Top) Hydrocortisone to cortisone; (middle) estradiol to estrone; (bottom) reduction of progesterone.

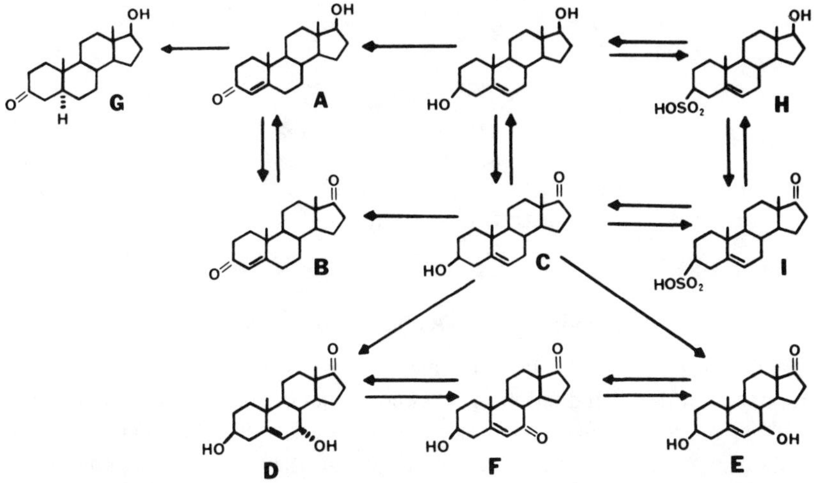

FIGURE 2 Metabolism of testosterone (A) and related steroids in human skin. (B) 4-Androstene-3,17-dione; (C) dehydroepiandrosterone (DHA); (D) 7α-hydroxy-DHA; (E) 7β-hydroxy-DHA; (F) 7-keto-DHA; (G) 5α-dihydrotestosterone; (H and I) sulfate conjugates (redrawn from Pannatier et al., 1978).

sterone (structure D in Fig. 2). A significant amount (16%) of the 7β-hydroxy metabolite (structure E) was generated, along with an equal amount of the 7-keto metabolite (structure F).

This example illustrates a well-known hepatic metabolic route in skin, the regioselective hydroxylation reaction at an allylic position. In contrast with the cutaneous metabolic route, human hepatic enzymes produced only the 7α-hydroxylated metabolite of DHA. A mechanistic interpretation of this metabolic route was difficult since two different mechanisms were possible. One mechanism involves the presence of both a 7α- and a 7β-hydroxylase, either or both of which could be oxidized to the ketone. The other mechanism involves only a 7α-hydroxylase. In this case, the 7α-hydroxy-DHA would be oxidized to 7-keto-DHA. Reduction of the 7-keto-DHA would then form a mixture of the two 7-hydroxy epimers. The mechanism has not been determined.

Carbonyl Reduction

The carbonyl groups of various steroids can be reduced by metabolic reactions in the skin. An example of this type of reaction is the reduction of 7-keto-DHA, mentioned in the last section. Two more definitive examples involve the cutaneous reduction of the 20-oxo group of hydrocortisone (Hsia et al., 1965) and progesterone (Frost et al., 1969). In both cases, the 20-oxo group (carbonyl) was reduced to a secondary alcohol and yielded two epimers. Figure 1 shows the reduction of progesterone by enzymes found in both human skin and vaginal mucosa.

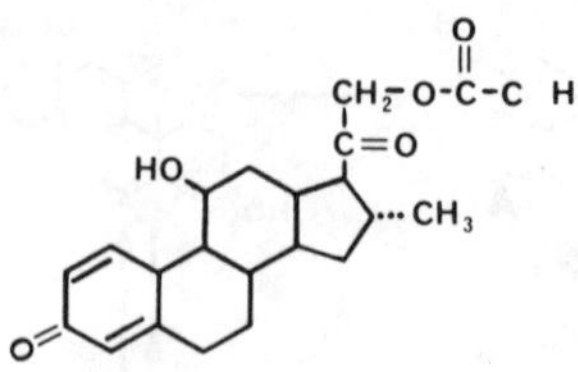

FIGURE 3   Structure of diflucortilone valerate.

Carbon-Carbon Double Bond Reduction

The hepatic metabolism of many steroids proceeds through carbon-carbon double bond reduction. The same reductase activity is present in skin. While hepatic microsomal systems often yield both α and β epimers, cutaneous metabolism exhibits more stereospecificity in that only the α epimers are produced. Some examples of cutaneous reductase activity have been shown for hydrocortisone, testosterone, and progesterone. Hydrocortisone (structure A in Fig 1) is reduced to allodihydrocortisol by human skin (Hsia et al., 1965), testosterone is reduced via a 5α-reductase to 5α-dihydrotestosterone (structure G in Fig. 2), and progesterone is reduced to 5α-pregnane derivatives by human skin (Frost et al., 1969).

Hydrolytic Reactions

Tauber and Toda (1976) investigated the biotransformation of diflu-cortolone valerate (DFV, shown in Fig. 3) in rat, guinea pig, and human skin. Guinea pig and rat skin hydrolyze DFV rapidly (half-life, 30–60 min) to diflucortilone (DF) and valeric acid. *In vitro* hydrolysis of DFV in human skin was much slower; only 5–15% DF was formed after 7 h. In this case, absorption of the drug into the skin was the rate-limiting step since it was found that the reaction proceeded more rapidly with injured skin.

Conjugation Reactions

The predominant phase II reaction with steroids involves sulfate conjugation. Berliner et al. (1968) isolated two water-soluble metabolites of [^{14}C]-DHA after incubation of [^{14}C]DHA (Fig. 2) with human abdominal skin (dermis and epidermis) for 5 d. These metabolites were identified as the sulfate conjugates (structures H and I in Fig. 2). In a similar study, Faredin et al. (1968) incubated [^{14}C]DHA with small pieces (1–2 mm "cubes") of normal human female abdominal skin. They too found the DHA-sulfate conjugate, from which they concluded that human skin contained sulfokinase activity. These studies show that skin cannot only participate in steroid biotransformation reactions but can eliminate polar materials through sulfate conjugation reactions.

EPIDERMAL METABOLISM OF POLYCYCLIC
AROMATIC HYDROCARBONS

Much work has been devoted to the effects of polycyclic aromatic hydrocarbons (PAHs) on the skin. As a group, PAHs induce skin carcinomas. Metabolic activation of these compounds is usually the first step toward the induction of skin cancer. Study of the cutaneous metabolism of PAHs can yield important data on the structure of the ultimate carcinogen responsible for tumor induction.

Cutaneous Metabolism of Benzo[a]pyrene

Phase I reactions. When benzo[a]pyrene (BP) is applied to human skin, it may be metabolized to several distinct metabolites. These metabolic reactions not only detoxify BP but also activate it to more reactive species, which may react with cell macromolecules. Figure 4 shows some of the metabolic products of BP formed during *in vitro* incubation with cultures of human epithelial cells.

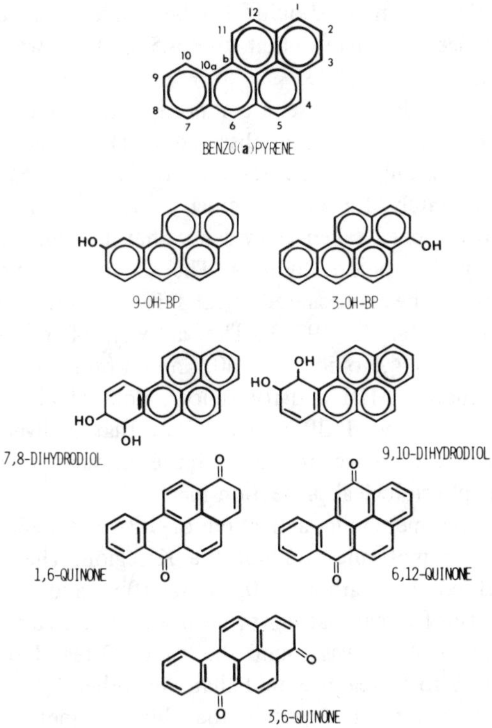

FIGURE 4 Metabolic products of benzo[a]pyrene formed *in vitro* during incubation with cultures of human epithelial cells (Fox et al., 1975).

These metabolites of BP fall into three classes: phenols, quinones, and dihydrodiols (Fox et al., 1975). The phenols formed were 3- and 9-hydroxy-BP and were products of a nonspecific cytochrome P-450 containing enzyme known as aromatic hydrocarbon hydroxylase (AHH). The two dihydrodiols formed were the 7,8- and 9,10-dihydrodiols (Fig. 4). Three quinones of BP (the 1,6-, and 3,6-, and 6,12-quinones) were isolated from the incubation medium. Although these quinones could be formed spontaneously in culture medium alone, the amounts formed were significantly greater than those in the blank.

An important observation was that cutaneous metabolism of BP in the "K region" (C 4, 5 in Fig. 4) was not detectable, although it had been detected in hepatic incubations. Neither the 4,5-dihydrodiol nor the 4,5-epoxide of BP was detected. It is possible that the 4,5-epoxide was unstable and was bound to cellular macromolecules before it could be converted to the dihydrodiol. Fox et al. (1975) were unable to show any significant binding to cells and were able to account for the remaining label [^{3}H] BP, which was not metabolized. Selkirt et al. (1975) isolated the 4,5-dihydrodiol as a product of the metabolism of BP by human hepatic microsomes. Since this metabolite was stable in a hepatic system, it should also be stable in a cutaneous enzyme system. Thus it seems unlikely that the 4,5-epoxide was formed by the cutaneous system.

The enzyme epoxide hydrase, a component necessary for the detoxification of the BP epoxides, has been observed in skin (Bentley et al., 1976). These epoxides are thought to be responsible for the alkylation of macromolecules and ultimately for carcinogenicity. The presence of dihydrodiol metabolites has often been taken as evidence that an epoxide was formed but was deactivated by the epoxide hydrase. The activity of this enzyme toward K-region epoxides has been measured in rat skin and compared to the activity from liver (Bentley et al., 1976). The activity of rat skin microsomal preparations toward BP-4,5-oxide was 60 times lower than that of rat liver preparations. Cutaneous AHH activity is low. Pohl et al. (1976) found the AHH activity in skin toward BP to be 2% of that in liver. Although these activities are low, the presence of these minute amounts of enzyme may still offer a significant physiological protection mechanism.

Studies of the metabolic activation of BP have been focused on the "bay region" of the molecule and not the K region. The bay region of BP would be identified by carbons 10, 10a, 10b, and 11 (Fig. 4). The tumorigenic activity of a material has often been correlated with the ability to covalently bind to DNA. It was found that metabolites of BP-7,8-dihydrodiol were bound to DNA to a greater extent than any other BP metabolite (Borgen et al., 1973). These studies suggested that BP was metabolized to BP-7,8-dihydrodiol-9,10-epoxide, which was the ultimate carcinogen. Carcinogenicity studies of BP and its metabolites have been performed in mouse skin (Levin et al., 1977). BP-7,8-dihydrodiol was more carcinogenic than BP but was not carcinogenic if the 9,10 double bond was reduced. Note that if the 9,10 double bond is reduced, formation of the epoxide diol is no longer possible in the bay region. BP-7,8-dihydrodiol-9,10-epoxide was a more potent carcinogen than BP (Kapitulunik et al., 1977).

Knowledge of the binding of BP metabolites to macromolecules has reached a higher level of sophistication. Binding of BP-dihydrodiol epoxides was found to occur with high stereoselectivity by Koreeda et al. (1978). These investigators isolated the polymer adducts that were formed when [³H]BP was applied to the skin of mice. Figure 5 shows that there are two stereochemical configurations for the BP-7,8-dihydrodiols and they may both be metabolized to the respective 9,10-epoxide. The epoxide may then react with cellular nucleophiles such as DNA, RNA, or proteins. For nucleic acids, the *in vivo* binding occurred preferentially to guanine at the 2-amino group (in both DNA and RNA). Both stereoisomers bound cellular components, but isomer A formed most of the covalently bound products.

Phase II reactions. In the hepatic system, once an aromatic has been oxidized to phenol, it can be conjugated by a phase II reaction and

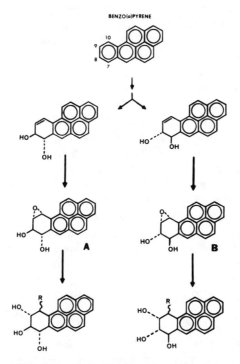

FIGURE 5 Metabolic activation of benzo[*a*]-pyrene in mouse skin with stereochemistry indicated; R = OH or cellular nucleophile (redrawn from Koreeda et al., 1978).

eliminated. Skin tissues oxidize BP via AHH to hydroxylated metabolites, which would be available to conjugating enzyme systems if they were present. Harper and Calcutt (1960) found that BP is metabolized *in vivo* and *in vitro* by mouse skin to a mixture of glucuronide conjugated benzpyrenols. In a separate study, they applied the same amount of either BP or 8-benzpyrenol to mouse skin and assayed the skin for metabolites. They found the same amount of glucuronide conjugate in both cases. They concluded that hydroxylation of BP in this system was not the rate-limiting step; instead, glucuronidation of the metabolites was rate-limiting. They attempted to detect the corresponding sulfate conjugates. Sulfate conjugation had been identified as a metabolic route of elimination for steroids. They were unable to detect these in *in vitro* studies with ATP supplementation. Thus, skin does not seem to be able to eliminate benzpyrenols as sulfate conjugates.

Cutaneous Metabolism of 3-Methylcholanthrene

3-Methylcholanthrene (3-MC) is a polycyclic aromatic hydrocarbon and a potent carcinogen. Experiments with BP indicated that diol epoxides, in which the epoxide was located in the bay region, were the ultimate carcinogenic metabolites. A similar mechanism (i.e., metabolic activation) may be applicable to 3-MC. Several oxygenated metabolites of 3-MC (Fig. 6) have been identified (Levin et al., 1979). The structures shown are rat liver metabolites but, as discussed in the previous section, skin also has the AHH activity necessary for such oxidations.

The metabolites in Fig. 6 were tested for tumor-initiating activity in mouse skin after single-dose applications (Levin et al., 1979) of 3–30 nmol. If metabolic activation was required before tumor initiation, those compounds structurally most similar to the ultimate carcinogen would have been most active in this *in vivo* test. At the 3-nmol dose, 2-hydroxy-3-MC was more tumorigenic than 3-MC; 1-hydroxy-9,10-dihydrodiol had very little activity. At the 10-nmol dose, 1-hydroxy-9,10-dihydrodiol was as active as both 3-MC and 2-hydroxy-3-MC. The dihydrodiol metabolite was two to three times as active as 3-MC in producing pulmonary tumors and up to 10 times as active in producing hepatic tumors. The results indicated that 2-keto-3-MC, 2-hydroxy-3-MC, and 1-hydroxy-9,10-dihydrodiol-3-MC were equipotent with 3-MC in tumor induction. Also, each of these was more active than the other metabolites (Fig. 6).

Woods et al. (1978) found 1-hydroxy-9,10-dihydrodiol-3-MC consistently the most active (*in vitro*) of the 3-MC metabolites, indicating that it may be a proximate carcinogen. Other studies in mouse skin indicated that the 9,10-dihydrodiol-7,8-epoxide of 3-MC may be the ultimate carcinogen (Vigny et al., 1977a). DNA-bound adducts were isolated and found to be saturated in the 7, 8, 9, and 10 positions, consistent with formation of the 7,8-epoxide-9,10-dihydrodiol of 3-MC.

As in the case of BP, metabolic activation of 3-MC is necessary for

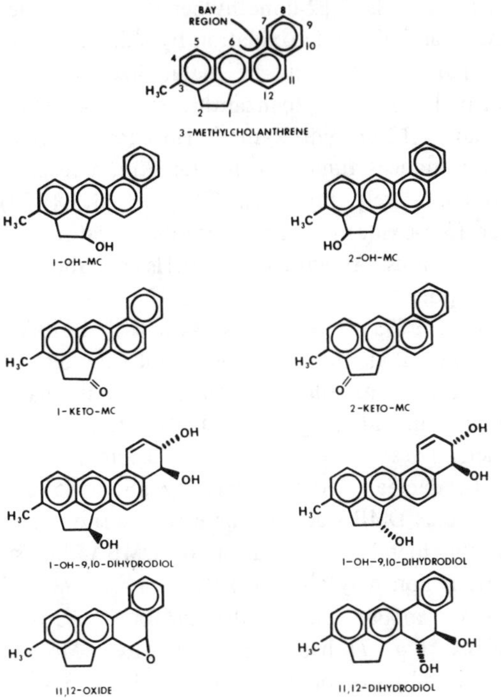

FIGURE 6 Structure of 3-methylcholanthrene and
several hepatic metabolites of 3-MC (redrawn from
Levin et al., 1979).

tumorigenic activity. Skin contains the necessary oxidative enzymes for
activation and deactivation. Epoxide hydrase was found to be present (Bentley
et al., 1976) and metabolized the 11,12-oxide of 3-MC to the corresponding
dihydrodiol. Although these cutaneous enzymes are responsible for detoxify-
ing most of the 3-MC, they are also responsible for the formation of reactive
(toxic) metabolites.

Benzanthracene Derivatives

Members of the benz[a]anthracene group of PAHs are among the most
potent PAH carcinogens. Two are shown in Fig. 7. One of the most important

FIGURE 7 Structures of 7,12-dimethylbenzanthracene
(left) and 7-methylbenzanthracene (right).

members of this group is 7,12-dimethylbenz[a]anthracene (DMBA). DMBA undergoes aromatic and aliphatic oxidation by skin enzymes. DiGiovanni et al. (1977) showed that DMBA could be metabolized to at least three metabolites: 7-hydroxymethyl-12-methylbenzanthracene, 12-hydroxymethyl-7-methylbenzanthracene, and 7,12-di(hydroxymethyl)benzanthracene.

Since DMBA induces tumors in mouse skin, a reactive metabolite (e.g., an epoxide) is most likely produced. Slaga et al. (1979) found that the K-region epoxide (5,6-oxide) was a poor tumor initiator and was probably not involved in tumorigenesis. As with other PAHs, metabolism at the bay region was most likely responsible for activity.

Vigney et al. (1977a) dosed mouse skin with DMBA and isolated DNA adducts. They found that the 3,4-dihydrodiol-1,2-oxide of DMBA was involved in adduct formation. Additional support for the bay region theory was provided by Huberman and Slaga (1979), who tested the activity of several fluoro-DMBA derivatives on mouse skin. Fluorination at the 1, 2, or 5 position of DMBA decreased the activity by about 85%, whereas 11-fluoro-DMBA was as active as DMBA alone. These results showed that the bay region was involved in the metabolic activation of DMBA, but suggested that substituents in the K region may also be able to affect the activation of DMBA.

The cutaneous metabolism of the DMBA derivative 7-methylbenz[a]-anthracene (7-MBA, Fig. 7) has been investigated. Mouse skin metabolized 7-MBA to several dihydrodiol metabolites (1,2-, 3,4-, 5,6-, and 10,11-dihydrodiols). In addition, adducts of 7-MBA have been isolated and were derived from 3,4-dihydrodiol-1,2-oxide of 7-MBA (Vigny et al., 1977b). Chouroulinkov et al. (1977) applied 7-MBA and each of the above dihydrodiols separately to mouse skin and found that the 3,4-dihydrodiol was the most active (tumor promoter) in this series. This result is in agreement with that for DMBA and with the bay region theory; the dihydrodiol is located next to the bay region (vicinal), yet leaves the region available for epoxide formation.

Bentley et al. (1976) found that microsome-bound epoxide hydrase was present in rat skin and capable of hydrating several different K-region epoxides from this PAH series. Epoxide hydrase activity was present but decreased in the following order: phenanthracene-9,10-oxide > 7-MBA-5,6-oxide > benz[a]anthracene-5,6-oxide > dibenz[a,h]anthracene-5,6-oxide. Values of the Michaelis constant K_m for this enzyme ranged from 2.0 to 4.6 μM. Bentley et al. concluded that these "low K_m values indicate that epoxide hydrase could be efficient at removing active epoxides at the low concentrations at which they would be produced metabolically from low levels of ubiquitous hydrocarbons."

MISCELLANEOUS CUTANEOUS METABOLIC REACTIONS

Oxidations

The ability of skin to deaminate organic amines was documented by Hakanson and Möller (1963b). They incubated norepinephrine with rat, rabbit, mouse, and human skin; it was metabolized to dehydroxymandelic acid (DHMA). Thus, they were able to demonstrate the presence of monoamine oxidase (MAO) in skin.

They also demonstrated (Hakanson and Möller, 1963a) both DOPA (3,4-dihydroxyphenylalanine) decarboxylase and dopamine-β-oxidase activity in skin (rabbit, mouse, rat, and human). Dopamine-β-oxidase is an enzyme that catalyzes the last reaction in the biosynthesis of norepinephrine. Mouse skin (which gave the highest yields) metabolized [^{14}C] DOPA and [^{14}C]-dopamine to epinephrine. The authors established that all of the enzymes involved in the biosynthesis of norepinephrine were present in skin.

Other dealkylations in skin were demonstrated by Pohl et al. (1976), who detected the presence of a mixed-function oxidase (MFO) that de-alkylated 7-ethoxycoumarin (7-EC). The activity of this enzyme in skin was only 2% of that in liver. Although deethylation of 7-EC was observed in skin, dealkylation of *d*-benzphetamine (*N*-demethylase activity) could not be detected.

Deaminase activity in skin was further demonstrated by Ando et al. (1977), who detected adenosine deaminase in viable epidermis. This enzyme metabolized the drug vidarabine (9-α-*d*-arabinofuranosyladenine) to 9-α-*d*-arabinofuranosylhypoxanthine.

Pohl et al. (1976) showed that a mouse skin microsomal preparation contained aniline hydroxylase. This enzyme was able to metabolize aniline to *p*-aminophenol. Thus, the cutaneous oxidation of aromatic rings was not restricted to polycyclic aromatic hydrocarbons.

Reductive Reactions

Cutaneous reductive metabolism is not restricted to the steroids. A nonsteroidal compound metabolized by the skin is croton oil, a tumor promoter in mouse skin. One of the most potent components of this oil is phorbol myristate acetate (PMA, Fig. 8). When 25 μg [^{3}H] PMA was painted on mouse skin (for 5 h), about 2% of the dose was metabolized to the hydroxylated metabolite (PHMA) in which the carbonyl at the 5 position (Fig. 8) was reduced to yield the 5β-hydroxy metabolite (Segal et al., 1975). This metabolite is a potent inflammatory agent on mouse skin. When

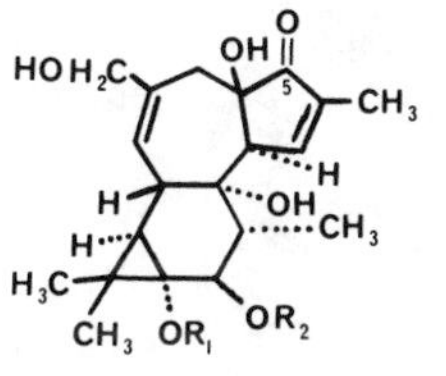

FIGURE 8 Structure of phorbol myristate acetate; R_1 = acetate, R_2 = myristate (redrawn from Segal et al., 1975).

[^{3}H]PHMA was painted on mouse skin, no PMA was formed, indicating that the reaction was not reversible. This study showed that cutaneous tissue contained the enzymes for reducing substances other than steroids. It is not known whether PHMA is the active tumor-producing agent (proximate carcinogen) in croton oil.

Conjugation Reactions

Glucuronidation. As mentioned for the hydroxylated metabolites of BP, the skin contains the enzymes necessary for glucuronidation (i.e., UDP glucuronyltransferase). Only a few substrates other than BP metabolites have been shown to be glucuronidated. Stevenson and Dutton (1960) showed glucuronide synthesis in the skin. They demonstrated that the conjugation of *o*-aminophenol in skin was similar to that in liver. Rugstad and Dybing (1975) investigated glucuronidation in cultures of whole human skin and homogenates of the same cells. The homogenates were supplemented with UDPGA (UDP glucuronic acid) to eliminate the possibility of a permeability barrier (through cell membranes). When *p*-nitrophenol (PNP), *p*-aminophenol (PAP), and bilirubin were used as substrates, only PNP and PAP were glucuronidated even though bilirubin was actively taken up by skin cells.

Methylation. Hakanson and Möller (1963a) found that catechol-*O*-methyltransferase (COMT) was present in cutaneous tissues. They incubated norepinephrine anaerobically with skin from four species (rat, rabbit, mouse, and human) and identified normetanephrine (Fig. 9) as a metabolite. This metabolic reaction was inhibited by pyrogallol, which is a specific COMT inhibitor. Bamshad (1969) observed that COMT was present in normal skin. He investigated the distribution of COMT between the dermis and epidermis compared to the whole skin and concluded that the activity of COMT was much greater in the epidermis than in either the dermis or whole skin.

CYTOCHROME P-450

Cytochrome P-450, which is present in skin at low concentrations, is inducible by topical application of some of the agents that induce hepatic metabolism (Alvares et al., 1973). Although phenobarbital is an inducer of P-450 in hepatic systems, it did not produce induction after topical administration to skin (Pohl et al., 1976). The authors applied phenobarbital for only 24 h, during which they monitored P-450 induction. Conney (1971)

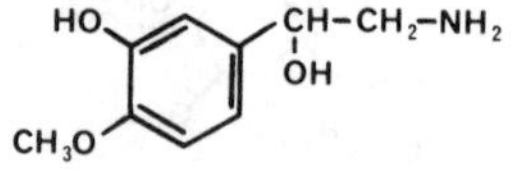

FIGURE 9   Normetanephrine formed as an *in vitro* metabolite of norepinephrine in skin.

observed that maximum phenobarbital induction of zoxazolamine hydroxylase in rat liver microsomes occurred after 3–4 d of phenobarbital injections. It is possible that phenobarbital induction of P-450 in skin takes much longer than 24 h; perhaps it should have been followed for 3–7 d.

Pohl et al. (1976) investigated the induction of cytochrome P-450 in skin after topical application of 3-MC and TCDD (2,3,7,8-tetrachlorodibenzo-*p*-dioxin) in skin. 3-MC caused a slight increase in cutaneous P-450 levels, but they returned to control values within 72 h. Percutaneous absorption of TCDD not only increased cutaneous P-450 levels but doubled the hepatic levels of P-450. These studies show that cutaneous tissues do contain cytochrome P-450 and that this cytochrome can be induced by at least two PAHs.

Many investigators have been unable to detect cytochrome P-450 in normal skin. Often the inconclusive results were due to one or a combination of the following factors. (1) The levels of P-450 in noninduced skin were low, often approaching the limits of the analytical methods available. (2) Cytochrome oxidase is present in skin and causes a distorted difference spectrum, often masking the presence of low concentrations of P-450. (3) Cytochrome P-420 was often found in skin when P-450 could not be detected (Pohl et al., 1976). Cytochrome P-420 is an artifact of the solubilization process. Cytochrome P-450 is unstable, and the small amount of P-450 present in skin may have been degraded to P-420 during the isolation procedure. Since these studies were performed, investigators have learned how to solubilize P-450 with minimal degradation. With these new techniques it should be possible to quantitate the levels of P-450 in induced and noninduced skin.

ENZYME INDUCTION/INHIBITION

Cytochrome P-450 is not the only component of skin that is inducible. Many other enzymes can be either induced or inhibited after topical administration of various agents. The PAHs are known to be hepatic enzyme inducers, and there is evidence that they are cutaneous enzyme inducers. Dutton and Stevenson (1962) found that topical application of BP increased the UDP glucuronyltransferase activity in skin. On the other hand, Rugstad and Dybing (1975) found that the glucuronidation rate of human skin epithelial cells (in culture) was not increased by either BP or benzanthracene. They suggested, however, that under the conditions used in their cell cultures the cells may already have been maximally induced.

Pohl et al. (1976) studied the induction of several cutaneous enzymes after topical application of 3-MC (3 mg) or TCDD (0.3 μg). Application of 3-MC caused a temporary 2-fold increase in AHH activity, but this activity returned to noninduced levels 72 h after dosing. After dosing with TCDD, the cutaneous AHH activity had increased 8-fold at 24 h and 30-fold at 72 h. They noted that 3-MC was unable to induce either 7-ethoxycoumarin deethylase or aniline hydroxylase in skin. TCDD increased the deethylase activity 4-fold after 24 h and 7-fold after 72 h.

Fox et al. (1975) observed that the cutaneous metabolism of BP was significant even without prior induction but was increased by induction. When hydrocortisone was applied simultaneously with the inducer, the metabolism of BP decreased significantly. The metabolic products that decreased were the quinone and dihydrodiol metabolites. Fox et al. showed that the cutaneous metabolism of BP could be either induced or inhibited under the proper conditions.

Bowden et al. (1974) studied the effects of topically applied MFO modifiers on the induction of AHH activity in skin. The modifiers used were phenobarbital, DBA (1,2,5,6-dibenzanthracene), DMBA, 5,6-BF (5,6-benzo-flavone), and 7,8-BF (7,8-benzoflavone). Although phenobarbital induces hepatic enzyme activity, no effect on cutaneous AHH activity was detected. Both AHH activity and induction were inhibited by 7,8-BF. DiGiovanni et al. (1977) noted that 7,8-BF inhibited AHH activity *in vitro*. The activity of AHH in cutaneous tissues was increased by 5,6-BF, DMBA, and DBA; the levels of induction were 350, 600, and 1200%, respectively.

Bowden et al. (1974) and DiGiovanni et al. (1977) investigated the effects of these modifiers on the initiating potential (tumorigenic) of DMBA and DBA. Both 5,6-BF and 7,8-BF inhibited DMBA skin tumorigenesis in mice. DMBA binding to DNA, RNA, and proteins was inhibited by 7,8-BF, while only its binding to DNA was inhibited by 5,6-BF. The effects of 7,8-BF on DBA were opposite to those on DMBA; that is, 7,8-BF increased the carcinogenicity of DBA. DiGiovanni et al. (1977) also studied the modifying effects of 17β-estradiol on DMBA activity. The formation of all detectable metabolites of DMBA was inhibited by 17β-estradiol, but it had no effect on tumor initiation by DMBA.

From these data, it may be concluded that inhibitors and inducers may affect the rates of activation and detoxification of drugs in the skin. For example, 7,8-BF inhibited the activation of DMBA to a greater extent than it inhibited the detoxification of DMBA; therefore the carcinogenicity of DMBA decreased. On the other hand, 7,8-BF inhibited the detoxification of DBA to a greater extent, resulting in increased carcinogenicity (Bowden et al., 1974). Therefore, a modifier may have different effects on different carcinogens, depending on the delicate balance between the activation and detoxification pathways.

PHARMACOLOGICAL AND TOXICOLOGICAL IMPLICATIONS OF SKIN METABOLISM

Where little or no skin metabolism occurs, the chemical that penetrates the skin barrier is introduced into the systemic circulation. The implication is that some chemicals may be more toxic after topical application than when administered orally. Topically applied hexachlorophene does not appear to be metabolized. It passes into the bloodstream unchanged. In contrast, orally ingested hexachlorophene quickly reaches the liver through the enterohepatic shunt system (portal) and is metabolized (Marzulli and Maibach, 1975). Thus the only barrier to topical hexachlorophene toxicity is the barrier to percutaneous absorption. The metabolic detoxification that occurs after oral absorption is not present with dermal administration.

Nevertheless, we know that skin metabolism of chemicals does occur. The question is which routes of metabolism occur for a particular chemical and to what extent. This is impossible to assess for every chemical because the information available is insufficient. It is known that the route of metabolism after dermal administration can be different from that after oral administration (Greaves, 1971). After oral administration of [^{3}H]cortisol the urinary metabolites were mainly corticosteroids, whereas after dermal administration they were mainly oxosteroids. However, cortisol (hydrocortisone) is clinically effective in either case, and this metabolic difference would not be important unless one of the metabolites was an active moiety.

It can probably be assumed that skin metabolism usually deactivates or detoxifies the applied chemical agent. Most skin metabolism studies seem to indicate this. The most notable exception is the case of skin AHH activating chemical agents into potent carcinogens.

It is important to discuss the implication of skin metabolism potential for clinical disease because in most situations the metabolically viable epidermis is situated between the applied pharmacological agent and the disease being treated. A recent study suggests that there may be a difference in drug-metabolizing potential between normal and diseased skin. AHH activity was the same in both psoriatic lesions and noninvolved skin, but lower than the activity in normal volunteers. Preincubation of tissue with benzanthracene increased the activity in both normal and noninvolved epidermis. However, no stimulation was observed in psoriatic lesions (Chapman et al., 1977). Unfortunately, more information like this is not available.

One area of study of percutaneous toxicity concerns infants. In preterm infants the skin (and hence the barrier function) is not completely developed. It is not known what role skin metabolism plays in the developing or full-term infant.

It is difficult to assess the amount of skin metabolism that occurs *in vivo* because most skin metabolism studies have been done *in vitro*. However, the lack of clinical effectiveness of cortisone suggests that there is not sufficient metabolism to hydrocortisone. With topically applied [^{14}C]benzoyl peroxide, all of the compound was metabolized to benzoic acid during *in vitro* absorption by human skin. Following *in vivo* topical application to rhesus monkeys, all of the radioactive material in the urine was benzoic acid. Renal clearance of the metabolite was sufficiently rapid to preclude hepatic conjugation with glycine to form hippuric acid (Nacht et al., 1981). When nitroglycerin was applied topically to rhesus monkeys the percutaneous first-pass metabolism was 16–20% of the applied dose (Wester et al., 1981). These data suggest that the amount of skin metabolism of a topically applied chemical *in vivo* may be related to the structure of the chemical. It can be low as suggested for cortisone, or significant as suggested for benzoyl peroxide.

DISCUSSION

It is obvious that skin is not a passive barrier that only restricts the diffusion of chemical agents into the body. The skin is a viable membrane that can metabolize an assortment of topically applied substances before they become systemically available.

Enzyme systems in skin are highly inducible. For example, after TCDD exposure, the activity of AHH increased up to 30-fold and that of 7-ethoxycoumarin deethylase increased 6-fold. Such changes in cutaneous metabolizing ability may alter the availability of topically applied drugs.

Since the skin has many of the same enzymes as the liver, it is of interest to compare their relative activities. This would be important if the activity of the skin were sufficient to allow it to serve as an alternative metabolic site for systemically (e.g., iv or orally) administered drugs. The activities of several cutaneous enzymes have been measured and compared to hepatic activities (Pohl et al., 1976). The activities of these enzymes in skin are low compared to those in liver, typically 2–6% of the hepatic values (Table 1). Although these data indicate that cutaneous metabolism is low, this may not be representative of the situation *in vivo*.

The distribution of metabolizing enzymes in skin is an important consideration. Laerum (1969) found that oxygen consumption was 5.4 times greater in the epidermis than the dermis. Bamshad (1969) noted that the activity of catechol-*O*-methyltransferase was 8.3 times greater in the epidermis. Weinstein et al. (1968) found that the epidermal metabolism of estradiol to estrone was greater than the dermal metabolism. Finally, Chapman et al.

TABLE 1   Enzyme Activity Ratios in Skin Compared to Liver

	Activity ratio (skin/liver)	
Enzyme	Whole skin[a]	Epidermis[b]
Aromatic hydrocarbon hydroxylase	0.02	0.80
7-Ethoxycoumarin deethylase	0.02	0.80
Aniline hydroxylase	0.06	2.40
NADP-cytochrome c reductase	0.06	2.40

[a]Calculated from data in Pohl et al. (1976).
[b]Assuming epidermis is 2.5% of whole skin.

(1977) showed that 96.5% of the AHH activity in skin was present in the epidermis. These results indicate that most of the enzyme activity of skin may be localized in the epidermal layer.

The epidermal thickness ranges from 0.06 to 0.1 mm. The dermis may be 2–4 mm thick. Therefore, the epidermis makes up only 2.5–3% of the total skin. The percentage may be even smaller if the subcutaneous layers are included. The cutaneous enzyme activities reported in the literature were based on enzyme activities in whole skin homogenates. Assuming that these enzymes are constrained to the epidermal layer, the real activities range from 80 to 240% of those in the liver (Table 1). Therefore, cutaneous enzymes are active and in the epidermis may equal or even exceed the activity of hepatic drug-metabolizing enzymes.

If the enzyme activity in the epidermis is high, perhaps the skin is an alternative site for the metabolism of systemically available drugs. The liver is normally assumed to be the major drug-metabolizing organ, responsible for the clearance of many drugs. Drug clearance from an organ depends on the blood flow to that organ, the tissue volume of the organ, and the extraction ratio of the drug. The liver volume is approximately 3.9 l and the blood flow is 1600 ml/min in humans. The total skin volume is 75% that of the liver (3 l) and the blood flow 10% (100 ml/min) that of the liver (Benet, 1978). Unless the extraction of a drug into the skin is high, the skin would not be expected to play a significant role as an alternative site of drug metabolism.

Since cutaneous metabolic activity has been shown to be high, these enzymes may have a first-pass metabolic effect on topically applied drugs. If a drug diffuses slowly through the epidermis, the skin may serve as a site of first-pass metabolism. Such metabolism may decrease both the amount of drug at the site of action (often the dermis) and the amount systemically available. If absorption is fast, the cutaneous enzymes may become saturated. In this case, a significant amount of drug may be absorbed into the systemic circulation without being metabolized. This was tested for nitroglycerin (glyceryl trinitrate, GTN), which is often administered topically for the treatment of angina pectoris. Wester et al. (1981) demonstrated that GTN may be metabolized as it is absorbed through the skin. [14C] GTN was administered iv and topically to rhesus monkeys. Plasma concentrations of unchanged GTN, total ^{14}C, and urinary excretion of ^{14}C were determined as a function of time and bioavailability was estimated. The difference in bioavailability between unchanged GTN and total ^{14}C was the fraction of the dose that was metabolized as it was absorbed. Wester et al. concluded that 16–21% of the dose was metabolized by the skin.

The skin is a highly active metabolic organ. It contains a multitude of different drug-metabolizing enzymes, including a cytochrome P-450 system. These enzymes may be highly inducible in much the same way as the liver enzymes. Some information suggests that there are pharmacological and toxicological implications of the cutaneous biotransformation of chemical agents that come in contact with the skin. When studying the availability of topically administered drugs or environmental contaminants, one must consider the metabolizing ability of the skin, which may affect the bioavailability during the first passage through the skin.

REFERENCES

Alvares, A., Bickers, D., and Kappas, A. 1973. Alteration of hepatic microsomal hemoprotein by polychlorinated biphenyls. *Fed. Proc.* 32:235.

Ando, H., Ho, H., and Higuchi, W. 1977. Skin as an active metabolizing barrier. I. Theoretical analysis of topical bioavailability. *J. Pharm. Sci.* 66:1525–1528.

Bamshad, J. 1969. Catechol-*O*-methyltransferase in epidermis and whole skin. *J. Invest. Dermatol.* 52:351–352.

Benet, L. Z. 1978. Effect of route of administration and distribution on drug action. *J. Pharmacokinet. Biopharm.* 6:559–585.

Bentley, P., Schuassmann, H., Sims, P., and Oesch, F. 1976. Epoxides derived from various polycyclic hydrocarbons as substrates of homogeneous and microsome bound epoxide hydratase. *Eur. J. Biochem.* 69:97–103.

Berliner, D., Pasqualini, J., and Gallegos, A. 1968. The formation of water soluble steroids by human skin. *J. Invest. Dermatol.* 50:220–224.

Borgen, A., Davey, H., Castagnoli, N., Crocker, T., Rasmussen, R., and Wang, I. 1973. Metabolic conversion of benzo(*a*)pyrene by Syrian hamster liver microsomes and binding of metabolites to deoxyribonucleic acid. *J. Med. Chem.* 16:502–506.

Bowden, G., Slaga, T., Shapas, B., and Boutwell, R. 1974. The role of aryl hydrocarbon hydroxylase in skin tumor initiation by 7,12-dimethylbenz(*a*)anthracene and 1,2,5,6-dibenzanthracene using DNA binding and thymidine-^{3}H incorporation into DNA as criteria. *Cancer Res.* 34:2634–2642.

Chapman, P. H., Rawlins, M. D., and Shuster, S. 1977. Activity of aryl hydroxylase in adult human skin. *Br. J. Clin. Pharmacol.* 4:393P.

Chapman, P. H., Rawlins, M. D., Rogers, S., and Shuster, S. 1977. Aryl hydroxylase activity in psoriatic skin. *Br. J. Clin. Pharmacol.* 4:644P.

Chouroulinkov, I., Gentil, A., Tierney, B., Grover, P., and Sims, P. 1977. The metabolic activation of 7-methylbenz(*a*)anthracene in mouse skin: High tumor initiating activity of the 3,4-dihydrodiol. *Cancer Lett.* 3:247–253.

Conney, A. H. 1971. Environmental factors influencing drug metabolism. In *Fundamentals of Drug Metabolism and Disposition*, eds. B. LaDu, H. Mandel, and E. Way, pp. 253–278. Baltimore, Md.: Williams & Wilkins.

DiGiovanni, J., Slaga, T., Berry, D., and Juchau, M. 1977. Metabolism of 7,12-dimethylbenz(*a*)anthracene in mouse skin with high pressure liquid chromatography. *Drug Metab. Dispos.* 5:295–301.

Dutton, G. and Stevenson, I. 1962. The stimulation by 3,4-benzpyrene of glucuronide synthesis in skin. *Biochim. Biophys. Acta* 58:633–634.

Faredin, I., Fazekas, A., Toth, I., Kokai, K., and Julesz, M. 1968. Transformation *in vitro* of (4-^{14}C)-dehydroepiandrosterone into 7-oxygenated epiandrosterone sulfate by normal human female skin slices. *J. Endocrinol.* 41:295–296.

Faredin, I., Fazekas, A., Toth, I., Kokai, K., and Julesz, M. 1969. Transformation *in vitro* of (4-^{14}C)-dehydroepiandrosterone into 7-oxygenated derivatives by normal human male and female skin slices. *J. Invest. Dermatol.* 52:357–361.

Fox, C., Selkirk, J., Price, F., Croy, R., Sanford, K., and Fox, M. 1975. Metabolism of benzo(*a*)pyrene by human epithelial cells in vitro. *Cancer Res.* 35:3551–3557.

Frost, P., Gomez, E., Weinstein, G., Lamas, J., and Hsia, S. 1969. Metabolism of progesterone-4-^{14}C *in vitro* in human skin and vaginal mucosa. *Biochemistry* 8:948–952.

Greaves, M. S. 1971. The *in vivo* catabolism of cortisol by human skin. *J. Invest. Dermatol.* 57:100–107.

Hakanson, R. and Möller, H. 1963b. On metabolism of noradrenaline in the skin: Activity of catechol-*O*-methyl transferase and monamine oxidase. *Acta Derm.-Venereol.* 43:552–555.

Hakanson, R. and Möller, H. 1963a. On formation of noradrenaline in the skin: Activity of dopamine-β-oxidase. *Acta Derm.-Venereol.* 43:548–551.

Harper, K. and Calcutt, G. 1960. Conjugation of 3:4-benzpyrenols in mouse skin. *Nature (Lond.)* 186:80–81.

Hsia, S., Mussallem, J., and Witten, V. 1965. Further metabolic studies of hydrocortisone-4-^{14}C in human skin. *J. Invest. Dermatol.* 45:384–390.

Hsia, S. L. 1971. Steroid metabolism in human skin. *Mod. Trends Dermatol.* 4:69–88.

Huberman, E. and Slaga, T. J. 1979. Mutagenicity and tumor-initiating activity of fluorinated derivatives of 7,12-dimethylbenz(*a*)anthracene. *Cancer Res.* 39:411–414.

Kapitulunik, J., Levin, W., Conney, A. H., Yagi, H., and Jerina, D. M. 1977. Benzo(*a*)pyrene 7,8-dihydrodiol is more carcinogenic than benzo(*a*)-pyrene in newborn mice. *Nature (Lond.)* 266:378–380.

Koreeda, M., Moore, P., Wislocki, P., Levin, W., Conney, A., Yagi, H., and Jerina, D. 1978. Binding of benzo(*a*)pyrene 7,8-diol-9,10-epoxides to DNA, RNA and protein of mouse skin occurs with high stereoselectivity. *Science* 199:778–781.

Laerum, O. D. 1969. Oxygen consumption of basal and differentiating cells from hairless mouse epidermis. *J. Invest. Dermatol.* 52:204–211.

Levin, W., Wood, Q., Wislocki, P., Kapitulunik, J., Yaki, H., Jerina, D., and Conney, A. 1977. Carcinogenicity of benzo-ring derivatives of benzo(*a*)-pyrene on mouse skin. *Cancer Res.* 37:3356–3361.

Levin, W., Buening, M. K., Wood, A., Chang, R., Thakker, D., Jerina, D., and Conney, A. 1979. Tumorigenic activity of 3-methylcholanthrene metabo-lites on mouse skin and in newborn mice. *Cancer Res.* 39:3549–3553.

Marzulli, F. N. and Maibach, H. I. 1975. Relevance of animal models: The hexachlorophene story. In *Animal Models in Dermatology*, ed. H. I. Maibach, pp. 156–167. Edinburgh: Churchill Livingstone.

Nacht, S., Yeung, D., Beasley, J. N., Jr., Anjo, M. D., and Maibach, H. I. 1981. Benzoyl peroxide: Percutaneous penetration and metabolic disposi-tion. *J. Am. Acad. Dermatol.* 4:31–37.

Pannatier, A., Jenner, P., Testa, B., and Etter, J. 1978. The skin as a drug-metabolizing organ. *Drug Metab. Rev.* 8:319–343.

Pohl, R., Philpot, R., and Fouts, J. 1976. Cytochrome P-450 content and mixed-function oxidase activity in microsomes isolated from mouse skin. *Drug Metab. Dispos.* 4:442–450.

Rugstad, H. and Dybing, E. 1975. Glucuronidation in cultures of human skin epithelial cells. *Eur. J. Clin. Invest.* 5:133–137.

Segal, A., Van Durren, B., and Maté, U. 1975. The identification of phorbolol myristate acetate as a new metabolite of phorbol myristate acetate in mouse skin. *Cancer Res.* 35:2154–2159.

Selkirk, J., Croy, R., and Gelboin, H. 1975. Isolation and characterization of benzo(*a*)pyrene-4,5-epoxide as a metabolite of benzo(*a*)pyrene. *Arch. Biochem. Biophys.* 168:322–326.

Singer, E. J., Wegmann, P. C., Lehman, M. D., Christensen, M. S., and Vinson, L. J. 1971. Barrier development, ultrastructure, and sulfhydryl content of the fetal epidermis. *J. Soc. Cosmet. Chem.* 22:119–137.

Shaw, J. and Chandrasekaran, S. 1978. Controlled topical delivery of drugs for systemic action. *Drug Metab. Rev.* 8:223–233.

Slaga, T., Gleason, G., DiGiovanni, J., Sukumaran, K., and Harvey, R. 1979. Potent tumor-initiating activity of the 3,4-dihydrodiol of 7,12-dimethylbenz(*a*)anthracene in mouse skin. *Cancer Res.* 39:1934–1936.

Stevenson, I. and Dutton, G. 1960. Mechanism of glucuronide synthesis in skin. *Biochem. J.* 77:19P.

Tauber, V. and Toda, T. 1976. Biotransformation of diflucortolone valerate in the skin of rat, guinea pig and man. *Arzneim.-Forsch.* (Drug Research) 26:1484–1487.

Vigny, P., Duquesne, M., Coulomb, H., Tierney, B., Grover, P., and Sims, P. 1977b. Fluorescence spectral studies on the metabolic activation of 3-methylcholanthrene and 7,12-dimethylbenz(*a*)anthracene in mouse skin. *FEBS Lett.* 82:278–282.

Vigny, P., Duquesne, M., Coulomb, H., Lacombe, C., Tierney, B., Grover, P., and Sims, P. 1977a. Metabolic activation of polycyclic hydrocarbons. *FEBS Lett.* 75:9–12.

Weinstein, G., Frost, P., and Hsia, S. 1968. *In vitro* conversion of estrone and 17β-estradiol in human skin and vaginal mucosa. *J. Invest. Dermatol.* 51:4–10.

Wester, R. C., Noonan, P. K., Smeach, S., and Kosobud, L. 1981. Estimate of nitroglycerin percutaneous first-pass metabolism. *Pharmacologist* 23:203.

Wood, A., Chang, R., Levin, W., Thomas, P., Ryan, D., Stoming, T., Thakker, D., Jerina, D., and Conney, A. 1978. Metabolic activation of 3-methylcholanthrene on its metabolites to products mutagenic to bacterial and mammalian cells. *Cancer Res.* 38:3398–3404.

Wotiz, H., Mescon, H., Doppel, H., and Lemon, H. 1956. The *in vitro* metabolism of testosterone by human skin. *J. Invest. Dermatol.* 26:113.

3

skin permeability theory in relation to measurements of percutaneous absorption in toxicology

■ Paul H. Dugard ■

INTRODUCTION

Because of the increasing emphasis on quantitative assessment of safety, measurements of the absorption of potentially harmful chemicals through the skin are being made more frequently. Our understanding of the factors involved in the passage of molecules across the skin has advanced considerably in recent years, and this knowledge should now be exploited by those interested in hazards resulting from absorption via the skin. The description that follows is intended to show how the theory of skin permeability processes may be interpreted to extend the usefulness of measured absorption parameters.

SKIN ABSORPTION MEASUREMENTS AND ASSESSMENTS OF HAZARD

Skin absorption or skin penetration is the passage of molecules from the medium in contact with one face of the stratum corneum to the medium outside the other face. When assessing the toxicological significance of *in vivo* or *in vitro* measurement of skin absorption several approaches may be taken, and the nature of the assessment is usually determined by the extent of the information on the fate of the chemical within the body.

Because of the continuous, usually "slow" release of a chemical into the body via intact skin, the best treatment is perhaps a comparison of the skin absorption *rate* with detoxification and/or elimination kinetics. This comparison of dynamic parameters permits an estimate of whether toxic material accumulates within the body in sufficient quantity to produce adverse effects. Alternatively, if a certain body burden of the chemical is known to produce symptoms of toxicity, this amount may be compared with the amount absorbed via the skin under given conditions and in a specified time. These may be regarded as absolute assessments of the systemic hazards associated with percutaneous absorption. In addition, measurements of absorption of a chemical from different formulations may indicate which of these is safest. As yet, the absorption of materials producing local skin responses may only be handled in this latter type of comparative assessment because no information is available on the local tissue concentrations that produce responses. The comparison of the absorption properties of different chemical substances does not indicate relative safety unless relative potencies and, preferably, detoxification and elimination kinetics are also known.

The treatment of skin permeability theory given here is directed toward the types of assessment briefly stated above and to obtaining predictions of absorption patterns for the widest range of situations from the minimum number of skin permeability experiments.

DIFFUSION BARRIER OF HUMAN SKIN

It is now generally accepted that the diffusion barrier properties of human skin are determined by the "keratinized" outermost layer, the stratum corneum (SC) (Berenson and Burch, 1951; Scheuplein and Blank, 1971). Because the SC, as a membrane, displays no indications of transport mechanisms involving metabolic processes (Tregear, 1966a), the relatively straightforward physical chemistry and mathematics that describe passive diffusion may be applied to absorption through skin.

Very complete descriptions of the biology and structure of skin in relation to its permeability properties have been included in recent reviews (Katz and Poulsen, 1971; Scheuplein and Blank, 1971) and this information will not be duplicated in this account. However, certain assumptions concerning the properties of the SC are required for some of the treatments that follow. These are stated briefly with references that should be consulted for fuller discussions:

1. The full thickness of the SC contributes to the overall diffusion barrier properties rather than just a discrete layer at its base (Blank, 1965).

2. If obviously not homogeneous, the SC is uniform in character for theoretical purposes (Tregear, 1966a).

3. Diffusion across the SC is the rate-limiting step for molecular movement across skin, and clearance within the body is sufficiently rapid not to affect absorption (Scheuplein and Blank, 1971).
4. Molecules diffuse across the SC by purely passive means (Tregear, 1966a).
5. There is not a limiting size above which molecules are excluded from the SC, and this membrane does not behave as though "porous" (Tregear, 1966b).
6. (a) Penetrant (the chemical whose absorption is being considered) and components of the vehicle (the medium in which the penetrant contacts the skin) diffuse as separate entities within the SC—convective transfer does not occur. (b) The SC behaves as a solution phase and the penetrant must dissolve in the SC in its passage into the body (Scheuplein, 1965).
7. The characteristics of the SC are not progressively altered by the penetrant or by changing concentrations of penetrant within the membrane.
8. The vehicle does not progressively alter the characteristics of the skin.
9. The driving force for the net transfer of material across the SC by diffusion is a concentration difference.

Many of the listed properties of the SC have been found to be generally true in practice. Several specific exceptions to these assumptions are considered later in this article.

PERCUTANEOUS ABSORPTION FROM SOLUTIONS AND THE BASIC LAWS OF DIFFUSION

The best understood skin absorption situation is that of penetration from a solution of unchanging composition where the penetrant is completely dissolved. Usually the inside face of the SC is effectively at zero penetrant concentration whether in an experimental or practical situation. Under these conditions, Fick's law of diffusion shows that, for a single vehicle, the absorption rate is proportional to the applied concentration, thus:

$$J \propto C_v$$

where J is the absorption rate per unit area (also known as the flux) and C_v is the concentration of penetrant in the vehicle.

A proportionality constant, k_p (the permeability constant), may be added

$$J = k_p C_v \tag{1}$$

In many cases this relationship holds and the permeability constant is independent of concentration over a very wide range of concentrations (Blank, 1964; Scheuplein and Ross, 1974).

The relationship breaks down if there is any concentration-dependent effect of the penetrant on the SC or if the penetrant concentration becomes high enough to alter the solvent properties of the vehicle (Blank, 1964). Deviations from ideality may often be expected to occur as penetrants approach saturation in the vehicle because the interaction between molecules increases.

The permeability constant provides a means of expressing absorption measurements for comparing different penetrants, different vehicles, and different experimental conditions, provided that no more than one parameter (other than penetrant concentration) is changed. For predictive purposes, the permeability constant permits calculation of the absorption rate from different concentrations in the same solvent system. Thus, an absorption rate measured, *in vivo* or *in vitro*, from a single known concentration is the basis for the calculation of a permeability constant (absorption rate divided by applied concentration). The rate of absorption from any other concentration is found by multiplying the permeability constant by that concentration. Note that when manipulating the various terms in any of the equations given here all units must be compatible. Thus, a permeability constant expressed as "cm/hr" requires concentration in terms of "amount/cm^3." Measured permeability constants for human skin range approximately from 1×10^{-6} to 5×10^{-2} cm/hr.

Blank (1964) and Scheuplein (1965) have expanded the permeability constant to show the parameters controlling the absorption process

$$k_p = \frac{K_m D_m}{\delta} \qquad (2)$$

where δ is the thickness of the SC membrane, D_m is the diffusion constant of the penetrant in the membrane, and K_m is the SC:vehicle partition coefficient. The diffusion constant is a measure of the mobility of the penetrant molecules within the SC and values range from 1×10^{-8} to 1×10^{-13} cm^2/sec for human SC. The partition coefficient, similar to that used in chemistry, is the ratio, at equilibrium, of penetrant concentration in the SC to that in the vehicle when isolated SC has been immersed. This partition term takes into account the fact that the driving force for net movement of penetrant across SC is, strictly, the difference in concentration *within* the tissue. The product of applied penetrant concentration and partition coefficient $(K_m C_v)$ gives the penetrant concentration in the outermost zone of the SC. Katz and Poulsen (1971) describe in depth the nature and importance of partition coefficients and absorption rates. Values for K_m may be less than one to several hundred.

Inserting the terms of Eq. (2) in Eq. (1) shows that the absorption rate depends on two easily controlled externally determined factors (penetrant concentration and partition coefficient) and two innate internal factors (diffusion constant and SC thickness) as follows:

$$J = \frac{K_m C_v D_m}{\delta} \tag{3}$$

As indicated in the "techniques" section of this account, partition coefficients and diffusion constants may be experimentally determined and SC thickness estimated.

EARLY TIME COURSE OF PERCUTANEOUS ABSORPTION

The foregoing section describes the condition of steady-state penetration. Before this maximum absorption rate is achieved, the rate builds up over a period of time following the initial contact between skin and the penetrant solution—a lag phase is apparent. A time course for penetration is shown in Fig. 1. The extrapolation of the steady-state, linear region of the graph of total amount absorbed versus time to zero absorption yields τ, the lag time

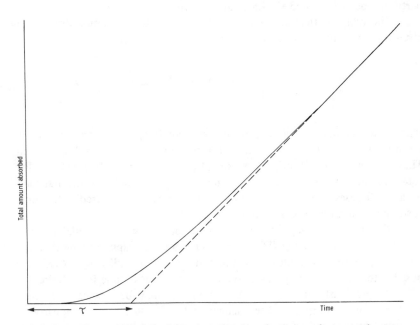

FIGURE 1 Time course of absorption showing the approach to steady-state penetration (achieved when solid line becomes linear) and the derivation of τ, the lag time (broken line).

(note that τ does not mark the time at which steady state is achieved). The equation for the linear region of this graph is given by Crank (1970):

$$Q_t = \frac{C_v K_m}{\delta} \left(t - \frac{\delta^2}{6 D_m} \right) \tag{4}$$

Where Q_t is the total amount absorbed by time t. This expression gives

$$\tau = \frac{\delta^2}{6 D_m} \tag{5}$$

Experimental determination of τ is a useful means of finding the membrane diffusion constant of a penetrant. Numerical values of τ for the absorption of different penetrants across general body surface SC range from a few minutes to several days. Thus, the pre-steady-state absorption phase is often significant when making safety evaluations. A mathematical approach provides information on the early pattern of absorption that may be impossible to establish experimentally. In this section complex equations have been converted into reference graphs, which may be used in a very straightforward manner for predicting the time course of absorption. These are suitable for any penetrant, vehicle, and type of membrane provided the membrane diffusion constant, partition coefficient, and thickness are known.

The mathematical expression that gives the total amount absorbed by a given time, and that covers early times, is (Crank 1970):

$$\frac{Q_t}{\delta C_v K_m} = \frac{D_m t}{\delta^2} - \frac{1}{6} - \frac{2}{\pi^2} \sum_{n=1}^{\infty} \frac{(-1)^n}{n^2} \exp\left(- \frac{D_m t}{\delta^2} \pi^2 n^2 \right) \tag{6}$$

Where the symbols are as before and n is an integer with values from 1 to infinity. This equation is the basis for the graphs shown in Figs. 2 and 3. These are graphs of $Q_t/\delta C_v K_m$ versus $D_m t/\delta^2$, which is effectively a plot of total amount absorbed against time, but in a dimensionless form that may be used in all cases. The graphs in Figs. 2 and 3 are used to predict the amount absorbed by a given time as follows:

The value of $D_m t/\delta^2$ for the time of interest is calculated and the corresponding value for $Q_t/\delta C_v K_m$ is read from the graph. Solving then shows that Q_t is given by multiplying the value for $Q_t/\delta C_v K_m$ by $\delta C_v K_m$. It is possible to replot the graph as amount absorbed versus time if so desired.

As previously stated, the absorption rate may be especially meaningful for toxicological purposes. The changing rate of absorption during early times is derived by differentiating Eq. (6) with respect to time:

Absorption rate at time $t = \dfrac{dQ}{dt} = \dfrac{D_m C_v K_m}{\delta}$

$$\times \left[1 - 2 \sum_{n=1}^{\infty} (-1)^{n+1} \exp \left(-\frac{D_m t}{\delta^2} \pi^2 n^2 \right) \right] \quad (7)$$

This equation also may be plotted as a graph, which may be used to predict the rate of absorption at any particular time. In this case the vertical axis carries the ratio of the rate of absorption at time t to the final steady-state rate and the horizontal axis is again time expressed as $D_m t/\delta^2$. This plot is shown in Figs. 4 and 5. When predicting an absorption rate at given time the treatment is as follows:

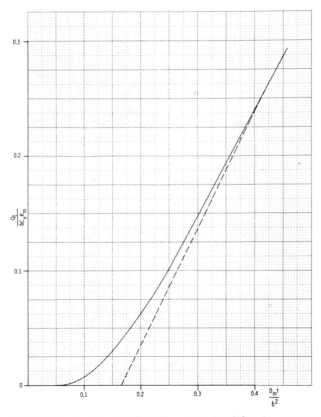

FIGURE 2 Graph of $Q_t/\delta C_v K_m$ versus $D_m t/\delta^2$ that permits calculation of the total amount having penetrated a unit membrane area (Q_t) at any time during the lag phase (see text for method). The early time period is expanded in Fig. 3.

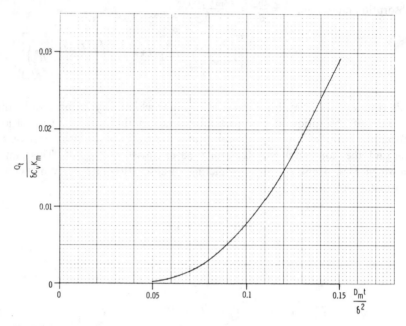

FIGURE 3 Graph of $Q_t/\delta C_v K_m$ versus $D_m t/\delta^2$ that permits calculation of the total amount having penetrated a unit membrane area at early times during the lag phase.

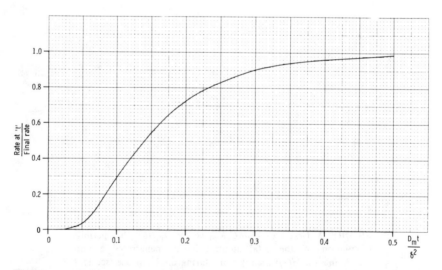

FIGURE 4 Graph that permits calculation of the rate of absorption per unit membrane area at any time during the lag phase (see text for method). The early time period is expanded in Fig. 5.

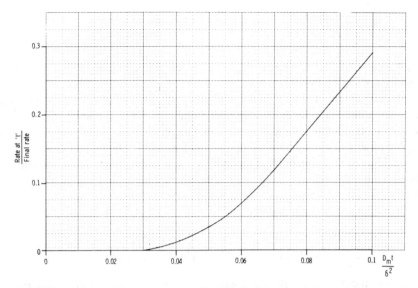

FIGURE 5 Graph that permits calculation of the rate of absorption per unit membrane area at early times during the lag phase.

The value of $D_m t/\delta^2$ for the time of interest is calculated and the corresponding value of rate of absorption at t over steady-state absorption rate read from the graph. Since the steady-state absorption rate is known, either from experiments or calculations based on Eq. (1) or (3), the unknown rate may be found. The graph may be replotted as the rate of absorption versus time.

Another factor of toxicological interest is the amount remaining dissolved within the SC at the end of a short period of contact with a solution. Material that is within the SC cannot be quickly washed away and, unless volatile or lost through desquamation of SC, will eventually enter the body. The "reservoir effect" reported for certain steroids is a special case, which is discussed later. Crank (1970) gives the following equation, which describes the buildup of material in a membrane during the lag phase:

$$\frac{M_t}{M_\infty} = 1 - \frac{8}{\pi^2} \sum_{n=0}^{\infty} \frac{1}{(2n+1)^2} \exp\left[-\frac{D_m t}{\delta^2} \pi^2 (2n+1)^2\right] \tag{8}$$

where M_t is the amount of penetrant per unit area at time t and M_∞ is the corresponding amount present once steady state has been achieved. The penetrant concentration profile across SC at steady state, assuming uniform properties across the membrane, is shown in Fig. 8. The linear concentration gradient indicates that

$$M_\infty = \frac{C_v K_m \delta}{2} \qquad (9)$$

The graphs of M_t/M_∞ versus $D_m t/\delta^2$ shown in Figs. 6 and 7 are used in a similar fashion to the previous reference graphs:

The value of $D_m t/\delta^2$ for the time of interest is calculated and the corresponding value of M_t/M_∞ is read from the graph. Since M_∞ is given by Eq. (9), the value of M_t is then readily calculated. This graph may be replotted as the amount dissolved per unit area of SC (M_t) versus time.

Figures 2–7 provide a means of establishing the time course of absorption and also of predicting absorption during and following a short period of contact between skin and a solution of penetrant.

ROLE OF HAIR FOLLICLES AND SWEAT DUCTS
IN PERCUTANEOUS ABSORPTION

No mention has yet been made of the possible role of hair follicles and sweat ducts as potentially "easy" routes for absorption through SC. The only direct measurement of absorption yielded no indication of rapid entry of tri-*n*-butyl phosphate via the hair follicles of pig skin (Tregear, 1961). Qualitative evidence for the importance of hair follicles and sweat ducts as pathways of penetration (Mackee et al., 1945; Shelley and Melton, 1949; Rutherford and Black, 1969; Fredriksson, 1961; Van Kooten and Mali, 1966) is less easily interpreted. Comparisons of absorption rates of several penetrants

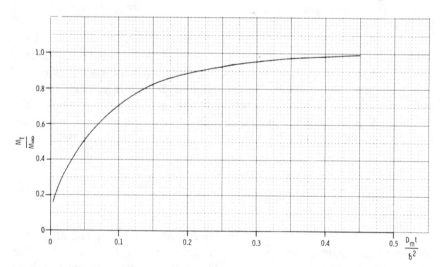

FIGURE 6 Graph that permits calculation of the amount of penetrant (M_t) dissolved in a unit area of the stratum corneum at any time during the lag phase (see text for method). The early time period is expanded in Fig. 7.

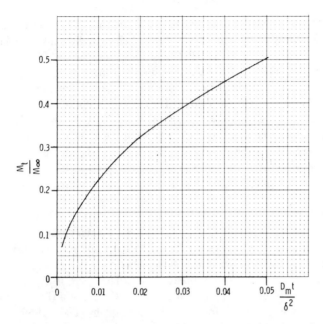

FIGURE 7 Graph that permits calculation of the amount of penetrant dissolved in a unit area of stratum corneum at early times during the lag phase.

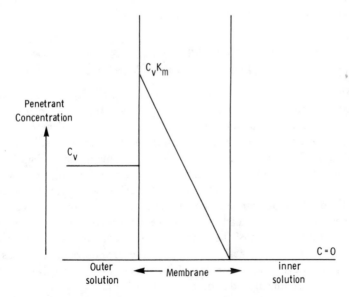

FIGURE 8 Diagram showing the concentration profile across stratum corneum during steady-state absorption.

through follicle-rich areas and areas with considerably lower hair density suggested importance for the appendageal route in humans (Maibach et al., 1971; Feldmann and Maibach, 1967) and the guinea pig (Wahlberg, 1968).

Scheuplein (1967) attacked this problem mathematically by taking the known geometry and distribution of appendages in humans and assuming diffusion constants for these routes. The approach chosen by Scheuplein was to take numbers deliberately biased in favor of the appendageal route of absorption, and he concluded that absorption via follicles and ducts could be significant for slower penetrants of SC. Because the diffusion constant for penetrant movement through the appendages may be several orders of magnitude faster than within SC, the lag phase for them may be virtually nonexistent. Absorption through appendages may achieve a steady rate very quickly and thus predominate at early times (line A, Fig. 9). The total area of the appendages is very small and, for most penetrants, absorption through the general skin surface eventually overwhelms appendageal absorption (line B, Fig. 9). In the case of some very slow penetrants of SC, the route through follicles and ducts may always predominate. The type of absorption pattern displayed by the addition of appendageal and SC diffusion (line A + B, Fig. 9) has been observed *in vitro* for steroids (Scheuplein et al., 1969) and such a graph may permit the separation of appendageal absorption by attributing any initial linear region to the follicles and ducts.

The full significance of appendageal absorption still awaits final experimental assessment. However, Scheuplein has shown that these routes predominate only in the very early stages of absorption. The possible exception could be "very slow" penetrants of SC.

PREDICTIONS OF PERCUTANEOUS ABSORPTION FROM VEHICLE TO VEHICLE

The treatments given above provide means of predicting absorption behavior of a specific penetrant applied in a single vehicle. In many cases it is desirable to be able to predict the absorption pattern of a penetrant for many vehicles from permeability properties measured for one vehicle. This would be possible if SC were to behave as an ideal membrane. Higuchi (1960) recognized that, rather than a difference in concentration, the true driving force for net transfer of material across SC is a difference in chemical potential (or thermodynamic activity). If the membrane diffusion constant for the penetrant and the thickness and solvent properties of the membrane are unchanged by the nature of the external vehicle, then the rate of absorption is proportional to the chemical potential in the various vehicles. Fick's law of diffusion is obeyed for a single vehicle when the chemical potential and concentration are linearly related.

The chemical potential of a solute is given by the product of the activity coefficient and the concentration of the solute (Glasstone, 1953). The

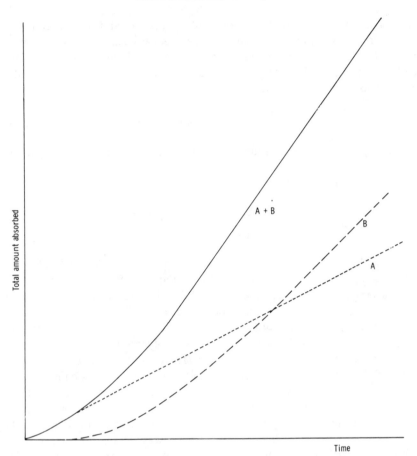

FIGURE 9 Contribution of diffusion through sweat ducts and hair follicles (line A) and across the general SC surface (curve B) to the early time course of absorption (curve A + B) if appendages are significant.

activity coefficient may not be known and may be difficult to measure. More accessible are manipulations based on the fact that, for equilibrium states, the chemical potential of a given material in the two phases is equal. This is true for equilibria of the partition system type, vapor-liquid equilibria, saturated solutions in contact with excess saturating agents, etc. One approach based on this property and which is easy to apply takes as a starting point the recognition that the chemical potential of a penetrant is maximal in saturated solution and hence a maximum absorption rate occurs from a saturated solution (also a corollary of Fick's law). The chemical potential of a particular chemical is the same in all saturated solutions—that is, that of the neat liquid or solid—regardless of solvent. This means that there is a single maximum absorption rate definable for any penetrant. In an ideal system the absorption rate is proportional to the degree of saturation and, for example, all half-saturated solutions of a penetrant have equal chemical potential and all give half the maximum possible absorption rate (Flynn and Smith, 1972; Hadgraft et al., 1973; Roberts and Anderson, 1975). The useful mathematical expressions from this treatment are

$$J_{max} = k_p S_v \qquad (10)$$

where J_{max} is the maximum achievable absorption rate for the penetrant and S_v is its solubility in the vehicle.

When considering two vehicles x and y:

$$\frac{k_{px}}{k_{py}} = \frac{K_{mx}}{K_{my}} = \frac{S_{vy}}{S_{vx}} \qquad (11)$$

The solubility of the penetrant in SC is equal to $K_m S_v$. Related to the solubility approach to predictions is that of Katz and Poulsen and co-workers, who attempted to manipulate drug absorption rates by modifying the partition coefficient (for example, Ostrenga et al., 1971b).

Knowledge of any physical equilibrium condition may be used to relate the chemical potential in one vehicle or physical state to that in another. The system described by Ostrenga et al. (1971a) is suitable for determining the chemical potential of a penetrant in complex vehicles by partitioning.

It should be stressed that the predictive treatments based on solubilities or on equilibria are largely untested. Because they depend on several systems behaving reasonably closely to the ideal, they should be regarded as providing only "range-finding" predictions at present. Reasons for the breakdown of solubility-derived predictions include solvent damage to SC, deviations from ideality near penetrant saturation in vehicles, variations in SC hydration in contact with different solvents, and entry of vehicle components into the SC to alter its solvent properties.

SITUATIONS WHERE DIFFUSION ACROSS STRATUM CORNEUM IS NOT RATE LIMITING

Although it is probably rare for the determinant of absorption rates via skin to be other than diffusion across SC, this does arise for a number of pharmaceutical preparations. Three possible cases will be considered: (1) the penetrant is entirely dissolved in the vehicle and its diffusion in this medium is slow; (2) the vehicle contains suspended penetrant whose dissolution is limiting; (3) the penetrant is dissolved in the dispersed phase of a two-phase emulsion. These have been treated theoretically and the mathematical expressions tested experimentally.

Higuchi (1962) has considered the first case and, assuming that any penetrant reaching the SC is instantly absorbed and that not more than 30% of the original amount of penetrant applied is absorbed, the following expression is approximately true.

$$Q_t = 2C_v \left(\frac{D_v t}{\pi} \right)^{1/2} \tag{13}$$

where D_v is the diffusion constant of the penetrant in the vehicle, and Q_t is the total amount of penetrant released from the vehicle by time t and, in this case, is the amount absorbed.

If the vehicle contains suspended penetrant whose dissolution is rate limiting, only material in true solution may enter unbroken SC and be absorbed. When the penetrant is in small particles dispersed evenly in the vehicle, the expression describing release and absorption is (Higuchi, 1960):

$$Q_t = (2A_v - S_v) \left[\frac{D_v t}{1 + 2(A_v - S_v)/S_v} \right]^{1/2} \tag{14}$$

where A_v is the total amount of penetrant, dissolved and suspended, in the vehicle per unit volume.

The rate of absorption at a given time t is yielded by differentiating Eq. (14) (Katz and Poulsen, 1971).

$$\text{Rate of absorption} = \frac{dQ}{dt} = \frac{1}{2} \left[\frac{D_v(2A_v - S_v)S_v}{t} \right]^{1/2} \tag{15}$$

Higuchi (1960) states that, if A_v is much greater than S_v, Eqs. (14) and (15) reduce to:

$$Q_t = (2A_v D_v S_v t)^{1/2} \tag{16}$$

and

$$\frac{dQ}{dt} = \left(\frac{A_v D_v S_v}{2t} \right)^{1/2} \tag{17}$$

It is possible to combine Eq. (17) with the permeability constant for SC if both release and SC control the rate of absorption (Katz and Shaikh, 1965):

$$\text{Rate of absorption} = \frac{dQ}{dt} = k_p \left(\frac{A_v D_v S_v}{2t} \right)^{1/2} \tag{18}$$

Katz and Poulsen (1971) state that Eqs. (14) to (18) do not take into account particle size, which appears to become important for very small particles such as micronized drugs.

For the third case, that of emulsion-type vehicles, Ostrenga et al. (1971a) quote an equation attributed to Higuchi giving an "effective diffusion constant", D_e, for penetrant movement in the vehicle:

$$D_e = \frac{D_1}{V_1 + KV_2}\left[1 + 3V_2\left(\frac{KD_2 - D_1}{KD_2 + D_1}\right)\right] \qquad (19)$$

where D_1 and D_2 are the diffusion constants in the bulk and dispersed phase, respectively, V_1 and V_2 are the volume fractions of these two phases, and K is the partition coefficient between the dispersed and bulk phase. If V_1 is much greater than V_2 and D_2 is much greater than D_1, then (Ostrenga et al., 1971a):

$$D_e = \frac{D_1}{KV_2}(1 + 3V_2) \qquad (19a)$$

Many more complex release situations have been analyzed (Higuchi, 1967; Higuchi and Higuchi, 1960).

ABSORPTION FROM SMALL QUANTITIES OF PENETRANT IN CONTACT WITH SKIN AND ABSORPTION FROM SOLID MATERIAL

The description that follows applies equally to small amounts of penetrant applied per unit area whether in the form of solid, neat liquid, or a small volume of solution. "Small" is interpreted here as meaning that the source of the penetrant is significantly reduced in quantity by the absorption process. This type of system has been used *in vivo* (Feldmann and Maibach, 1970) and *in vitro* (Franz, 1975; Scheuplein and Ross, 1974) and is one that may be relevant to toxicological situations.

When depletion of the external source of penetrant occurs, curves A and B in Fig. 10 indicate the manner in which the absorption rate changes with time. As may be seen, a maximum rate is achieved followed by falling rates. Scheuplein and Ross (1974) have analyzed this pattern and established certain relationships. The time taken to reach the maximum rate, τ_{max}, is predicted as follows:

$$\tau_{max} = \frac{\delta^2 - h^2}{6D_m} \qquad (20)$$

The thickness of the penetrant layer, h, is usually small in comparison with δ, the SC thickness, and therefore

$$\tau_{max} \cong \frac{\delta^2}{6D_m} \tag{21}$$

These authors also state that the peak rate of absorption is directly proportional to the amount of penetrant applied per unit area, designated the "specific dose." This relationship permits calculation of the maximum rate of absorption from any specific dose following measurement of the maximum absorption rate at a single specific dose. A further relationship exists for this situation:

$$\text{Peak absorption rate} = \frac{1.85\, D_m A}{\delta^2} \tag{22}$$

where A is the specific dose. The proportionality relationship and Eq. (22) are only suitable for cases where depletion of the external penetrant is marked, and they cannot be applied when an effectively infinite source exists.

Measurements of the area under a plot of absorption rate per unit area versus time, such as in Fig. 10, yields the amount of material absorbed. The

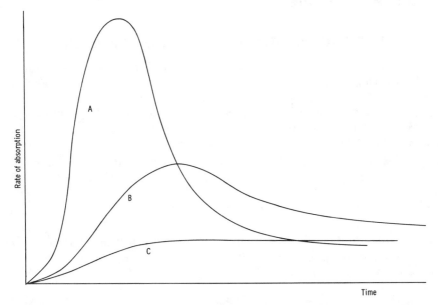

FIGURE 10 The pattern of changing absorption rate for small amounts of penetrant per unit area of skin. Curve A, moderately fast penetrant; curve B, slower penetrant; curve C, very slow penetrant. Curves A and B show the effect of the depletion of penetrant source.

amount accumulating within the body once a detoxification plus elimination rate has been exceeded may be found by measuring the area contained above this rate. The slower the penetrant, the broader and lower will be the maximum rate peak (see lines A and B, Fig. 10). For the very slow penetrant cortisone, the rate of absorption was found by Scheuplein and Ross (1974) to be constant for a relatively long period (line C, Fig. 10). This rate was shown to be approximately proportional to the specific dose, permitting an expression similar to Eq. (1) to be used:

$$J = k_t A \tag{23}$$

where k_t is the transfer coefficient, which may be expressed in percentage dose terms:

$$J = \frac{k_t A}{100} \tag{24}$$

Unlike the permeability constant, as A increases k_t gradually decreases because the source of penetrant eventually comes to contain excess material where additions cause no further increase in absorption rate. Equations (23) and (24) are of limited usefulness but do widen the predictive scope of measurements made using small amounts of very slow penetrants.

PERCUTANEOUS ABSORPTION OF GASES AND VAPORS

In many ways the absorption of a chemical from the gaseous or vapor state is analogous to that from solution. There is no evidence to suggest that even the lightest gases pass through SC via pores, and solution in the membrane is a prerequisite for absorption (Scheuplein and Blank, 1971). The skin permeability properties in relation to gases have been investigated by Scheuplein (1970).

The rate of absorption of a gas is proportional to the concentration of penetrant and a gas phase permeability constant (k_{pg}) may be defined:

$$J = k_{pg} C_{vg} \tag{25}$$

Instead of C_{vg}, the gas concentration in parts per million or amount per volume, the partial pressure (p) of the gas or vapor may be used:

$$J = k_{pg} \frac{p}{RT} \tag{26}$$

where R is the appropriate gas constant and T the absolute temperature. Equations (25) and (26) may be manipulated as Eq. (1) to predict rates of absorption from any atmosphere of a gaseous penetrant once a rate is known for a given atmosphere.

The gas phase permeability constant may be expanded as follows:

$$k_{pg} = \frac{K_{mg}D_m}{\delta} \tag{27}$$

hence $$J = \frac{K_{mg}C_{vg}D_m}{\delta} = \frac{K_{mg}pD_m}{\delta RT} \tag{28}$$

Notice that D_m and δ are the same terms as Eq. (2) but that a gas phase partition term K_{mg} is used. The gas phase partition coefficient is the ratio of the concentration of the penetrant in the tissue to the external concentration if the SC is totally immersed and equilibrated in the gas system. The numerical values of the gas phase partition coefficient, and hence permeability constant, are considerably higher than solution phase values for the same penetrant. This is compensated by the very much lower concentration term used in Eqs. (26) and (28) for calculations of absorption rate.

Although volatile materials and gases tend to be the more rapid type of penetrant, the nature of any lag phase will depend on SC thickness and membrane diffusion constant as for absorption from solution. Predictions of the early time course of penetration thus follow the lines already described.

A useful relationship exists between the absorption of a penetrant as a gas or vapor and its absorption from a solution or liquid phase. The gas or vapor in equilibrium with dissolved or condensed gas has the same chemical potential in each phase and thus the penetration rate from each phase should be the same (see above). Once details of a vapor-liquid equilibrium state are known, the absorption rate from one phase may be used to predict penetration rates from the other.

FACTORS AFFECTING THE APPLICATION OF SKIN PERMEABILITY THEORY

If the SC behaved as an ideal membrane, its thickness, and the solubility and diffusion constant of a penetrant within it, would be unchanged by the nature of the vehicle or the concentration of penetrant applied. Only temperature would alter the values of the membrane diffusion constant and partition coefficient. Solution pH may change the latter factor through alteration of the degree of dissociation of the penetrant, but ideally the partition for the individual charged and uncharged moieties should remain constant in this special case. Although SC behaves reasonably closely to the ideal in most instances, there are exceptions. Some of the more common situations where deviations occur are summarized below.

Stratum corneum hydration. It has long been known that occlusion of the site of application of a penetrant increases the absorption rate—probably by a combination of a temperature and a hydration effect. Perhaps the most dramatic indications of the importance of hydration to diffusion in SC are manifest for steroid absorption (Scheuplein and Ross, 1974; Vickers, 1969). At least two factors are known to be altered through varying the degree of hydration of the statum corneum: both SC thickness (Scheuplein and Morgan, 1967) and membrane diffusion constants (Scheuplein, 1975) increase with rising SC hydration. These factors oppose one another [Eq. (3)], but for water itself (Scheuplein, 1975), steroids (Scheuplein and Ross, 1974; Vickers, 1969) and acetylsalicylic acid (Fritsch and Stoughton, 1963) the increases in diffusion constants are dominant. The degree of hydration may also affect the solubility of the penetrant in the membrane and thereby raise or lower the anticipated partition coefficient. In practical situations, the nature of the vehicle or penetrant or atmospheric conditions may affect SC hydration.

Stratum corneum damage by vehicle or penetrant. It is perhaps obvious that components of vehicles or penetrants themselves may decrease the barrier properties of SC through any destructive mechanism. Many of the theoretical relationships described become difficult to apply if progressive or concentration-dependent changes in membrane properties occur. Damage may be apparent in the nature of the time course for the absorption process, from "before and after" measurements of the absorption of test penetrants, or from recordings of the conductance of the skin (Dugard and Scheuplein, 1973).

Solvent uptake by stratum corneum. Components of vehicles, or the penetrant itself, may enter SC in sufficient quantities to reversibly alter the properties of the membrane. The diffusion constant, partition coefficient, and perhaps rarely even SC thickness may be affected in this way. The final steady-state penetration in such cases may be treated as though ideal, but the early phase of absorption may be complex. Predictions of absorption rates from vehicle to vehicle based on solubility or on a thermodynamic activity foundation are not possible if the vehicle alters SC properties.

Temperature effects on absorption rates. Because the activation energies for diffusion across SC tend to be high (Scheuplein and Blank, 1971) the absorption rate is highly temperature dependent and increases exponentially with rising temperature. The temperature effect is largely due to changes in the membrane diffusion constant (Blank et al., 1967).

Binding of penetrant to stratum corneum. If a finite number of binding sites that effectively immobilize penetrant molecules exist in the SC, the steady state is unchanged. However, the lag phase is extended and is approximately described by (Ostrenga et al., 1971b):

$$\tau = \frac{\delta^2}{4D_m} + \frac{\delta^2 A_b}{2k_p} \tag{29}$$

where A_b is the amount bound per unit volume of SC. Equation (29) becomes inaccurate for small values of A_b. Falsely high partition coefficients may be obtained when measured directly if penetrant binding occurs. To establish the presence of and to quantitate binding, partition coefficients should always be determined for a range of penetrant concentrations.

Broken or diseased skin. The idiosyncratic properties of physically damaged or disease-affected SC preclude accurate predictions of absorption rates, which may be increased in these cases (Grice et al., 1975; Spruit and Malten, 1966). The factor by which the penetration rate is increased above normal will vary from penetrant to penetrant even for the same site of diseased or damaged skin.

Regional variations in skin permeability properties. Scheuplein and Blank (1971) have summarized the existing information on the regional variations in skin permeability to water and other penetrants and show that, for water, the variations are not simply due to differences in SC thickness. If the diffusion constant varies from skin site to skin site it is probable that the relative permeability between areas will vary with the penetrant being considered; there will not be a constant factor difference between absorption rates through two different sites, and thickness will not be a reliable guide to relative permeability.

EXPERIMENTAL TECHNIQUES

Many variations of several main *in vivo* and *in vitro* techniques have been used to measure the amount of, or rate of, absorption through skin (Katz and Poulsen, 1971; Marzulli et al., 1969; Grasso and Lansdown, 1972; Idson, 1975). Many workers hesitate to use *in vitro* techniques since they feel that information representative of the *in vivo* skin properties will not be given. Although there is no reason to believe that SC properties are altered by removal from the body, there are certain differences between the two experimental modes (Franz, 1975): Shedding of superficial SC cells does not occur *in vitro*, whereas *in vivo*, over a period of time, superficial (slow) penetrant may be lost from the body. This applies to material outside the SC or dissolved within the shed cells. If the penetrant or components of the vehicle affect the activities of viable epidermal cells in any way, an abnormal SC may eventually result whose permeability properties may be altered. Thus, *in vivo*, prolonged or repeated applications of a penetrant may modify absorption rates in a manner not possible *in vitro*. The role of hair follicles or sweat ducts may well be different *in vitro* and *in vivo*. The rate of blood flow is probably not an important controlling factor of absorption rates because clearance below the SC is rapid (Scheuplein and Blank, 1971) although it may be important in relation to local effects of the penetrant.

Overall, *in vitro* techniques are easier to perform, more precise, conditions are more easily controlled, and human tissues may be used. There are probably no reasons against use of *in vitro* experiments for all but slow penetrants (Franz, 1975). However determined, absorption rates provide a basis for the calculation of a permeability constant.

SC diffusion constants may be determined from the lag phase observed in absorption experiments by applying Eq. (5) or from steady-state absorption values if the SC:vehicle partition coefficient is known [Eq. (3)]. Sorption experiments (Roberts et al., 1975; Scheuplein, 1975; Scheuplein and Dugard, 1973), although difficult to perform, may yield membrane diffusion constants. These experiments follow the time course of the penetrant dissolving in SC or, in cases where the partition coefficient is low, desorption of material previously sorbed into the tissue to a state of equilibrium.

Stratum corneum:vehicle partition coefficients may be determined directly by immersing isolated SC (prepared by the methods of Kligman and Christophers, 1963) in penetrant solution and allowing equilibration. The calculation may be based on either the loss of penetrant from solution (Scheuplein et al., 1969) or the penetrant content of the SC. Sorption experiments also give partition coefficients at the final equilibrium and, if the diffusion constant is known, the partition coefficient may be calculated from Eq. (2) or (3).

Evaluation of SC thickness is often problematic because it depends on the degree of hydration of this tissue (Scheuplein and Morgan, 1967). Estimates of thickness of SC for various body regions *in vivo* under "normal" ambient conditions are listed by Scheuplein and Blank (1971). In *in vitro* experiments or under occlusion *in vivo*, SC may become greatly hydrated and, dependent on time, may swell considerably. Human abdominal SC may be less than 10 μm thick when dry and 40–50 μm when well hydrated. Prolonged immersion in aqueous systems may result in even greater values for hydrated thickness. The release properties of vehicles may be measured *in vitro* by the technique described by Ostrenga et al. (1971a).

All the equations and graphical treatments described above are in terms of unit area of skin surface. Thus scaling up to an area appropriate to any particular assessment may be necessary. Since absorption is proportional to the area of contact, this is achieved by multiplication of the absorption rate per unit area, for example, by the practical area of contact. In the extreme, the whole body surface may be available for absorption, as would often be the case for gaseous penetrants, and the total area may be estimated using the relationship of Dubois and Dubois (quoted in Leider, 1949):

$$\text{Body surface area, cm}^2 = (\text{weight, kg})^{0.425} \times (\text{height, cm})^{0.725} \times 71.8$$

For the average adult the whole body area is approximately 18,000 cm^2. The estimate based on total body area takes no account of regional variations in permeability properties, whose significance may vary from situation to situation.

CONCLUSION

Even performed *in vitro*, measurements of absorption through skin require considerable effort and consistent results are difficult to obtain. However, meaningful information may be generated in this manner and, by applying treatments based on theory, the results may be used in a comprehensive fashion. The equations and graphical treatments described in this chapter simply require insertion of the appropriate values, although care must be exercised in the choice of units to ensure their compatibility.

Absorption experiments and the theoretical relationships used for predictions divide into two levels of complexity. The lower level involves the determination of a rate of absorption which permits calculation of a proportionality constant such as the permeability constant. This constant is then the basis for predictions of absorption rate for the full range of penetrant concentrations in a given vehicle or all possible gas concentrations. The majority of skin absorption measurements, even as performed at present, are suitable for the calculation of a permeability constant, and the remainder require only minor modifications to make this possible. Apart from predictions that may be made using the permeability constant, this term also provides the best means of comparing various skin absorption measurements, and it is to be hoped that it will be used more widely in the future. More complex experiments give the diffusion constant of the penetrant in SC and a solubility parameter such as the SC:vehicle partition coefficient. These terms allow a very wide range of absorption situations to be analyzed mathematically. Deviations from the ideal do occur, but, in my experience, theory may be successfully applied in many instances.

NOMENCLATURE

J	Absorption rate per unit area at steady state. Also known as the flux.
C_v	Concentration of penetrant in the vehicle.
k_p	Permeability constant.
K_m	Stratum corneum: vehicle partition coefficient.
δ	Stratum corneum thickness.
D_m	Diffusion constant of penetrant in stratum corneum.
t	Time after initial contact between penetrant and skin surface.
Q_t	Total amount absorbed per unit area by time t.
τ	Lag time.
n	An integer with values as shown in the equations.
π	Numerically 3.1416 ....
dQ/dt	Instantaneous absorption rate per unit area at time t.
M_t	Amount of penetrant in stratum corneum per unit area at time t.
M_∞	Amount of penetrant in stratum corneum per unit area once steady-state absorption has been achieved.

J_{max} Maximum absorption rate per unit area possible for a given penetrant.

S_v Solubility of the penetrant in the vehicle.

D_v Diffusion constant of penetrant in the vehicle.

A_v The total amount of penetrant, dissolved or suspended in unit volume of vehicle.

D_e Effective diffusion constant of penetrant in an emulsion-type vehicle.

D_1 Diffusion constant of penetrant in the bulk phase of an emulsion.

D_2 Diffusion constant of penetrant in the disperse phase of an emulsion.

V_1 Volume fraction of the bulk phase in an emulsion.

V_2 Volume fraction of the disperse phase in an emulsion.

K Disperse: bulk phase partition coefficient for penetrant in an emulsion.

h Thickness of penetrant layer on the skin surface.

A Specific dose, the amount of penetrant initially applied per unit area of skin surface.

k_t Transfer coefficient.

k_{pg} Gas phase permeability constant.

C_{vg} Gas phase penetrant concentration.

p Partial pressure.

R Gas constant.

T Absolute temperature.

K_{mg} Gas phase stratum corneum: atmosphere partition coefficient.

A_b Amount of penetrant bound per unit volume of stratum corneum.

REFERENCES

Berenson, G. S. and Burch, G. E. 1951. Studies of diffusion through dead human skin. *Am. J. Trop. Med. Hyg.* 31:842–853.

Blank, I. H. 1964. Penetration of low molecular weight alcohols into skin. *J. Invest. Dermatol.* 43:415–420.

Blank, I. H. 1965. Cutaneous barriers. *J. Invest. Dermatol.* 45:249–256.

Blank, I. H., Scheuplein, R. J. and Macfarlane, D. J. 1967. Mechanism of percutaneous absorption III. The effect of temperature on the transport of non-electrolytes across skin. *J. Invest. Dermatol.* 49:582–589.

Crank, J. 1970. *The mathematics of diffusion.* London: Oxford Univ. Press.

Dugard, P. H. and Scheuplein, R. J. 1973. Effects of ionic surfactants on the permeability of human epidermis: An electrometric study. *J. Invest. Dermatol.* 60:263–269.

Feldmann, R. J. and Maibach, H. I. 1967. Regional variation in percutaneous penetration of ^{14}C cortisol in man. *J. Invest. Dermatol.* 48:181–183.

Feldmann, R. J. and Maibach, H. I. 1970. Absorption of some organic compounds through the skin in man. *J. Invest. Dermatol.* 54:399–404.

Flynn, G. L. and Smith, R. W. 1972. Membrane diffusion III: Influence of solvent composition and permeant solubility on membrane transport. *J. Pharm. Sci.* 61:61–66.

Franz, T. J. 1975. Percutaneous absorption. On the relevance of *in vitro* data. *J. Invest. Dermatol.* 64:190–195.

Fredriksson, T. 1961. Studies on the percutaneous absorption of parathion and paraoxon. II Distribution of ^{32}P-labelled parathion within the skin. *Acta Derm. Venereol. (Stockh.)* 41:344–352.

Fritsch, W. C. and Stoughton, R. B. 1963. The effect of temperature and humidity on the penetration of ^{14}C acetylsalicylic acid in excised human skin. *J. Invest. Dermatol.* 41:307–312.

Glasstone, S. 1953. *Textbook of physical chemistry*, London: Macmillan.

Grasso, P. and Lansdown, A. B. G. 1972. Methods of measuring and factors affecting, percutaneous absorption. *J. Soc. Cosmet. Chem.* 23:481–521.

Grice, K., Sattar, H., Baker, H. and Sharratt, M. 1975. The relationship of transepidermal water loss to skin temperature in psoriasis and eczema. *J. Invest. Dermatol.* 64:313–315.

Hadgraft, J., Hadgraft, J. W. and Sarkany, I. 1973. The effect of thermodynamic activity on the percutaneous absorption of methyl nicotinate from water glycerol mixtures. *J. Pharm. Pharmacol.* 25(Suppl.):122P and 123P.

Higuchi, T. 1960. Physical chemical analysis of percutaneous absorption process from creams and ointments. *J. Soc. Cosmet. Chem.* 11:85–97.

Higuchi, W. I. 1962. Analysis of data on the medicament release from ointments. *J. Pharm. Sci.* 51:802–804.

Higuchi, W. I. 1967. Diffusional models useful in biopharmaceutics; drug release rate processes. *J. Pharm. Sci.* 56:315–324.

Higuchi, W. I. and Higuchi, T. 1960. Theoretical analysis of diffusional movement through heterogeneous barriers. *J. Am. Pharm. Assoc. Sci. Ed.* 49:598–606.

Idson, B. 1975. Percutaneous absorption. *J. Pharm. Sci.* 64:901–924.

Katz, M. and Poulsen, J. B. 1971. Absorption of drugs through the skin. In *Concepts in biochemical pharmacology*, part I, eds. B. B. Brodie and J. R. Gillette *Handbook of experimental pharmacology*, vol. 28. Berlin: Springer-Verlag.

Katz, M. and Shaikh, Z. I. 1965. Percutaneous corticosteroid absorption correlated to partition coefficients. *J. Pharm. Sci.* 54:591–594.

Kligman, A. M. and Christophers, E. 1963. Preparation of isolated sheets of human stratum corneum. *Arch. Dermatol.* 88:702–705.

Leider, M. 1949. On the weight of skin. *J. Invest. Dermatol.* 12:187–191.

Mackee, G. M., Sulzberger, M. B., Herrmann, F. and Baer, R. L. 1945. Histologic studies on percutaneous penetration with special reference to the effect of vehicles. *J. Invest. Dermatol.* 6:43–61.

Maibach, H. I., Feldmann, R. J., Milby, T. H. and Serat, W. F. 1971. Regional variation in percutaneous penetration in man. *Arch. Environ. Health* 23:208–211.

Marzulli, F. N., Brown, D. W. C. and Maibach, H. I. 1969. Techniques for studying skin penetration. *Toxicol. Appl. Pharmacol. Suppl.* 3:76–83.

Ostrenga, J., Haleblian, J., Poulsen, B., Ferrell, B., Mueller, N. and Shastri, S. 1971a. Vehicle design for a new topical steroid, fluocinonide. *J. Invest. Dermatol.* 56:392–399.

Ostrenga, J., Steinmetz, C., Poulsen, B. and Yett, S. 1971b. Significance of vehicle composition II: Prediction of optimal vehicle composition. *J. Pharm. Sci.* 60:1180–1183.

Roberts, M. S. and Anderson, R. A. 1975. Percutaneous absorption of phenolic compounds: The effect of vehicles on the penetration of phenol. *J. Pharm. Pharmacol.* 27:599–605.

Roberts, M. S., Triggs, E. J. and Anderson, R. A. 1975. Permeability of solutes through biological membranes measured by a desorption technique. *Nature (Lond.)* 257:225–227.

Rutherford, T. and Black, J. G. 1969. The use of autoradiography to study the localization of germicides in skin. *Br. J. Dermatol.* 81(Suppl. 4):75–87.

Scheuplein, R. J. 1965. Mechanism of percutaneous absorption. I Routes of penetration and the influence of solubility. *J. Invest. Dermatol.* 45:334–346.

Scheuplein, R. J. 1967. Mechanism of percutaneous absorption. II Transient diffusion and the relative importance of various routes of skin penetration. *J. Invest. Dermatol.* 48:79–88.

Scheuplein, R. J. 1970. The permeability of the skin to gases. *Annual Report No. 1.* Arlington, Va.: Army Research Office, Life Sciences Division.

Scheuplein, R. J. 1975. Sorption and retention of substances in the surface layers of the skin. *Final Technical Report.* Arlington, Va.: Army Research Office.

Scheuplein, R. J. and Blank, I. H. 1971. Permeability of the skin. *Physiol. Rev.* 51:702–747.

Scheuplein, R. J. and Dugard, P.H. 1973. Sorption and retention of substances by the skin. *J. Invest. Dermatol.* 60:252.

Scheuplein, R. J. and Morgan, L. J. 1967. "Bound water" in keratin membranes measured by a microbalance technique. *Nature (Lond.)* 214:456–458.

Scheuplein,R. J. and Ross, L. W. 1974. Mechanism of percutaneous absorption. V Percutaneous absorption of solvent deposited solids. *J. Invest. Dermatol.* 62:353–360.

Scheuplein, R. J., Blank, I. H., Brauner, G. T. and MacFarlane, D. J. 1969. Percutaneous absorption of steroids. *J. Invest. Dermatol.* 52:63–70.

Shelley, W. B. and Melton, F. M. 1949. Factors accelerating the penetration of histamine through normal intact human skin. *J. Invest. Dermatol.* 13:61–71.

Spruit, D. and Malten, K. E. 1966. The regeneration rate of the water vapour loss of heavily damaged skin. *Dermatologica* 132:115–123.

Tregear, R. T. 1961. Relative penetrability of hair follicles and epidermis. *J. Physiol. (Lond.)* 156:307–313.

Tregear, R. T. 1966a. *Physical functions of skin.* London: Academic Press.

Tregear, R. T. 1966b. The permeability of skin to albumin, dextrans and polyvinyl pyrrolidone. *J. Invest. Dermatol.* 46:24–27.

Van Kooten, W. J. and Mali, J. W. H. 1966. The significance of sweat ducts in permeation experiments on isolated cadaverous human skin. *Dermatologica* 132:141–151.

Vickers, C. F. H. 1969. Stratum corneum reservoir for drugs. In *Advances in biology of skin,* vol. 12, *Pharmacology and skin,* eds. W. Montague, E. J. Van Scott, and R. B. Stoughton. New York: Appleton-Century-Crofts.

Wahlberg, J. E. 1968. Transepidermal or transfollicular absorption. *In vitro* studies on hairy and non-hairy guinea pig skin with sodium (^{22}Na) and mercuric (^{203}Hg) chlorides. *Acta Derm. Venereol. (Stockh.)* 48:336–344.

4

in vitro percutaneous absorption

Robert L. Bronaugh ■ Howard I. Maibach

INTRODUCTION

It is sometimes desirable to measure percutaneous absorption by *in vitro* techniques. Since absorption through the barrier of the skin is thought to be a passive diffusion process, no elaborate conditions to maintain the physiological state are required. The effect of metabolism on the absorption of compounds is only beginning to be studied (Chapter 3, Chapter 20), but it seems likely that in many cases it will not be rate-determining. The keratinization process in the epidermis leads to formation of the unique stratum corneum structure. This lipid-protein matrix serves as an effective barrier, particularly for hydrophilic compounds.

In vitro methods are useful for the study of percutaneous absorption separated from the other pharmacokinetic factors associated with the uptake of compounds by the topical route. Large numbers of diffusion cells can be run simultaneously and sampling is performed directly under the surface of the skin (in contrast to *in vivo* studies). Only *in vitro* methods can be used to obtain permeability data with highly toxic compounds on human skin.

METHODOLOGY

Diffusion Cells

There have been many variations of a few basic types. Historically, physical chemists have preferred a two-chambered cell in which a similar fluid (often water or saline) is placed on both sides of a membrane and the diffusion of a compound from one side to the other is observed. More representative of human use or exposure conditions is the one-chambered cell (Fig. 1) with the stratum corneum surface of the skin exposed to the environment. This permits application of the compound to the skin in a vehicle of choice and also allows evaporation of volatile compounds. The cells can be closed to prevent evaporation if desired.

The receptor fluid is continually mixed and maintained at a physiological temperature. The receptor is sampled at various intervals through a side-arm to determine absorption.

Preparation of Skin

Freshly obtained skin is desirable but, if necessary, skin can be stored frozen for 1–2 mo with no significant increase in permeability. Since there is some variability in the effectiveness of storing skin in this manner, it is highly recommended that the integrity of the skin be verified before use. For this purpose we find permeability to tritiated water extremely useful as a standard (Bronaugh et al., 1981).

The hair on the skin of animals should be lightly shaved with electric clippers (Wester and Maibach, 1975) to permit efficient application of compounds to the skin. Leaving some stubble is preferable to attempting complete removal of hair and thereby damaging the barrier. Chemical depilatories are

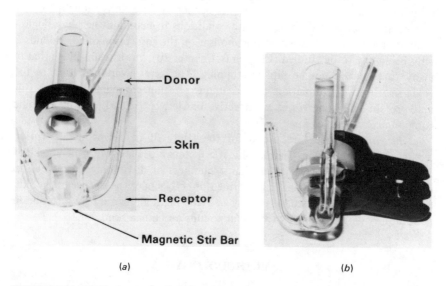

(a)   (b)

FIGURE 1 (a) Diffusion cell used in percutaneous studies. The components and the location where the skin sample is placed between the halves of the cell are shown. (b) The halves are joined by a pinch clamp, which is tightened and then attached to a holder in the water bath.

known to enhance skin absorption (Wahlberg, 1973; Andersen et al., 1980). With human skin and the skin of animals with a thick dermal layer, use of full-thickness skin should be avoided. Compounds absorbed *in vivo* enter the systemic circulation in the highly vascular region of the upper dermis and are not required to diffuse through the remainder of this layer. The aqueous dermal tissue does have some barrier properties (particularly for lipoidal compounds) since it is many times thicker than the stratum corneum. A dermatome slice at the level of the upper dermis provides a convenient preparation. With nonhairy skin, it is possible to separate readily the epidermis from the dermis by heat treatment at 60°C (Bronaugh et al., 1981) or by chemical means. This separation is difficult to perform without leaving holes when it is attempted with hairy (shaved) skin.

Calculations

Data are most frequently expressed in terms of the steady-state rate of penetration (permeability constant) or the percent of the applied dose absorbed.

For comparison of absorption data with data for other compounds and from other laboratories, a measurement of steady-state absorption can be useful. Normalization of the absorption rate by the concentration (C) of applied compound results in a permeability constant (k_p):

$$\frac{\text{Rate}}{C} = k_p$$

In practice, it is sometimes difficult to determine the steady-state rate with compounds that penetrate extremely rapidly or slowly. It can be impossible to measure this rate when vehicles are used that alter the stratum corneum.

Data expressed as a percent of the applied dose measure more practical aspects—how much is absorbed in a given time, regardless of lag time and linear absorption rate. The investigator must select the method of data expression that is most appropriate.

COMPARISON OF *IN VITRO* AND *IN VIVO* RESULTS

Based on the limited number of compounds that have been examined to date, very good agreement can usually be expected between *in vitro* and *in vivo* results. Burch and Winsor (1944) found excellent agreement in transepidermal water loss between excised human skin and that of human volunteers. Ainsworth (1960) reported a similarity between *in vivo* and *in vitro* absorption measurements with tributyl phosphate in rat, rabbit, and pig skin. Sekura and Scala (1972) obtained the same results for the penetration of two alkyl methyl sulfoxides with either type of absorption measurement in the rabbit.

Franz (1975, 1978) determined the absorption of 12 organic compounds through excised human skin and compared the results to the *in vivo* values obtained by Feldmann and Maibach (1970). In both studies, compounds were applied in an acetone vehicle and results were expressed as percent of the dose absorbed. In general, good agreement was found and the few dissimilarities could be explained by experimental differences.

The largest *in vivo* to *in vitro* comparison of human skin done in the same laboratory with standardized methods over a period of two decades was summarized by Anjo et al. (1980). *In vivo* flux was determined from urinary excretion data (with correction for incomplete urinary excretion); and *in vitro* rates were measured with a flow-through system (Crutcher and Maibach, 1969). A direct correlation was obtained between the two methods when a plot of the log transformations was employed. Careful examination of each compound shows that with some a good correlation of the methods does not exist. In some cases differences could be explained by a lack of solubility of the compound in the dermal perfusate; other differences are not presently explainable.

Bronaugh et al. (1982a) compared three compounds, using a petrolatum vehicle, for *in vivo* and *in vitro* absorption in the rat. Benzoic acid, acetylsalicylic acid, and urea were selected because of the expected differences in rate of permeability caused by their solubility differences. The *in vivo* absorption (Fig. 2) compares well with the *in vitro* absorption (Fig. 3), with data expressed as percent of the applied dose. Permeability constants were calculated *in vivo* for caffeine and acetylsalicylic acid from the sum of rates of accumulation in the body and excretion. Blood was sampled hourly from the tail vein to determine the rate of compound accumulation in the body (using the volume of distribution). Urine was collecting by bladder cannula to measure the rate of excretion

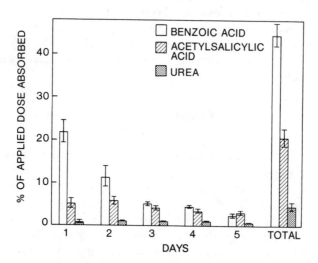

FIGURE 2 Percutaneous absorption in the rat *in vivo*. Values are the means ± SE of 5–8 determinations.

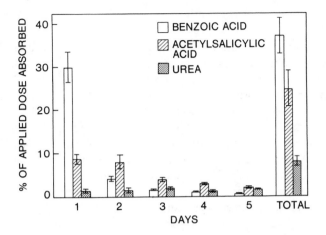

FIGURE 3 Percutaneous absorption in the rat *in vitro*. Values are the means ± SE of 4-8 determinations.

during the same time periods. Permeability constants obtained *in vivo* were similar to those obtained in diffusion cells (Table 1).

ANIMAL MODELS FOR HUMAN SKIN

It is not always feasible to use human skin in the evaluation of percutaneous absorption. Particularly for research or developmental studies, it is useful to work out procedures with skin that is in plentiful supply. It is obviously advantageous to use animal skin with permeability properties similar to those of human skin.

In a number of studies the weanling pig or miniature pig has proved to be a good animal model. This conclusion is based on results of permeability tests with tributyl phosphate (Ainsworth, 1960), chemical warfare agents (Marzulli et al., 1969), hexachlorophene (Marzulli and Maibach, 1975; Chow et al., 1978),

TABLE 1 Comparison of *in Vivo* and *in Vitro* Percutaneous Absorption through Rat Skin[a]

	Rate (ng/h·cm^2)		Permeability constant	
Compound	Body	Urine	*In vivo*	*In vitro*
Caffeine	16.3	27.8	2.1×10^{-4} (7)	3.1×10^{-4} (6)
Acetylsalicylic acid	0	11.4	5.2×10^{-5} (7)	6.5×10^{-5} (5)

[a]Compounds applied in a petrolatum vehicle to a 2.0-cm^2 area of skin on the living animals and in diffusion cells. Results are the means of the number of determinations in parentheses.

water (Galey et al., 1976), and other compounds (Tregear, 1966; Bartek et al., 1972).

Laboratory rodents are more convenient than the pig for dermal toxicity studies because they are easy to handle and inexpensive. The hairless mouse has been increasingly used because of the reported similarity of its skin to human skin in the absorption of anti-inflammatory steroids (Stoughton, 1975) and C_1 to C_8 alcohols (Durrheim et al., 1980). The skin of the rat has been considered more permeable than human or pig skin (Tregear, 1966; Marzulli and Maibach, 1975; Bartek et al., 1972). However, in studies of caffeine, N-acetylcysteine, and butter yellow (Bartek et al., 1972), rat skin seemed to be at least as good a model for human skin as pig skin.

The permeability properties of the skin of the miniature pig, hairless mouse, rat, and Swiss mouse were compared, by in vitro techniques, to those of human skin (Bronaugh et al., 1982b). Full-thickness back skin from female rodents was used. Human skin and pig skin were from either sex; the epidermis and a 350-μm dermatome slice were the preparations used, respectively. Figure 4 shows the permeability constants calculated from steady-state rate measurements; a tenfold smaller scale is used for the benzoic acid data. Similar results were obtained for human, pig, and rat skin in the measurements of acetylsalicylic acid permeation. With benzoic acid a greater difference was observed; permeability increased in the order pig < rat < human. For both of these compounds the skin of the mouse and hairless mouse was more permeable than that of the other species. With the more slowly penetrating urea, pig, human, and hairless mouse skin gave similar slow results; rat and mouse skin were the most permeable.

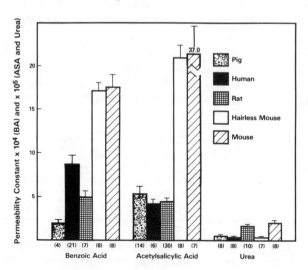

FIGURE 4 Permeability constants obtained with human and animal skin. Values are means ± SE of the number of determinations in parentheses.

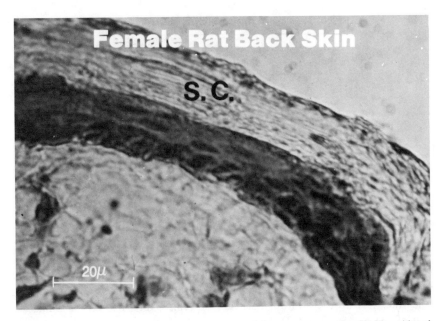

FIGURE 5 Microtome section of frozen rat skin. S.C., stratum corneum. Viable epidermis (layer below S.C.) is stained with Mayer's hematoxylin to facilitate thickness measurements.

It has been recognized that the stratum corneum thickness of different areas of skin should be known for proper interpretation of comparative permeability data (Baker and Kligman, 1967; Holbrook and Odland, 1974). Other factors besides thickness (for instance, lipid composition) are also important. Knowledge of the stratum corneum thickness in addition to permeability data can indicate possible structural differences in the skin at different sites.

Measurements of the thickness of stratum corneum, epidermis, and whole skin were made with frozen sections of skin to overcome the destructive effect on the stratum corneum of standard embedding and fixative procedures. A photomicrograph of a cross section of rat skin is shown in Fig. 5 to illustrate a typical preparation of skin. The viable epidermis layer was stained with Mayer's hematoxylin to facilitate microscopic measurements with an eyepiece micrometer. Table 2 shows the values for the thickness of the stratum corneum, whole epidermis, and whole skin. Of most interest in relation to permeability are the stratum corneum measurements. The thickest stratum corneum (and also whole skin) was that of the pig. The thicknesses of rat (18.4 μm) and human (16.8 μm) stratum corneum were similar to but less than that of pig skin. Rat epidermis and whole skin were only two-thirds as thick as human skin; the relatively thick stratum corneum was due to the composition of the epidermis, which was more than 50% stratum corneum. The stratum corneum of the Swiss mouse was the most permeable barrier and the thinnest (5.8 μm). The thickness of the stratum corneum of the hairless mouse was intermediate between that of human and Swiss mouse skin.

TABLE 2   Human and Animal Skin Thickness Measurements[a]

Type of skin	Stratum corneum (μm)	Epidermis (μm)	Whole skin (mm)
Human (16)	16.8 ± 0.7	46.9 ± 2.3	2.97 ± 0.28
Pig (35)	26.4 ± 0.4	65.8 ± 1.8	3.43 ± 0.05
Rat (9)	18.4 ± 0.5	32.1 ± 1.3	2.09 ± 0.07
Hairless mouse (12)	8.9 ± 0.4	28.6 ± 0.9	0.70 ± 0.02
Mouse (9)	5.8 ± 0.3	12.6 ± 0.8	0.84 ± 0.02

[a]Values are means ± SE for the number of sections shown in parentheses. Three to six sections were taken from each skin sample.

Comparative permeability data from a number of studies are shown in Table 3. Permeability is expressed relative to the absorption found with human skin in each study. Pig skin often gives permeability values similar to those for human skin. Fewer studies have been done with monkey skin, but it also appears similar to human skin. When the skin of the rat has been found to be more permeable than human skin, the differences have not been large. The thickness of the stratum corneum of female rat back skin is similar to that of the human (Table 2).

SEX-RELATED AND REGIONAL
VARIATIONS IN THE RAT

Horhota and Fung (1978) observed that nitroglycerin applied topically to male Sprague-Dawley rats was absorbed more readily through abdominal than back skin. This regional variability in skin permeation was confirmed by Bronaugh et al. (1982c) in Osborne-Mendel rats. These authors also observed a sex-related difference in the permeability properties of rat back skin.

The permeability constants of cortisone, caffeine, water, and urea (water vehicle) were 2–3 times greater when female back skin was used (Table 4). When benzoic acid was examined in a petrolatum vehicle (Table 5), k_p value and lag time differences in male and female rat back skin resulted in substantially increased absorption through female skin in a short-term experiment, where lag times are most important.

The thickness of layers of skin was measured with frozen sections (Table 6). Regional differences in absorption in the male rat and sex-related differences were explained in terms of stratum corneum thickness. Male rat back stratum corneum was twice as thick as that of the female, and an even greater difference was found between the thickness of male back and abdominal stratum corneum. Castration of weanling male rats prevented the sex-related difference in stratum corneum thickness seen in adults, which can therefore be explained in terms of differences in androgen levels.

Other factors besides barrier thickness are likely to be important in determining the site dependence of percutaneous absorption in the rat. Lipids in the stratum corneum are a major factor in absorption, and it is conceivable that their concentrations vary in a regional or sex-related manner. The difference in permeation of water and salicylic acid between human leg and abdominal epidermis has been attributed to differences in lipid content of the stratum corneum of these tissues (Elias et al., 1981).

TABLE 3 Permeability of Animal Skin Relative to Human Skin[a,b]

Reference and compound	Species						
	Pig	Monkey	Rat	Guinea pig	Hairless mouse	Mouse	Rabbit
Bartek et al. (1972)							
N-Acetylcysteine	2.5		1.4				0.8
Benzoic acid[c]		1.4					
Butter yellow	1.9		2.2				4.6
Caffeine	0.7		1.1				1.5
Cortisone	1.2		7.3				9.0
Haloprogin	2.6		3.7				4.4
Hydrocortisone[c]		1.6					
Testosterone[c]	2.2	1.4	3.6				5.3
Tregear (1966)							
Ethylene bromide	0.8		2.3	1.5			
Paraoxon	1.4		3.3	3.0			
Thioglycolic acid	3.3		3.0	2.3			
Water	1.4			1.0			3.3
Andersen et al. (1980)							
Benzoic acid				0.7			
Hydrocortisone				1.3			
Testosterone				2.6			
Chowhan and Pritchard (1978)							
Naproxin			2.3				3.5
Durrheim et al. (1980)							
Butanol					1.8		
Ethanol					1.5		
Octanol					0.6		
Stoughton (1975)							
Betamethasone					1.3		
5-Fluorouracil					1.1		
Hydrocortisone					1.5		
Bronaugh et al. (1982b)							
Acetylsalicylic acid	1.2		1.0		4.9	8.7	
Benzoic acid	0.2		0.6		2.0	2.0	
Urea	1.5		4.8		0.9	5.8	

[a]Human skin in all studies was assigned the value 1.0.
[b]Values from Bartek et al. (1972) and Andersen et al. (1980) were obtained *in vivo*. Other results are from experiments with excised skin.
[c]Data taken completely or in part from Wester and Maibach (1975).

TABLE 4   Effect of Sex and Body Site on Permeability of Rat Skin

	Male		Female	
Compound	k_p (cm/h $\times$ 10⁴)	Lag time (h)	k_p (cm/h $\times$ 10⁴)	Lag time (h)
Caffeine	(B) 3.0 ± 1.2 (A) 6.8 ± 1.0	22.6 ± 5.1 (8) 14.7 ± 1.7 (4)	7.0 ± 1.3	27.2 ± 1.4 (4)
Water	(B) 4.9 ± 0.4 (A) 13.1 ± 2.1	2.4 ± 0.1 (7) 1.7 ± 0.2 (4)	9.3 ± 1.1	2.0 ± 0.1 (4)
Urea	(B) 1.6 ± 0.5 (A) 18.8 ± 5.5	15.0 ± 1.8 (6) 16.5 ± 4.3 (4)	4.8 ± 1.3	11.1 ± 0.6 (3)
Cortisone	(B) 1.7 ± 0.4 (A) 12.2 ± 0.6	33.4 ± 4.4 (8) 32.9 ± 2.4 (4)	4.7 ± 1.1	20.0 ± 2.6 (3)

[a]Each value is the mean ± SE of the number of determinations in parentheses. Compounds were applied to excised skin in a water vehicle; (B), back; (A), abdomen.

Regional differences in permeation were also observed in the monkey (Wester et al., 1980). As in humans (Feldmann and Maibach, 1967), the ventral forearm had low permeability and the scalp was 2–3 times as permeable. The back and abdominal regions were not examined. With male hairless mouse skin, Behl et al. (1980) found similar absorption in the back and abdominal regions. Little difference was observed in the permeability of human skin in these two regions (Feldmann and Maibach, 1967; Maibach et al., 1971).

PREDICTION OF PERCUTANEOUS ABSORPTION FROM PHYSICAL CHEMICAL DATA

Certain chemical properties are important for good absorption of a compound. Awareness of these properties is important even for percutaneous absorption studies, since it can help in designing the sampling regimen and evaluating experimental results.

Best absorption is obtained with smaller molecules (molecular weight < 400). Solubility in the barrier is extremely important to facilitate the diffusion process. Lipoidal compounds are absorbed well, but they encounter hydrophilic regions in the skin—the keratin matrix of the stratum corneum and the viable tissue of the epidermis and dermis. Best absorption is therefore obtained with compounds that also have some water solubility.

Lipid:water partition coefficients have been correlated with permeation of the skin. This was observed by Scheuplein et al. (1969) with steroids in (1) amyl caproate and water and (2) hexadecane and water. Michaels et al. (1975) found a good correlation between the permeability constants of 10 drugs and their mineral oil:water partition coefficients. Hansch and Dunn (1972) preferred

TABLE 5 Regional and Sex-Related Differences in Absorption
of Benzoic Acid

Type of skin	Permeability constant (cm/h)	Lag time (h)	Percent of applied dose (after 5 h)
Male			
Back (10)	$3.0 \pm 0.3 \times 10^{-4}$	6.0 ± 0.2	0.5 ± 0.07
Abdomen (13)	$2.9 \pm 0.4 \times 10^{-4}$	1.0 ± 0.1	5.1 ± 0.9
Female			
Back (7)	$4.5 \pm 0.8 \times 10^{-4}$	3.5 ± 0.1	2.5 ± 0.6
Abdomen (13)	$4.4 \pm 0.6 \times 10^{-4}$	1.2 ± 0.2	6.5 ± 0.9

[a]Each value is the mean ± SE of the number of determinations in parentheses.

octanol as the model liquid for membrane lipids, in part because of the OH group, which permits hydrogen bonding. An extensive list of compounds and their octanol:water partition coefficients has been published (Leo et al., 1971).

Anjo et al. (1980) found an excellent correlation between the *in vivo* half-life of penetration in humans and benzene solubility with a series of steroids. It is important to relate penetration to its actual solubility in model lipid solvents and water. The ratio (partition coefficient) will be misleading—until a certain minimum solubility occurs.

CONCLUSION

The studies summarized present the current data base that permits or limits the extrapolation from the *in vitro* experiment to penetration in the

TABLE 6 Rat Skin Thickness Measurements
from Frozen Sections

Type of skin	Skin thickness		
	Stratum corneum (μm)	Whole epidermis (μm)	Whole skin (mm)
Male			
Back	34.7 ± 2.3	61.1 ± 3.0	2.80 ± 0.08
Abdomen	13.8 ± 0.7	30.4 ± 1.5	1.66 ± 0.06
Female			
Back	18.2 ± 1.0	31.2 ± 1.5	2.04 ± 0.05
Abdomen	13.7 ± 0.6	34.8 ± 1.8	0.93 ± 0.02

[a]Each value is the mean ± SE of 36 measurements for each layer of skin.

living animal and human. When one considers the complexity of steps involved in penetration (Chapter 3), it is surprising that we have as many reasonable correlations as we do. *In vitro* absorption measurements can be used with greatest confidence when they can be correlated with *in vivo* studies.

REFERENCES

Ainsworth, M. 1960. Methods for measuring percutaneous absorption. *J. Soc. Cosmet. Chem.* 11:69–78.

Andersen, K. E., Maibach, H. I., and Anjo, M. D. 1980. The guinea pig: An animal model for human skin absorption of hydrocortisone, testosterone and benzoic acid? *Br. J. Dermatol.* 102:447–453.

Anjo, D. M., Feldmann, R. J., and Maibach, H. I. 1980. Methods for predicting percutaneous penetration in man. In *Percutaneous Absorption of Steroids*, eds. P. Mauvis-Jarvis, C. F. H. Vickers, and J. Wepierre, pp. 31–51. London: Academic.

Baker, H. and Kligman, A. M. 1967. A simple *in vivo* method for studying the permeability of the human stratum corneum. *J. Invest. Dermatol.* 48:273–274.

Bartek, M. J., Labudde, J. A., and Maibach, H. I. 1972. Skin permeability *in vivo*: Comparison in rat, rabbit, pig and man. *J. Invest. Dermatol.* 58:114–123.

Behl, C. R., Flynn, G. L., Kurihara, T., Harper, N., Smith, W., Higuchi, W. I., Ho, N. F. H., and Pierson, C. L. 1980. Hydration and percutaneous absorption. I. Influence of hydration on alkanol permeation through hairless mouse skin. *J. Invest. Dermatol.* 75:346–352.

Bronaugh, R. L., Congdon, E. R., and Scheuplein, R. J. 1981. The effect of cosmetic vehicles on the penetration of *N*-nitrosodiethanolamine through excised human skin. *J. Invest. Dermatol.* 76:94–96.

Bronaugh, R. L., Stewart, R. F., Congdon, E. R., and Giles, A. L. 1982a. Methods for *in vitro* percutaneous absorption studies. I. Comparison with *in vivo* results. *Toxicol. Appl. Pharmacol.* 62:474–480.

Bronaugh, R. L., Stewart, R. F., and Congdon, E. R. 1982b. Methods for *in vitro* percutaneous absorption studies. II. Animal models for human skin. *Toxicol. Appl. Pharmacol.* 62:481–488.

Bronaugh, R. L., Stewart, R. F., and Congdon, E. R. 1982c. Methods for *in vitro* percutaneous absorption studies. III. Differences in permeability of rat skin related to sex and body site. *Toxicol. Appl. Pharmacol.*, in press.

Burch, G. E. and Winsor, T. 1944. Rate of insensible perspiration locally through living and through dead human skin. *Arch. Intern. Med.* 74:437–444.

Chow, C., Chow, A. Y. K., Downie, R. H., and Buttar, H. S. 1978. Percutaneous absorption of hexachlorophene in rats, guinea pigs and pigs. *Toxicology* 9:147–154.

Crutcher, W. and Maibach, H. I. 1969. The effect of perfusion rate on *in vitro* percutaneous penetration. *J. Invest. Dermatol.* 53:264–269.

Chowhan, Z. T. and Pritchard, R. 1978. Naproxin I: Comparison of rabbit, rat and human skin. *J. Pharm. Sci.* 67:1272–1274.

Durrheim, H., Flynn, G. L., Higuchi, W. I., and Behl, C. R. 1980. Permeation of hairless mouse skin. I. Experimental methods and comparison with human epidermal permeation by alkanols. *J. Pharm. Sci.* 69:781–786.

Elias, P. M., Cooper, E. R., Korc, A., and Brown, B. E. 1981. Percutaneous transport in relation to stratum corneum structure and lipid composition. *J. Invest. Dermatol.* 76:297–301.

Feldmann, R. J. and Maibach, H. I. 1967. Regional variation in percutaneous penetration of ^{14}C-cortisol in man. *J. Invest. Dermatol.* 48:181–183.

Feldmann, R. J. and Maibach, H. I. 1970. Absorption of some organic compounds through the skin in man. *J. Invest. Dermatol.* 54:399–404.

Franz, T. J. 1975. Percutaneous absorption. On the relevance of *in vitro* data. *J. Invest. Dermatol.* 64:190–195.

Franz, T. J. 1978. The finite dose technique as a valid *in vitro* model for the study of percutaneous absorption. *Curr. Probl. Dermatol.* 7:58–68.

Galey, W. R., Lansdale, H. K., and Nacht, S. 1976. The *in vitro* permeability of skin and buccal mucosa to selected drugs and tritiated water. *J. Invest. Dermatol.* 67:713–717.

Hansch, R. and Dunn, W. J. 1972. Linear relationships between lipophilic character and biological activity of drugs. *J. Pharm. Sci.* 61:1–19.

Holbrook, K. A. and Odland, G. F. 1974. Regional differences in the thickness (cell layers) of the human stratum corneum: An ultrastructural analysis. *J. Invest. Dermatol.* 62:415–422.

Horhota, S. T. and Fung, H. L. 1978. Site dependence for topical nitroglycerin absorption in rats. *J. Pharm. Sci.* 67:1345–1346.

Leo, A., Hansch, C., and Elkins, D. 1971. Partition coefficients and their uses. *Chem. Rev.* 71:525–616.

Maibach, H. I., Feldmann, R. J., Milby, T. H., and Serat, W. F. 1971. Regional variation in percutaneous penetration in man: Pesticides. *Arch. Environ. Health* 23:208–211.

Marzulli, F. N. and Maibach, H. I. 1975. Relevance of animal models: The hexachlorophene story. In *Animal Models in Dermatology*, ed. H. I. Maibach, pp. 156–167. Edinburgh: Churchill Livingstone.

Marzulli, F. N., Brown, D. W. G., and Maibach, H. I. 1969. Techniques for studying skin penetration. *Toxicol. Appl. Pharmacol.* 3 (Suppl.):76–83.

Michaels, A. S., Chandrasekaran, S. K., and Shaw, J. E. 1975. Drug permeation through human skin: Theory and *in vitro* experimental measurements. *AIChE J.* 21:985–996.

Scheuplein, R. J., Blank, I. H., Brauner, G. J., and MacFarlane, D. J. 1969. Percutaneous absorption of steroids. *J. Invest. Dermatol.* 52:63–70.

Sekura, D. and Scala, J. 1972. The percutaneous absorption of alkyl methyl sulfoxides. In *Pharmacology and the Skin*, eds. W. Montagna, E. Van Scott, and R. Stoughton, pp. 257–269. New York: Appleton-Century-Crofts.

Stoughton, R. B. 1975. Animal models for *in vitro* percutaneous absorption. In *Animal Models in Dermatology*, ed. H. I. Maibach, pp. 121–132. Edinburgh: Churchill Livingstone.

Tregear, R. T. 1966. Molecular movement, the permeability of skin. In *Physical Functions of Skin*, pp. 1–52. New York: Academic.

Wahlberg, J. E. 1973. Percutaneous absorption. *Curr. Probl. Dermatol.* 5:1.

Wester, R. C. and Maibach, H. I. 1975. Percutaneous absorption in the rhesus monkey compared to man. *Toxicol. Appl. Pharmacol.* 32:394–398.

Wester, R. C., Noonan, P. K., and Maibach, H. I. 1980. Variations in percutaneous absorption of testosterone in the rhesus monkey due to anatomic site of application and frequency of application. *Arch. Dermatol. Res.* 267:229–235.

5

in vivo percutaneous absorption

Ronald C. Wester ■ Howard I. Maibach

INTRODUCTION

Percutaneous absorption is a primary focal point for dermatotoxicology and dermatopharmacology. Local and systemic toxicity depend on a chemical penetrating the skin. The skin is both a barrier to absorption and a primary route to the systemic circulation. The skin's barrier properties are impressive. Fluids and precious chemicals are reasonably retained within the body, while at the same time hundreds of foreign chemicals are restricted from entering the systemic circulation. Many pharmacologists and physicians have been frustrated in their attempts to deliver drugs to and through the skin.

Even with these impressive barrier properties, the skin is a primary body contact with the environment and the route by which many chemicals enter the body. In most instances the toxicity of the chemical is slight and/or the bioavailability (rate and amount of absorption) of the chemical is too low to cause an immediate response. However, some chemicals applied to the skin have proved to be toxic. In addition, potentially toxic chemicals that come in contact with the skin continue to be discovered.

This chapter deals with the methods used to study *in vivo* percutaneous absorption and the many factors affecting it. The interpretation of such studies should be restricted to the limits of the study design. The methodology and supportive information discussed here should help formulate good study design.

METHODS USED TO DETERMINE *IN VIVO*
PERCUTANEOUS ABSORPTION

Percutaneous absorption *in vivo* is usually determined by the indirect method of measuring radioactivity in excreta following topical application of the labeled compound. In human studies, plasma levels of the compound are extremely low following topical application, often below assay detection level, so it is necessary to use tracer methodology. The labeled compound, usually carbon-14 or tritium, is applied to the skin. The total amount of radioactivity excreted in urine (or urine plus feces) is then determined. The amount of radioactivity retained in the body or excreted by some route not assayed (CO_2, sweat) is corrected by determining the amount of radioactivity excreted following parenteral administration. This final amount of radioactivity is then expressed as the percent of the applied dose that was absorbed (Feldmann and Maibach, 1969a).

The equation used to determine percutaneous absorption is:

$$\text{Percent} = \frac{\text{total radioactivity following topical administration}}{\text{total radioactivity following parenteral administration}} \times 100$$

Determination of percutaneous absorption from urinary radioactivity excretion does not account for metabolism by skin. The radioactivity in urine is a mixture of parent compound and metabolites. Plasma radioactivity can be measured and the percutaneous absorption determined by the ratio of the areas under the plasma concentration versus time curves following topical and intravenous administration (Wester and Noonan, 1978). Radioactivity in blood and excreta can include both the applied compound and metabolites. If the metabolism by skin is extensive and different from that of other systemic tissues, then this method is not valid because the pharmacokinetics of the metabolites can be different from that of the parent compound. However, in practice, this method has given results similar to those obtained from urinary excretion (Wester et al., 1981).

The only way to determine the absolute bioavailability of a topically applied compound is to measure the compound by specific assay in blood or urine following topical and intravenous administration. This is difficult to do since plasma concentrations after topical administration are often very low. However, as more sensitive assays are developed, estimates of absolute topical bioavailability will become a reality.

A comparison of the above methods was performed by using [14C]-nitroglycerin in rhesus monkeys (Table 1). Bioavailability estimated from urinary excretion of radioactivity was $72.7 \pm 5.8\%$. This was similar to the $77.2 \pm 6.7\%$ estimated from plasma total radioactivity AUC (area under the plasma concentration versus time curve). The absolute bioavailability estimated

TABLE 1 Bioavailability of Topical Nitroglycerin
Determined from Plasma Nitroglycerin, Plasma
^{14}C, and Urinary Excretion of ^{14}C[a]

Method	Mean bioavailability (%)
Plasma nitroglycerin AUC[b]	56.6 ± 2.5
Plasma total radioactivity AUC[b]	77.2 ± 6.7
Urinary total radioactivity[c]	72.7 ± 5.8

[a]See Wester et al. (1981) for details.
[b]Absolute bioavailability of nitroglycerin and ^{14}C:

$$\text{Percent} = \frac{\text{AUC (ng·h/ml)/topical dose}}{\text{AUC (ng·h/ml)/iv dose}} \times 100$$

[c]Percent = (total ^{14}C excretion following topical administration)/(total ^{14}C excretion following iv administration) × 100.

from plasma nitroglycerin unchanged compound AUCs was 56.6 ± 2.5%. The difference between the estimate of absolute bioavailability (56.6%) and that of ^{14}C (72.7-77.2%) is the percent of compound metabolized in the skin as the compound was being absorbed. For nitroglycerin this is about 20% (Wester et al., 1981).

Another approach used to determine *in vivo* percutaneous absorption is to measure the loss of radioactive material from the surface as it penetrates the skin. Recovery of an ointment or solution following skin application is difficult because total recovery from the skin is never assured. With topical application of a transdermal delivery device, the total unit can be removed from the skin and the residual amount of drug in the device can be determined. The difference between the applied and the residual dose is assumed to be the amount of drug absorbed. One must be aware that the skin may act as a reservoir for unabsorbed material.

Another *in vivo* method of estimating absorption is to use a biological/pharmacological response (McKenzie and Stoughton, 1962). Here, a biological assay is substituted for a chemical assay and absorption is estimated. An obvious disadvantage to the use of a biological response is that it is only good for compounds that will elicit an easily measurable response. An example of a biological response would be the vasoconstrictor assay when the blanching effect of one compound is compared to that of a known compound. This method is perhaps more qualitative than quantitative.

Other qualitative methods of estimating *in vivo* percutaneous absorption include whole body autoradiography and fluorescence. Whole body autoradiography will given an overall picture of dermal absorption followed by the involvement of other body tissues with the absorbed compound.

PARAMETERS THAT AFFECT *IN VIVO* PERCUTANEOUS ABSORPTION

Drug Concentration and Surface Area

When a compound comes in contact with skin the amount of absorption will depend on many parameters. Foremost among these parameters are concentration of applied dose and surface area. As the concentration of applied dose increases, the efficiency of absorption (percent) can change. However, a more relevant point is that as the amount applied is increased the total amount absorbed into the body increases (Wester and Maibach, 1976; Scheuplein and Ross, 1974). The other parameter, closely associated with dose, is surface area. Increasing the area of surface on which the dose is applied increases the absorption (Noonan and Wester, 1980). Therefore, the greatest potential for percutaneous absorption can occur when a high concentration of compound is spread over a large part of the body.

Skin Site of Application

Variation in absorption occurs depending on the anatomic site of application. This is true for both humans (Feldmann and Maibach, 1967; Maibach et al., 1971) and animals (Wester et al., 1980b). Presented in Table 2 is a brief outline of some data derived from *in vivo* absorption of hydrocortisone after application to various anatomic sites (Feldmann and Maibach, 1967). The data are of obvious practical significance in that increased total absorption is found for head, neck, and axilla, where both cosmetic and environmental exposure are greater. Preliminary results indicate that the female genitalia show greater absorption than forearm skin surfaces (not mucosa), but less absorption than scrotal skin. Similar anatomic variation has been shown for pesticides (Maibach et al., 1971). With the wide variety of chemical moieties examined (steroids, pesticides, and antimicrobials) the general pattern of regional varia-

TABLE 2 Penetration of Hydrocortisone in Humans at Various Anatomic Sites

Anatomic site	Penetration ratio
Forearm (ventral)	1.0
Forearm (dorsal)	1.1
Foot (plantar)	0.14
Ankle (lateral)	0.42
Palm	0.83
Back	1.7
Scalp	3.5
Axilla	3.6
Forehead	6.0
Jaw angle	13.0
Scrotum	42.0

TABLE 3   Penetration of Hydrocortisone
through Modified Skin

Treatment	Penetration ratio
None	1
Strip	4
Occlude	10
Cantharidine blister	15
Strip plus occlude	20

tion holds. One exception was carbaryl, which was extensively absorbed from the forearm, although other sites were not significantly higher. This suggests that carbaryl is extensively absorbed from all body sites.

Occlusion

Percutaneous absorption is increased if the site of application is occluded. Occlusion is a covering of the application site, either intentionally as with bandaging or unintentionally as by putting on clothing after applying a topical compound. A vehicle such as an ointment can also have occlusive properties. Occlusion results in a combination of many physical factors affecting the skin and the applied compound. It changes the hydration and temperature of the skin, and these physical factors affect absorption. It also prevents the accidental wiping off or evaporation (volatile compound) of the applied compound.

Skin Condition

There are skin conditions other than hydration and temperature that affect percutaneous absorption. The most obvious is loss of barrier function of the stratum corneum through disease or damage. Skin also changes with age. The genesis of the stratum corneum occurs during gestation and is probably concluded by birth (Singer et al., 1971). Preterm infants probably do not have a fully developed stratum corneum and therefore may have increased skin permeability (Nachman and Esterly, 1971). The skin of the elderly also undergoes change and this may influence absorption. Virtually any type of change in skin condition, especially in the barrier function of the stratum corneum, whether natural or inflicted, may change the percutaneous absorption of the skin.

Shown in Table 3 are the results of removal of the stratum corneum with cellophane tape stripping, occlusion with plastic film, removal of the epidermis with cantharidin, and the combination of stripping and occlusion (Feldmann and Maibach, 1965). Stripping the skin with tape until it glistens removes the stratum corneum and causes damage to the upper layers of the epidermis; this is a model for damaged and diseased skin. Stripped skin shows a fourfold increase in penetration of hydrocortisone. Occluding the hydrocortisone with a plastic film during the first 24 h causes a 10-fold increase in absorption over that of unoccluded skin. Recent work (unpublished) at our laboratory indicates that trapping of water under the occlusive layer is necessary for this increased penetration. Removal of the epidermis by topical application of a cantharidin solution leaves a denuded skin site, which absorbs 15 times more hydrocortisone than untreated skin. The greatest absorption was obtained by stripping followed by a 24-h occlusion, yielding penetration 20 times the value for normal skin.

It is commonly stated that the stratum corneum is the major barrier to percutaneous penetration. This is generally true for intact skin. Fortunately, when the stratum corneum is damaged the other layers function as barriers to penetration, as evidenced by these data; none of the damages inflicted on the skin caused 100% absorption. Presumably, each epidermal cell membrane, the basement membrane, and other cellular structures must also have barrier properties.

Vehicle

Percutaneous absorption of a drug from a vehicle depends on the partitioning of the drug between the vehicle and the skin and the solubility of the drug in the vehicle. In addition to drug solubility, factors such as drug concentration and pH may influence the interaction between vehicle, drug, and skin. The vehicle may change the integrity of the skin and this will influence absorption. An example would be an occlusive vehicle, which would alter skin hydration. Vehicles can contain an agent such as urea that will enhance percutaneous absorption, or the vehicle itself will enhance absorption. The best example of the latter is dimethyl sulfoxide (DMSO), which readily permeates skin and causes enhanced absorption. In most cases the vehicle disappears quickly, and its destination is not determined. The increase in absorption observed with DMSO may be due to changes in the horny layer, shown by significant decreases in electrical resistance after treatment. Others have attempted to enhance penetration by employing bases with lower solvency for the active compound than the skin lipids. With lower solubility in the carrier it is expected that the compound would preferentially diffuse into the skin. This effect was not observed with mineral oil and propylene glycol, which are poor hydrocortisone solvents but produced no significant change in penetration effects (Anjo et al., 1980).

Multiple Dose Application

Percutaneous absorption studies are usually conducted with a single application. By some analytical means the amount absorbed is determined and the percentage of absorption of that compound is calculated. This is a standard absorption study. Some question remains as to its relevance to the clinical situation, where a topically administered compound (prescribed or exposed contamination) is usually applied more frequently than once per day

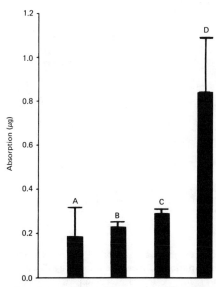

FIGURE 1 Effect of frequency of application on percutaneous absorption of hydrocortisone from ventral forearm of rhesus monkey. Ordinate is micrograms absorbed. Bar A, 13.3 μg/cm^2 applied once at 9:00 a.m. Bars B and C, 40 μg/cm^2 applied in divided doses of 13.3 μg/cm^2 at 9:00 a.m., 2:30 p.m., and 9:00 p.m. The site of application was washed between divided doses for C, but not for B. Bar D, 40 μg/cm^2 applied at 9:00 a.m.

and the topical exposure is usually on a chronic basis. This is a new area in the pharmacokinetics of skin absorption.

Figure 1 shows the percutaneous absorption of hydrocortisone following a single application of 40 μg/cm^2 and the same amount applied in divided doses. The total amounts absorbed per 24-h application are different. Absorption from one application of the high concentration was greater than absorption from the same concentration applied in equally divided doses (Wester et al., 1977b, 1980b). This suggests that the absorption from subsequent applications was influenced by the first topical application.

Skin has been referred to as a reservoir. Compounds will reside in skin for days or weeks and continue to release material into the general circulation (Vickers, 1980). Perhaps in the above study the first application saturated or altered the reservoir capacity, and this in turn changed the absorption of subsequent applications. A practical consideration based on the above study is that in clinical practice, one daily application of a topical drug may be all that is needed for some disease entities.

The other relevant deviation from acute administration studies is that of

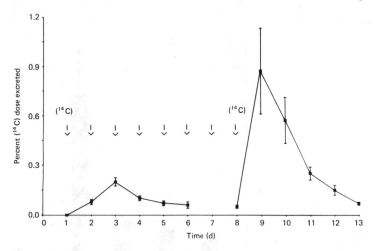

FIGURE 2 Percutaneous absorption of hydrocortisone following acute and chronic administration. Arrows represent application of hydrocortisone (13.3 μg/cm²), and ¹⁴C indicates where [¹⁴C] hydrocortisone was applied.

chronic administration. Absorption of hydrocortisone can significantly increase during chronic administration (Wester et al., 1980a) (Fig. 2). Hydrocortisone causes atrophy, which is a thinning of the skin. Since the stratum corneum is the main barrier to percutaneous absorption, chronic administration of hydrocortisone may decrease the barrier function, resulting in enhanced absorption. The relevance to *in vivo* percutaneous absorption is that the skin is a viable tissue, able to change or respond to topical administration. Similarly, with chronic administration of salicylic acid, the penetration flux increased during the first 5 d of application, then decreased with weekly application (Roberts and Horlock, 1978). The authors suggested that the initial applications altered the skin's barrier function, which resulted in the different absorption for subsequent applications.

Metabolism

Skin metabolism is discussed in Chapters 1 and 2. However, there is a relation between metabolism and percutaneous absorption that can be discussed here. A single chemical entity is applied to the skin, but what enters the systemic circulation is that chemical entity and its metabolites. Percutaneous first-pass metabolism is defined as the metabolism of the compound as it is absorbed through the skin. This is about 16–20% for topical nitroglycerin (Wester et al., 1981) and about 100% for benzoyl peroxide (Nacht et al., 1981).

In both *in vitro* and *in vivo* percutaneous absorption studies, amounts and rates of absorption are determined from radioactivity counting. The implication is that the rates and amounts represent the applied compound, whereas in fact they represent the applied compound and its metabolites. Unless the applied parent compound is measured by a specific assay, the existence of metabolites must be assumed.

In the preceding section the capacity of the skin to change or respond to the applied compound was discussed. This also applies to skin metabolism and the subsequent percutaneous absorption. Skin metabolic enzymes, like other metabolic enzymes, can be induced. For example, chronic administration of coal tar products can change the metabolic activity of skin. This or other inducing products can be applied as part of the treatment course or added in the vehicle used to deliver a particular compound. What this means for *in vivo* percutaneous absorption is that the ratio of parent compound to metabolites may be different in single and in chronic administration.

COMPARATIVE *IN VIVO* STUDIES

The basic data for *in vivo* human percutaneous absorption, to which animal models are compared, were obtained by Feldmann and Maibach (1969a, 1969b, 1974). In these clinical studies a specific concentration of radioactive compound was applied to a specific nonoccluded anatomic site and the subjects were requested not to wash the area for 24 h.

Bartek et al. (1972) undertook a comparative study of percutaneous absorption in rats, rabbits, miniature swine, and humans. The methodology used with animals was similar to that used with humans, except that in animals the compounds were applied to the back and the skin was shaved. Radioactive compounds were applied to the skin in the same manner that had been used with humans. A nonoccluding device was used to keep the animal from removing the applied compound.

Haloprogin, a topical antifungal agent, was completely absorbed in the rat and the rabbit. Penetration through the skin of pigs and humans was similar and much slower than it was through rat and rabbit skin. Penetration of acetylcysteine was minimal in all species. Cortisone, a minimal penetrant through the skin of humans and miniature swine, was well absorbed in the rat and rabbit. Caffeine readily penetrated the skin of all species. With butter yellow (dimethylaminoazobenzene), penetration through rabbit skin was much greater than through the skin of the other three species. Testosterone penetration was greatest in the rabbit, followed closely by the rat and then the pig, which was closest to humans. The results of this study showed rabbit skin to be the most permeable to topically applied compounds, followed closely by rat skin. In contrast, it appears that the permeability of the skin of the miniature swine is closer to that of human skin. Clearly, percutaneous absorption in the rabbit and rat would not be predictive of that in humans. It is not known whether the subtle differences seen between pig and human skin were due to methodology (site of application, shaving) or the skin itself. However, in general the pig appears to be a good predictor of percutaneous absorption in humans.

Bartek and La Budde (1975) also studied the percutaneous absorption of pesticides in the rabbit, pig, and squirrel monkey and compared the results with the absorption observed in humans. The compounds were applied to the backs of animals and compared with application to the human ventral forearm. DDT was a minimal penetrant in humans, whereas in the rabbit and pig penetration rates were considerably greater. Absorption in the squirrel monkey was very low; however, the value reported was uncorrected with parenteral control data. Penetration of lindane, parathion, and malathion in the rabbit exceeded that in the other species. With lindane, penetration in the squirrel monkey was closer to that in humans, whereas with parathion, penetration in the pig was closest to that in humans. Penetration of malathion was similar in the squirrel monkey and the pig and could be predictive of that in humans. It appears that the *in vivo* percutaneous absorption of pesticides in the rabbit was again much greater than in humans, whereas penetration in the pig and squirrel monkey was closer to that in humans.

Several comparisons of percutaneous absorption in the rhesus monkey and in humans have been made (Wester and Maibach, 1975a, 1975b, 1976, 1977; Wester and Noonan, 1980; Wester et al., 1979). The methodology and site of application (ventral forearm) were the same for both species. The site of application was lightly clipped in the monkey. [A direct comparison of unshaven and lightly clipped skin showed no difference in absorption (Wester and Maibach, 1975a).] The *in vivo* percutaneous absorption and dose response for hydrocortisone, testosterone, and benzoic acid were similar for rhesus monkeys and humans.

Hunziker et al. (1978) studied the percutaneous absorption of ^{14}C-labeled benzoic acid, progesterone, and testosterone in the Mexican hairless dog and compared the absorption with that observed in humans. Total absorption and maximum absorption rates were greater in humans than in the hairless dog. Surface counting experiments showed that benzoic acid and progesterone persisted on the dog skin far longer than on human skin.

In several of the preceding studies the percutaneous absorption of testosterone was determined. In these studies the same topical concentration (4 mcg/cm^2) and method of analysis (determination of urinary ^{14}C excretion) were used. Table 4 summarizes the results. Absorption of testosterone in the rat and rabbit was high compared to that in humans. Absorption in the pig was approximately twice that in humans, and the rhesus monkey was closest to humans. The site of application for the rat, rabbit, and pig was the back, whereas for the rhesus monkey and human the site of application was the ventral forearm. Percutaneous absorption of testosterone in the rhesus monkey and human varies with site of application. What proportions of the variation in the above comparison are due to species and to site of application are not known. However, the comparison points out that when a difference is found, it could be a sum of the many variabilities in the study.

The comparative *in vivo* data that have been reviewed demonstrate that

TABLE 4 Percutaneous Absorption of Testosterone
in Several Species

Species	Percent of dose absorbed	Ratio
Human	13.2	1.0
Rhesus monkey	18.4	1.4
Pig	29.4	2.2
Guinea pig	34.9	2.6
Rat	47.4	3.6
Rabbit	69.6	5.3

percutaneous absorption in the pig and monkey (rhesus and squirrel) is similar to that in humans, whereas in the rat, and especially in the rabbit, skin penetration is greater than that observed in humans. The skin of the Mexican hairless dog has significantly different permeability characteristics than human skin.

This discussion does not mean that a suitable animal model has been developed. In fact, old models are continually being evaluated and new models are being pursued. Andersen et al. (1980) determined the percutaneous absorption of hydrocortisone, testosterone, and benzoic acid in the guinea pig. Absorption of hydrocortisone and benzoic acid was similar to that in humans, but testosterone was absorbed to a greater extent in the guinea pig. The absorption value for testosterone was closer to the human value if the excretion of radioactivity in urine and feces was measured rather than that in urine alone. If a large proportion of the radioactivity is excreted in feces, a more accurate estimate of the percutaneous absorption can be obtained by determining the radioactivity excretion in both urine and feces. Another animal model available for percutaneous absorption studies is the hairless mouse, with and without a thymus. With thymus-deficient hairless mice, skin from other species (including humans) can be transplanted and the percutaneous absorption through the transplanted skin determined (Kruger and Shelby, 1981).

IN VIVO AND *IN VITRO*
PERCUTANEOUS ABSORPTION

Franz (1975) evaluated the permeability of 12 organic compounds *in vitro* in excised human skin and compared the results to those obtained previously by Feldmann and Maibach in living humans. Care was taken to ensure that the *in vitro* conditions closely followed those used *in vivo*, although it was necessary to use human abdominal skin for the *in vitro* studies. Also, the doses employed ranged from 4 to 40 mcg/cm^2, with the assumption that the percent of applied dose absorbed would not be dose dependent. Quantitatively, the *in vitro* and *in vivo* data did not agree. The *in vitro* method was of value to the extent that it tended to distinguish compounds of low permeability from those of high permeability. However, there are notable differences, suggesting that the *in vitro* method alone would not always be a reliable or accurate predictor of percutaneous absorption in living humans. A more recent presentation by Franz (1979) suggested that many of the differences in the above studies were due to technical reasons. Future work in this area may prove the *in vitro* method to be predictive of *in vivo* absorption.

PERCUTANEOUS ABSORPTION
IN THE NEONATE

Little is known about percutaneous absorption in the infant. Yet it is in the infant where the greatest toxicological response has been seen following topical administration.

In studies with animals (rat and guinea pig) the development of the stratum corneum was observed through fetal life (Singer et al., 1971). The genesis of the permeability barrier starts in the last quarter of gestation and is concluded just before term. At birth, the ultrastructure of the stratum corneum is indistinguishable from that of the adult. We do not know when barrier function is complete in the human infant. However, a normal full-term infant probably has a fully developed stratum corneum with complete barrier function (Rasmusseñ, 1979).

The preterm infant does not have intact barrier function. Nachman and Esterly (1971) suggested that preterm infants have increased skin permeability. This was evaluated by observing the blanching response to topically applied Neo-Synephrine. Infants at 28–34 wk gestational age had a rapid response, infants at 35–37 wk responded less dramatically, and infants at 38–42 wk in most instances failed to respond. This is indirect evidence of skin permeability; however, it is consistent with the animal data. Preterm infants probably do not have intact barrier function and would show enhanced skin permeability.

If preterm infants are susceptible to enhanced skin penetration, they would also be more susceptible to systemic toxicity from a topically applied compound. Greaves et al. (1975) determined the concentration of hexachlorophene in serial blood samples from seven premature infants washed with pHisohex. Systemic absorption was detected at 4 h. Peak blood levels occurred between d 2 and d 4 after a single application on the first day of life. Peak blood levels of hexachlorophene were in the range 0.75–1.37 mcg/ml. These levels were considerably higher than those observed in full-term infants who had undergone the same washing procedure. Greaves et al. concluded that dermal absorption of hexachlorophene was greater in premature than in full-term infants. If this is true for hexachlorophene, it might be true for other toxic material applied to the skin of premature infants.

Percutaneous absorption in the newborn rhesus monkey was assessed (Wester et al., 1977a). The study showed that absorption of testosterone in the full-term newborn was the same as that in the adult. With one other newborn rhesus, a topical dose of 40 mcg/cm^2 testosterone was applied to the ventral forearm and the area was occluded with Saran wrap and adhesive tape for 24 h. Percutaneous absorption was 14.7%, which was twice the value for nonoccluded absorption.

The study showed that a high percentage of a steroid can be absorbed through the skin of an infant. It also suggested an interesting relation between the skin surface area of a newborn and the systemic availability of the applied compound. Once the compound (and/or metabolites) is absorbed, it is available systemically. In the newborn the ratio of surface area (square centimeters) to body weight (kilograms) is three times that in the adult. Therefore, given an equal application area of skin in the newborn and adult, the systemic absorption seen in the newborn can be much more when based on kilograms of body weight. After topical application of the same strength of compound to both the adult and the newborn, the systemic availability in the newborn is 2.7 times that in the adult (Table 5). With a different ratio of skin surface to body weight, the therapeutic ratio is probably lower in the newborn than in the adult when the compound is applied topically. This increased systemic availability in the newborn would also be related to any differences in systemic metabolism between the newborn and the adult.

PHARMACOKINETICS OF PERCUTANEOUS ABSORPTION

Most of the preceding discussion of percutaneous absorption has, in fact, been a discussion of pharmacokinetics. In particular, it has been a discussion of bioavailability from a percutaneous route of administration. Bioavailability can be defined as the rate and extent to which the administered drug ingredient or therapeutic moiety is absorbed from a drug formulation and becomes available at the site of drug action and/or reaches the general circulation. We have extensively discussed this for a topically applied chemical. Other pharmacokinetic parameters are the distribution, metabolism, and excretion of the applied chemical. Distribution can be in the layers of skin or in all tissues of

TABLE 5 Systemic Availability in Newborn
and Adult following Topical Application

Parameter	Adult[a]	Infant[b]
Surface area, cm^2	17,000	2,200 (13% of adult)
Topical dose, mg	100	13 (13% of adult)
Patient weight, kg	70	3.4 (neonate)

[a] Systemic dose = (100 mg × 0.2)/(70 kg) = 0.28 mg/kg (0.2 represents 20% of compound absorbed).
[b] Systemic dose = (13 mg × 0.2)/(3.4 kg) = 0.76 mg/kg.

the body through the general circulation. Metabolism can be a two-way street. A toxic chemical can be detoxified by metabolism. Skin and other tissue enzymes can also be induced. The enzymes can then form toxic metabolites. The rate of excretion is important, for it also determines the steady-state concentration of chemical within the body. For example, the absorption of hexachlorophene is slow; however, excretion from the body is also very slow. As a result, steady-state blood levels can quickly reach toxic values (Marzulli and Maibach, 1975).

Therefore, with percutaneous absorption we focus on the bioavailability potential of a chemical. However, the potential toxicity or effective therapeutic dose may depend on the total pharmacokinetics of the chemical.

DISCUSSION

In vivo percutaneous absorption is a complex biological process. The skin is a multilayered biomembrane that has certain absorption characteristics. If the skin were a simple inert membrane, absorption parameters could easily be measured and they would be fairly constant provided there was no change in the chemistry of the membrane. However, skin is a dynamic living tissue, and its absorption parameters are susceptible to constant change. Factors such as occlusion, vehicles, and skin condition can rapidly change the absorption characteristics. Also, the skin will change through its own growth patterns. With percutaneous absorption, the skin should not be viewed as an inert membrane but as a dynamic living biomembrane with unique properties.

Animals are used in experiments with substances that cannot be used in humans. No one animal, with its complex anatomy and biology, will simulate the penetration in humans for all compounds. We found that rhesus monkeys and miniature domestic pigs yield the best correlation with human penetration. Physical studies and *in vitro* models yield useful information about the mechanism of penetration and its theoretical implications, but they have not duplicated human *in vivo* rates or total penetration. We feel that the best estimate of human percutaneous absorption is determined by *in vivo* studies in humans or animals.

The key to good data is the design at the start of the study. The interpretation of results should not go beyond the limits of the study. We have summarized many complex aspects of percutaneous absorption. Each of these should be carefully considered. The results will lead to a better understanding of percutaneous absorption.

REFERENCES

Andersen, K. E., Maibach, H. I., and Anjo, D. M. 1980. The guinea pig: An animal model for human skin absorption of hydrocortisone, testosterone and benzoic acid. *Br. J. Dermatol.* 102:447–453.

Anjo, D. M., Feldmann, R. J., and Maibach, H. I. 1980. Methods for predicting percutaneous penetration in man. In *Percutaneous Absorption of Steroids*, eds. P. Mauvais-Jarvis, C. F. H. Vickers, and J. Wepierre, pp. 31-51. New York: Academic.

Bartek, M. J. and La Budde, J. A. 1975. Percutaneous absorption *in vitro*. In *Animal Models in Dermatology*, ed. H. Maibach, pp. 103-120. New York: Churchill Livingstone.

Bartek, M. J., La Budde, J. A., and Maibach, H. I. 1972. Skin permeability *in vivo*: Comparison in rat, rabbit, pig and man. *J. Invest. Dermatol.* 58:114-123.

Feldmann, R. J. and Maibach, H. I. 1965. Penetration of ^{14}C hydrocortisone through normal skin: The effect of stripping and occlusion. *Arch. Dermatol.* 91:661-666.

Feldmann, R. J. and Maibach, H. I. 1967. Regional variation in percutaneous penetration of ^{14}C cortisone in man. *J. Invest. Dermatol.* 48:181-183.

Feldmann, R. J. and Maibach, H. I. 1969a. Absorption of some organic compounds through the skin in man. *J. Invest. Dermatol.* 54:339-404.

Feldmann, R. J. and Maibach, H. I. 1969b. Percutaneous penetration of steroids in man. *J. Invest. Dermatol.* 52:89-94.

Feldmann, R. J. and Maibach, H. I. 1974. Percutaneous penetration of some pesticides and herbicides in man. *Toxicol. Appl. Pharmacol.* 28:126-132.

Franz, T. J. 1975. Percutaneous absorption. On the relevance of *in vitro* data. *J. Invest. Dermatol.* 64:190-195.

Franz, T. J. 1979. The finite dose technique as a valid *in vitro* model for study of percutaneous absorption in man. Presented at the Annual Scientific Seminar, *Society of Cosmetic Chemists*, May, Dallas, Texas.

Greaves, S. J., Ferry, D. G., McQueen, E. G., Malcolm, D. S., and Buckfield, P. M. 1975. Serial hexachlorophene blood levels in the premature infant. *N.Z. Med. J.* 81:334-336.

Hunziker, N., Feldmann, R. J., and Maibach, H. I. 1978. Animal models of percutaneous penetration: Comparison in Mexican hairless dogs and man. *Dermatologica* 156:79-88.

Kruger, G. G. and Shelby, J. 1981. Biology of human skin transplanted to the nude mouse. I. Response to agents which modify epidermal proliferation. *J. Invest. Dermatol.* 76:506-510.

Maibach, H. I., Feldmann, R. J., Milby, T. H., and Serat, W. F. 1971. Regional variation in percutaneous penetration in man. *Pestic. Arch. Environ. Health* 23:208-211.

Marzulli, F. N. and Maibach, H. I. 1975. Relevance of animal models: The hexachlorophene story. In *Animal Models in Dermatology*, ed. H. Maibach, pp. 156-167. New York: Churchill Livingstone.

McKenzie, A. W. and Stoughton, R. B. 1962. Method for comparing percutaneous absorption of steroids. *Arch. Dermatol.* 86:608-610.

Nachman, R. L. and Esterly, N. B. 1971. Increased skin permeability in pre-term infants. *J. Pediatr.* 79:628-632.

Nacht, S., Yeung, D., Beasley, J. N., Jr., Anjo, D. M., and Maibach, H. I. 1981. Benzoyl peroxide: Percutaneous penetration and metabolic disposition. *J. Am. Acad. Dermatol.* 4:31-37.

Noonan, P. K. and Wester, R. C. 1980. Percutaneous absorption of nitroglycerin. *J. Pharm. Sci.* 69:365-366.

Rasmussen, J. E. 1979. Percutaneous absorption in children. In *1979 Year Book of Dermatology*, ed. R. L. Dobson, pp. 15-38. Chicago, Ill.: Year Book Medical.

146 · · · · · *R. C. Wester and H. I. Maibach*

Roberts, M. S. and Horlock, E. 1978. Effect of repeated skin application on percutaneous absorption of salicylic acid. *J. Pharm. Sci.* 67:1685–1687.

Scheuplein, R. J. and Ross, L. W. 1974. Mechanism of percutaneous absorption. V. Percutaneous absorption of solvent deposited solids. *J. Invest. Dermatol.* 62:353–360.

Singer, E. J., Wegmann, P. C., Lehman, M. D., Christensen, S., and Vinson, L. J. 1971. Barrier development, ultrastructure, and sulfhydryl content of the fetal epidermis. *J. Soc. Cosmet. Chem.* 22:119–137.

Vickers, C. F. H. 1980. Reservoir effect of human skin: Pharmacological speculation. In *Percutaneous Absorption of Steroids,* eds. P. Maurais-Jarvis, C. F. H. Vickers, and J. Wepierre, pp. 19–30. New York: Academic.

Wester, R. C. and Maibach, H. I. 1975a. Percutaneous absorption in the rhesus monkey compared to man. *Toxicol. Appl. Pharmacol.* 32:394–398.

Wester, R. C. and Maibach, H. I. 1975b. Rhesus monkey as an animal model for percutaneous absorption. In *Animal Models in Dermatology,* ed. H. Maibach, pp. 133–137. New York: Churchill Livingstone.

Wester, R. C. and Maibach, H. I. 1976. Relationship of topical dose and percutaneous absorption in rhesus monkey and man. *J. Invest. Dermatol.* 67:518–520.

Wester, R. C. and Maibach, H. I. 1977. Percutaneous absorption in man and animal: A perspective. In *Cutaneous Toxicity,* eds. V. Drill and P. Lazar, pp. 111–126. New York: Academic.

Wester, R. C. and Noonan, P. K. 1978. Topical bioavailability of a potential anti-acne agent (SC-23110) as determined by cumulative excretion and areas under plasma concentration time curves. *J. Invest. Dermatol.* 70:92–94.

Wester, R. C. and Noonan, P. K. 1980. Relevance of animal models for percutaneous absorption. *Int. J. Pharmacol.* 7:99–110.

Wester, R. C., Noonan, P. K., Cole, M. P., and Maibach, H. I. 1977a. Percutaneous absorption of testosterone in the newborn rhesus monkey: Comparison to the adult. *Pediatr. Res.* 11:737–739.

Wester, R. C., Noonan, P. K., and Maibach, H. I. 1977b. Frequency of application on percutaneous absorption of hydrocortisone. *Arch. Dermatol.* 113:620–622.

Wester, R. C., Noonan, P. K., and Maibach, H. I. 1979. Recent advances in percutaneous absorption using the rhesus monkey model. *J. Soc. Cosmet. Chem.* 30:297–307.

Wester, R. C., Noonan, P. K., and Maibach, H. I. 1980a. Percutaneous absorption of hydrocortisone increases with long-term administration: *In vivo* studies in the rhesus monkey. *Arch. Dermatol.* 116:186–188.

Wester, R. C., Noonan, P. K., and Maibach, H. I. 1980b. Variations in percutaneous absorption of testosterone in the rhesus monkey due to anatomic site of application and frequency of application. *Arch. Dermatol. Res.* 267:229–235.

Wester, R. C., Noonan, P. K., Smeach, S., and Kosobud, L. 1981. Estimate of nitroglycerin percutaneous first-pass metabolism. *Pharmacologist* 23:203.

6

skin irritation testing in animals

Arthur H. McCreesh ▪ Marshall Steinberg

INTRODUCTION

In the past, soaps, cosmetic materials, and pest control chemicals were recognized as potential sources of cutaneous irritation. More recently, a multitude of occupational and environmental factors, such as organic dyes, solvents, and industrial waste materials, some predictably and some not, have been contributing greatly to the mounting list of topical skin disorders. Recognition has long been given by industrial hygienists and toxicologists to the impact of topical skin effects on the usefulness of a particular chemical in the workplace. The threshold limit values of the American Conference of Governmental Industrial Hygienists provide for a skin notation when effects on the skin contribute to the hazard involved in the use of an industrial chemical.

As the potential for wider varieties of materials to cause cutaneous damage has become recognized, an increasing effort has been made by industry and environment protection groups to characterize this potential in areas previously not considered. Lubowe (1972) commented on the dermatologic effects of industrial air pollutants, which can lead to impaired keratinization and the development of pyogenic infective reactions. Terrell and Lee (1977), who tested the inhalation toxicity of phenylglycidyl ether (PGE) in rats, came to the same conclusion as Hine et al. (1956), that the greatest hazard to workers exposed to PGE is not systemic toxicity but dermal irritation. Federal legislative agencies and commercial manufacturers must consider such risks when developing, registering, or certifying materials or systems that affect individuals or environments.

In reviewing these problems, responsible organizations and their staffs must differentiate among toxicity, hazard, and risk. In the context of this chapter, toxicity refers to the inherent irritancy of a material; hazard refers to the potential of an inherently irritant material or formulation to cause irritation under conditions of a proposed use situation; and risk refers to the chance that an individual in a specific situation will suffer some form of skin damage. Of these factors, only toxicity is inherent, and this factor is the least important facet of topical insult. A toxic material can readily be replaced, diluted, neutralized, or deleted to reduce hazard and risk. When this is impossible, as in the case of environmental waste, the toxic irritant must be avoided, buried, or otherwise disposed of, taking great care to prevent current and future exposures.

The major varieties of topical localized primary irritation responses for which predictive animal tests are routinely employed are:

1. Acute primary irritation, defined as a local reversible inflammatory response of normal living skin to direct injury caused by a single application of a chemical agent without the involvement of an immunologic mechanism. Its important manifestations in standard animal testing are erythema and edema [National Academy of Sciences (NAS), 1977].
2. Cumulative irritation (also reversible), consisting of primary irritation resulting from repeated exposures to materials that do not in themselves cause acute primary irritation, as reviewed by Finkelstein et al. (1965) and Guillot et al. (1977).
3. Corrosion, defined as direct chemical action on normal living skin that results in its disintegration and irreversible alteration at the site of contact. Its important manifestations in standard animal testing are ulceration, necrosis, and, in time, the formation of scar tissue (NAS, 1977).
4. Photochemically induced irritation, consisting of a primary irritation resulting from light-induced molecular changes in the structure of chemicals applied to the skin.

DEVELOPMENT OF STANDARDIZED TESTS

Standardized tests have been used, with various levels of confidence, to establish degrees of risk based on suitable warning, labeling, and formulation. The validation of these tests has depended on feedback from clinical exposures. The development of newer tests, too, has relied on retrospective comparisons with effects on humans. Because confidence in a specific test may be related to the chemical properties of materials involved, such feedback has been essential in hazard assessment.

The test most widely used for predicting potential skin irritation in humans from results obtained with animal models was published by Draize et al. (1944). The test was designed to identify chemicals that would not cause primary irritation when applied to people. It is singularly effective in this regard. However, in designing a test that would eliminate false negatives (type 2 errors), the authors, by the nature of the design of the model, permitted the introduction of a significant number of false positives (type 1 errors).

Depending on the intended use of a candidate chemical, a model permitting type 1 errors but not allowing type 2 errors is acceptable. The experimental design is predicated on options being available to the investigator. For example, there may be other compounds that can be substituted for the offending material; it may be possible to protect people from the material; the compound may not be so irritating as to preclude skin tests in humans; or the requirement for the material may be such that the potential for skin irritation is an acceptable risk.

However, when these conditions do not exist and options are limited or not available, the Draize test with animal models can be too restrictive. The development of materials with a beneficial commercial or public health use has been prevented because of ultraconservative animal test models, a situation not unique to skin irritation predictive testing.

The standard skin irritation test [Code of Federal Regulations (CFR), 1980a] legislated under provisions of the Federal Hazardous Substances Act is described below; terms that are in dispute are italicized.

> Primary irritation to the skin is measured by a patch test technique on the *abraded* and intact skin of the *albino rabbit, clipped* free of hair. A minimum of *six* subjects are used in *abraded and intact* skin tests. *Insert under a square patch* such as surgical gauze measuring 1 inch by 1 inch and two single layers thick 0.5 *milliliter* (in the case of liquids) or 0.5 *gram* (in the case of solids and semisolids) of the test substance. Dissolve solids *in an appropriate solvent* and apply the *solution* as for liquids. The animals are immobilized with patches secured in place by *adhesive tape*. The entire trunk of the animal is then wrapped with *an impervious material* such as rubberized cloth, for the *24 hour period of exposure*. This material aids in maintaining the test patches in position and retards the evaporation of volatile substances. After 24 hours of exposure, the patches are removed and the resulting reactions are evaluated *on the basis of the designated values shown in Table 1.*
> Readings are again made at the end of *72 hours*. An equal number of exposures are made on areas of skin that have been previously abraded. The abrasions are minor incisions through the stratum corneum, but not sufficiently deep to disturb the derma or to produce bleeding.

The many variables and disputed terms noted above have led, not surprisingly, to internally developed modifications of the method. Thus the term "modified Draize method" has often replaced "Draize method" in reports of primary irritation. The modifications generally reflect attempts to

TABLE 1 Grading Values for Skin Reactions in Albino Rabbits
following Topical Application of Potential Primary Irritants[a]

Skin reaction	Value[b]
Erythema and eschar formation	
No erythema	0
Very slight erythema (barely perceptible)	1
Well-defined erythema	2
Moderate to severe erythema	3
Severe erythema (beet redness) to slight eschar formations (injuries in depth)	4
Edema formation	
No edema	0
Very slight edema (barely perceptible)	1
Slight edema (edges of area well defined by definite raising)	2
Moderate edema (raised approximately 1 mm)	3
Severe edema (raised more than 1 mm and extending beyond the area of exposure)	4

[a]Code of Federal Regulations, 1980a.
[b]The value recorded for each reading is the average value for the six or more animals subject to the test.

improve interpretations because inconsistent results were obtained with the standard method or because of special production needs of the testing laboratories. In attempting to "parallel" accidental exposure situations, the Department of Transportation recommends that the occlusion-exposure periods be shortened to 4 h (CFR, 1980b). Four-hour and even shorter application periods, at the time of this writing, have been recommended by the Advisory Center on Toxicology, National Academy of Sciences–National Research Council, in revising NAS publication 1138 (NAS, 1977). Tables 2 and 3 reflect the types of warnings sometimes developed from modified tests.

While properly applied quality control procedures can ensure intralaboratory reproducibility, they do not in themselves indicate whether results agree with those of other laboratories or whether they reflect potential hazard better than a more arbitrary reference method. To test the precision and predictability of laboratories and the reference method, Weil and Scala (1971) developed and supervised a collaborative test program in which 25 highly rated laboratories evaluated 16 materials for their ability to cause primary irritation to skin, using the Draize method as well as their own modified Draize methods. The results led to some interesting conclusions concerning the variability and predictability of skin irritation tests with albino rabbits.

1. Intralaboratory variability in both scoring and rating was great; some laboratories characteristically graded more severely and others less severely than the "norm."

2. Individual irritation responses varied considerably within some laboratories and were much more uniform in others; this may be attributable to training in grading of irritant effects or in animal handling.
3. There was little intralaboratory variation between the reference test and modifications developed by individual laboratories.
4. Most laboratories rated relatively nonirritating materials similarly; it was in the testing of moderate to severe irritants that the greatest variability, both between and within laboratories, occurred.

The authors concluded that the extremes of variability could not be explained by any one factor and that a change of standard tests would probably not improve results. They recommended that "courses or clinics" in methodology be established and that, until uniformity could be improved, skin (and eye) irritation evaluation procedures not be recommended specifically by legislative agencies.

The Draize method, as legislatively modified, has become a "reference procedure" despite multitudinous objections, because of its uniformity, simplicity, and reported effectiveness in identifying strong irritants. Currently it exists legislatively under the provisions of the Federal Hazardous Substance Act. The method has some serious flaws, however, particularly in its inability to identify mild or moderate irritants (Philips et al., 1972) and the propensity of rabbits to demonstrate irritant effects greater than demonstrated in humans (Nixon et al., 1975; Philips et al., 1972). These false positive responses, although they are undesirable in the development of new soaps and cosmetics, for example, are infinitely preferable to false negative responses, which could

TABLE 2   National Institute for Occupational Safety and Health
Interpretation of Skin Test Ratings[a]

Rating		Interpretation
Intact skin	Abraded skin	
0–0.9		Nonirritant; probably safe for intact human skin contact
1–1.9		Mild irritant; may be safe for use, but appropriate protective measures are recommended during contact
2–4		Too irritant for human skin contact; avoid contact
	0–0.9	Nontoxic to cellular components of abraded skin; probably safe for human skin contact
	1–1.9	Mild cellular toxins; may be safe for abraded skin contact provided protective measures are employed
	2–4	Cellular toxins too irritant for abraded skin contact; avoidance of contact is advised

[a]Campbell et al., 1975.

TABLE 3   Environmental Protection Agency Labeling Guidelines
for Pesticides Applied to Skin or Eyes[a]

Toxicity category	Precautionary statements
I. Irreversible corneal opacity at 7 d; severe irritation or damage at 72 h	Corrosive, causes eye and skin damage (or skin irritation). Do not get in eyes or on skin or clothing. Wear goggles or face shield and rubber gloves when handling. Harmful or fatal if swallowed. (Appropriate first aid statement required).
II. Corneal opacity reversible within 7 d; irritation persisting for 7 d	Causes eye and skin irritation. Do not get in eyes or on skin or clothing. Harmful if swallowed. (Appropriate first aid statement required)
III. No corneal opacity; irritation reversible within 7 d	Avoid contact with skin, eyes, or clothing. In case of contact, immediately flush eyes or skin with plenty of water. Get medical attention if irritation persists
IV. No irritation	No precautionary statements required

[a]Code of Federal Regulations, 1980c.

lead to misevaluating hazardous materials before or after exposure to the consumer or the environment.

The many variables referred to earlier in describing the reference primary irritation test procedures have been reviewed previously and are mentioned briefly below.

Abrasion

The effect of breaks in the skin surface on primary irritation hazard is determined by testing on abraded skin. The method for abrading is not specified, other than that the stratum corneum should be incised but this incision should not cause bleeding. The abrader most used for animal tests is the tip of a syringe needle, and the procedure requires some experience to ensure uniformity. Other abraders are the Berkeley Scarifier,[1] which is used frequently in human skin abrasion but is difficult to use on more hirsute skin, and the disposable abrader first used at the National Center for Toxicological Research (Haley and Hunziger, 1974). The last item is a disposable plastic scraper designed to permit readily repeatable abrasions.

To test abraders and abrasion, we (unpublished data) used the three procedures in primary irritation testing of five materials, including acetone, 95% ethanol, a solid dissolved in acetone, a liquid irritant (Table 4), and a liquid nonirritant. No difference in effects between the abrasion materials was noted. Neither was there a difference, in these tests, between abraded and

[1] Trademark of Berkeley Biologicals, Berkeley, Calif.

unabraded skin. A review of over 100 materials recently tested in our laboratory failed to show any pattern of response attributable to abrasion of the skin. Nixon et al. (1975) reported no correlation between testing on abraded skin of rabbits and potential for primary skin irritation in people, and concluded that testing on abraded skin is unnecessary and misleading in the interpretation of test results.

Animal Species

The albino rabbit is the animal of choice and has been used for many years in Draize-type testing. The albino guinea pig has been frequently studied (Roudabush et al., 1965; Nixon et al., 1975) and its use has become more accepted by federal agencies (Campbell et al., 1975; CFR, 1980c). The National Academy of Sciences–National Research Council (NAS, 1977), while commenting on the limited repertoire of responses from rabbits and guinea pigs, recommended the latter species (Hartley strain) over the rabbit, because the response of guinea pig skin is more like that of humans over a wide range of test materials and because of testing economies.

Many studies compare different animal species for ability to predict human responses. Davies et al. (1972) tested a variety of cosmetic ingredients on six species (and various strains) of test animals. They reported considerable interspecies variability, but no better predictor than the albino rabbit. Motoyoshi et al. (1979) tested 40 cosmetic components by dermal application to rabbits, guinea pigs, albino rats, humans, and swine and found that the degree of responsiveness of the species decreased in that order. Unfortunately, the testing procedures were not uniform and the interspecies comparisons are difficult to evaluate. Their comparisons, however, are in agreement with those of many other authors. Kastner (1977), using 24-h patch procedures, tested 40 fat-derived cosmetics in rabbits, guinea pigs, hairless mice, and humans and recommended hairless mice as the test animal of choice. He also recommended that no final indication of human irritant response should be made without

TABLE 4 Effects of Abrasion Techniques on Total Irritation Values for Carboranyl Methylpropyl Sulfide (5% in Ethanol)

	Irritation values (±1 SD)[a] after abrasion		
Abrasion technique	24 h	72 h	7 d
No abrasion	1.5 ± 0.5	2.1 ± 1.0	2.8 ± 1.1
Hypodermic needle	1.5 ± 0.5	2.0 ± 1.1	2.6 ± 1.0
Berkeley Scarifier	1.5 ± 0.5	1.9 ± 0.8	2.5 ± 1.1
Maryland Plastics skin abrader	1.4 ± 0.5	1.9 ± 0.8	2.5 ± 1.1

[a]Methodology and scoring are described in Code of Federal Regulations (1980a). Each value is the mean of irritation scores for six rabbits determined by three independent evaluators.

some human testing or knowledge of the mechanism of reaction in different species. MacMillan et al. (1975) compared a variety of cosmetic products on albino rabbits, guinea pigs [by the immersion technique described by Opdyke and Burnett (1965)], beagle dogs, and humans. They reported a fair degree of correlation between rabbits and guinea pigs but found the beagles "most unresponsive to known irritants."

Albino rabbits are still used for most skin irritation testing because of their relative uniformity of response, ease of handling, and documented history of exposure, with the recognition that rabbits are more responsive than other species (including humans) to mild or moderate irritant insult.

Method of Application

Sullivan and Strausburg (1975) demonstrated the effects of this factor on primary irritation test results by using five different but acceptable methods of administering test material to clipped rabbit backs beneath a patch. Six powdered detergents were applied either dry to dry patches, dry to premoistened skin, dry and covered with a moistened patch, dry and "injected" beneath a preapplied patch to which 1.5–2.0 ml of distilled water was added, or as a slurry made on glassine paper, applied to the skin, and covered with a patch. The areas were covered for either 4 or 24 h and reactions were graded after 4, 24, and 48 or 72 h. Significant differences in effect were reported, although all techniques comply with legislated procedural guidelines.

Gilman et al. (1978), disturbed by the lack of specificity in describing application procedures, tested various sample preparation systems, durations of exposure, and degrees of occlusivity of patch coverings and found that these factors made great differences in irritation scoring of a variety of detergent products. This study, performed to assess the effects of incidental or unplanned (i.e., short-term) exposure to dry skin irritants, stressed the importance of relating the actual situation in life to the test procedure.

Experience in our laboratory, considering relative readings of a series of chemicals rather than scoring or classification results, showed less inconsistency when different application procedures were used. In one study 12 compounds were evaluated (Steinberg et al., 1975). It is apparent that the physiochemical nature of the applied material is more important than the method of application. The degree of occlusion greatly modifies epidermal penetration (Bartek et al., 1971; Feldmann and Maibach, 1966) and this penetration, at least through the keratinized layer, is necessary for gross irritant effects (Frosch and Kligman, 1977).

Volume Applied

Although 0.5 ml of test material applied under a 1 X 1 in patch is specified in the standard test procedure, smaller volumes are often used for various reasons, including availability of the test material (particularly for early screening studies), systemic toxicity, or limitations of available skin surface for application. When a smaller volume is applied, the application should be confined to an equivalently smaller test area for uniformity of exposure. For example, skin testing procedures employed at the National Institute for Occupational Safety and Health specify application of 0.1 ml of a liquid to a 20-mm^2 test site (Campbell et al., 1975). While this procedure would not affect intralaboratory precision and might be desirable in many testing situations, the relatively more dilute skin site application could result in increased interlaboratory variation in test results, particularly when the compounds tested penetrate epidermal layers and cause inflammatory responses throughout the epidermal-dermal system.

Occlusion

Occlusive covering, which is required to increase the test insult by preventing loss by evaporation and by increasing tissue penetration, also subjects the test site to thermal insult through exothermic reactions between test materials and tissues and to increased tissue hydration. Such variations would depend primarily on the material being tested, rather than the method of test. In addition, effects of chemical-tissue interactions resulting from irritant adhesive materials, effects of various "appropriate solvents," variations in sites of application, and so forth can all contribute to variability in responses.

Repetitive Application

The use of repeated applications to animal skin for 5–7 d was reported by Ingram and Grasso (1975), Brown (1970), and MacMillan et al. (1975). Repeated-application tests were compared to patch tests on human skin by Finkelstein et al. (1963) and Kligman and Woodring (1967). These studies were expanded by Marzulli and Maibach (1975), who tested a variety of readily available drugs and cosmetic materials on humans, comparing 14 daily applications (weekend applications were not made) with 21 consecutive day occluded patch testing as described by Philips et al. (1972). Visual assessment of irritation was also compared with changes in skinfold thickness. Since the data permitted statistical comparison, the grade degree of agreement between those parameters could be quantitated ($N = 0.96$; therefore the probability of this correlation being accidental was less than 0.1%). The correlation between repeated-application results and human irritation results was good.

Steinberg et al. (1975) compared the relative irritancy of 12 chemicals in rabbits and humans. Results of 21 consecutive daily applications of predetermined threshold irritant concentrations to clipped rabbit backs were statistically compared to results of 21-d patch testing in humans (Table 5). Irritant reactions at graded concentrations were subjected to regression analysis, which indicated positive dose-response relation over a broad range of chemical and irritant effects (Table 6). Rankings of primary chemical irritation on rabbit backs produced by various occlusive techniques were compared nonparametrically to give an indication of the loss of predictability related to these factors (Table 7). These analyses indicted an excellent correlation between the effects of repeated applications to rabbits (at threshold concentrations) and cumulative irritancy to human skin. The repeated-application test on rabbits, although economically heroic, appeared to be better able to predict irritant effects on the skin of many people, particularly if the material, when used, will remain in contact with the skin or multiple exposures will be experienced. Inspections of the laboratory data generated indicated that satisfactory relative ranking and prediction of irritant hazard might be attempted after 10 d of testing, but many more compounds should be tested before such conclusions can be made. The methodologies for the major repeated-application techniques were reviewed by Hood (1976).

With most animal models and experienced personnel, it is possible to predict whether compounds will be severe irritants or nonirritants. The problem is with compounds that are mild or moderate irritants to animals but do not produce a demonstrable effect when applied to humans. Part of this

TABLE 5 Comparison of Irritant Rankings for 12 Compounds Applied Daily for 21 d under Saran Wrapping (Occluded) or Elastic Cloth (Partially Occluded) at Threshold Irritant Concentrations[a]

	Irritant ranking (1 = most irritating)		
Test compound	A To people (occluded)	B To rabbits (partially occluded)	C To rabbits (occluded)
Salicylic acid	3	2	1
N-Butylsulfonimidocyclo-hexamethylene	6	4	4
N-Hexadecylpyridinium	12	12	10
Benzoic acid	2	1	2
Formaldehyde	4	10	8
Resorcinol monoacetate	5	8	11
Cyclohexamethylene carbamide	9	11	12
Triethyleneglycol-N-hexyl ether	7	7	9
Resmethrin	10	6	6
Benzalkonium chloride	11	5	5
Diethyltoluamide	1	3	3
Triethanolamine	8	9	7

Relative irritant ranking[b]
A vs. B   Rank coeff. = 0.61 $p < 0.05$
A vs. C   Rank coeff. = 0.53 $p < 0.05$
B vs. C   Rank coeff. = 0.90 $p < 0.001$

[a]Steinberg et al., 1975.
[b]Spearman rank order analysis (Siegel, 1956).

TABLE 6 Regression Analysis of Irritant Response Score (24 h) versus Concentration for Seven Compounds Applied Topically to Albino Rabbits (One Application)[a,b]

Irritant compound	Skin covering	Slope	Y intercept[c]	Correlation coefficient
Salicylic acid	Open[d]	0.01	0.39	0.17
	Occluded[e]	0.05	0.19	0.95
N-Hexadecylpyridinium	Open	0.21	0.57	0.96
	Occluded	0.10	3.36	0.70
Formaldehyde	Open	0.09	0.77	0.87
	Occluded	0.12	1.09	0.81
Cyclohexamethylene carbamide	Open	0.02	0.67	0.85
	Occluded	0.02	0.81	0.85
Triethyleneglycol-N-hexyl ether	Open	0.16	0.16	0.98
	Occluded	0.25	0.59	0.91
Benzalkonium chloride	Open	0.41	0.75	0.94
	Occluded	0.49	2.41	0.72
Triethanolamine	Open	0.01	0.28	0.82
	Occluded	0.04	1.09	0.84

[a] Steinberg et al., 1975.

[b] Each compound was tested at four or more concentrations ranging between 100 and 0.01%.

[c] Y-intercept units are irritant scores.

[d] Open, no covering other than gauze pad over application area.

[e] Occluded, area covered with gauze pad and Saran seal.

problem has been testing of compounds with an occluded animal model; when the compounds were tested on humans, the humans were often not occluded. The results of the tests on humans would indicate that the animal model was not reliable, despite the difference in the techniques. Attention should be directed to the potential use concentration when conducting tests in animals. It was observed with humans that in a series of dissimilar primary irritant compounds, increasing the concentration over time decreased the irritation potential (unpublished results), possibly due to a decrease in penetration as the skin responded to the continuing presence of the irritant. This is in contrast to the fatigue theory (Finkelstein et al., 1965) and to the response observed with single applications. Steinberg et al. (1975) demonstrated that the method of occlusion in the animal model (e.g., Saran wrap, elastic bandage, stockinette) did not alter the response (Table 6). The responses of an occluded series and a nonoccluded series were different; however, because of variation in the nonoccluded model, no definitive judgment could be made. The nonoccluded series appeared to have a lesser response than the occluded one, but not consistently. More consistent results are obtained with occluded models. Care should be exercised when testing materials that are potential

TABLE 7   Comparison of Application Methods for Single Applications
of Eight Irritant Compounds to Intact Rabbit Skin;
Relative Irritant Ranking after 24 h[a]

	Relative ranking (1 = most irritating)		
Compound	A Covered by gauze and elastic bandage	B Covered by gauze, elastic bandage, and stockinette	C Covered by gauze, elastic bandage, stockinette, and Saran wrap
Salicylic acid	6	5	7
N-Butylsulfonimidocylohexa- methylene	8	6	5
N-Hexadecylpyridinium	2	2	3
Benzoic acid	7	7	6
Formaldehyde	4	8	8
Cyclohexamethylene carbamide	3	1	1
Benzalkonium chloride	1	3	2
Diethyltoluamide	5	4	4

Relative irritant ranking[b]
A vs. B   Rank coeff. = 0.60 $p < 0.05$
A vs. C   Rank coeff. = 0.64 $p > 0.05$
B vs. C   Rank coeff. = 0.90 $p < 0.01$

[a] Steinberg et al., 1975.
[b] Spearman rank order analysis (Siegel, 1956).

tissue fixatives. Solvent controls are needed whenever aqueous or acetone-alcohol solutions are used. It is important to note the hair patterns on test animals; animals with extremely patchy or dense hair patterns are not good subjects. Variations can be demonstrated when animals of different strains or from different sources are used. The variability of animal response with site hair pattern, strain, species, depilation technique, and other factors is well documented (Rony et al., 1953). It is most important that each laboratory routinely testing potential skin irritants develop predetermined repetitive techniques and use well-trained personnel.

Guillot et al. (1977), as part of a program to assess the ocular and cutaneous hazards of a large number of cosmetic formulations, compared primary cutaneous irritation to cumulative (60 d) treatment on rabbits. The procedures generally followed official French guidelines, although scoring was modified. Cumulative results were evaluated macroscopically and histologically. The study exemplified problems associated with repetitive animal testing, for example, the appearance of allergy-associated vesicular eruptions in rabbits (but not in normal or hairless rats tested) using test materials that were known not to be sensitizers. The severity of irritant reactions to some materials that were at most slightly irritating in primary testing prevented the continuation of all applications to their planned conclusion.

OTHER TESTING APPROACHES

The desire to add parameters to primary irritant evaluations has resulted in the continued modification of tests and their interpretation. Ingram and Grasso (1975) employed histological evaluation of irritant-induced tissue changes. After three test compounds were applied, visual irritant evaluation scores were compared with histopathologic evaluations of fixed, stained sections from test areas on rabbit backs. Changes in the epidermal layers, ranging from epidermal destruction through isolated dermal infiltration, were rated. Good correlations between tissue and visual estimates of damage were possible, but the development of irritation, maximal degree of damage, and recovery could not be followed by this procedure without greatly increasing the number of test animals. Similar testing procedures have been discussed by Lansdown (1972) and Brown (1970), among others, and, for a somewhat different purpose, by Du Vivier and Stoughton (1975), who screened for topical effects of drugs with hairless mice.

Brown (1970), in addition to performing a histological review of mice, rabbits, and guinea pigs, examined the test animals for irritation stress-induced biochemical changes by measuring phosphogluconate dehydrogenase, glucose-6-phosphate dehydrogenase, acid phosphatase, and alkaline phosphatase, monoamine oxidase, succinic dehydrogenase, and DNA, but found no changes attributable to testing. In a broadly based comparison of animal tests Brown (1970) measured dye extravasation (sulfan blue), using single and repeated applications and various modes of application. There appeared to be no correlation between test methods with the diluted surfactants chosen, although visual examination of rabbit and guinea pig skin again showed good correlation. Brown concluded that such biochemical studies do not at present offer much hope for simplified predictive testing. Similarly, Marzulli and Maibach (1975), using radioimmunoassay of skin prostaglandin E in rabbits, found no differences attributable to application of irritant chemicals.

Imokawa (1980) studied the effects of a series of highly purified monoalkyl phosphate surfactants on a variety of biological systems, including surface protein adsorption, enzyme inhibition, and lysosomal labilizing effects. He concluded that irritation was related to action in the biomembrane system, and he stressed the importance of adsorption on skin surfaces in the initiation of skin roughness, a response to chemical insult that may or may not be related to the inflammatory responses usually scored. Penetration through human skin has been measured (i.e., impedance, water vapor loss, chloride transport) to provide a better theoretical understanding of the factors that control the penetration of irritants below the keratinized skin surface (Malten and Den Arend, 1978; Grice et al., 1975). Similar testing with animal models may provide better and more predictable indices of irritant potency for newly developed chemicals.

Campbell and Bruce (1981) reported a rabbit skin test procedure to account for variation caused by vehicles, doses, and occlusion durations. An incomplete Latin square experimental design was employed to minimize variations between animals and different stain sites. A similar design was used in parallel human testing. The authors reported little site-to-site variation as long as the back was used, abdominal applications having been shown (e.g., Vinegar, 1979) to produce greater variability in response. These studies may lead to a more rational testing scheme, but they also point out the hazard of overextending parametric analysis of irritation scores. It must be stressed that Draize scoring is nonparametric (i.e., nonlinear) and not suitable to more than minimal mathematical manipulation.

Many authors endeavored to relate primary irritant test results to sensory irritation, but with little success. Shanchau and Ward (1975) used this test to evaluate the sting potential of shampoos, and Finkelstein et al. (1965) reported using the procedure with better results. Ballantyne and Swanston (1973, 1974) concluded that sensory irritant tests in animals may not be reliable for predicting irritant effects in humans and that human testing is still necessary, but only after topical damage levels have been determined.

It appears from the multiplicity of irritant testing procures, most of which show some merit in reflecting human cutaneous irritation, that materials "causing primary irritation or corrosive effects are not selective in their action. They will affect animal and human skin alike after sufficient time and appropriate concentrations" (NAS, 1975). This conclusion, reached by a select group of scientists after a review of irritant test procedures, should act as a stimulus to refine available procedures and, when possible, to elucidate the types of potential irritants that might not be expected to show predictable effects in standard tests.

The good correlation between tests results obtained by using modifications of the Draize procedure with albino rabbits (and, in more limited testing, with albino guinea pigs) indicates that modifications of the reference method may provide more acceptable information than the many other novel procedures explored over the past 20 yr. For example, Philips et al. (1972), among others, found that test data for rabbits were capable of assessing the human irritant potential of nonirritants or severe irritants (including corrosives), but not the many mild to moderate irritants to which people are exposed. When single-application procedures yielded inconclusive data, they concluded that human patch testing would be necessary to separate mildly and moderately irritating materials.

The Organization for Economic Cooperation and Development (OECD) released a series of guidelines for the testing of chemicals (OECD, 1981), including a guideline for acute dermal irritation/corrosion which established a procedure and provided international standards for such testing. These differ in many respects from those in the U.S. Federal Hazardous Substances Act (FHSA) (i.e., the Draize tests). The OECD procedure recommends a minimum of three animals, suggesting the albino rabbit, and does not demand a fixed test duration; covering may be occlusive or semiocclusive as appropriate, the exposure duration should usually be 4 h, and skin abrasion is not required. Irritant scoring is that recommended in standard Draize testing. In addition, husbandry and reporting requirements are noted. The guideline states specifically that extrapolation of the results of irritancy/corrosivity studies from animals to humans has only limited validity and addition of results for several animal species may give more weight to such extrapolations.

A comparison of test guidelines proposed by the OECD, FHSA (CFR, 1980a), Department of Transportation (DOT) (CFR, 1980b), and Environmental Protection Agency (EPA) (CFR, 1980d, 1980e) demonstrated several similarities and differences. Table 8 shows some of the major requirements of the various guidelines. All the tests call for application of 0.5 g or 0.5 ml, depending on the physical form of the substance. They call for some form of wrapping and either animal restraint or some mechanism for preventing ingestion or inhalation of the test material. Albino rabbits are used in all tests and the sites of application are similar. All use the Draize scoring system, although not always in the same way. Controls are required when a vehicle of unestablished irritant potential is used.

DISCUSSION AND CONCLUSIONS

There is no single-all-inclusive predictive model for primary irritation. The physicochemical nature of the test materials; anticipated duration and location of skin contact; conditions of use, temperature, and humidity; degree of occlusion, presence of other chemicals, condition and histochemical makeup of the skin; and presence of other modifiers influence the nature of predictive testing and its reliability.

The modified Draize skin irritancy tests are valuable because of their ability to separate severe from moderate irritants and identify materials with little or no potential for causing skin irritation in humans. The Draize test and modifications demonstrate little ability to predict the reaction of humans to a compound that produces moderate or mild irritation in rabbits. Experience indicates that the Draize skin irritancy test in rabbits tends to be too conservative in its predictions (Nixon et al., 1975; Philips et al., 1972).

At least in regard to employing a modified Draize test, one should choose a technique and raters and standardize them. We prefer a modification in which the animal is wrapped with an elastic bandage and then placed in a stockinette sleeve (vest). The main reasons are that the occlusive bandage stays in place and the results are not different from those obtained with a more impermeable occlusive bandage. This technique lends itself to use for longer term (21, 24, or 90 d) studies, which require the bandage to remain in place for 6 or 7 d on an unrestrained rabbit.

TABLE 8 Comparison of Regulatory Requirements

Source	Test material		Exposure time (h)	Number of rabbits	Sites per animal intact/abraded	Action at end of exposure	Scoring periods after exposure
	Solid	Liquid					
OECD, 1981	Moisten	Undiluted	4	3[a]	1/0	Wash with water or solvent	30–60 min, 24, 48, 72 h, or until obviously irreversible; no longer than 14 d
FHSA (CFR, 1980a)	Dissolve	Neat	24	6	1/1	Not specified	24 and 72 h
DOT (CFR, 1980b)	Not specified	Not specified	4	6	1/0	Wash with appropriate solvent	4 and 48 h
EPA (CFR, 1980d)	Solid	Not specified	24	6	2/2	Skin wiped, not washed	24 and 48 h; may continue until irritation subsides or is obviously irreversible
EPA (CFR, 1980e)	Moisten with saline	Undiluted					

[a]Additional animals may be required to clarify equivocal results.

The determination of a threshold irritation concentration (TIC), which is part of a dose-response relation, could offer guidance regarding the acute application of a material to human skin (Smyth et al. 1949; Steinberg et al., 1975). This test should be particularly useful if the intended use concentration is known and the anticipated skin contact is incidental or accidental. The TIC test would not be useful if prolonged or deliberate contact with human skin is foreseen or intended. A 21-d continuous application test in rabbits appears better able to predict the irritant effects of a candidate chemical on human skin, particularly if the material is to remain in contact with the skin or multiple exposures are anticipated. Materials that have minimal or no effects in rabbits may be expected to produce no response in the human assay technique. Compounds that produce a significant response in rabbits will probably elicit a response in humans.

An irritant response with the Draize test in rabbits should not automatically exclude a candidate chemical from human testing or potential use. Concentration and conditions of use, acceptable risk, professional judgment, and the results of other test techniques should enter into the decision.

Animal models have a high degree of reliability for predicting when a compound will not cause primary irritation in humans. With forethought, careful training, and attention to details, animal models may be used reliably to predict when a candidate material will produce irritation.

REFERENCES

Ballantyne, B. and Swanston, D. W. 1973. Screening tests for assessing the relative potency of sensory irritant materials. *Br. J. Pharmacol.* 48:367.

Ballantyne, B. and Swanston, D. W. 1974. The irritant effects of dilute solutions of dibenzoxazepine (CR) on the eye and tongue. *Acta Pharmacol. Toxicol.* 35:412–423.

Bartek, M., LaBudde, J., and Maibach, H. I. 1971. Skin permeability *in vivo*: Rat, rabbit, pig and man. *J. Invest. Dermatol.* 56:409 (abstract).

Brown, V. 1970. A comparison of predictive irritation tests with surfactants on human and animal skin. *J. Soc. Cosmet. Chem.* 20:411–420.

Campbell, K. I., George, E. L., Hall, L. L., and Stara, J. F. 1975. Dermal irritancy of metal compounds. *Arch. Environ. Health* 30:168–170.

Campbell, R. L. and Bruce, R. D. 1981. Comparative dermatotoxicology. 1. Direct comparison of rabbit and human skin initiation responses to isopropylmyristate. *Toxicol. Appl. Pharmacol.* 59:555–563.

Code of Federal Regulations. 1980a. Title 16, part 1500.41.

Code of Federal Regulations. 1980b. Title 49, part 173.240.

Code of Federal Regulations. 1980c. Title 40, part 162.10.

Code of Federal Regulations. 1980d. Title 40, part 771.

Code of Federal Regulations. 1980e. Title 40, part 163.31.

Davies, R. E., Harper, K. H., and Kynoch, S. R. 1972. Interspecies variation in dermal reactivity. *J. Soc. Cosmet. Chem.* 23:371–381.

Draize, J. H., Woodard, G., and Calvery, H. O. 1944. Methods for the study of irritation and toxicity of substances applied topically to the skin and mucous membranes. *J. Pharmacol. Exp. Ther.* 82:377–390.

DuVivier, A. J. and Stoughton, R. B. 1975. An animal model for screening topical and systemic drugs for protective use in the treatment. *J. Invest. Dermatol.* 65:235–237.

Feldman, R. and Maibach, H. I. 1966. Percutaneous penetration of ^{14}C hydrocortisone in man. *Arch. Dermatol.* 94:649–651.

Finkelstein, P., Laden, K., and Miechowski, W. 1963. New methods for evaluating skin irritancy. *J. Invest. Dermatol.* 40:11–16.

Finkelstein, P., Laden, K., and Miechowski, W. 1965. Laboratory methods for evaluating skin irritancy. *Toxicol. Appl. Pharmacol.* 7:74–78.

Frosch, P. J. and Kligman, A. M. 1977. The chamber scarification test for assessing irritancy of topically applied substances. In *Cutaneous Toxicology,* edited by V. A. Drill and P. Lasar, pp. 127–144. New York: Academic Press.

Gilman, M. R., Evans, R. A., and De Salva, S. J. 1978. The influence of concentration, exposure duration, and patch occlusivity upon rabbit primary dermal initiation indices. *Drug Chem. Toxicol.* 1:391–400.

Grice, K., Sattar, H., Casey, T., and Baker, H. 1975. An evaluation of Na, Cl and pH ion specific electrodes in the study of the electrolyte contents of epidermal transudate and sweat. *Br. J. Dermatol.* 92:511.

Guillot, J. P., Martini, M. C., and Giauffret, J. Y. 1977. Safety evaluation of cosmetic raw materials. *J. Soc. Cosmet. Chem.* 28:377–393.

Haley, T. and Hunziger, J. 1974. Instrument for producing standardized skin abrasions. *J. Pharm. Sci.* 63:106.

Hine, C. H., Kodama, J. K., Wellington, J. S., Dunlap, M. S., and Anderson, H. M. 1956. The toxicology of glycidol and some glycidol ethers. *Arch. Ind. Health* 14:250–264.

Hood, D. B. 1977. Practical and theoretical considerations in evaluating dermal safety. In *Cutaneous Toxicology,* edited by V. A. Drill and P. Lazar, pp. 15–30. New York: Academic Press.

Imokawa, G. 1980. Comparative study on the mechanism of irritation by sulfate and phosphate types of anionic surfactants. *J. Soc. Cosmet. Chem.* 31:45–66.

Ingram, A. J. and Grasso, P. 1975. Patch testing in the rabbit using a modified patch test method. *Br. J. Dermatol.* 92:131–142.

Kastner, W. 1977. Zur Speziesabhangigheit der Hautvertgleichbeit von Kosmetik-Grundstoffen. *J. Soc. Cosmet. Chem.* 28:741–784.

Kligman, A. M. 1976. New procedures for appraising irritants in humans. Conference on Cutaneous Toxicity, Proceedings.

Kligman, A. M. and Woodring, W. M. 1967. A method for the measurement and evaluation of irritants on human skin. *J. Invest. Dermatol.* 49:78–80.

Lansdown, A. B. 1972. An appraisal of methods for detecting primary skin irritants. *J. Soc. Cosmet. Chem.* 23:739–772.

Lubowe, I. I. 1972. Dermatitis urbis. *Soap Perfum. Cosmet.* 45:35–38.

MacMillan, F. S., Raft, R. R., and Cloers, W. B. 1975. A comparison of the skin irritation produced by cosmetic ingredients and formulations in the rabbit, guinea pig and beagle dog to that observed in the human. In *Animal Models in Dermatology,* ed. H. I. Maibach, pp. 12–22. Edinburgh: Churchill Livingstone.

Malten, K. E. and Den Arend, J. 1978. Topical toxicity of various concentrations and DMSO recorded with impedance measurements and water vapor loss measurements. *Contact Dermatitis* 4:80–92.

Marzulli, F. N. and Maibach, H. I. 1970. Perfume phototoxicity. *J. Soc. Cosmet. Chem.* 21:685–715.

Marzulli, F. N. and Maibach, H. I. 1975. The rabbit as a model for evaluating skin irritants: A comparison of results obtained on animals and man using repeated skin exposure. *Food Cosmet. Toxicol.* 13:533–540.

Motoyoshi, K., Toyoshima, Y., Sato, M., and Yoshimura, M. 1979. Comparative studies on the irritancy of oils and synthetic perfumes to the skin of rabbit, guinea pig, rat, miniature swine and man. *Cosmet. Toiletries* 94:41–42.

National Academy of Sciences. 1964. *Principles for Evaluating the Toxicity of Household Products*, bull. 1138. Washington, D.C.: National Academy of Sciences.

National Academy of Sciences, Committee for the Revision of NAS Publication 1138. 1977. *Principles and Procedures for Evaluating the Toxicity of Household Substances.* Washington, D.C.: National Academy of Sciences.

Nixon, G. A., Tyson, C. A., and Wertz, W. C. 1975. Interspecies comparisons of skin irritancy. *Toxicol. Appl. Pharmacol.* 31:481–490.

Opdyke, D. L. and Burnett, C. M. 1965. Practical problems in the evaluation of the safety of cosmetics. *Proc. Sci. Sect. Toilet Goods Assoc.* 44:3–4.

Organization for Economic Cooperation and Development. 1981. *OECD Guidelines for Testing of Chemicals*, sect. 404, *Acute Dermal Irritation/Corrosion*. Paris: OECD. In press.

Philips, L., Steinberg, M., Maibach, H. I., and Akers, W. A. 1972. A comparison of rabbit and human skin response to certain irritants. *Toxicol. Appl. Pharmacol.* 21:369–382.

Rony, H. R., Cohen, D. M., and Schaffner, I. 1953. Patterns of hair growth cycle in the colored rabbit and their modification by experimental means. *J. Invest. Dermatol.* 21:313.

Roudabush, R. A., Terhaar, C. J., Fassett, D. W., and Dziuba, S. P. 1965. Comparative acute effects of some chemicals on the skin of rabbits and guinea pigs. *Toxicol. Appl. Pharmacol.* 7:559–565.

Shanchau, R. W. and Ward, C. D. 1975. An animal model for estimating the relative sting potential of shampoos. *J. Soc. Cosmet. Chem.* 26:581–592.

Siegel, S. 1956. *Nonparametric Statistics for the Behavioral Sciences.* New York: McGraw-Hill.

Smyth, H. F., Carpenter, C. P., and Weil, C. S. 1949. Range finding toxicity data list III. *J. Ind. Hyg. Toxicol.* 31:60.

Steinberg, M., Akers, W. A., Weeks, M. H., McCreesh, A. H., and Maibach, H. I. 1975. A comparison of test techniques based on rabbit and human skin responses to irritants with recommendations regarding the evaluation of mildly or moderately irritating compounds. In *Animal Models in Dermatology*, ed. H. I. Maibach, pp. 1–11. Edinburgh: Churchill Livingstone.

Sullivan, J. B., Strausburg, K., and Kapp, R. W., Jr. 1975. A comparative study of dermal reactions using the intact rabbit skin. *Toxicol. Appl. Pharmacol.* 33:165–166.

Terrell, J. B. and Lee, K. P. 1977. The inhalation toxicity of phenylglycidyl ether. 1. 90-day inhalation study. *Toxicol. Appl. Pharmacol.* 42:263–269.

Vinegar, M. 1979. Regional variation in primary skin irritation and corrosivity potentials in rabbits. *Toxicol. Appl. Pharmacol.* 49:63–69.

Weil, C. S. and Scala, R. A. 1971. Study of intra- and interlaboratory variability in the results of rabbit eye and skin irritation tests. *Toxicol. Appl. Pharmacol.* 19:276–360.

7

clinical and experimental aspects of cutaneous irritation

■ C. G. Toby Mathias ■

INTRODUCTION

Cutaneous irritation (toxicity) accounts for almost 80% of all cases of contact dermatitis, either domestic or occupational in origin. *Irritation* has been defined as "the evocation of a normal or exaggerated reaction in a tissue by application of a stimulus" (Stedman's Medical Dictionary, 1976). The words *reaction* and *stimulus* lack specificity, which limits the usefulness of this definition. Several different reactions may be observed; likewise, a wide range of stimuli may evoke them.

The most common reaction consists of a local inflammatory response characterized by erythema and/or edema, or a corrosive reaction characterized by local tissue destruction or necrosis. Other reactions, sometimes referred to as irritation, do not involve an inflammatory response. Subtle increases in epidermal thickness, without visible or histological inflammation, may be produced by a variety of substances usually thought to be nonirritating: yellow soft paraffin and polyethylene glycol (Sarkany and Gaylarde, 1973); olive oil (Butcher, 1951; Schaaf and Gross, 1953); and liquid paraffin, sorbitol, cocoa butter, and Carbowax 6000 (Schaaf and Gross, 1953). Some reactions may appear morphologically quite different from an inflammatory response; foreign body granuloma, pigmentary changes, and chloracne are among the variations encountered. Reactions may be subjective as well as objective; *subjective irritation* refers to transient pruritus, stinging, burning, or related sensations without subsequent visible inflammation (e.g., alcohol on an open wound).

A wide range of stimuli may evoke the above reactions. Chemical substances, ultraviolet radiation, heat, friction, and mechanical trauma may all produce an identical inflammatory response, although different mechanisms may be involved. To qualify as an *irritant*, a chemical substance should evoke inflammation on initial exposure (*primary irritation* or on repeated exposure to an identical site (*cumulative irritation*). An important concept is that virtually any chemical, including water, may qualify as an irritant; this depends largely on the circumstances of exposure to the chemical substance (Kligman and Wooding, 1967).

To avoid confusion, an operational definition of irritation is needed. For the purpose of this review, irritation is defined as "a nonimmunologic local *inflammatory reaction*, characterized by erythema, edema, or corrosion, following single or repeated application of a *chemical substance* to the identical cutaneous site." This definition is purely descriptive and does not define the mechanism. This review thus excludes noninflammatory, non-immunologic cutaneous reactions evoked by some chemical substances (e.g., chloracne) and nonchemical stimuli capable of inducing local inflammation.

Since virtually any chemical substance, under certain conditions of exposure, may provoke an inflammatory response, a thorough understanding of the factors that may influence the cutaneous response to potential chemical irritants is essential. Although animal and human screening tests (discussed in detail elsewhere in this text) provide some measure of the inherent irritant potential of chemical substances, no simple "test" exists that will easily identify a specific chemical irritant under all conditions of exposure (use). This is particularly important in the evaluation of *occupational* contact dermatitis, where exposure to the same chemical substance may often occur under different conditions. In these situations, the best test for irritation often becomes the identification of conditions of exposure known to increase the irritant potential of chemical substances.

Using the operational definition of irritation given above, the conditions of exposure influencing the clinical response to chemical irritants may be divided as follows: (1) extrinsic factors, which influence the ability of a chemical substance to penetrate the skin barrier and produce an inflammatory reaction, and (2) intrinsic (constitutional) factors, which influence an individual's capacity to react with an inflammatory response.

EXTRINSIC FACTORS

The *sine qua non* of cutaneous irritation, as defined above, is the penetration of a chemical substance through the skin barrier; if the chemical does not penetrate through the barrier, no inflammation can occur. Conceptually, an irritant response (IR) results from the interaction of membrane permeability factors (K_p), amount of exposure (A), inherent irritant potential (IP) of the penetrating chemical, and individual capacity to react (R)

with inflammation. These variables may be related by the expression $IR = K_p \times A \times IP \times R$. The first portion of this equation is analogous to the Fick equation, $J = K_p \, \Delta C$ (see Chapter 3, p. 91), describing rate of penetration (flux) across a membrane.

Membrane Permeability Factors

Membrane diffusibility. Diffusibility of a chemical substance through the stratum corneum membrane depends on a complex interaction of several variables: temperature of the membrane, degree of membrane hydration, regional anatomic variations in the chemical composition of the membrane, physical properties of the penetrating chemical substance, and damage to the structural or chemical integrity of the membrane itself. Skin hardening, where the resistance of the membrane to penetration by a chemical substance apparently increases after repeated skin application, may also occur.

Diffusibility through a membrane increases as the *temperature* of the membrane increases. Cutaneous exposure to a heated chemical substance might therefore be expected to increase the probability of an irritant response. This can be demonstrated experimentally. Strong irritant reactions were provoked by a perfume component (citral) heated to 43°C and applied to forearm skin; little or no inflammation was observed following exposure at 25°C (Rothenberg et al., 1977). The intensity of the inflammatory response to certain irritants (e.g., sodium lauryl sulfate) may be enhanced by environmental elevation of skin temperature (Malten and Thiele, 1973b).

Increasing the water content of the stratum corneum (*membrane hydration*) generally enhances percutaneous absorption. Occlusion of the skin surface with a water-impermeable material (e.g., plastic wrap) prevents evaporative water loss from the skin, increasing the degree of hydration of the stratum corneum; skin maceration may result if the skin is left occluded for more than 8-12 h. Occlusion of a topical corticosteroid with plastic wrap increases its absorption and efficacy 10-100 times; soaking or compressing the skin with water 10-15 min prior to application of a topical steroid further increases its effect (McKenzie, 1972). Clinical irritation may be enhanced when chemical substances are inadvertently trapped and occluded against the skin surface (e.g., inside rubber gloves, shoes, or protective clothing).

Environmental humidity may influence the cutaneous response to irritants. The incidence of positive irritant reactions to propylene glycol in the New York City area was shown to be greatest during the winter months (Warshaw and Hermann, 1952), when the seasonal incidence of chapping was greatest. The same seasonal variation in reactivity to propylene glycol has been observed in Finland (Hannuksela et al., 1975). Presumably, climatic factors that dehydrate the stratum corneum and induce chapping alter cutaneous permeability, increasing susceptibility to irritants.

Sweating may increase hydration of the stratum corneum. Although the transeccrine route may be important in the percutaneous absorption of some substances, the absence of sweating per se does not appear to increase susceptibility to irritants. Bettley and Grice (1966) were unable to demonstrate any difference in reactivity to irritating concentrations of toilet soap, lauryl sulfate, or potassium palmitate between normal skin and skin rendered anhydrotic by the topical application of poldine methosulfate. Active sweating (e.g., during the summer months) may decrease irritant reactions to propylene glycol (Warshaw and Hermann, 1952); whether this is due to increased hydration of the stratum corneum with improved barrier function, to surface dilution and "washout" of topically applied substances, or to other unidentified factors is not known.

Percutaneous absorption is influenced by anatomic *regional variation*, and the response to irritants may likewise vary, depending on the particular region of the body to which the irritant is applied. Percutaneous penetration of histamine (Cronin and Stoughton, 1962), hydrocortisone (Feldmann and Maibach, 1967), and pesticides (Maibach et al., 1971) is greater over the face, upper back, and presternal region than over the forearm and thigh skin. Regional variations in absorption are not directly proportional to differences in stratum corneum thickness and undoubtedly also reflect regional differences in membrane composition. Increased reactivity to irritating concentrations of benzalkonium chloride over the upper back, compared with other body regions (Magnusson and Hersle, 1965), has been demonstrated. The upper back is the site currently recommended for patch testing by the North American Contact Dermatitis Group (NACDG) and should be the standard test site for future research on irritancy. Previous publications should be carefully evaluated in light of these known regional variations in percutaneous absorption.

After a chemical penetrates the skin, regional variations in cutaneous reactivity must also be considered. The size of wheal and flare reactions to various allergens introduced through the normal skin barrier, by prick or scarification techniques, may vary on different regions of the back, the midback giving the largest reactions (Gallant and Maibach, 1973). Similar data are not available for irritant reactions.

Diffusibility through the stratum corneum is affected by the *physical properties of the penetrating chemical substance*. These properties include *molecular size and volume, polarity,* and *state of ionization*. Large, polar, ionized molecules are poorly absorbed in general, while small, nonpolar molecules that are not ionized are absorbed more readily. Consideration of pH is particularly important where the skin is exposed to potential ionizable irritants.

Physical or chemical damage to the stratum corneum increases membrane permeability. Physical trauma (cuts, abrasions) to the skin has enhanced accidental poisoning with paraquat (Newhouse et al., 1978). Experimental tape stripping of the stratum corneum also increases the subsequent response to a topical chemical irritant. Certain solvents may gradually damage the structural and chemical integrity of the stratum corneum, increasing their own absorption and irritant potential. Skin inflamed with preexisting dermatitis is more susceptible to chemical irritation.

Skin hardening refers to the ability of the skin to adapt to substances that provoke irritation (or allergic dermatitis) so that repeated exposures to irritating concentrations at the identical skin site no longer provoke inflammation (Mitchell, 1969). Acquired tolerance of the skin may be specific for a particular irritant, or nonspecific. Specific hardening has been demonstrated with sodium lauryl sulfate; when it was reapplied (e.g., 10 d later) to previously inflamed skin and adjacent normal skin, only the normal skin reacted with inflammation (Rothenborg et al., 1977). On challenge with other irritants, the "hardened" skin may again become inflamed (McOsker and Beck, 1967). The biological basis of this phenomenon is not known. Experimental work with guinea pigs suggested that it is not entirely due to decreased percutaneous absorption in the irritated site (McOsker and Beck, 1967). Nonspecific hardening to a wide variety of irritants may occur after exposure to a single irritant; an example is the hardening of skin in leather workers following exposure to tanning solutions, presumably secondary to thickening of the horny layer (Mitchell, 1969).

Vehicle. The stratum corneum:vehicle partition coefficient influences percutaneous absorption; the more soluble a chemical substance is in the stratum corneum, compared with its vehicle, the greater the percutaneous penetration. Van Ketel (1978, 1979) demonstrated the unsuitability of petrolatum as a vehicle in the experimental evaluation of nickel and chromate allergies; positive patch tests were elicited only when water was used as a vehicle. Similar vehicle problems existed in a patient who was allergic to *p*-aminobenzoic acid (PABA) in a commercial sunscreen (Mathias et al., 1978); a positive photopatch test response could be obtained only when alcohol was used as a vehicle in place of petrolatum. These discrepancies were presumably due to differences in percutaneous absorption, influenced by different vehicles.

Selection of vehicles for experimental evaluation of irritants has largely depended on only two considerations: the solubility of the irritant in the vehicle, and the absence of clinical inflammation when the vehicle is tested alone. The influence of the vehicle on absorption of the irritant is most often ignored. Some vehicles may also produce subclinical reactions of their own (e.g., acanthosis) in the absence of clinical inflammation (Sarkany and Gaylarde, 1973; Schaaf and Gross, 1953). It is not known whether these subclinical responses facilitate or suppress irritant reactions. The addition of various "nonirritating" emulsifiers may either facilitate or suppress the subsequent allergic response to potassium dichromate in petrolatum (Rudzki et al., 1976).

The influence of vehicles on clinical irritant reactions is largely unknown. A 10% frequency of irritant responses to 0.1% thimerosal in water (included in a routine preservative patch test series) was observed at the Mayo Clinic (Iden and Shroeter, 1977). No irritant response to thimerosal at the same concentration was observed in the International Contact Dermatitis Research Group preservative patch test series; this was presumably due to the use of petrolatum as a vehicle.

Membrane thickness. Percutaneous absorption varies inversely with the thickness of the stratum corneum. Regional anatomic variations in stratum corneum thickness explain, in part, regional differences in percutaneous absorption. The anatomic areas most susceptible to clinical irritation are those where the stratum corneum is relatively thinnest: the scrotum, eyelids, and face. Membrane thickness does not completely account for differences in permeability; absorption of hydrocortisone is 40 times greater on scrotal skin than on the palm, whereas there is only about a 5- to 10-fold difference in stratum corneum thickness (Feldmann and Maibach, 1967).

Amount of Exposure

The amount or degree of exposure to a given chemical irritant is determined by the volume of material in contact with the skin, concentration of the irritant, duration and frequency of skin contact, and surface area of the skin actually contacted. The larger the total exposure, the more likely are irritant reactions to develop.

Concentrations. Higher concentrations of a chemical irritant are more likely to cause irritation than lower ones; dilution of a strong irritant may completely eliminate the irritant effect. Despite the disadvantages involved, concentrations of substances used in investigations of irritancy have traditionally been expressed as percent by volume or weight. It is often assumed that substances that produce inflammation at lower concentrations are more irritating. This conclusion may be erroneous; biological effect is probably dependent on the *number of molecules* available for reaction, not on the *weight*. Chemists have long appreciated this fact and express concentrations as moles or millimoles per liter. No equivalent terminology exists with which to define the number of moles of a particular substance in a nonaqueous vehicle. Precedent appears in the German literature (Schaaf, 1961) for expressing such concentrations in terms of moles per kilogram of vehicle. When comparing irritant effects of different chemical substances, equimolar amounts or concentrations should be compared.

Amount applied to skin surface. The total amount of irritant applied to the skin surface influences the subsequent inflammatory response. Few experimental studies have carefully controlled this variable. Liquids may be applied with the aid of a micropipette. Irritants incorporated into petrolatum are more difficult to dispense accurately; the best method available is to use a calibrated glass or plastic tuberculin syringe containing the irritant-petrolatum suspension.

Duration and frequency of exposure. In general, longer periods of cutaneous exposure to a given chemical irritant produce more intense, longer lasting inflammatory responses. Frequent skin contact also enhances the inflammatory response when individual exposures are of short duration.

Surface area. The total surface area over which an irritant is applied is of critical importance. The irritant response to pentadecylcatechol (rhus) depends on a critical surface area; it cannot be elicited in some patients if the test site is too small (W. Epstein, personal communication). The popular Al-test patches may be too small to detect responses to some irritants. The larger Finn chamber provides a larger surface area and may be more suitable.

Confinement of the chemical to the application site poses a further problem in experimental irritation studies. Cloth, gauze, or fabric units do not form a tight seal with the skin and probably allow lateral diffusion of the chemical from the application site. Greater control of the dose per unit area is obtained with various chambers (e.g., Finn chambers), which form a tight seal with the skin, limiting lateral diffusion (Pirila, 1975).

Specific Chemical Irritant Potential

The ability of a chemical substance to provoke irritation is related to chemical *stability, purity,* and unique *chemical properties.* Little information is available about the chemical stability of the substances traditionally selected for irritancy studies. Several factors, such as sunlight, temperature, and air oxidation, may alter chemical composition, concentration, or shelf life; although carefully considered by cosmetic and pharmaceutical industries, these factors have been largely ignored in dermatologic investigations. Unless such information is available, the investigator should employ freshly prepared materials. The chemical purity of the irritant is a separate problem, and commercially supplied materials frequently contain impurities that may confuse results. Further laboratory purification may be necessary to achieve reliable results. This point is illustrated by a case in which allergic sensitization developed to commercial stearyl alcohol; complete purification of the alcohol eliminated the reaction, implicating an impurity (Shore and Shelley, 1974) as the cause of the sensitivity. Some irritants (e.g., croton oil) may be heterogeneous mixtures of chemicals; if they are obtained from different sources the chemical composition may also vary, making extrapolation of results difficult. Finally, it must be remembered that irritants have unique chemical properties and may produce unique irritant responses.

Evaluation of Irritant Responses

Experimental evaluation of irritant potential depends, in no small measure, on the indices and methods used to grade the irritant response. Numerous methods for evaluating the irritant response have been developed. Most experimental reports on irritancy are concerned with the intensity and morphology of the inflammatory response, which is assigned a numerical "weight." Despite attempts at standardization, the evaluation of intensity and morphology is still largely subjective, and agreement between investigators is difficult to obtain. Photobiologists have avoided this problem by employing a minimal erythema threshold at 24 h after exposure to a light source as an index of photosensitivity; much higher concordance is achieved when evaluating barely perceptible erythema than when evaluating intensity of inflammation. Kligman and Wooding (1967) suggest that a minimal erythema threshold be used as a visual index of irritation. In this way, an irritant concentration (dose) that produces perceptible erythema in 50% of the subjects (ID50) may be calculated.

The time when experimental irritant reactions are evaluated is equally important. Irritant reactions are commonly said to arise within minutes to hours following exposure, to become maximum at 24 h, and to fade or completely disappear between 48 and 72 h. In general, for a given concentration of irritant, longer exposure times will produce quicker, more intense, and longer lasting inflammatory responses. Certain chemicals may characteristically produce an irritant reaction of delayed onset. Malten et al. (1979) recently demonstrated a delayed irritant reaction to two diacrylates employed as part of a paint coating operation in a door manufacturing plant. Experimentally induced irritant reactions did not appear for 15 h and were dependent on the initial length of exposure to the irritants. Chemical burns produced by hydrofluoric acid may also have a delayed onset (Shewmake and Anderson, 1979).

It has become customary to evaluate irritant reactions 24 h after the initial application. However, inflammatory irritant reactions may disappear by 24 h or increase in intensity through 48 h (Malten et al., 1979). Because of the extreme variability in the time course of inflammatory reactions, negative reactions at 24 h should be interpreted with caution, if no other readings are recorded.

INTRINSIC FACTORS

The inflammatory reaction following cutaneous exposure to irritants depends not only on the extrinsic conditions of exposure, as outlined above, but also on the capacity of an individual to react with inflammation. Intrinsic (constitutional) factors that may influence the irritant response include *genetic background, age, sex, race,* concomitant *systemic or cutaneous disease, neurological influences,* and *systemic medication.*

Genetic Background

Genetic factors have been implicated in the cutaneous response to irritants. Holst and Moller (1975) studied the irritant responses to benzalkonium chloride, sodium lauryl sulfate, and sapo kalinus among matched pairs of monozygotic and dizygotic twins and controls. Concordance of response was much greater in monozygotic twins, while controls had significantly greater variations in individual responses. These observations support a genetic basis for the well-recognized biological phenomenon that the response to a given concentration of a specific irritant may vary widely from individual to individual.

Age

Susceptibility to irritants appears to be enhanced in children and diminished in the elderly. An increased incidence of positive reactions to nonirritating concentrations of standard patch test tray chemicals (potassium dichromate, mercury bichloride, Formalin, nickel sulfate, turpentine, Benzocaine) has been observed in children, compared with adults (Rockl et al., 1966). Peak incidence of reactivity in this study occurred between the ages of 4 mo and 3 yr. These results more likely reflect a lower threshold to irritation than an increased incidence of allergic sensitization; in fact, a decreased capacity for allergic sensitization to pentadecylcatechol (rhus) has been demonstrated in children of the same age group (Epstein, 1961). The incidence of irritant reactions to croton oil decreases with age (Coenraads et al., 1975); this correlation was not demonstrated with thymoquinone or crotonaldehyde. Thus, increasing resistance to irritancy with increasing age may depend, in part, on the specific chemical properties of irritants as well as nonspecific age factors.

Sex

Women are frequently alleged to have more reactive or irritable skin than men. Early studies showed that women had stronger irritant reactions than men to alkalies (Wagner and Purschel, 1962) and detergents (Seeberg, 1955). These observations were not confirmed by Bjornberg (1975), who, in a scrupulously matched and controlled study of subjects both with and without hand eczema, failed to identify any consistent sex difference in response to 11 different irritants. Data on the influence of the menstrual cycle or pregnancy on cutaneous reactivity are confusing and inconclusive; changes, if they occur at all, would appear to be premenstrual or in the third trimester of pregnancy (Bjornberg, 1968).

Race

A commonly held belief is that Negro skin is less reactive or irritable than Caucasian skin; few studies convincingly validate this claim. Early experimentation with the irritant mustard gas (dichloroethyl sulfide) showed that a 1% solution in mineral oil elicited erythema in 58% of Caucasians but in only 15% of Negroes (Marshall et al., 1919). Similar results were obtained with the lacrimator CS (*o*-chlorobenzylidene malononitrile) (Weigand and Mershon, 1970). Since it is more difficult to detect slight changes in erythema in dark skin than in light skin, these results are open to question. Weigand and Gaylor (1974) studied the minimal erythema threshold response of black skin to irritating concentrations of DNCB (dinitrochlorobenzene). Although concentrations of DNCB required to elicit minimal erythema were significantly higher in intact black skin than in Caucasian skin, this difference disappeared if the stratum corneum was stripped with cellophane tape prior to application of the DNCB. Arguing that a significant difference should have persisted if it were due to pigmentation alone, these investigators concluded that Negro skin was truly less reactive than Caucasian skin, possibly due to a more effective barrier function of the stratum corneum. An increased resistance to irritation in black skin was also noted by Frosh and Kligman (1977a, 1977b), using a chamber scarification procedure and an ammonium hydroxide blister formation technique.

The basis of the decreased susceptibility of black skin to irritation is poorly understood. Weigand et al. (1974) claimed that the stratum corneum in Negroes, while not thicker than that in Caucasians, contained more cells and was a more efficient skin barrier. Others have supported this idea by demonstrating a higher resistance of black skin than of Caucasian skin (Johnson and Corah, 1960). Nevertheless, no racial differences in percutaneous penetration of corticosteroid could be demonstrated *in vivo* (Wickrema Sinha et al., 1978) or *in vitro* (F. N. Marzulli, personal communication).

Concomitant Disease

Generalized wasting and debilitation in patients with advanced carcinoma have been associated with decreased reactivity to croton oil and DNCB (Johnson et al., 1971). Decreased reactivity to croton oil (Weidenfeld, 1912) and increased susceptibility to alkali (Ziierz et al., 1960) were reported in patients with ichthyosis vulgaris. Other investigators noted increased reactivity to phenol (Schultz, 1912) but decreased reactivity to croton oil (Halter, 1941) on the depigmented skin in patients with vitiligo. The literature on patch test reactions to irritants in the presence of eczema is conflicting. This subject has been partly clarified by Bjornberg (1968), who showed that an increased susceptibility to irritants may be demonstrated in eczematous patients with some but *not all* irritants. Susceptibility to irritation has also been correlated with the extent of the eczema. Patients with *localized* hand eczema had increased reactivity to sodium lauryl sulfate; patients with *generalized* eczema had increased reactivity to four additional irritants (croton oil, trichloroacetic acid, mercury bichloride, and sapo kalinus). Bjornberg (1974) further demonstrated that patients with healed hand eczema have no greater susceptibility to irritants than noneczematous controls. The type of eczema may also influence the response to irritants. Skog (1960) showed an increased incidence of primary irritant reactions to pentadecylcatechol in patients with preexisting allergic contact eczema but not in patients with preexisting irritant eczema or atopic dermatitis. Although clinical observations have strongly suggested that individuals with atopic dermatitis or an atopic diathesis are more susceptible to skin irritation, experimental proof is mostly lacking.

Neurologic Influence

Neurologic factors may influence cutaneous reactivity. Biberstein (1940) reported an increased inflammatory response to mustard oil on sympathectomized ears in rabbits, compared with nonsympathectomized contralateral control ears. Others reported decreased reactivity to phenol in areas of peripheral paralysis but increased reactivity to phenol in areas of central paralysis (Schaefer, 1921), decreased reactivity to tincture of iodine in areas of peripheral anesthesia (Kaufman and Winkel, 1922), and a generalized increase in reactivity in areas of peripheral neuritis (Halter, 1941).

The nervous system is obviously involved in the subjective response to irritants. A specific somatosensory receptor, selectively stimulated by certain irritants (e.g., lacrimators), has been identified in cat skin (Foster and Ramaze, 1976).

Medication

Corticosteroids in sufficient dose administered either topically or systemically may suppress subsequent irritant responses to croton oil (Nilzen and Wikstrom, 1955), but not to turpentine or cantharidin (Goldman et al., 1952). In general, there appears to be a limiting dose of systemically administered corticosteroid below which the inflammatory response is not inhibited. Although there is not universal agreement, the limiting dose appears to be in the range of 15 mg of prednisone or equivalent (Feuerman and Levy, 1972). Antihistamines in any dose probably do not impair responses to irritants. No data exist on the cutaneous response to irritants in patients with Addison's or Cushing's disease.

PREDICTIVE IRRITANCY TESTING

Predictive irritancy testing involves specific tests for the irritant potential of individual chemicals as well as tests for individual susceptibility to irritation.

Predictive Testing for Chemical Irritant Potential

Predictive testing is widely performed to determine the irritant potential of various chemicals. The most popular methods are bioassays with human or animal subjects. Most procedures employ a single application of a test substance, with evaluation of the response in 24–48 h. The oldest of these assays is the Draize rabbit test, in which test substances are applied for 24 h under occlusion to abraded and nonabraded skin. While this procedure detects severe irritants for human skin, it is unsatisfactory for mild to moderate irritants (Phillips et al., 1972). Numerous modifications adaptable to special situations have been developed. The reader is referred to Chapter 6 of this text or to a National Research Council (1977) special publication that discusses the principles and practices involved.

Because of species variability, correlation of irritancy studies of animal skin with human skin has not been entirely satisfactory. A rabbit cumulative irritancy test has been described which compares favorably with a cumulative human irritancy assay (Marzulli and Maibach, 1975; Steinberg et al., 1975).

Bioassays involving human subjects are patterned after those involving animal models. Frosh and Kligman (1977b) introduced a chamber-scarification test, which enhances the capacity to detect mild irritants. The forearm is scarified in a crisscross pattern; the suspected irritant is applied to this area in a large aluminum chamber once daily for 3 d.

To date, bioassays have utilized visible degrees of erythema and edema as indices of irritancy; this method is simple and convenient. The development of physical techniques for measuring subtle degrees of noninflammatory skin damage has improved our understanding of this area. Skin permeability to water vapor (transepidermal water loss) was the first physical measurement to be used for this purpose. Early investigations clearly established that chemicals that provoked inflammation increased transepidermal water loss (Rollins, 1978; Spruit, 1970, 1971). Malten and Thiele (1973a) subsequently showed that increases in transepidermal water loss occurred *before* visible inflammation when ionic, polar, water-soluble substances (e.g., sodium hydroxide, soaps, detergents) were used as irritants. Malten and den Arend (1978) showed that an unionized, polar irritant (dimethyl sulfoxide) did not provoke increased water vapor loss until visible inflammation had already occurred. Similarly, two unionized nonpolar (water-insoluble) irritants, hexanediol diacrylate and butanediol diacrylate, did not provoke increased skin water vapor loss until visible inflammation occurred (Malten et al., 1979). Thus, transepidermal water loss measurements may detect the irritant capacity of certain chemicals in the absence of visible inflammation, but only for ionizable, polar, water-soluble substances.

Measurements of the electrical impedance (resistance) of human skin also detect subtle degrees of skin damage before skin inflammation occurs (Thiele and Malten, 1973). This method has the advantage over water loss measurements that it is capable of detecting subtle changes produced by unionizable or nonpolar substances as well as ionizable, polar ones (Malten et al., 1979).

Measurements of carbon dioxide emission from human skin have been developed (Malten and Thiele, 1973a). Rates of carbon dioxide emission from irritated skin increase roughly in proportion to the degree of irritation (Thiele, 1974).

Electrolyte flux through the skin barrier may be measured with the aid of ion-specific skin electrodes (Grice et al., 1975; Anjo et al., 1978). Measurements of chloride ion flux through psoriatic or eczematous skin indicate that, despite the dramatic increases in permeability to water vapor, the electrolyte barrier remains relatively intact (Grice et al., 1975). Chloride ion flux may provide another noninflammatory index of cutaneous irritation.

Predictive Testing for Susceptibility to Irritation

The ability to predict which individuals are more prone to irritant skin reactions has practical significance as a preemployment screening test. The ability of the skin to neutralize solutions of sodium hydroxide was first proposed as a screening test for susceptibility to irritation by Gross et al. (1954). Bjornberg (1968) reviewed previous attempts to predict general susceptibility by determining irritant responses to selected irritants. He was unable to corroborate earlier claims that inability to neutralize alkaline solutions, decreased resistance to alkaline irritation, or increased susceptibility to common experimental irritants could be used to predict susceptibility to irritation in a preemployment setting.

Frosh and Kligman (1977a) used the length of time to slight blister formation after experimental exposure to ammonium hydroxide as a predictive index. They found that short times were highly correlated with the intensity of inflammation produced by irritating concentrations of sodium lauryl sulfate. They also found that patients with atopic dermatitis (who were presumably more susceptible to irritation) had shortened times to blister formation than controls (Frosh, 1978).

SUMMARY

Adequate evaluation of clinical irritant reactions to chemical substances depends on a thorough understanding of all the variables influencing the irritant response. This is particularly important in the evaluation of occupational dermatitis, where precise identification of the offending irritant is often required but no simple test exists. Virtually any chemical substance may be an irritant under conditions of exposure that predispose to the occurrence of an irritant response. Conversely, irritant reactions to any chemical substance may be diminished or eliminated by reversing or correcting the factors of exposure predisposing to the irritant response. Application of the principles discussed above at the experimental and clinical levels will improve the understanding and management of cutaneous irritant reactions.

REFERENCES

Anjo, D. M., Cunico, R. L., and Maibach, H. I. 1978. Transepidermal chloride diffusion in man. *Clin. Res.* 26:208A.

Basmajian, J. V. et al., eds. 1982. *Stedman's Medical Dictionary,* 24th ed., p. 727. Baltimore: Williams & Wilkins.

Bettley, F. R. and Grice, K. A. 1966. The effect of sweating on patch test reactions to soap. *Br. J. Dermatol.* 78:636.

Biberstein, H. 1940. The effects of unilateral cervical sympathectomy on reactions of the skin. *J. Invest. Dermatol.* 3:201.

Bjornberg, A. 1968. *Skin Reactions to Primary Irritants in Patients with Hand Eczema.* Goteborg, Sweden: Oscar Isacsons Tryckeri AB.

Bjornberg, A. 1974. Skin reactions to primary irritants and predisposition to eczema. *Br. J. Dermatol.* 91:425.

Bjornberg, A. 1975. Skin reactions to primary irritants in men and women. *Acta Derm. Venereol. (Stockh.)* 55:191.

Butcher, E. 1951. The effects of applications of various substances on the epidermis of the rat. *J. Invest. Dermatol.* 16:85.

Coenraads, P. J., Bleumink, E., and Nater, J. P. 1975. Susceptibility to primary irritants. Age dependence and relation to contact allergic reactions. *Contact Dermatitis* 1:377.

Cronin, E. and Stoughton, R. B. 1962. Percutaneous absorption. Regional variations and the effect of hydration and epidermal stripping. *Br. J. Dermatol.* 74:265.

Dahl, M. V. and Trancik, R. J. 1977. Sodium lauryl sulfate irritant patch tests: Degree of inflammation at various times. *Contact Dermatitis* 3:263.

Epstein, W. R. 1961. Contact-type delayed hypersensitivity in infants and children: Induction of rhus sensitivity. *Pediatrics* 27:51.

Feldmann, R. J. and Maibach, H. I. 1967. Regional variation in percutaneous penetration of ^{14}C cortisol in man. *J. Invest. Dermatol.* 48:181.

Feuerman, E. and Levy, A. 1972. A study of the effect of prednisone and an antihistamine on patch test reactions. *Br. J. Dermatol.* 86:68.

Foster, R. W. and Ramaze, A. G. 1976. Evidence for a specific somatosensory receptor in the cat skin that responds to irritant chemicals. *Br. J. Pharmacol.* 57:436P.

Frosh, P. J. 1978. Rapid blister formation in human skin with ammonium hydroxide. Presented before the Society of Investigative Dermatology, San Francisco, Calif. May, 1978.

Frosh, P. J. and Kligman, A. M. 1977a. Rapid blister formation in human skin with ammonium hydroxide. *Br. J. Dermatol.* 96:461.

Frosh, P. J. and Kligman, A. M. 1977b. The chamber scarification test for assessing irritancy of topically applied substances. In *Cutaneous Toxicity*, eds. V. A. Drill and P. Lazar, p. 150. New York: Academic.

Gallant, S. P. and Maibach, H. I. 1973. Reproducibility of allergy epicutaneous test techniques. *J. Allergy Clin. Immunol.* 51:245.

Goldman, L., Preston, R., and Rockwell, E. 1952. The local effect of 17-hydroxycorticosterone-21-acetate (compound F) on the diagnostic patch test reaction. *J. Invest. Dermatol.* 18:89.

Grice, K., Sattar, H., Casey, T., and Baker, H. 1975. An evaluation of Na$^+$, Cl$^-$, and pH ion-specific electrodes in the study of the electrolyte contents of epidermal transudate and sweat. *Br. J. Dermatol.* 92:511.

Gross, P., Blade, M. O., Chester, J., and Sloane, M. B. 1954. Dermatitis of housewives as a variant of nummular eczema. A study of pH of the skin and alkali neutralization by the Burckhart technique. Further advances in therapy and prophylaxis. *Arch. Dermatol.* 70:94.

Halter, K. 1941. Zur pathogenese des ekzems. *Arch. Dermatol. Syph.* 181:593. Cited in Bjornberg (1968), p. 21.

Hannuksela, M., Pirila, V., and Salo, O. P. 1975. Skin reactions to propylene glycol. *Contact Dermatitis* 1:112.

Holst, R. and Moller, H. 1975. One hundred twin pairs patch tested with primary irritants. *Br. J. Dermatol.* 93:145.

Iden, D. L. and Schroeter, A. L. 1977. The vehicle tray revisited. The use of the vehicle tray in assessing allergic contact dermatitis by a 24-hour application method. *Contact Dermatitis* 3:122.

Johnson, M. A., Maibach, H. I., and Salmon, S. E. 1971. Skin reactivity in patients with cancer-impaired delayed hypersensitivity of faulty inflammatory response. *N. Engl. J. Med.* 284:1255.

Johnson, R. C. and Corah, N. L. 1960. Racial differences in skin resistance. *Science* 139:766.

Kaufmann, F. and Winkel, M. 1922. Entzundung und nervensystem. *Klin. Wochenschr.* 1:12. Cited in Bjornberg (1968), p. 35.

Kligman, A. M. and Wooding, W. M. 1967. A method for the measurement and evaluation of irritants on human skin. *J. Invest. Dermatol.* 49:78.

Magnusson, B. and Hersle, K. 1965. Patch test methods. II. Regional variations of patch test responses. *Acta Derm. Venereol. (Stockh.)* 45:257.

Maibach, H. I., Feldmann, R. J., Milby, T. H., and Serrat, W. F. 1971. Regional variation in percutaneous penetration in man. Pesticides. *Arch. Environ. Health* 23:208.

Malten, K. E. and den Arend, J. A. C. J. 1978. Topical toxicity of various concentrations of DMSO recorded with impedance measurements and water vapor loss measurements. Recording of skin's adaptation to repeated DMSO irritation. *Contact Dermatitis* 4:80.

Malten, K. E. and Thele, F. A. J. 1973a. Evaluation of skin damage. II. Water loss and carbon dioxide release measurements related to skin resistance measurements. *Br. J. Dermatol.* 89:565.

Malten, K. E. and Thiele, F. A. J. 1973b. Some theoretical aspects of orthoergic (irritant) dermatitis. *Arch. Belg. Dermatol.* 28:9.

Malten, K. E., den Arend, J. A. C. J., and Wiggers, R. E. 1979. Delayed irritation: Hexanediol diacrylate and butanediol diacrylate. *Contact Dermatitis* 5:178.

Marshall, E. K., Lynch, V., and Smith, H. W. 1919. Variations in susceptibility of the skin to dichloroethylsulfide. *J. Pharmacol. Exp. Ther.* 12:291. Cited in Weigand and Gaylor (1974), p. 548.

Marzulli, F. N. and Maibach, H. I. 1975. The rabbit as a model for evaluating skin irritants: A comparison of results in animals and man using repeated skin exposures. *Food Cosmet. Toxicol.* 13:533.

Mathias, C. G. T., Maibach, H. I., and Epstein, J. H. 1978. Allergic contact photodermatitis to *para*-aminobenzoic acid. *Arch. Dermatol.* 114:1665.

McKenzie, A. W. 1972. Percutaneous absorption of steroids. *Arch. Dermatol.* 86:911.

McOsker, D. E. and Beck, L. W. 1967. Characteristics of accommodated (hardened) skin. *J. Invest. Dermatol.* 48:372.

Mitchell, J. C. 1969. Hardening in allergic contact dermatitis and immunological tolerance. *Trans. St. John's Hosp. Dermatol. Soc.* 55:141.

National Research Council. 1977. *Principles and Procedures for Evaluating the Toxicity of Household Substances.* Washington, D.C.: National Academy of Sciences.

Newhouse, M., McEvoy, D., and Rosenthal, D. 1978. Percutaneous paraquat absorption. *Arch. Dermatol.* 114:1516.

Nilzen, A. and Wikstrom, K. 1955. Factors influencing the skin reaction in guinea pigs sensitized with 2,4-dinitrochlorobenzene. *Acta Derm. Venereol. (Stockh.)* 35:415.

Phillips, L., Steinberg, M., Maibach, H. I., and Akers, W. A. 1972. A comparison of rabbit and human skin responses to certain irritants. *Toxicol. Appl. Pharmacol.* 21:369.

Pirila, V. 1975. Chamber test versus patch test for epicutaneous testing. *Contact Dermatitis* 1:48.

Rockl, H., Muller, E., and Haltermann, W. 1966. Zum aussagewert positiver epicutantest bei sauglingen und kindern. *Arch. Klin. Exp. Dermatol.* 226:407.

Rollins, T. G. 1978. From xerosis to nummular dermatitis: The dehydration dermatosis. *J. Am. Med. Assoc.* 206:637.

Rothenborg, H. W., Menne, T., and Sjolin, K. E. 1977. Temperature dependent primary irritant dermatitis from lemon perfume. *Contact Dermatitis* 3:37.

Rudzki, E., Zakrzewski, Z., Prokopczyk, G., and Kozlowska, A. 1976. Application of emulsifiers in the patch test. *Dermatologica* 153:333.

Sarkany, L. and Gaylarde, P. M. 1973. Thickening of guinea pig epidermis due to application of commonly used ointment bases. *Trans. St. John's Hosp. Dermatol. Soc.* 59:241.

Schaaf, F. 1961. Chemische konstitution und wirkung im akanthosetest. *Dermatologica* 123:361.

Schaaf, F. and Gross, F. 1953. Tierexperimentelle untersuchungen mit salben und salbengrundlagen. *Dermatologica* 106:357.

Schaefer, W. 1921. Beitrage zum klinischen studium und der quantitativen prufung der hautreaktion auf chemische reize. II. Uberdie chemische hautreakition bei peripheren und zentralen lahmungen. *Arch. Dermatol. Syph.* 132:87. Cited in Bjornberg (1968), p. 35.

Schultz, I. H. 1912. Beitrage zum klinischen studium und der quantitativen prufung der hautreaktion auf chemische reize. I. Mitteilung: Uber das verhalten normaler und leukopathischer hautstellen hautranker und hautreaktion bei peripheren und zentralen lahmungen. *Arch. Dermatol. Syph.* 113:987. Cited in Bjornberg (1968), p. 21.

Seeberg, G. 1955. Hudens reactivitet for tvattmedel i deras egenskap av primart hudretande amnen. *Sven. Laekartidn.* 52:3081. Cited in Bjornberg (1968), p. 24.

Shewmake, S. W. and Anderson, B. G. 1979. Hydrofluoric acid burns. *Arch. Dermatol.* 115:593.

Shore, R. N. and Shelley, W. B. 1974. Contact dermatitis from stearyl alcohol and propylene glycol in fluocinonide cream. *Arch. Dermatol.* 109:397.

Skog, E. 1960. Primary irritant and allergic eczematous reactions in patients with different dermatoses. *Acta Derm. Venereol. (Stockh.)* 40:307.

Spruit, D. 1970. Evaluation of skin function by the alkali application technique. *Curr. Probl. Dermatol.* 3:148.

Spruit, D. 1971. Interference of some substances with water vapor loss of human skin. *Am. Perfum. Cosmet.* 8:27.

Steinberg, M., Akers, W. A., Weeks, M., McCreesh, A. H., and Maibach, H. I. 1975. A comparison of test techniques based on rabbit and human skin responses to irritants with recommendations regarding the evaluation of mildly or moderately irritating compounds. In *Animal Models in Dermatology*, ed. H. I. Maibach. New York: Churchill Livingstone.

Thiele, F. A. J. 1974. *Measurements on the Surface of the Skin*, p. 81. Nijmegen, Netherlands: Drukkeij van Mammeren B. V.

Thiele, F. A. J. and Malten, K. E. 1973. Evaluation of skin damage. I. Skin resistance measurements with alternating current (impedance measurements). *Br. J. Dermatol.* 89:373.

Van Ketel, W. G. 1978. Patch testing with nickel sulfate in DMSO. *Contact Dermatitis* 4:167.

Van Ketel, W. G. 1979. Petrolatum again: An adequate vehicle in cases of metal allergy? *Contact Dermatitis* 5:192.

Wagner, G. and Purschel, W. 1962. Klinisch-analytische studie zum neuro-dermitisproblem. *Dermatologica* 125:1. Cited in Bjornberg (1968), p. 24.

Warshaw, T. G. and Hermann, F. 1952. Studies of skin reactions to propylene glycol. *J. Invest. Dermatol.* 19:423.

Weidenfeld, St. 1912. Beitrage zur pathogenese des ekzems. *Arch. Dermatol. Syph.* 111:891. Cited in Bjornberg (1968), p. 21.

Weigand, D. A. and Gaylor, J. R. 1974. Irritant reactions in Negro and Caucasian skin. *South. Med. J.* 67:548.

Weigand, D. A. and Mershon, M. M. 1970. The cutaneous irritant reaction to agent *o*-chlorobenzylidene malononitrile (CS). I. Quantitation and racial influence in human subjects. Edgewood Arsenal Tech. Rept. 4332. Cited in Weigand and Gaylor (1974), p. 548.

Weigand, D. A., Haygood, C., and Gaylor, J. R. 1974. Cell layers and density of Negro and Caucasian stratum corneum. *J. Invest. Dermatol.* 62:563.

Wickrema Sinha, W. J., Shaw, S. R., and Weber, O. J. 1978. Percutaneous penetration and excretion of tritium-labelled diforasone diacetate, a new corticosteroid, in the rat, monkey, and man. *J. Invest. Dermmtol.* 7:372.

Ziierz, P., Kiessling, W., and Berg, A. 1960. Experimentelle prufung der hautfunktion bdi ichthyosis vulgaris. *Arch. Klin. Exp. Dermatol.* 209:592. Cited in Bjornberg (1968), p. 21.

8

in vitro tests for delayed skin hypersensitivity: lymphokine production in allergic contact dermatitis

■ John E. Milner ■

INTRODUCTION

Skin tests for assessment of delayed hypersensitivity in sensitized subjects have been primarily of two deliveries: intradermal injections of products of systemic infections such as tuberculin, histoplasmin, and coccidioidin, and epicutaneous testing of chemicals that cause allergic contact dermatitis.

Patch testing, developed by Jadassohn (1895), has been the method most often employed by dermatologists and allergists to chemically assess allergic contact hypersensitivity in patients. The tests are simple to perform and are based on decades of experience with the thousands of chemicals that are known as contact allergens. Patch testing has its drawbacks, however: the tests require repeated examinations of the patch sites because they may become positive from 1 to 7 d after testing; they may sensitize previously unsensitized patients; they may be difficult to interpret; and they can exacerbate a quiescent dermatitis.

In an effort to solve the problems of patch testing and to study allergic contact dermatitis in a setting that eliminates problems with percutaneous absorption, sensitization, and so on *in vitro*, studies of allergic contact hypersensitivity have been pursued by investigators for approximately two decades. Their methodology is based on *in vitro* methods of assessing delayed hypersensitivity to systemic infections, but it has now progressed to the point where their work stands alone and deserves an independent evaluation.

This chapter is concerned with *in vitro* tests for delayed hypersensitivity, specifically allergic contact hypersensitivity.

LYMPHOKINES

The earliest reports of *in vitro* responses of delayed hypersensitivity were concerned with hypersensitivity to tuberculin in animals. In 1932 Rich and Lewis demonstrated that tuberculin in culture medium would diminish the migration of cells from splenic and lymph node tissue.

Three decades later, George and Vaugh (1962) studied peritoneal exudate cells from sensitized guinea pigs and found that migration of these cells from capillary tubes was inhibited by antigen to which the donors had been sensitized.

Later, Bloom and Bennett (1966) discovered a soluble factor in supernatants of tissue cultures of sensitized lymphocytes and tuberculin which inhibited the migration of guinea pig peritoneal exudate cells. David (1966) reported similar findings with conjugated serum proteins as the antigen.

Dumonde et al. (1969) pointed out four transferable phenomena of cell-mediated immunity: production of delayed-type hypersensitivity, lymphocyte transformation, cytotoxicity of target cells by sensitized lymphocytes, and inhibition of macrophage migration. They presented evidence that in the guinea pig the four phenomena were mediated by cell-free soluble factors produced by sensitized lymphocytes in contact with specific antigen but were expressed without immunologic specificity. The term "lymphokine" was suggested to encompass the mediators of the four phenomena.

A variety of lymphokines has been studied by a number of investigators. Four have been evaluated for their participation in or ability to detect allergic contact hypersensitivity. They are migration (or macrophage) inhibition factor (MIF), mitogenic factor (MF), lymphotoxin (LT), and leukocyte inhibition factor (LIF). Early investigations established that the lymphocyte was the source of lymphokines, but later investigators probed for the specific lymphocyte type responsible—T or B lymphocytes.

Rocklin et al. (1974) obtained highly purified populations of T and B lymphocytes by affinity column separation, stimulated them with antigen, and assayed their ability to produce MIF and MF. They reported that both T and B cells made MIF, and that the T cells that produced MIF were proliferating cells, whereas the B cells were not. In contrast, they reported that MF was made only by T cells, not B cells, when stimulated by antigen.

Similar findings were reported by Geha and Merler (1974), who obtained MF from human lymphocytes stimulated by tetanus toxoid. Their data also implicated the T cell as the unique source of MF.

Yoshida et al. (1973), using sensitized guinea pigs, found that pure soluble protein antigens or hapten-protein conjugates would cause only T lymphocytes to produce MIF. Purified protein derivative (PPD) elicited MIF production from both T and B cells. They also found that PPD could produce MIF from unsensitized donors, but only in B cells, not T cells. They attributed this to the role of PPD as a cell mitogen that functions in an antigenically nonspecific manner.

Other work by Korszun et al. (1981) indicated that lymphokines could affect epidermal cells in ways that did not manifest obvious injury. They injected guinea pigs intradermally with antigen-stimulated lymphocyte culture supernatants and a partially purified lymphokine preparation. Test animals showed significantly higher epidermal cell mitotic rates than controls. They concluded that lymphokines induce an alteration in epidermal kinetics and keratinization directly without necessary inflammation.

MIGRATION INHIBITION FACTOR

The most studied of the lymphokines is MIF, which has a molecular weight of 25,000 to 60,000. It has been shown to aggregate macrophages, to increase their adherence to glass surfaces, and to decrease their mobility (David and Remold, 1976).

In studying MIF and allergic contact hypersensitivity, Nishioka and Amos (1973) sensitized guinea pigs with dinitrofluorobenzene (DNFB) and prepared suspensions of lymph node cells. Epidermal cells were treated to obtain subcellular fractions, which were conjugated with dinitrochlorobenzene (DNCB). The DNFB-sensitized lymph node cells and DNCB-conjugated epidermal subcellular fractions were cultured together and the supernatant was added to normal guinea pig peritoneal exudate cells that were migrating. Nishioka and Amos detected significant inhibition of migration with supernatants from sensitized guinea pig cells but not with supernatants from unsensitized animals.

Another investigation of MIF and allergic contact MIF sensitivity was carried out by Miyagawa et al. (1977). They sensitized guinea pigs with picryl chloride and studied the inhibition of migration of their peritoneal exudate cells compared with those from normal controls. A soluble extract of picryl chloride-treated epidermis was able to inhibit the migration of peritoneal exudate cells in sensitized donors but not in normal controls. The substance that elicited MIF was a fraction of water-soluble conjugates containing six antigenic fragments of epidermal origin. Miyagawa et al. were unable to demonstrate MIF-inducing activity in any studies of free hapten or non-epidermal-conjugated hapten.

MITOGENIC FACTOR

In 1955 Osgood and Brooke described a method for continuous tissue culture of leukocytes by the application of "gradient" principles. This technique was modified by Hungerford et al. (1959), who were able to obtain high frequencies of mitosis of lymphocytes for the purpose of karyotyping humans. The lymphocytes enlarge prior to division and resemble "blast cells" of leukemia, hence the term "blast transformation" or "lymphocyte transformation." Nowell (1960) later reported that a mucoprotein plant extract, phytohemagglutinin (PHA), was a specific initiator of mitotic activity and blast transformation.

While investigating the mitogenic effect of PHA, Pearmain et al. (1963) substituted tuberculin for PHA in peripheral blood leukocyte cultures of "sensitive" patients and found mitotic rates similar to those obtained with PHA. Cultures of leukocytes from unsensitized patients did not demonstrate mitoses. Later workers reported that other substances such as pokeweed mitogen, periodate, and concanavalin A could produce similar effects.

This work was extended to contact allergens by Aspergren and Rorsman (1962), who found that nickel could transform lymphocytes *in vitro*. Unfortunately, the transformation was nonspecific and not an indicator of nickel hypersensitivity. Schöpf et al. (1969), Pappas et al. (1970), and Pauly et al. (1969) also found that nickel could nonspecifically transform lymphocytes *in vitro*. Nevertheless, in 1970 MacLeod et al. found that transformation as measured by [^{14}C] thymidine uptake could be demonstrated in 7 of 12 nickel-sensitive patients and not in any controls.

Geczy and Baumgarten (1970) sensitized guinea pigs to DNCB and then incubated the sensitized animals' lymphocytes with DNFB, thus attaching the dinitrophenyl group to cells. These cells then transformed to a greater degree than did those from unsensitized hosts.

Milner (1970) reported that lymphocytes from guinea pigs sensitized to DNFB would transform in culture, as measured by the incorporation of tritiated thymidine, when exposed to epidermal proteins conjugated with DNFB. This work was later extended to guinea pigs sensitized to *p*-phenylenediamine. Milner (1971) later found that his method was capable of detecting allergic contact hypersensitivity to DNFB in humans when he used human lymphocytes from sensitized donors and human epidermal extracts conjugated with DNFB.

Miller and Levis (1973) reported the *in vitro* detection of allergic contact hypersensitivity to DNCB conjugated to leukocyte and erythrocyte cellular membranes; this indicated that the reaction was not specifically directed toward epidermal cell conjugates.

Work with Langerhans cells has demonstrated their pivotal role in the allergic contact hypersensitivity process and indicated that it is these cells to which the contact allergens conjugate in the epidermis and to which the lymphocytes in Milner's work responded. The work of Miller and Levis shows that there may be other cellular receptors to which allergens can bind and trigger the release of lymphokines when contacted by sensitized lymphocytes.

LYMPHOTOXIN

Granger and Kolb (1968) were the first investigators to report on lymphokines that could damage antigen-coated cells. Ruddle and Waksman

(1968) reported similar findings. This lymphokine has been termed LT. Delescluse and Turk (1970) studied this phenomenon in allergic contact hypersensitivity by sensitizing guinea pigs to DNFB and incubating their peripheral blood lymphocytes with chicken erythrocytes conjugated with DNFB. Cytotoxicity was measured by the release of an isotopically labeled substance from the damaged erythrocytes. They found that this method was effective in assessing allergic contact hypersensitivity.

Tamaki et al. (1981) studied LT in a system in which epidermal cells were the targets. They sensitized mice by topically applying trinitrochlorobenzene (TNCB). These mice were donors for spleen cells that were stimulated *in vitro* to trinitrophenylated (TNP-conjugated) syngeneic spleen cells, whose responses were compared to those of cells from unsensitized donors. Effector cell activity was assayed with TNP-conjugated syngeneic epidermal cells and conjugated epidermal cells. Hapten-specific cytotoxic activity was detected, suggesting that epidermal damage in allergic contact dermatitis may be contributed to by sensitized cytotoxic effector cells.

LEUKOCYTE INHIBITION FACTOR

LIF was first reported by Soborg and Bendixen (1967), who developed a counterpart of the MIF test that used only human cells. Their system was used to assay the inhibition of migration of human peripheral blood lymphocytes from capillary tubes that contained leukocytes from sensitized donors into chambers containing specific antigen. The test involved patients with positive delayed skin sensitivity to brucellin. Rosenberg and David (1970) demonstrated leukocyte migration inhibition in humans sensitive to tuberculin. The test was extended to studies of schistosomiasis by Wolfson et al. (1972) and candidiasis by Bidtz-Jorgenson (1972).

This technique was extended to allergic contact hypersensitivity by Thulin and Zacharian (1972), who studied chromium hypersensitivity. They employed chromium complexed with albumin as the antigen. Mirza et al. (1974) reported similar findings with nickel complexed with albumin.

Jordan and Dvorak (1976) carried out similar work with nickel-sensitive subjects by a direct assay technique employing uncomplexed nickel as the antigen. They agreed with other investigators that the concentration of nickel should be just below the toxic dose.

Not all leukocyte migration inhibition is related to cell-mediated immunity. Packalen and Wasserman (1971) sensitized guinea pigs with thyroglobulin and demonstrated that only buffy coat leukocytes coated with gamma 1 or gamma 2 fractions of serum were inhibited in their migration in the presence of thyroglobulin. Brostoff (1974) concluded from this work that "cell-mediated immunity played no part in migration inhibition" in that particular system.

CONCLUSIONS

In vitro testing for delayed skin hypersensitivity is progressing. The various cellular and noncellular components of delayed hypersensitivity are being elucidated with the sophisticated techniques now available to the great number of investigators in this field. Yet in the whole area of study related to allergic contact hypersensitivity there remain many unanswered questions and avenues of investigation as yet unexplored.

The primary question to be addressed is whether or not haptens must be conjugated to elicit an immune reaction *in vitro*. Some of the studies mentioned in this chapter indicate that conjugates are necessary but that the carriers are diverse: erythrocytes, leukocytes, bovine and human albumin, lymphocyte membranes, and so on. Is it true that free haptens remain free, or have they conjugated with tissue culture-soluble proteins or cell membranes of participating cells?

A fertile area of exploration concerns the lymphokines and their applicability to the study of allergic contact hypersensitivity *in vitro*. One must recall, however, that tuberculin hypersensitivity is not the same as allergic contact hypersensitivity and that the various lymphokines may not wax and wane synchronously in the evolution of allergic contact dermatitis.

REFERENCES

Aspergren, N. and Rorsman, H. 1962. Short-term culture of leucocytes in nickel hypersensitivity. *Acta Derm. Venereol. (Stockh.)* 42:412–417.

Bidtz-Jorgenson, E. 1972. Delayed hypersensitivity to *Candida albicans* in man: Demonstration *in-vitro*: The capillary tube migration test. *Acta Allergol. (Kbh.)* 27:41–49.

Bloom, B. R. and Bennett, B. 1966. Mechanism of a reaction *in vitro* associated with delayed-type hypersensitivity. *Science* 153:80–82.

Brostoff, J. 1974. Critique of present *in-vitro* methods for the detection of cell-mediated immunity. *Proc. R. Soc. Med.* 67:514–516.

David, J. R. 1966. Delayed hypersensitivity *in vitro*: Its mediation by cell-free substances formed by lymphoid cell-antigen interaction. *Proc. Natl. Acad. Sci. U.S.A.* 56:72–77.

David, J. R. and Remold, H. G. 1976. Macrophage activation by lymphocyte mediators and studies on the interaction of macrophage inhibitory factor (MIF) with its target cell. In *Immunobiology of the Macrophage,* ed. D. S. Nelson, pp. 401–427. New York: Academic.

Delescluse, J. and Turk, J. L. 1970. Lymphocyte cytotoxicity: A possible *in vitro* test for contact dermatitis. *Lancet* ii:75–77.

Dumonde, D. C., Wolstencroft, R. A., Panayi, G. S., Matthew, M., Morley, J., and Howson, W. T. 1969. Lymphokines: Non-antibody mediators of cellular immunity generated by lymphocyte activation. *Nature (Lond.)* 224:38–43.

Geczy, A. F. and Baumgarten, A. 1970. Lymphocyte transformation in contact sensitivity. *Immunology* 19:189–203.

Geha, R. S. and Merler, E. 1974. Human lymphocyte mitogenic factor: Synthesis by sensitized thymus-derived lymphocytes, dependence of expression on the presence of antigen. *Cell. Immunol.* 10:86–104.

George, M. and Vaughan, J. H. 1962. *In-vitro* cell migration as a model for delayed hypersensitivity. *Proc. Soc. Exp. Biol. Med.* 111:514–521.

Granger, G. A. and Kolb, W. P. 1968. Lymphocyte *in vitro* cytotoxicity: Mechanisms of immune and non-immune small lymphocyte mediated target L-cell destruction. *J. Immunol.* 101:111–120.

Hungerford, D. A., Donnelly, A. J., Nowell, P. C., and Beck, S. 1959. The chromosome constitution of a human phenotypic intersex. *Am. J. Hum. Genet.* 11:215–236.

Jadassohn, J. 1896. Zur kenntnis medicamentosen dermatosen. *Verh. Dtsch. Dermatol. Ges.* 5:103.

Jordan, W. P. and Dvorak, J. 1976. Leucocyte migration inhibition assay (LIF) in nickel contact dermatitis. *Arch. Dermatol.* 112:1741–1744.

Korszun, A.-K., Wilton, J. M., and Johnson, N. W. 1981. The *in-vitro* effects of lymphokines on mitotic activity and keratinization in guinea pig epidermis. *J. Invest. Dermatol.* 76:433–437.

MacLeod, T. M., Hutchinson, F., and Raffle, E. J. 1970. The uptake of labelled thymidine by leucocytes of nickel sensitive patients. *Br. J. Dermatol.* 82:487–492.

Miller, A. E., Jr. and Levis, W. R. 1973. Studies on the contact sensitization of man with simple chemicals. I. Specific lymphocyte transformation in response to dinitrochlorobenzene sensitization. *J. Invest. Dermatol.* 61:261–269.

Milner, J. E. 1970. *In vitro* lymphocyte responses in contact hypersensitivity. *J. Invest. Dermatol.* 55:34–38.

Milner, J. E. 1971. *In vitro* lymphocyte responses in contact hypersensitivity II. *J. Invest. Dermatol.* 56:349–352.

Mirza, M., Perera, M. G., and Bernstein, I. L. 1974. Leukocyte migration inhibition in nickel dermatitis. *Fed. Proc.* 33:728.

Miyagawa, N., Miyagawa, S., Ashizawa, T., Sakamato, K., and Aoki, T. 1977. Studies on carrier protein in contact dermatitis: Macrophage migration inhibition by soluble epidermal substances as carrier proteins. *Acta Derm. Venereol. (Stock.)* 57:23–28.

Nishioka, K. and Amos, H. E. 1973. Contact sensitivity *in vitro.* The production of macrophage migration inhibition factors from DNCB sensitized lymphocytes by subcellular organelles obtained from DNCB-epidermal tissue. *Immunology* 25:423–432.

Nowell, P. C. 1960. Phytohaemagglutinin: An initiator of mitoses in cultures of normal human leucocytes. *Cancer Res.* 20:462–468.

Osgood, E. E. and Brooke, J. H. 1955. Continuous tissue culture of leucocytes from human leukemic bloods by application of "gradient" principles. *Blood* 10:1010–1022.

Packalen, T. and Wasserman, J. 1971. Inhibition of migration of normal guinea pig blood leucocytes in homologous gamma 2-globulin in the presence of specific antigen. *Int. Arch. Allergy Appl. Immunol.* 41:790–796.

Pappas, A., Orfanos, C. E., and Bertram, R. 1970. Non-specific lymphocyte transformation *in vitro* by nickel acetate. *J. Invest. Dermatol.* 55:198–200.

Pauly, J. L., Caron, G. A., and Suskind, R. R. 1969. Blast transformation of lymphocytes from guinea pigs, rats, and rabbits induced by mercuric chloride *in vitro. J. Cell Biol.* 40:847–850.

Pearmain, G. E., Lycette, R. R., and Fitzgerald, P. H. 1963. Tuberculin-induced mitoses in peripheral blood lymphocytes. *Lancet* i:637–638.

Rich, A. R. and Lewis, M. R. 1932. The nature of allergy in tuberculosis as revealed by tissue culture studies. *Bull. Johns Hopkins Hosp.* 50:115–131.

Rocklin, R. E., MacDermott, R. P., Chess, L., Schlossman, S. F., and David, J. R. 1974. Studies on mediator production by highly purified human T and B lymphocytes. *J. Exp. Med.* 140:1303–1316.

Rosenberg, S. A. and David, J. R. 1970. Inhibition of leucocyte migration: An evaluation of this *in vitro* assay of delayed hypersensitivity in man to a soluble antigen. *J. Immunol.* 105:1447–1452.

Ruddle, N. H. and Waksman, B. H. 1968. Cytotoxicity mediated by soluble antigen and lymphocytes in delayed hypersensitivity. *J. Exp. Med.* 128:1237–1279.

Schöpf, E., Schulz, K. H., and Isensee, I. 1969. Untersuchungen uber den lymphocytentrans formationstest be: Quecksilberallergie. *Arch. Klin. Exp. Dermatol.* 234:420.

Soborg, M. and Bendixen, G. 1967. Human lymphocyte migration as a parameter of hypersensitivity. *Acta Med. Scand.* 181:247–256.

Tamaki, K., Fujiwara, H., Levy, R. B., Shearer, G. M., and Katz, S. I. 1981. Hapten specific TNP-reactive cytotoxic effector cells using epidermal cells as targets. *J. Invest. Dermatol.* 77:225–229.

Thulin, H. and Zacharian, H. 1972. The leukocyte migration test in chromium hypersensitivity. *J. Invest. Dermatol.* 58:55–58.

Wolfson, R. L., Maddison, S. E., and Kaggan, I. G. 1972. Migration inhibition of peripheral leucocytes in human schistosomiasis. *J. Immunol.* 109:123–128.

Yoshida, T., Sonozak, H., and Cohen, S. J. 1973. The production of migration inhibition factor by B and T cells of the guinea pig. *J. Exp. Med.* 138:784–797.

9

identification of contact allergens: predictive tests in animals

■ Georg Klecak ■

INTRODUCTION

The objective of this chapter is to describe the experimental animal procedures that are claimed to be appropriate for predictive testing of the allergenic potential of chemicals and finished formulations as well as for calculating the risk of sensitization associated with skin contact with these substances. Before concentrating on the experimental strategy of individual test procedures, however, some essential aspects of dermatology and experimental immunology should be recalled.

Human modes of behavior in industrial society essentially determine the conditioning data of exposure to allergens and thus the rise of sensitization risk (Turk, 1966, 1967; Rostenberg, 1957). The skin has, among other functions, that of protecting against all insults to the organism from the environment (Stüttgen et al., 1965; Blank and Scheuplein, 1969; Jarrett, 1973). The chemical industry introduces a multiplicity of new substances and products, some of which, in case of accidental or intentional contact with the skin surface, may cause an allergic contact dermatitis (Baer, 1964; Bandman et al., 1972; Calnan, 1962; Calnan et al., 1970; Cruickshank, 1969; Department of Health, Education and Welfare, 1975; Ferguson and Rothman, 1959; Fisher, 1967; Fisher et al., 1971; Fregert et al., 1969a, 1969b; Hjorth, 1959, 1961; Hjorth and Fregert, 1972; Magnusson and Möller, 1979; Miescher, 1962; Rantuccio and Meneghini, 1970; Rostenberg, 1953, 1954; NACDG, 1973). The increasing frequency of allergic dermatitis in occupational diseases (Cronin and Wilkinson, 1973) reflects the effect on humans of chemical pollution in the environment (Agrup, 1969a, 1969b; Andersen and Maibach, 1980; Cronin, 1980; Epstein, 1962; Ferguson and Rothman, 1959; Foussereau and Benezra, 1970; Grimm and Gries, 1968; Lüders, 1976; Magnusson and Mobacken, 1972; Malten et al., 1964, 1969, 1971; Malten, 1979; Marcussen, 1962; Pirilä, 1947, 1962; Rudner et al., 1973; Rudzki and Kleiniewsak, 1970; Schubert et al., 1973; Schwartz and Peck, 1940; Schwartz et al., 1957).

In addition to the relatively small group of substances that are obligatory allergens (Paschoud, 1967), there is a large and steadily growing group of facultative allergenic agents (Baer et al., 1973; Epstein, 1962; Epstein et al., 1968; Fregert et al., 1969b; Meneghini et al., 1971; Mitchell, 1975; Schwartz and Peck, 1944). As their allergenic potential is variable, it is necessary to have a reliable predictive method for determining the risk of contact sensitization to these substances. Because of their selective skin pathogenicity, only part of the population is at risk. Whether an individual is affected is related to immune responsiveness as well as momentary skin condition. A dysfunction of the skin barrier, with or without overt skin manifestations, favors contact sensitization. To comprehend a broad spectrum of potential allergens is thus of interest not only from a clinical (Coombs and Gell, 1968) but also from an occupational-medical and industrial-hygienic viewpoint (Malten, 1975). The complexity of this problem reaches far beyond the purely medical aspects; it also has economic and sociopolitical dimensions. A number of measures within the compass of technology and occupational and preventive medicine have been taken and regulations have been issued (Bär, 1969; Behrbohm, 1975; Federal Register Amendment, 1964; Hopf, 1971).

"Absolute innocuousness" does not exist. Most products are neither wholly innocuous nor very dangerous. There are opportunities for injury through misuse or inadequate exposure (Gloxhuber, 1976; Opdyke, 1975; Rand, 1972). The risk of injury resulting from product exposure must be kept as low as possible; it should be restricted to such a degree that no special measures for users' protection are necessary (Anderson, 1975; Bär, 1974; Goldemberg, 1962; Weil, 1972). Practical experience is the best guide for determining which biological properties are relevant to consumer safety (Idman, 1976; Siegel and Melther, 1948). For new substances, experimental investigations provide a reliable basis for estimating hazards (Calnan et al., 1964; Carter and Griffith, 1965; Dohr-Lux and Lietz, 1965; Draize et al., 1944; Gloxhuber, 1974; Gloxhuber et al., 1974; Rowe and Olson, 1965). However, not every test procedure succeeds in doing this. Laboratory experiments may be conducted under extreme or unrealistic conditions. When evaluating the results, one considers how the relevant dermatotoxicologic and allergologic data should be interpreted for humans and what other factors—such as form of application and conditions of exposure—must be considered (Rand, 1972; Rostenberg, 1959; Weil, 1972).

Numerous biological test procedures in humans and animals have been devised, both for research related to eczema and to help the physician recognize the etiologic agents involved (Hardy, 1973; Steigleder, 1975). Various test procedures with a predictive character have been described (Calnan et al., 1964; Epstein and Kligman, 1964; Griffith, 1969; Holland et al., 1950; Maibach and Epstein, 1965; Newcomer and Landau, 1964; Rostenberg, 1959). These methods determine mainly allergenic capability, and seldom sensitizing capacity (Gloxhuber, 1976; Idson, 1968; Maibach, 1975; Rowe and Olson, 1965). Their development was motivated by clinical experience (Schwartz, 1951). The patch test of Jadassohn (1896a, 1896b) is still used with many variants for both induction and elicitation of contact sensitization (Magnusson et al., 1962, 1965, 1966; Schwartz and Peck, 1944).

In principle, predictive sensitization studies in humans are of two types: the "prophetic" patch test (Brunner and Smiljanic, 1952; Epstein and Kligman, 1964; Schwartz and Peck, 1944, 1946; Traub et al., 1954) and the "repeated-insult" patch test. The repeated-insult test (Draize, 1955, 1959; Shelanski and Shelanski, 1953) was a modification of the Landsteiner technique (Landsteiner and Jacobs, 1935, 1936; Landsteiner and Chase, 1937, 1941; Landsteiner and Di Somma, 1938) for guinea pigs and was intended to evaluate finished formulations. Simultaneous use of mild irritants such as sodium lauryl sulfate (SLS), allergens, and occlusive application potentiates penetration and enhances sensitization (Kligman and Epstein, 1959).

The "maximization provocative patch test" of Kligman (1966a, 1966b, 1966c, 1966d) is intended to classify substances according to the sensitizing capacity they elicit under arbitrarily defined sets of experimental conditions. This method is justifiable from an experimental point of view (Brunner, 1967; Giovacchini, 1972; Greif, 1967; Kligman and Epstein, 1975; Marzulli and Maibach, 1974). With respect to the risk of injury to persons involved in the test, Kligman's maximization test is controversial and is inadmissible in many countries (Agrup, 1968). The experience of many years suggests that humans as well as guinea pigs are suitable for experimental studies on allergic contact dermatitis (Magnusson and Kligman, 1970; Maguire, 1975; Maibach, 1975; Marzulli et al., 1968). The sequence for predictive testing should be: animal first, human afterwards.

After Jadassohn in 1896 differentiated between toxic and allergic reactions in an eczematous patient by means of a patch test, experimental studies of delayed-type allergy flourished. With the successful sensitizing assay of Bloch and Steiner-Wourlisch in humans in 1926 and in guinea pigs in 1930 by means of a *Primula veris* extract, experimental studies of the mechanism of contact allergy in animals gained importance. The systematic studies of Landsteiner and co-workers (1935, 1936, 1937) brought about the most significant understanding of incubation period, sensitization routes, dosage dependence, group specificity, technique of application, and duration of sensitization. The later findings of Landsteiner and Chase (1941, 1942) on the formation of antigens by interaction of simple chemical substances with protein carriers in exposed guinea pig skin were corroborated by Sulzberger and Baer (1938) and Simon et al. (1934; Simon, 1936). Chase (1941, 1950, 1953) closely examined genetics in guinea pigs in relation to susceptibility to skin sensitization. Landsteiner and Chase (1941) noted the influence of adjuvants. Frey and Wenk (1956, 1958) verified the role of regional lymph nodes in the mechanism of delayed-type allergy. In reviewing the innumerable experimental studies of contact dermatitis, we see that only the test object (guinea pig or human) and the application of generally strong allergens such as dinitrochlorobenzene (DNCB) and picryl chloride were common features until the middle of the 1950s (Chase, 1950, 1954; Chase and Maguire, 1974). This methodological arbitrariness was tolerable in basic research on immunologic processes. Shelanski and Shelanski (1953) and Draize et al. (1944; Draize, 1959), took the first step toward standardizing the test methods in humans and animals for predictive purposes.

The factors that most influence the occurrence of allergic contact dermatitis can be divided into physiological and physiochemical ones (Federal Register Amendment, 1964; Katz and Poulsen, 1971; Kligman, 1966a; La Du, 1965; Meyer and Ziegenmeyer, 1975; Rockwell, 1955; Wagner, 1961; Scheuplein, 1965; Stoughton, 1965). When animal models are used as a substitute for experiments in humans in dermatotoxicology, the differences and similarities between species represent the most important physiological factors. The structural and biochemical differences between human and animal skin (Bartek et al., 1972; Davies et al., 1972; Dvorak et al., 1974; Justice et al., 1961; Oberste-Lehn and Wiemann, 1950; Roudabush et al., 1965) influence penetration. Eczematous sensitization occurs in species other than humans and guinea pigs (Asherson and Ptak, 1968; Crowle and Crowle, 1961; Frey and Geleick, 1959; Nobréus et al., 1974; Rostenberg and Haeberlin, 1950; Roudabush et al., 1965; Strauss, 1937). Guinea pigs have proved especially suitable for experimental sensitization. Handling and economy are decisive factors in their choice for screening procedures (Asherson and Ptak, 1968; Ginsburg et al., 1937; Hood et al., 1965; Hunziker, 1969; Jadassohn et al., 1955; Landsteiner and Chase, 1941; Lane-Petter and Porter, 1963; Maguire, 1974a, 1974b; Maibach and Mitchell, 1975; Malten et al., 1966a, 1966b; Middleton, 1978; Nicholas, 1978; Oberste-Lehn and Wiemann, 1950; Paterson, 1966; Polak et al., 1973; Poole et al., 1970; Rackemann and Simon, 1934; Ritz et al., 1975; Rostenberg, 1947; Sulzberger, 1930; Thorgeirsson et al., 1975; Voss, 1958; Ziegler et al., 1972).

Guinea pigs stem from a strain endowed genetically with the property of homogeneously reacting upon antigenic exposure. Appropriate strains include the Hartley and Pirbright ones; animals of either sex are used. Even among the commonly used strains there are striking differences, which Chase (1941, 1953) and Polak and co-workers (Polak et al., 1968a; Polak and Turk, 1968b) attributed to a Mendelian dominant characteristic. The proclivity to sensitization must be verified from time to time by using strong sensitizers. Strains with a low allergic aptitude are inappropriate for determining the allergic potential of chemicals. Utilization of climatic chambers at $20 \pm 1°C$, a relative humidity of $40 \pm 5\%$, artificial light 12 h/d, and a uniform dry food complemented by carrots and water *ad libitum* is generally accepted (Magnusson and Kligman, 1969). Some of the physicochemical factors that are important in sensitization are identical with those enhancing skin penetration. How much of a potential allergen can pass the skin barrier is of paramount theoretical and practical importance (Calvery et al., 1946; Cameron and Short, 1966; Idson, 1971; Jungermann and Silberman, 1972; Katz and Poulsen, 1971; Landsdown and Grasso, 1972; Smeenk and Rijnbeek, 1969; Schaefer et al., 1975; Scheuplein, 1965; Schumacher, 1967; Stoughton, 1965; Stüttgen, 1972; Vinson et al., 1965; Wagner, 1961). The physicochemical properties of the vehicle (Bronaugh et al., 1981; Coldman et al., 1969; Higuchi, 1960; Hjorth and Trolle-Lassen, 1963; Katz and Poulsen, 1972; Katz and Shaikh, 1965; Mikkelsen and Trolle-Lassen, 1969; Ostrenga, 1971; Poulsen et al., 1968; Ritschel, 1969; Schaefer, 1974; Schaefer et al., 1975; Stemann, 1965; Wurster, 1968; Zesch, 1974) and of chemicals (Baer et al., 1967; Bleumink et al., 1976; Chulz, 1962; Johnson et al., 1972; Katz and Shaikh, 1965; Lieu and Tong, 1973; Nilzen and Wikström, 1955; Treherne, 1956; Wolter et al., 1970) and the concentration (Marzulli and Maibach, 1974), duration of exposure, and condition of the skin surface are determining for the occurrence of contact sensitization (Baker, 1968; Bettley, 1961; Blank, 1952; Brauer, 1974; Katz and Poulsen, 1972; Landsdown and Grasso, 1972; Lippold, 1974; Marzulli, 1962; Ritschel, 1969; Scheuplein, 1965; Stemann, 1965; Vinson et al., 1965; Wurster, 1968). The intradermal route passes natural barriers and in no way resembles real conditions of handling and consuming chemicals.

This chapter describes in detail the test procedures most frequently used in guinea pigs, including the Draize test (DT), the optimization test (OT), Freund's complete adjuvant test (FCAT), the guinea pig maximization test (GPMT) of Magnusson and Kligman, Maguire's modified "split adjuvant" technique, the Bühler test, and the open epicutaneous test (OET) (see Fig. 1). The test methods may be divided, according to the application route used for induction, into three groups:

1. Epicutaneous methods (Bühler test and OET)
2. Intradermal methods (DT, OT, and FCAT)
3. Methods using both application routes (Maguire split adjuvant technique and GPMT)

DRAIZE TEST

In 1944, 1955, and 1959 Draize published the first animal test with a predictive character for determining the allergenicity of new chemical substances. This technique is a variant of the classical Landsteiner and Jacobs technique, which was used in the 1930s for the determination of the

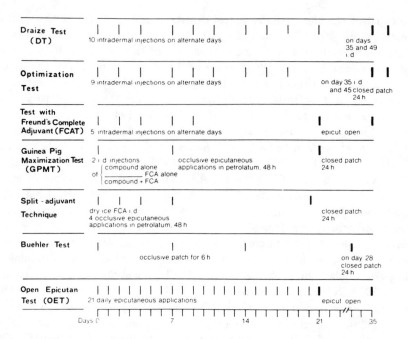

Draize Test (DT) — 10 intradermal injections on alternate days — on days 35 and 49 i.d.

Optimization Test — 9 intradermal injections on alternate days — on day 35 i.d. and 45 closed patch 24 h

Test with Freund's Complete Adjuvant (FCAT) — 5 intradermal injections on alternate days — epicut. open

Guinea Pig Maximization Test (GPMT) — 2 i.d. injections of { compound alone / FCA alone / compound + FCA } — occlusive epicutaneous applications in petrolatum, 48 h — closed patch 24 h

Split - adjuvant Technique — dry ice FCA i.d. — 4 occlusive epicutaneous applications in petrolatum, 48 h — closed patch 24 h

Buehler Test — occlusive patch for 6 h — on day 28 closed patch 24 h

Open Epicutan Test (OET) — 21 daily epicutaneous applications — epicut. open

Days 0 — 7 — 14 — 21 — 35

FIGURE 1 Techniques for detecting the capacity of low-molecular-weight compounds to induce contact hypersensitivity in guinea pigs.

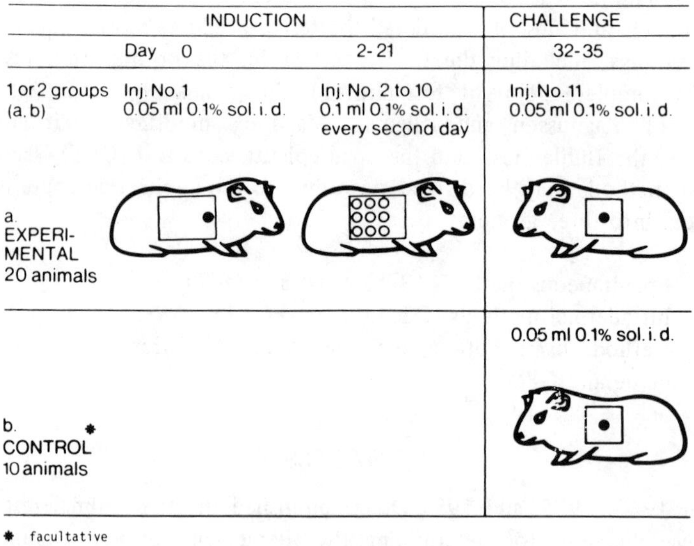

	INDUCTION		CHALLENGE
	Day 0	2-21	32-35
1 or 2 groups (a, b)	Inj. No. 1 0.05 ml 0.1% sol. i. d.	Inj. No. 2 to 10 0.1 ml 0.1% sol. i. d. every second day	Inj. No. 11 0.05 ml 0.1% sol. i. d.
a. EXPERI- MENTAL 20 animals			
b. CONTROL* 10 animals			0.05 ml 0.1% sol. i. d.

* facultative

FIGURE 2 The Draize test.

allergenicity of simple chemicals in guinea pigs. The Draize test is carried out as follows (see Fig. 2).

Materials and Methods

Animals. One or two groups of albino guinea pigs are used: (1) the experimental group (20 animals) and (2) the control group (facultative; 10 animals).

Materials. The test substance is applied intradermally (id) as a 0.1% solution, suspension, or emulsion in 0.85% NaCl, paraffin oil, or polyethylene glycol.

Induction

Before starting the treatment, an area of the back and the upper anterior flank of the animal is shaved with an electric clipper. Shaving is repeated before each reading and before any further injection. During about 3 wk the animals of the experimental group are given one id injection every second day, a total of 10 injections.

Day 0: Each animal of the experimental group is injected with 0.05 ml of the 0.1% solution, suspension, or emulsion of the test substance.

Day 1: Reading of skin reactions is performed.

Days 2–21: The remaining nine injections are administered as follows: Within an area of 3 × 4 cm on the back and the upper anterior flank, every second day, 0.1 ml of the test material is applied id at different spots; the skin reactions are read 24 h after each id injection.

Challenge

Days 32–35: The challenge is carried out on the contralateral flank of the experimental animal on a skin site that corresponds to the one subjected to the first injection. Control animals, if used, are treated in the same way and simultaneously, with 0.05 ml of the 0.1% test solution injected id in each animal.

Days 36–37: Animals of both groups are shaved and later are investigated. The intensity of erythema and occurrence and size of edema of the test reaction are evaluated and recorded.

Evaluation

To determine whether a test substance has sensitizing properties, the reactions of all animals after the first id injection (0.05 ml) are compared with the challenge test reactions among themselves and, if negative controls are used, among the control animals. If there are extreme differences between the reactions within a group, the averages of the mean values for the induction and test phases within the group are compared. The same holds for the mean values of the eliciting tests within the experimental and control groups.

Discussion

The Draize test can be carried out by simple means. Accordingly, the expenditures for materials and operations are small. However, the test has several drawbacks. The route of application is in many cases unrealistic in comparison with the actual conditions under which the substance or preparation is likely to come in contact with the skin surface. The induction concentration (0.1%) was chosen for the id route of application without considering the use concentration. Furthermore, the readings are not clear-cut and the subjective factor plays a role that should not be underestimated in evaluating the results.

Experience shows that this method is not sensitive enough for the identification of substances with a weak allergenic potential (Bühler, 1964; Klecak et al., 1977; Magnusson and Kligman, 1970; Maguire, 1973a, 1973b; Maurer, 1974). It is applicable for chemicals but not for finished preparations. Although recognized by the Food and Drug Administration (FDA) as a standard method, it does not meet the present standards for a predictive test for determining the allergenic potential of chemical substances and finished products. Because of its limitations, the Draize test is being replaced by other techniques.

FREUND'S COMPLETE ADJUVANT TEST

The FCAT is a further variant of the id test method for screening single chemical substances that are components of medical, cosmetic, and other products for their immunogenic properties. It has been routinely performed for 20 years in the Dermatotoxicological Department of Hoffmann-La Roche. It is a semiquantitative method by which the minimal eliciting concentration can be determined in sensitized animals (see Fig. 3).

Materials and Methods

Animals. Two groups of 10–20 guinea pigs each are used: (1) the experimental group and (2) the control group. An additional four guinea pigs are needed for the primary skin irritation study.

Materials. For the induction, performed by id application, oil-soluble test material is incorporated in Freund's (FCA) complete adjuvant mixed with an equal amount of twice-distilled water so that the final concentration in the emulsions is usually 5%. This depends on the physicochemical properties and the toxicity of the material to be tested. When incorporated in FCA, water-soluble test material is dissolved in the water phase before emulsification. For the challenge, performed by open epicutaneous application, the test material is diluted, emulsified, or suspended in the most appropriate vehicle

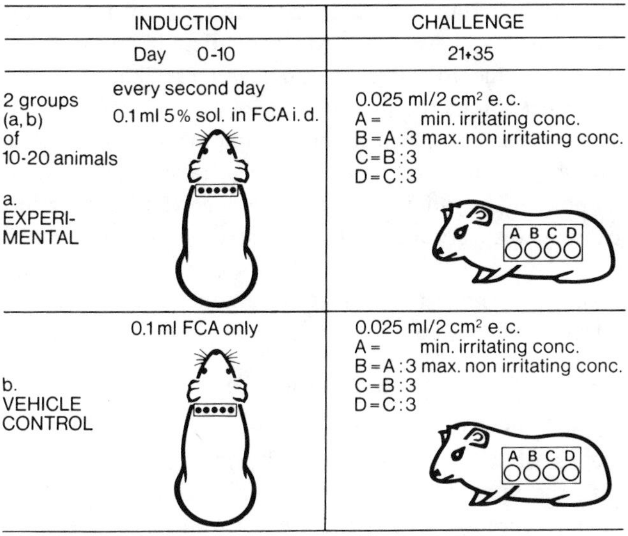

	INDUCTION	CHALLENGE
	Day 0-10	21+35
2 groups (a, b) of 10-20 animals a. EXPERI- MENTAL	every second day 0.1 ml 5% sol. in FCA i. d.	0.025 ml/2 cm² e. c. A = min. irritating conc. B = A : 3 max. non irritating conc. C = B : 3 D = C : 3
b. VEHICLE CONTROL	0.1 ml FCA only	0.025 ml/2 cm² e. c. A = min. irritating conc. B = A : 3 max. non irritating conc. C = B : 3 D = C : 3

FIGURE 3   Freund's complete adjuvant test (FCAT).

(water, acetone, alcohol, petrolatum, polyethylene glycol, and so on). The challenge concentrations vary in steps of three, so that any test substance can be tested epicutaneously undiluted as well as at concentrations of 30, 10, and 3% or less.

Induction

Shortly before the pretreatment, the shoulder region of both test and control animals is shaved.

Days 0-10: 0.1 ml of the test material in FCA is applied id in the shoulder region of the animals of the experimental group every second day (i.e., five times in all) on an area of 4×2 cm. The first injection is at the midline and the remaining four are alternately on the left and right sides. Animals of the control group are treated with 0.1 ml of FCA only.

Primary Irritation Study

One day before starting the challenge, a group of four guinea pigs is used to determine the threshold toxic concentration after a single topical application. Four different concentrations (e.g., 100, 30, 10, and 3%) are applied simultaneously to the left flank; 0.025 ml of each test concentration is spread homogeneously on a 2 cm² area of the flank skin, which was previously clipped and marked with a circular stamp. The highest concentration of a compound used in this test is limited by its solubility. The application site is left uncovered. It is necessary to rotate the various concentrations of the test substance across the different skin sites to minimize variation in response due to different skin locations. Skin reactions are read 24 h after the application of the test substance.

The minimal irritant concentration (A) and maximal nonirritant concentration (B) (threshold concentrations of each substance) are determined by an all-or-none criterion. The minimal irritant concentration is defined as the lowest one causing weak erythema on the test site. The maximal nonirritant concentration is defined as the highest one not causing macroscopic reactions in any of the animals. Estimation of these threshold concentrations is essential for the evaluation of allergic capacity on the basis of end point determination.

Challenge and Rechallenge

Days 21 and 35: To determine whether contact allergy was induced, both groups of animals (experimental and control) are tested on the flank with the same compound at the minimal irritant and some lower (nonirritant) concentrations. Tests are performed by pipetting 0.025 ml of each concentration to skin areas measuring 2 cm². To minimize site-to-site variations in skin reaction, the application of different concentrations of the test material is alternated on the four test sites. For rechallenge on d 35 the contralateral flank can be used.

Days 22-24 and 36-38: The skin sites are always read 24, 48, and 72 h after challenging for erythema, edema, and scaling.

This procedure makes it possible to determine the sensitizing capability of the material tested and the minimal concentration necessary to elicit an allergic reaction. The test material is considered allergenic when animals of the experimental group show positive reactions to nonirritant concentrations used for challenge.

Discussion

This test method is simple to perform and involves low material and operating expenses. It is not applicable for testing finished products. In our experience, this technique is at least as sensitive as the guinea pig maximization test and the optimization test (Stampf and Benezra, 1982).

However, there are some drawbacks related to the method used for induction of sensitization, namely the id application of the test material incorporated in Freund's complete adjuvant to enhance the immune response in experimental animals. Intradermal application bypasses the stratum corneum, thus excluding one of the most important variables determining the acquisition of contact sensitization. Like the maximization test and the optimization test, the FCAT procedure provides experimental conditions representing the very rare situation of skin exposure to a potential allergen.

Moreover, the adjuvant may convert chemicals with pure allergenic potential into good sensitizers. Consequently, the FCAT can establish the allergenicity of the test material, but not the actual risk of contact sensitization under conditions of use.

GUINEA PIG MAXIMIZATION TEST

By determining carefully all factors favoring contact sensitization and combining them in a single procedure, Magnusson and Kligman (1969, 1970, 1975) developed the guinea pig maximization test (GPMT). Assaying known human allergens in the GPMT and the human maximization test, Magnusson and Kligman found a high degree of correlation between the results. Discrepancies were found when the incidences of sensitization by some substances were compared. But agents that sensitized humans invariably sensitized guinea pigs as well. Therefore the GPMT can be considered a reliable procedure for screening of contact allergens and extrapolating the results to humans.

Materials and Methods

Animals. About equal numbers of male and female guinea pigs are used for (1) the experimental group (10–20 animals), (2) the control or vehicle group (10–20 animals), and (3) the primary irritation group (4 animals).

Materials. Application is id as well as epicutaneous. For id injections the test material is incorporated into FCA as well as diluted, suspended, or emulsified in NaCl. The concentration of material destined for id application may elicit neither strong local nor systemic toxic reactions in experimental animals. The concentration is generally between 1 and 5% and seldom, if ever, exceeds 5%. For topical application water-soluble substances are dissolved in water; for oil-soluble ones ethanol or other appropriate vehicles are used. Liquid materials are applied as such or diluted, if necessary. Solids are micronized or reduced to fine powder and then incorporated in a vehicle, usually petrolatum, at a maximum concentration of 25%. If the test agent is an irritant, a concentration is chosen that causes mild to moderate inflammation. If it is not an irritant, the area is pretreated with 10% sodium lauryl sulfate in petrolatum 24 h before the topical induction exposure. The concentrations of test material used for induction are adjusted to the highest one that can be well tolerated systematically.

Induction

Intradermal application. Experimental group: on d 0 an area of 4 × 6 cm over the shoulder region is clipped short with an electric clipper. Three pairs of id injections are made simultaneously, so that on each side of the midline there are two rows of three injections each. The injection sites are just within the boundaries of the 2 X 4 cm patch, which is applied 1 wk later. Injections are (1) 0.1 ml FCA alone (adjuvant blended with equal amount of water or saline), (2) 0.1 ml test material in saline, and (3) 0.1 ml test material in FCA. Injections 1 and 2 are given close to each other and nearest to the head, injection 3 most caudally (see Fig. 4).

Control group: The animals are given the same injections but without the test agent, that is, FCA and vehicle.

Topical application. Experimental group: on d 7 the same area over the shoulder region is again clipped and shaved with an electric razor. The test agent in petrolatum is spread over a 2 X 4 cm filter paper in an even, rather thick layer or, if liquid, to saturation. The patch is covered by overlapping, impermeable plastic adhesive tape. This, in turn, is firmly secured by an elastic adhesive bandage, which is wound around the torso of the animal. The dressing is left in place for 48 h.

Control group: the animals are exposed to the vehicle without the test agent in the same way as the experimental group. On d 9 the dressings are removed.

The treatment with FCA and occlusive bandage may lower the threshold level for skin irritation. The control group should therefore be exposed to the same maneuvers as the experimental group to exclude any false positive classifications when reading the challenge responses.

Primary Irritation Study

Before the challenge phase is started, the primary irritation study is performed with four fresh animals. Depending on the test material, up to three different concentrations and the vehicle can be applied to the flank skin with a patch, using four aluminum chambers. To minimize site-to-site variations in skin reactivity, the application of different concentrations of test material and vehicle is alternated on the test sites.

Challenge

Day 21: *Patch testing.* In experimental and control animals 5 X 5 cm areas of the flanks are shaved on both sides. Pieces of filter paper measuring 2 X 2 cm are sealed to the flanks for 24 h with the same occlusive bandage as for topical induction: (1) on the left side, a patch with the test agent in the highest nonirritant concentration and the same vehicle as for topical induction, and (2) on the right side, a patch with the vehicle alone. By using smaller ready-made test units, such as aluminum chambers (Finn chambers), challenge with the test agent at different concentrations and the vehicle can be performed on the same flank. If indicated, the contralateral flank can be used for rechallenge.

Days 23 and 24: *Readings.* At 21 h after removing the patches the flank skin is cleaned and shaved, if necessary, and 3 h later the first reading of

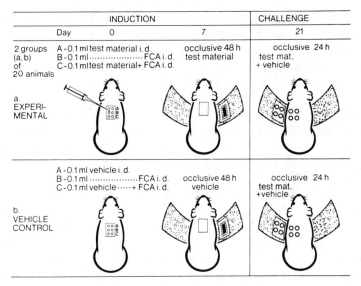

FIGURE 4 Guinea pig maximization test (GPMT).

the reactions is performed. The second reading is made the next day. For evaluation of skin reactions a four-point scale is used:

0 = No reaction
1 = Scattered reactions
2 = Moderate and diffuse reaction
3 = Intense reddening and swelling

Strength and duration of the skin reactions are compared within the experimental group and between the experimental and control groups. The allergic potential of the substance or finished formulation tested is considered proved only when the skin reactions to the challenge with the test material clearly outweigh those to the challenge with the vehicle and are greater than the reactions of the controls.

Using the scoring system of Kligman (1966c), an individual chemical or finished product may be classified according to its allergic potential as follows:

Sensitization rate (%)	Grade	Class
0–8	I	Weak
9–28	II	Mild
29–64	III	Moderate
65–80	IV	Strong
81–100	V	Extreme

Magnusson and Kligman (1969, 1970) do not regard sensitization of grade I as significant. Material so graded is not considered likely to present a hazard in use. Presumably, this would depend on the type of material, because a final product eliciting a weak reaction would be more hazardous than an individual chemical used as an ingredient in a substantially lower concentration than was tested.

Use of FCA and occlusion may cause some nonspecific effects. Guinea pigs pretreated with FCA have stronger irritant reactions to an occlusive patch of croton oil or other irritant than those not pretreated (B. Magnusson, personal communication). Potential sensitizers, which are also irritants, may show a lower concentration threshold for irritation than for sensitization. To overcome this problem and exclude the nonspecific FCA effect, it is necessary to use a control group pretreated with FCA and vehicle. This is the only way to exclude false positive results. Furthermore, we should point out the influence of the material used for the patch, of the vehicle, and of the tape used (Fernström, 1954, 1955; Magnusson et al., 1962, 1965).

The thickness of the patch is important since it may increase the pressure and therefore the penetration of the sensitizer. Usually, cellulose patches are not thicker than paper disks and are equally effective, but performing the challenge test with aluminum chambers gives slightly stronger responses (Pirilä, 1971, 1974). This agrees with clinical data from human patch tests. Finally, only Elastoplast should be used for the "booster" and challenge occlusive patches. It exerts pressure and holds the patch in position. Pressure is necessary for sensitization and elasticity is necessary for the comfort of the animal.

We have frequently observed strong skin reactions during induction of sensitization by id injection in the neck region, especially when FCA is applied. These sites may ulcerate, bleed, and/or form scales. On removal of the booster patch the scales are frequently pulled off and bleeding may occur. The animals tolerate the formation of ulcers, which generally heal in a few days.

Discussion

The GPMT is an excellent diagnostic procedure; however, it is less adequate for predicting reactions to finished formulations. Important criteria are lacking, such as the use of different concentrations and a form of application related to general use. Evaluation of the challenge reactions may be difficult, particularly when finished products are tested, because even the control animals and placebo sites may show weak to moderate skin reactions. According to Magnusson, "The maximization procedure only establishes the allergenic potentiality or sensitizing capacity of a substance, and not the actual risk of sensitization" (Magnusson, 1975).

The GPMT is used in many departments of dermatology in connection with research projects (Bourrinet et al., 1979; Campolmi et al., 1978; Kero et al., 1980; Nethercott, 1981; Senma et al., 1978; Skog and Wahlberg, 1970; Schubert and Ziegler, 1971; Schubert et al., 1973; Stampf et al., 1978; Thorgeirsson et al., 1975; Wahlberg et al., 1978; van der Walle et al., 1982; Ziegler et al., 1972; Ziegler, 1975, 1977). The U.S. Food and Drug Administration recommends the GPMT along with the split adjuvant technique (Marzulli and Maibach, 1976) and the Draize test as standard procedures for screening of new chemicals and finished products.

SPLIT ADJUVANT TECHNIQUE

Maguire and co-workers (1972, 1973b, 1975) utilized an adjuvant technique that enhances the processes leading to sensitization in the guinea pig, so that even weak and moderately weak contact allergens in humans can be identified in small groups of experimental animals (Maguire, 1975). It is derived from the split adjuvant test procedure (Maguire and Chase, 1967, 1972), in which FCA is injected into or near the skin site exposed to the allergen. In his predictive variant of the split adjuvant technique, Maguire used the observations of Bühler (1965) and Magnusson and Kligman (1970) that various adjuvant means can be used to render the guinea pig nonspecifically more susceptible to sensitization. The methodology of the split adjuvant technique is the following (see Fig. 5).

Materials and Methods

Animals. Two groups of 10-20 guinea pigs each are used for the experimental group and the control group, and at least four animals are used for the primary irritation test. The toenails and distal parts of both rear feet are wrapped with adhesive tape to prevent skin injuries.

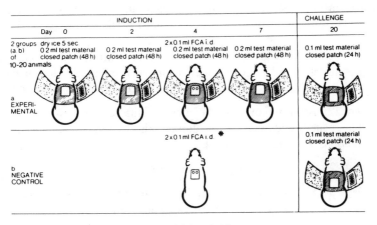

✱ essential supplement to the original sensitizing schedule

FIGURE 5   Split adjuvant technique.

Materials. Preparations are tested as such or, if necessary, diluted in accordance with use concentrations. Single components of the test material can also be examined in different concentrations by using adequate vehicles (e.g., petrolatum).

Induction

Day 0: Before starting the treatment, the skin on the back behind the shoulder girdle of the experimental animals is shaved to remove all the hair and some of the loose keratin. A window dressing is put on the animal, with the window over the shaved area (2 X 2 cm), and fixed in place with adhesive tape. Dry ice is applied for 5 s to this skin site. Then 0.2 ml ointment or 0.1 ml liquid is spread over the sensitization site and covered with Whatman filter paper. Finally, the whole area is covered with an occlusive tape, which is held in place with adhesive tape.

Day 2: The window is opened, the test material reapplied, and the window covered again.

Day 4: The window is opened, 0.1 ml FCA is injected id twice into the sensitization site, the test material is applied epicutaneously, and the window is closed again.

Day 7: Same procedure as on d 2.

Day 9: All wrappings are removed.

Challenge

The challenge is usually performed with a closed-patch test to a new (nonexposed) skin site with various exposure times (maximum, 24 h) and/or with an open test, depending on the toxicity of the test material. The challenge material should not produce substantial irritation in untreated animals. Therefore primary irritation tests must be done before the challenge.

Day 20: In both groups (experimental and control) a 2 X 2 cm area on the dorsal back is closely shaved, and 0.1 ml of the test material is applied to the skin site and covered with an occlusive dressing (patch).

Day 22: After removal of the dressing, the test area is marked with a skin pencil and the whole dorsal skin shaved atraumatically. Skin reactions are read for the first time.

Days 23 and 24: Readings are repeated.

Days 34 and 44: Rechallenging at a different (nonexposed) skin site in the same way as on d 21 may occasionally be performed.

The intensity of the skin reaction is classified according to the rating scale:

0 = Normal skin
± = Very faint, nonconfluent pink
+ = Faint pink
++ = Pale pink to pink, slight edema
+++ = Pink, moderate edema
++++ = Pink and thickened
+++++ = Bright pink, markedly thickened

The estimation of whether a preparation is sensitizing is based on a comparison of the frequency, intensity, and duration of skin reactions in the experimental and control animals.

Discussion

This test method, from a theoretical point of view, has most of the essential features of a predictive procedure. Finished preparations are tested as such and other substances are tested with regard to the use concentration. The mode of application is close to conditions of use. The application of dry ice, FCA, and the occlusive patch makes it possible to detect even weak sensitizers. As in the Bühler test, the closed patch is important, since occlusion enhances penetration and sensitization. Nevertheless, there is a difference between the methods in the duration of exposure, in the number of patches applied during the induction phase, and especially in the utilization of both dry ice and FCA in the split adjuvant technique. The Maguire technique is more sensitive and more effective for the detection of substances and products with a weaker allergic potential. To exclude false positive results in the split adjuvant technique it is essential that even the control animals be pretreated with FCA (as discussed in relation to the GPMT). The split adjuvant technique is applicable for screening numerous chemicals in which the dose dependence of presumed allergenic properties is to be checked, but it is time- and material-consuming. In the case of finished products, preparations of the same class or range—one with allergenic properties and the other devoid of them—may be included in the screening strategy as additional controls.

A modification of the Maguire procedure that is used in Japan by Dr. Okamoto is called the cumulation contact enhancement test (CCET). The test material is applied by means of an occlusive patch to the same skin site four times during 2 wk, and just before the third application 0.1 ml FCA is administered id on each side of the patch used for induction. The pretreatment with dry ice is omitted. For challenge, open application of the test material is preferred. If rechallenge is indicated, a closed patch test is recommended. In our experience the sensitivity of this method seems to be equal to that of Maguire's split adjuvant technique and the GPMT. The CCET and the Maguire technique have the same predictive value. They are both much more appropriate than the GPMT for screening of finished preparations that are externally applied to the human skin (toiletries and cosmetics) for their allergenic potential. In our experience, however, the FCA used during induction can convert chemicals with a pure allergenic potential into good sensitizers.

The U.S. Food and Drug Administration recommends the split adjuvant technique (Marzulli and Maibach, 1976) with the Draize test and the GPMT as standard procedures for screening new chemicals and finished products.

BÜHLER TOPICAL CLOSED-PATCH TECHNIQUE

Bühler (1965) and Griffith and Bühler (1969) at Procter & Gamble presented a predictive animal method that resembles the human repeated-insult patch test (RIPT), allows variation of screening conditions to optimize the detection of allergenic chemicals and finished formulations, and avoids unnecessary sensitization of human subjects. They have a number of years of successful experience with this closed-patch technique. Less than 3% of the materials that did not sensitize the guinea pig in the Bühler test were found to sensitize humans in the RIPT. Griffith and Bühler state that the test is sensitive enough to detect a moderate to strong sensitizer and that the probability of false positive results, which might lead to the rejection of an otherwise safe compound or formulation, is very low. The methodology has been modified and adapted several times. At present, experimental skin sensitization in guinea pigs according to Bühler and Griffith (1975) is carried out as follows (see Fig. 6).

Materials and Methods

Animals. About equal numbers of male and female guinea pigs are used for (1) the experimental group (at least 20 animals), (2) the control group(s) (10 animals), and (3) the primary irritation group (4 animals).

Materials. The test substance is diluted, emulsified, or suspended in a suitable vehicle. The concentration used for induction is allowed to provoke only weak skin irritation in the guinea pig and is calculated with respect to the use concentration.

Induction Phase for Primary Sensitization

The animals of the experimental and the vehicle group, if used, are shaved on the left shoulder in an area of about 2 × 2 cm on the day before exposure.

Week 1: Closed patches for the experimental group are prepared as follows: 0.4 ml of freshly prepared test material is applied on a 20 × 20 mm Webril pad on a 37 × 40 mm Parke-Davis reading bandage. The concentration chosen for induction of sensitization is usually 10 times higher than that calculated for human exposure. If it is found to be too irritating, the concentration may be decreased during the induction

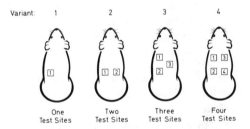

closed patch 6h 0.4 ml test mat.	INDUCTION	CHALLENGE	
	Week 1+2+3	5	6-7

animal groups :

EXPERIMENTAL
(20 animals)

VEHICLE
CONTROL
(10 animals)

NEGATIVE   CONTROL

- primary challenge -
(10 animals)
- rechallenge -
(10 animals)

• facultative

Various Schedules for Primary Irritation Studies

Variant: 1   2   3   4

One
Test Sites

Two
Test Sites

Three
Test Sites

Four
Test Sites

FIGURE 6   Bühler topical closed-patch technique.

phase. After the animal is placed in a special restrainer, the patch is applied to the clipped skin sites as soon as possible. The patch then is occluded with a rubber dental dam pulled tight and fastened to the bottom of the restrainer with binder clips. The restrainer is adjusted to minimize movement of the animal during the 6 h of exposure. Then the dental dam and patch are taken off. The residual material can be washed off with warm water before returning the animals to their cages.

Weeks 2 and 3: The 6-h closed patch with test material or vehicle is repeated (see d 0).

Primary Irritation Study

Before the induction phase is completed, the primary irritation study is performed with four previously unexposed animals. Depending on the test material, up to four different concentrations can be applied by the technique discussed above to various sites on the guinea pig's back. To minimize site-to-site variations in the skin reaction, concentrations of test material are alternated on the various test sites. The 24-h skin response is read and the highest nonirritant concentration determined. The day before challenge one or more virgin skin sites of about 2 X 2 cm are shaved on the backs of animals of the experimental and control groups.

Challenge

Week 5: The challenge test is performed on freshly clipped skin sites in the same way as the 6-h occlusive patch test of the induction phase. The test concentration is chosen such that the guinea pig skin tolerates it without any reaction. Vehicles commonly used for challenging are water and acetone. When other vehicles are chosen, the animals must also be tested with these. Multiple samples may be used to obtain as much data as possible. In principle, the control group is challenged in the same way as the experimental one.

At 24 h after application the patches are removed. The area of the challenge is marked and the skin of the whole back is shaved and depilated. At least 2 h after depilation the test site is examined for erythema and edema for the first time. The reaction is graded according to the following scale:

0   = No reaction
0.5 = Very faint erythema, usually confluent
1   = Faint erythema, usually confluent
2   = Moderate erythema
3   = Strong erythema with or without edema

Reading of the skin area is repeated 48 and 72 h after challenge and the skin reactions are graded.

The results of the challenge are expressed in terms of the incidence and severity of the skin response. An incidence index is calculated by dividing the number of animals with responses of grade 1 or more at 24 or 48 h by the number of animals tested. The severity index is the sum of the test grades divided by the number of animals tested. A comparison of the reactions elicited in terms of incidence, severity, and duration between all animal groups is made to determine whether a test substance induces sensitization.

Rechallenge

Sensitized animals can be rechallenged 1 and 2 wk after the primary challenge. For this purpose the animals can be divided into groups of at least

5 each, if more than three components of the sensitizing test material must be tested simultaneously. New control animals must be used for this rechallenge phase.

If the results of primary challenge or rechallenge do not allow clear conclusions and allergenicity of the test material is suspected, a rerun of the test material under aggravated conditions (higher concentrations) is indicated. A special situation occurs if a study with the maximum concentration for both induction and challenge indicates sensitization in animals, but of very low incidence. In this case an additional test is performed involving induction of sensitization by a single id injection of the test material (three concentrations with 10 animals per concentration group) in FCA and a closed-patch test for challenging 14 d later.

Discussion

The authors emphasize the predictive character of their method for determining the allergenic potential of substances and products (dermatologics, cosmetics, household products, etc.). This animal model allows variations in both the induction and the challenge phase. It mimics the conditions of use in that the epicutaneous mode of application is employed, induction concentrations in most cases correspond to the use concentration, and a solvent or vehicle can be chosen that is identical or similar to the end formulation. Finished preparations are tested as such or, if appropriate, diluted (e.g., shampoos).

The sensitivity of this method seems to be comparable to that of the RIPT in humans (Poole et al., 1970). The validity of the results of the Bühler test and the RIPT in humans for raw materials or single chemicals is, however, limited, inevitably depending on the test concentrations used. Accordingly, a substance tested at a concentration of 10% could not be declared a nonsensitizer because it did not provoke allergic sensitization in guinea pigs or humans, since the possibility exists that the test concentration was below the minimal dose engendering sensitization.

Even an experienced investigator has some difficulty reading and evaluating the challenge test reactions in this procedure. The spots on the controls as well as the experimental animals often show inflammatory reactions, whose strength, duration, and character must be evaluated subjectively. Further, the method requires a relatively large technical and material expenditure. Nevertheless, the technique in many respects satisfies the criteria for a predictive test method. The best recommendation for this technique is that it has been used satisfactorily for more than 15 yr by Procter and Gamble for the detection of substances and products with allergenic capability.

OPEN EPICUTANEOUS TEST

Procedures used with guinea pigs to detect sensitizing substances and select compounds that will be tolerated by humans should be simple and reliable, and the results obtained should be valid for humans. Taking into account all the variables that can influence the induction of contact sensitization in humans and guinea pigs, Klecak et al. (1977) developed an animal model, the open epicutaneous test (OET) (see Figs. 7 and 8). With this method one can screen many chemicals and finished formulations under conditions similar to those of human use and obtain quantitative results expressed in terms of a threshold concentration for skin tolerance. In contrast, in current methods compounds are tested at one concentration and the results are expressed in terms of frequency of sensitized animals and grade of intensity of lesions.

Materials and Methods

Animals. Up to six experimental groups and one control group of 8 guinea pigs are used. One group of 20 animals is used for finished formulations.

Materials. Substances are applied topically uncovered, undiluted, and, if possible and relevant, dissolved, suspended, or emulsified, in concentrations of 30, 10, 3, and 1% or lower in ethanol, acetone, water, petrolatum, polyethylene glycol, and/or other suitable vehicles. Finished products are tested as such or diluted according to use (shampoos). Constant volumes of each concentration are applied with a pipette or syringe on standard areas of the clipped animal flank.

Skin Irritation

When single chemicals and preparations used in dissolved form for testing are investigated, 1 d before starting the induction procedure the experimental group is used to determine the threshold toxic concentration by simultaneously applying the different concentrations (e.g., 100, 30, 10, and 3%) to the left flank skin. A 0.025-ml portion of each test concentration is homogeneously spread on a 2-cm^2 area of flank skin that was clipped and marked with a circular stamp. The highest concentration of a compound used is determined by its solubility and (for challenge) by its skin irritating capacity. The application site remains uncovered. It is necessary to rotate the various concentrations of test substance across the different application sites to minimize variations in response due to different skin locations.

Skin reactions are read 24 h after application. The minimal irritant concentration (A) and the maximal nonirritant concentration (B) (threshold concentrations) of the test substance are determined by an all-or-none criterion. The minimal irritant concentration is defined as the lowest one causing mild erythema in at least 25% of a group of animals. The maximal nonirritant concentration is the highest one not causing a macroscopic reaction in any animal. Estimation of the threshold concentrations is essential for evaluation of the allergenic capacity of the test material, based on the end point determination.

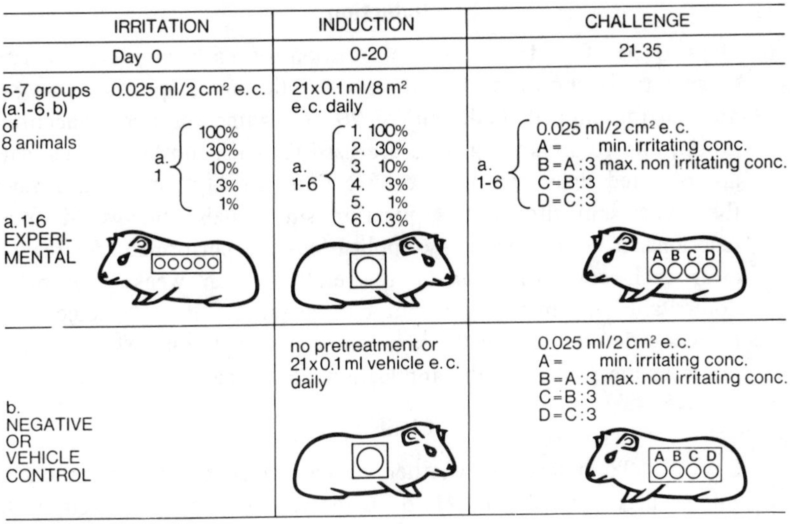

	IRRITATION	INDUCTION	CHALLENGE
	Day 0	0-20	21-35
5-7 groups (a.1-6, b) of 8 animals a.1-6 EXPERI-MENTAL	0.025 ml/2 cm² e.c. a.1 { 100% 30% 10% 3% 1%	21 × 0.1 ml/8 m² e.c. daily a.1-6 { 1. 100% 2. 30% 3. 10% 4. 3% 5. 1% 6. 0.3%	0.025 ml/2 cm² e.c. a.1-6 { A = min. irritating conc. B = A : 3 max. non irritating conc. C = B : 3 D = C : 3 A B C D
b. NEGATIVE OR VEHICLE CONTROL		no pretreatment or 21 × 0.1 ml vehicle e.c. daily	0.025 ml/2 cm² e.c. A = min. irritating conc. B = A : 3 max. non irritating conc. C = B : 3 D = C : 3 A B C D

FIGURE 7 Open epicutaneous test.

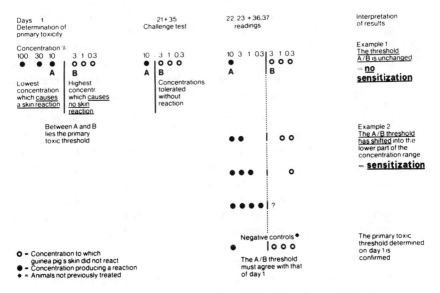

FIGURE 8 Schematic representation of the open epicutaneous test.

Induction

Days 0–20: On d 0, a 0.1-ml portion of each undiluted substance (preparation) and/or of its progressive dilutions is applied to an 8-cm^2 area on the clipped flank skin of 20 or 8 guinea pigs per concentration group; one to six such groups are used for each substance. Applications are repeated daily for 3 wk or five times weekly for 4 wk, always on the same skin site. The application site remains uncovered and the reactions, if continuous daily applications are performed, are read 24 h after each application or at the end of each week. The maximal nonirritant and minimal irritant concentrations after repeated applications are determined by the same all-or-none criterion. When strong skin reactions are provoked, the application site is changed.

Challenge

Day 21: To determine whether contact sensitization was induced, all guinea pigs treated for 21 d as described above, as well as 8–10 untreated controls for each substance, are tested on d 21 on the contralateral flank with the same substance at the minimal irritant and some lower concentrations. The minimal irritant concentration is used to confirm the primary irritant capacity determined before starting the induction (d −1) and to exclude false results due to instability of the test material. These tests are performed by pipetting 0.025 ml of each concentration on skin areas measuring 2 cm^2. It is necessary to rotate the concentrations of test substance across the different application sites to minimize variations in response at different skin locations. Skin reactions are read after 24, 48, and/or 72 h. In sensitized animals this procedure permits determinations of the *minimal sensitizing concentration* necessary for inducing allergic contact hypersensitivity and the *minimal eliciting concentration* necessary to cause a positive reaction. A concentration is considered allergenic when at least one animal in the concentration group shows a positive reaction with nonirritant concentrations.

Day 35: Rechallenge of all experimental animals as well as of old and new controls is performed with the same or lower challenge concentrations to reach the absolute threshold. Readings are made 24, 48, and 72 h after challenging and the results are analyzed. Rechallenge must be performed when finished formulations (shampoos, creams, ointments, etc.) are used for induction and the influence of phenomena such as angry-back syndrome on the results of the first challenge cannot be excluded. False positive results will thereby be avoided.

Discussion

It is important to know how well the OET compares with the tests in use—in other words, how reliably it detects substances with allergenic properties and how accurately it predicts the sensitizing potential of contact allergens. Therefore studies were performed to compare the predictive value of OET results with those of the GPMT, Freund's complete adjuvant test, and the Draize guinea pig test. In addition, the results for the animal models were compared with those of the human maximization test.

Instead of substances with pronounced allergenicity in humans, we chose substances with weak allergenicity for comparative studies with the OET. We selected fragrance materials that are present in most cosmetic, household, and some pharmaceutical products in order to study their biological effects with respect to skin toxicity and/or sensitizing power, determined by clinical investigations and under use conditions (Baer, 1935; Cronin, 1971; Epstein, 1969; Fisher, 1975; Fregert, 1970; Hjorth, 1967; Kahn, 1971; Kastner, 1968; Koch et al., 1971; Larsen, 1975; Mitchell, 1975; Ostbourne et al., 1956; Rothenborg and Hjorth, 1968).

Initially, we studied 32 fragrance materials that had been described in the literature as allergenic in humans. These compounds were tested concurrently in the four animal tests. The results are summarized in Table 1, which shows a high degree of correlation between clinically verified allergenicity and the results from the OET, GPMT, and FCAT. The Draize test was again found to be less sensitive than the other animal models. The seven substances for which we lacked confirmative data, such as positive history, positive patch test, or reexposure, were negative in all the animal tests. Their allergenicity is questionable or may be due to a cross-sensitizing capacity.

In the next stage, we performed comparative animal tests with 21 concentrated perfume compositions used for commercial products, such as perfumes, toilet waters, colognes, soaps and shampoos, all of which had already passed the test of time—that is, they were found to be harmless in consumer tests. The results are summarized in Table 2, which shows that clinically innocuous substances usually do not sensitize experimental animals

TABLE 1 Number of Compounds Described as Allergenic in Humans and Detected as Allergenic by the Four Animal Tests

Total number of compounds		Epicutaneous OET	Intradermal tests		
			DT	MT	FCAT
Positive					
In OET and id tests	18	18	7	15	17
In OET only	4	4	0	0	0
In id only	3	0	1	3	3
Total positive	25	22	8	18	20
Negative in all tests	7				
Total	32				

TABLE 2   Allergenicity in Four Animal Tests of 21
Perfume Compositions Harmless in Human Use

Total number of compounds	Epicutaneous OET	Intradermal tests		
		DT	MT	FCAT
Positive				
In all tests	1	1[a]	1	1	1
In OET only	1	1[a]	0	0	0
In id only	11	0	1	5	11
Total positive	13	2	2	6	12
Negative in all tests	8				
Total	21				

[a]Undiluted, positive; at user concentration, negative.

by the epicutaneous route. The achievement of sensitization by id procedures may not have clinical relevance and does not correspond to conditions of use.

Both these studies showed a high degree of correlation between clinical innocuousness as well as clinically estimated allergenicity and the results of the OET.

In addition, 194 fragrance materials, which are simple chemical compounds or substances of vegetable origin, were tested with the OET and the results were compared with those of the human maximization test and the repeated-insult patch test (Marzulli and Maibach, 1976; Nakayama et al., 1974; Opdyke, 1974, 1976). For most of these substances there is a high degree of agreement between the test results, as shown in Table 3. The OET results are correlated with those of the HMT and also those of the RIPT when

TABLE 3   Comparison of Test Results for 194
Substances Investigated for Their Allergenic
Potential in the Human Maximization Test
and in the Guinea Pig Open Epicutaneous Test

Human maximization test	Guinea pig OET	Number of preparations
Negative	Negative	185
Positive	Positive	7
Negative	Positive	1[a]
Positive	Negative	1[b]

[a]Hexen-2-al: humans, 4% negative; animals, 1% positive.

[b]Ethyl acrylate: humans, 4% positive; animals, 10% negative.

substances of the same origin and the same physical and chemical quality were used (Fisher and Dooms-Goossens, 1976). When these conditions were not fulfilled, differences in skin tolerance and/or allergenic capacity were observed. This may explain the discrepancies between results published by different authors, but it raises the question of the predictive value of such test results.

The results mentioned above should not be taken to indicate that the OET represents an ideal animal model. Like other techniques, the OET also has some weak points. For instance, it is not suitable for testing substances that color the skin, since this makes reading of skin reactions difficult, if not impossible. Furthermore, it did not indicate the allergenic potential of epoxy resins, perhaps because these chemicals have a low penetration rate through the intact guinea pig skin. Therefore new chemicals found to be nonallergenic under the test conditions of the OET should also be studied using id application with FCA, such as with Freund's complete adjuvant test. Conclusions concerning their allergenic potential can then be made.

In conclusion, I will summarize the reasons that lead us to favor and recommend the OET as a predictive technique for estimating the allergenic potential of chemicals and finished formulations:

1. Epicutaneously sensitized guinea pigs appear to be more appropriate models for allergic contact dermatitis in humans than guinea pigs sensitized by other methods. The id routes are likely to produce more heterogeneous forms of sensitization. The question arises whether sensitization induced by nonepicutaneous routes produces an immune response corresponding to that of contact allergy in humans.
2. Mode, frequency, and duration of exposure in the OET are compatible with the texture or consistency of most cosmetic products.
3. The OET allows variations in experimental strategy for the induction and elicitation of contact dermatitis. Moreover, it can be modified by stripping and by ultraviolet (UV-A and UV-B) light exposure.
4. The OET has adequate sensitivity and specificity. When used to test cosmetics, there is little likelihood of missing weak sensitizers or misidentifying substances as potent sensitizers when their allergenic potential is weak.
5. The OET results, not only in tests with fragrance materials, agree with those of the HMT, RIPT, and the consumer test.

OPTIMIZATION TEST

In 1974 Maurer published a variant of the Landsteiner-Draize guinea pig test which is highly sensitive (desirable for determining the allergenicity of substances) and easily reproducible. The motivation for developing the optimization test was the failure of the original Draize test (1955, 1959) to detect weak and moderate human sensitizers and the discovery of some drawbacks of the guinea pig maximization test. Moreover, Maurer assumed that humans may be more sensitive than animals to a range of substances with contact allergenic properties. Therefore, to enhance the sensitivity of guinea pig skin, Freund's complete adjuvant is used. In Maurer's opinion, the aim of the animal experiment is not to study the biological effect of a substance when applied by natural means, but to enhance the sensitivity of the animal skin so that substances with a sensitization rate of 1% or less in humans will sensitize a considerably higher percentage of animals in a small experimental group.

Materials and Methods

Animals. Forty guinea pigs of either sex are divided into two groups of 20 animals each (10 females and 10 males) as follows (see Fig. 9): (1) experimental group and (2) vehicle group (negative control).

Test material. In addition to repeated id injections with and without FCA, a single epicutaneous patch is applied. For the id application, solutions,

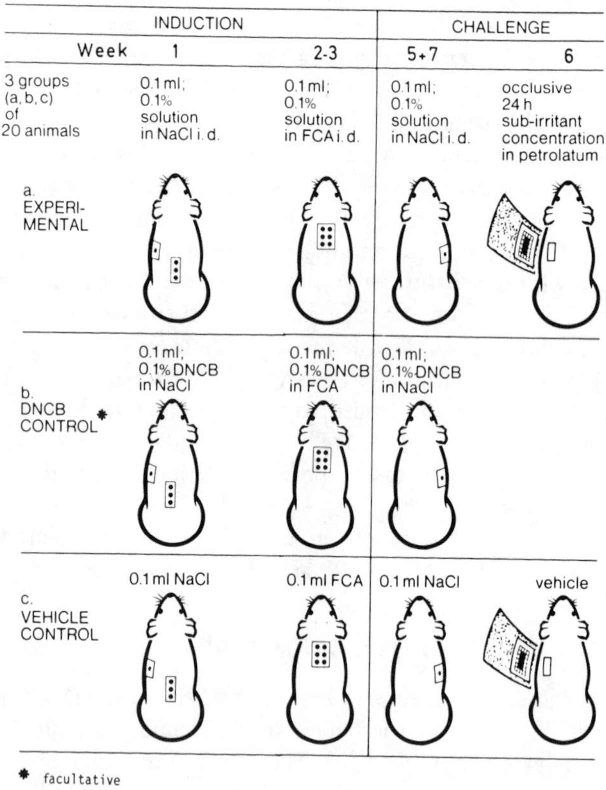

	INDUCTION		CHALLENGE	
Week	1	2-3	5+7	6
3 groups (a, b, c) of 20 animals	0.1 ml; 0.1% solution in NaCl i. d.	0.1 ml; 0.1% solution in FCA i. d.	0.1 ml; 0.1% solution in NaCl i. d.	occlusive 24 h sub-irritant concentration in petrolatum
a. EXPERI- MENTAL				
b. DNCB CONTROL *	0.1 ml; 0.1% DNCB in NaCl	0.1 ml; 0.1% DNCB in FCA	0.1 ml; 0.1% DNCB in NaCl	
c. VEHICLE CONTROL	0.1 ml NaCl	0.1 ml FCA	0.1 ml NaCl	vehicle

* facultative

FIGURE 9 Optimization test.

emulsions, or suspensions of the test substance in 0.9% saline and a mixture of FCA and saline containing the test material are prepared. Oil-soluble materials are mixed with FCA before saline is added. The end concentration used is 0.1%. For epicutaneous application (i.e., for the second challenge test), the substance, in subirritant concentrations for guinea pig skin, is dissolved or incorporated in appropriate solvents or vehicles (e.g., water, alcohol, diethyl phthalate, or petrolatum). Test material is always applied to freshly shaved new skin sites.

Induction

Induction is divided into two phases:

Week 1: On d 0 the test material in 0.9% saline is injected id (0.1 ml) into the flank and the dorsal skin sites. On d 2 and d 4 one id injection is made into the dorsal skin toward the region of the neck sites. During the first week, the skin sites are depilated 21 h after application and the 24-h skin reactions are evaluated under standard light conditions. The two largest diameters (in millimeters) of the erythematous reaction in vertical alignment are measured and the skinfold thickness (in millimeters) is determined with a skinfold gauge. Finally, the individual reaction volume (in microliters) is calculated for each reaction for individual animals.

Weeks 2 and 3: On d 7–21 six id injections (0.1 ml each of the test substance in a 1:1 mixture of FCA and saline are applied every second day in the region of the neck on both sides of the midline. During this period there is no reading of skin reactions.

Challenge

Challenge is performed in two steps, intradermally and epicutaneously.

First challenge step. On d 35 the animals of the experimental and control groups are tested with test material at the same dose and volume used for induction (without adjuvant) at a fresh site on the right shaved flank. On d 36 the test sites and surroundings are shaved and depilated 21 h after challenging. Readings are made 3 h later to measure the skin reactions (diameter and increase in skinfold thickness) and determine the reaction values.

Assessment: The average extent of the reaction to the first four induction doses (wk 1) and the standard deviation are calculated for each animal. The means and standard deviations are then added up and the sum used as an individual threshold value for each animal. The reactions to the challenge dose and the induction dose are compared in each animal. If the reaction volume on challenge exceeds the corresponding threshold value, the animal is considered sensitized. The number of positive animals in each group is counted and the significance of differences between the treated and control groups is assessed by the exact Fisher test for comparison of the basic probability of two binominal distributions (Sachs, 1971).

Second challenge step. Epicutaneous challenge is performed on d 45. Care must be taken that the test material is applied in nonirritating concentrations. The test substance in vehicle ($0.05 \ ml/cm^2$) is fixed during 24 h by means of an occlusive patch, using a 2×2 cm filter paper (Whatman 3M) on a shaved area of flank skin. On d 47, about 21 h after removing the patch, the reaction sites are chemically depilated (Butoquick for about 5 min); 3 h later the reactions are evaluated for intensity, size of erythema, and increase in thickness of the skin (edema). A distinctly visible redness within the field of application is considered an allergic reaction. The significance of differences in the number of positive animals between the treated group and the controls is again assessed by the Fisher test.

The number of positively reacting animals in the experimental group is compared with that in the control group, and the test material is classified according to its allergenicity and according to Kligman's system (1966b, 1966c) as shown in the table on p. 115.

Discussion

There is little experience with this technique except that of its authors (Maurer et al., 1975, 1978, 1979). In principle, this method is a modification of the Landsteiner-Draize guinea pig technique designed to detect moderate and weak sensitizers. According to (Maurer et al., 1975), the optimization test has the following significant advantages: "The measurement of the reaction occurring during the first week of induction, the calculation of the standard deviation and the comparison of induction and challenge in one and the same animal individually makes certain that the effective reaction is objectively measured, the assessment of intradermal reaction by calculation independent of the irritant effect of the substance and the solvent applied."

This seems to be the only appropriate procedure for exact evaluation of results obtained with experimental animals when id application of the test material is used for challenging. The sensitivity and reproducibility of the optimization test were proved in comparative studies with strong, moderate, and weak human sensitizers for which clinical data are available. The results indicate that the optimization test has about the same predictive value as a screening procedure for allergenicity testing as the guinea pig maximization test (Maurer et al., 1975, 1978, 1979) and Freund's complete adjuvant test (Maurer, unpublished data). However, of the three the optimization test seems to be the most complicated and time-consuming.

The main disadvantages of the optimization test are the following:

1. There is little evidence concerning the correlation between results of the optimization test and those of predictive human tests.
2. The use of id application limits the applicability of the optimization

test to single chemicals and a few formulations. For testing most finished formulations the test seems unsuitable.

3. The natural pathway of the contact allergen and other factors likely to influence the occurrence of contact allergy are not considered.

4. The optimization test (like the GPMT and FCAT) can only establish the allergenic potential or sensitizing capacity of a substance, not the actual risk of sensitization under use conditions.

Nevertheless, this method is a viable alternative to the GPMT or FCAT, particularly for testing synthetic dyes or skin coloring chemicals, since both of them allow no reading of skin reactions with the naked eye during challenge if applied epicutaneously.

CONCLUDING REMARKS

This chapter is meant to give an overview of the predictive animal tests most frequently used for evaluating the allergenic potential of chemicals and finished formulations and to discuss the merits and demerits of these methods. All these tests have been proposed to aid in predicting the probable incidence of adverse effects on the skin caused by contact sensitizers. When critically examined, none of these tests is entirely capable of doing this and none of them is universally applicable to all chemicals and types of formulations. Each substance poses its own unique problems, a fact ignored in recommendations of uniformity in predictive testing.

In practice, experienced dermatologists and toxicologists choose the test that they consider suitable for a specific problem (Benezra, 1980; Blomberg et al., 1978; Brulos et al., 1977; Forslind and Wahlberg, 1978; Hunziker, 1969; Ischy et al., 1969; Jadassohn et al., 1955; Lachapelle and Tennstedt, 1979; Meyer et al., 1979; Schäfer et al., 1978; Stampf et al., 1978). The assumption that a predictive test procedure is reliable is justified when the test technique corresponds to its purpose and the evaluation is sufficiently objective. In this respect, experts must take into account factors related to usage and induction of contact allergy.

The results of animal predictive testing will, of course, serve as guidelines rather than as absolute criteria for safety evaluation of materials and finished formulations before controlled testing on human subjects is indicated. (See Chapter 10 for additional information on contact dermatitis in animals.) There are some critics who incriminate the use of animal tests. We feel that the *in vitro* studies recommended by them are not suitable alternatives for prediction of safety in use.

REFERENCES

Agrup, G. 1968. Sensitization induced by patch testing. *Br. J. Dermatol.* 82:631–634.

Agrup, G. 1969a. Hand eczema. *Acta Derm. Venereol. (Stockh.)* 49(Suppl.): 40–41.

Agrup, G. 1969b. Hand eczema and other hand dermatoses in south Sweden. *Acta Derm. Venereol. (Stockh.)* 49(Suppl. 61):5–91.

Agrup, G. and Cronin, E. 1969. Contact dermatitis X. *Br. J. Dermatol.* 82:428–433.

Anderson, D. W. 1975. Cosmetic safety substantiation. In *5th Annual SCC Seminar, Los Angeles, November 15.* Hollywood, Calif.: Max Factor & Co.

Asherson, G. L. and Ptak, W. 1968. Contact and delayed hypersensitivity in the mouse. I. Active sensitization and passive transfer. *Immunology* 15:405–416.

Baer, R. L. 1935. Perfume dermatitis. *J. Am. Med. Assoc.* 104:1926.

Baer, R. L. 1964. Allergic eczematous sensitization in man 1936 and 1964. *J. Invest. Dermatol.* 43:223–229.

Baer, H., Watkins, R. C., Kurtz, A. P., Byck, J. S. and Dawson, C. R. 1967. Delayed contact sensitivity to catechols. III. The relationship of side-chain length to sensitizing potency of catechols of poison ivy. *J. Immunol.* 99:370–375.

Baer, R. L., Ramsey, D. L. and Biondi, E. 1973. The most common contact allergens 1968–1970. *Arch. Dermatol.* 108:74–78.

Bär, F. 1969. Höchstmengen-Verordnung–Pflanzenschutz unter dem Blickpunkt des Gesundheitsschutzes. *Bundesgesundheitsblatt* 2:21–27.

Bär, F. 1974. Die toxikologische Bewertung (Sicherheitsspannen, Höchstmengen) im Rahmen des Lebensmittelgesetzes (Lebensmittel-Zusatzstoffe und Pestizidrückstände). *Arch. Toxikol.* 32:51–62.

Baker, H. 1968. The effects of dimethylsulfoxide, dimethylformamide and dimethylacetamide on the cutaneous barrier to water in human skin. *J. Invest. Dermatol.* 50:282–288.

Bandmann, H. J., Calnan, C. D., Cronin, E., Fregert, S., Hjorth, N., Magnusson, B., Maibach, H., Malten, K. E., Meneghini, C. L., Pirilä, V. and Wilkinson, D. S. 1972. Dermatitis from applied medicaments. *Arch. Dermatol.* 106:335–337.

Bartek, M. J., LaBudde, J. A. and Maibach, H. I. 1972. Skin permeability in vivo: Comparison in rat, rabbit, pig and man. *J. Invest. Dermatol.* 58:114–123.

Behrbohm, P. 1975. Legislation on prevention of occupational dermatoses. *Contact Dermatitis* 1:207–210.

Benezra, C. 1980. Allergic contact dermatitis to alantolactone: The use of lymphocyte transformation test in experimentally sensitized guinea-pigs. *Abst. 5th Symp. Contact Dermatitis*, Barcelona, p. 76.

Bettley, F. R. 1961. The influence of soap in the permeability of the epidermis. *Br. J. Dermatol.* 73:448–454.

Blank, I. H. 1952. Factors which influence the water content of stratum corneum. *J. Invest. Dermatol.* 18:433–439.

Blank, I. H. and Scheuplein, R. J. 1969. Transport into and within the skin. *Br. J. Dermatol.* 81(Suppl. 4):4–10.

Bleumink, E., Mitchell, J. C., Geissman, T. A. and Towers, G. H. N. 1976. Contact hypersensitivity to sesquiterpene lactones in chrysanthemum dermatitis. *Contact Dermatitis* 2:81–88.

Bloch, B. and Steiner-Wourlisch, A. 1926. Die willkürliche Erzeugung der Primelüberempfindlichkeit beim Menschen und ihre Bedeutung für das Idiosynkrasieproblem. *Arch. Dermatol.* 52:283–303.

Bloch, B. and Steiner-Wourlisch, A. 1930. Die Sensibilisierung des Meerschweinchens gegen Primeln. *Arch. Dermatol.* 162:349–378.

Blomberg, M. V., Boerrigter, G. H., and Scheper, R. J. 1978. Interference of simultaneous skin tests in delayed hypersensitivity. *Immunology* 35:361–367.

Bourrinet, P., Puchault, P., Sarrazin, G., and Bercovic, A. 1979. Etude comparée de quelques substances allergéniques chez l'homme et chez le cobaye. *J. Pharm. Belg.* 34(1):21–26.

Brauer, E. W. 1974. The commission of skin through the medium of the skin patch test. *J. Soc. Cosmet. Chem.* 25:153–158.

Bronaugh, R. L., Congdon, E. R., and Scheuplein, R. J. 1981. The effect of cosmetic vehicles on the penetration of N-nitrosodiethanolamine through excised human skin. *J. Invest. Derm.* 76:94–96.

Brulos, M. F., Guillot, J. P., Martini, M. C., and Cotte, J. 1977. The influence of perfumes on the sensitizing potential of cosmetic bases. I. A technique for evaluating sensitizing potential. *J. Soc. Cosmet. Chem.* 28:357–365.

Brunner, M. J. 1967. Pitfalls and problems in predictive testing. *J. Soc. Cosmet. Chem.* 18:323–331.

Brunner, M. J. and Smiljanic, A. 1952. Procedure for evaluation of skin-sensitizing power of new materials. *Arch. Dermatol.* 66:703–705.

Bühler, E. V. 1964. A new method for detecting potential sensitizers using the guinea pig. *Toxicol. Appl. Pharmacol.* 6:341.

Bühler, E. V. 1965. Delayed contact hypersensitivity in the guinea pig. *Arch. Dermatol.* 91:171–177.

Bühler, E. V. and Griffith, F. 1975. Experimental skin sensitization in the guinea pig and man. In *Animal models in dermatology*, ed. H. Maibach, pp. 56–66. Edinburgh: Churchill Livingstone.

Calnan, C. D. 1962. Contact dermatitis from drugs; symposium on drug sensitization. *Proc. R. Soc. Med.* 55:39.

Calnan, C. D., Epstein, W. L. and Kligman, A. M. 1964. Methods of evaluating contact sensitizers. In *Evaluation of therapeutic agents and cosmetics*, eds. T. H. Sternberg and F. C. Newcomer. New York: McGraw-Hill.

Calnan, C. D., Bandmann, H. J., Cronin, E., Fregert, S., Hjorth, N., Magnusson, B., Malten, K., Meneghini, C. L., Pirilä, V. and Wilkinson, D. S. 1970. Hand dermatitis in housewives. *Br. J. Dermatol.* 82:543–548.

Calvery, H. O., Draize, J. H. and Lung, E. P. 1946. The metabolism and permeability of normal skin. *Physiol. Rev.* 26:495–540.

Cameron, G. R. and Short, R. H. D. 1966. Physiology and functional pathology of the skin. In *Modern trends in dermatology*, ed. R. M. B. McKenna. London: Butterworth.

Campolmi, P., Sertoli, A., Fabbri, P., and Panconesi, E. 1978. Alantolactone sensitivity in chrysanthemum contact dermatitis. *Contact Dermatitis* 4:93–102.

Carter, R. O. and Griffith, J. F. 1965. Experimental bases for the realistic assessment of safety of topical agents. *Toxicol. Appl. Pharmacol.* 7(Suppl. 2):60–73.

Chase, M. W. 1941. Inheritance in guinea pigs of the susceptibility to skin sensitization with simple chemical compounds. *J. Exp. Med.* 73:711–726.

Chase, M. W. 1950. A method for the enhancement of hypersensitivity to a simple chemical substance (picryl chloride). *Fed. Proc.* 9:379.

Chase, M. W. 1953. The inheritance of susceptibility to drug allergy in guinea pigs. *Trans. N.Y. Acad. Sci.* 15:79–82.

Chase, M. W. 1954. Experimental sensitization with particular reference to picryl chloride. *Int. Arch. Allergy* 5:163–191.

Chase, M. W. and Maguire, H. C. 1974. Further studies on sensitization to picric acid. *Monogr. Allergy* 8:1–12.

Chulz, K. H. 1962. *Chemische Struktur und allergene Wirkung*, p. 94. Aulendorf, Wurttemberg: Cantor.

Coldman, M. F., Poulsen, B. J. and Higuchi, T. 1969. Enhancement of percutaneous absorption by the use of volatile-nonvolatile systems as vehicles. *J. Pharm. Sci.* 58:1098–1102.

Coombs, R. R. A. and Gell, P. G. H. 1968. Classification of allergic reactions responsible for clinical hypersensitivity and disease. In *Clinical aspects of immunology*, 2nd ed., pp. 575–596. Oxford: Blackwell.

Cronin, E. 1971. Contact dermatitis from cinnamate. *Contact Dermatitis Newslett.* 9:216.

Cronin, E. and Wilkinson, D. S. 1973. Contact dermatitis. In *Recent advances in dermatology*, ed. A. J. Rook, vol. 3, pp. 134–192. New York: Churchill Livingstone.

Cronin, E. 1980. *Contact Dermatitis*. London: Churchill Livingstone.

Crowle, A. J. and Crowle, C. M. 1961. Contact sensitivity in mice. *J. Allergy* 23:302–320.

Cruickshank, C. N. D. 1969. Contact allergy. *J. Soc. Cosmet. Chem.* 20:479–485.

Davies, R. E., Harper, K. H. and Kynoch, S. R. 1972. Inter-species variation in dermal reactivity. *J. Soc. Cosmet. Chem.* 23:371–381.

Department of Health, Education and Welfare. June 1975. Investigation of consumer's perception of adverse reactions to consumer products. Contracted to Westat, Inc., Rockville, Md., contract 223738052. Rockville, Md.: Consumer Safety Statistic Staff, Office of Planning and Evaluation, Office of the Commissioner, *Food and Drug Administration.*

Dohr-Lux, R. and Lietz, G. 1965. Pharmakologisch-toxikologische und dermatologische Untersuchungsmethoden. *Parfüm. Kosmet.* 46:1:256–259; 2:289–293; 3:232–326.

Draize, J. H. 1955. Dermal toxicity. *Food Drug Cosmet. Law J.* 10:722–732.

Draize, J. H. 1959. Appraisal of the safety of chemicals in foods, drugs and cosmetics. In *Dermal toxicity*, p. 46. Austin, Tex.: Association of Food and Drug Officials of the United States, Texas State Department of Health.

Draize, J. H., Woodgard, G. and Calvery, H. O. 1944. Methods for the study of irritation and toxicity of substances applied topically to the skin and mucous membranes. *J. Pharmacol. Exp. Ther.* 82:377–390.

Dvorak, H. F., Dvorak, A. M. and Mihm, M. C., Jr. 1974. Morphological studies on cellular hypersensitivity in guinea pigs and man. *Monographs in Allergy* 8:54–65.

Epstein, E. 1969. Perfume dermatitis in mem. *J. Am. Med. Assoc.* 209:911–913.

Epstein, E., Rees, W. J. and Maibach, H. I. 1968. Recent experience with routine patch test screening. *Arch. Dermatol.* 98:18–22.

Epstein, S. 1962. Newer contact sensitizors in the home. In *Dermatoses due to physical and environmental factors*, ed. C. Rees. Springfield, Ill.: Thomas.

Epstein, W. L. and Kligman, A. M. 1964. Improved methods of prophetic patch testing. In *The evaluation of therapeutic agents and cosmetics*, eds. T. H. Sternberg and V. Newcomer, pp. 160–170. New York: McGraw-Hill.

Evans, D. A. P. 1963. Pharmacogenetics. *Am. J. Med.* 34:639–662.

Federal Register Amendment. 1964. 29 F.R. 13009.

Ferguson, E. H. and Rothman, S. 1959. Synthetic detergents and eczematous hand eruptions. *Arch. Dermatol.* 80:300–310.

Fernström, A. I. B. 1954. Patch-test studies. I. A new patch-test technique. *Acta Derm.-Venereol. (Stockh.)* 34:203–215.

Fernström, A. I. B. 1955. Patch-test studies. II. Details of the pressure test. *Acta Derm.-Venereol. (Stockh.)* 35:420–428.

Fisher, A. A. 1967. *Contact dermatitis.* Philadelphia: Lea & Febiger.

Fisher, A. A. 1975. Patch testing with perfume ingredients. *Contact Dermatitis* 1:166–168.

Fisher, A. A. and Dooms-Goossens, A. 1976. The effect of perfume "ageing" on the allergenicity of individual perfume ingredients. *Contact Dermatitis* 2:155–159.

Fisher, A. A., Pascher, F. and Kanof, N. B. 1971. Allergic contact dermatitis due to ingredients of vehicles. *Arch. Dermatol.* 104:286–290.

Forslind, B. and Wahlberg, J. E. 1978. The morphology of chromium allergic skin reactions at electron microscopic resolution: Studies in man and guinea pig. *Acta Derm.-Venereol. Suppl.* 79:43–51.

Foussereau, J. and Benetra, C. 1970. *Les eczémas allergiques professionnels.* Paris: Masson.

Fregert, S. 1970. Sensitization to phenylacetaldehyde. *Dermatologica* 141:11–14.

Fregert, S. and Hjorth, N. 1969. Results of standard patch tests with substances abandoned. *Contact Dermatitis Newslett.* 5:85–86.

Fregert, S., Hjorth, N., Magnusson, B., Bandmann, H. J., Calnan, D. C., Cronin, E., Malten, K. E., Meneghini, C. L., Pirilä, V., and Wilkinson, D. S. 1969b. Epidemiology of contact dermatitis. *Trans. St. John's Hosp. Dermatol. Soc.* 55:17.

Frey, J. R. and Geleick, H. 1959. Experimentelles Kontaktekzem durch Dinitrochlorbenzol an Ratten und Kaninchen. *Dermatologica* 119:294–300.

Frey, J. R. and Wenk, P. 1956. Experimentelle Untersuchungen zur Pathogenese des Kontaktekzems. *Dermatologica* 112:265–305.

Frey, J. R. and Wenk, P. 1958. Ueber die Funktion der regionalen Lymphknoten bei der Entstehung des Dinitrochlorbenzol-Kontaktekzems am Meerschweinchen. *Dermatologica* 116:243–259.

Ginsburg, J. E., Becker, F. T. and Becker, S. W. 1937. Sensitization of guinea pigs to poison ivy. *Arch. Dermatol.* 36:1165–1170.

Giovacchini, R. P. 1972. Old and new issues in the safety evaluation of cosmetics and toiletries. *CRC Crit. Rev. Toxicol.* 361–378.

Gleason, M. N., Gosselin, R. E., Hodge, H. C. and Smith, R. P. 1969. *Clinical toxicology of commercial products,* 3rd ed., sect. II, p. 80. Baltimore: Williams & Wilkins.

Gloxhuber, C. 1967. Toxikologische Prüfung von Kosmetika. *J. Soc. Cosmet. Chem.* 18:737–750.

Gloxhuber, C. 1974. Toxikologische und dermatologische Bewertung von chemischen Haushaltprodukten. *Fette Seifen Anstrichm.* 76:504–509.

Gloxhuber, C. 1976. Bewertung der gesundheitlichen Unbedenklichkeit von chemischen Haushaltprodukten und Kosmetika. *Seifen Oele Fette Wachse* 102:173–178.

Gloxhuber, C., Potokan, M., Braig, S., van Raay, H. G. and Schwarz, G. 1974. Untersuchungen über das Vorkommen eines sensibilisierenden Bestandteils in einem technischen Alkyläthersulfat. *Fette Seifen Anstrichm.* 76:126–129.

Goldemberg, R. L. 1962. Cosmetics and the general population: Safety aspects. *Proc. Sci. Sect. Toilet Goods Assoc.* 38:34–39.

Greif, N. 1967. Cutaneous safety of fragrance material as measured by the maximization-test. *Am. Perfum. Cosmet.* 82:54–57.

Griffith, J. F. 1969. Predictive and diagnostic testing for contact sensitization. *Toxicol. Appl. Pharmacol.* (Suppl. 3):90–102.

Griffith, J. F. and Bühler, E. V. 1969. *Experimental Skin Sensitization in the Guinea Pig and Man.* Cincinnati, Ohio: Procter and Gamble Co. (Presentation at the 26th Annual Meeting, American Academy of Dermatologists, Bal Harbour, Maine.)

Grimm, W. and Gries, H. 1968. Untersuchungen über die Terpentinöl-Allergie. *Berufsdermatosen* 16:190–203.

Hardy, J. 1973. Allergy, hypersensitivity and cosmetics. *J. Soc. Cosmet. Chem.* 24:423–468.

Higuchi, T. 1960. Physical chemical analysis of percutaneous absorption process from creams and ointments. *J. Soc. Cosmet. Chem.* 11:85–97.

Hjorth, N. 1959. Cosmetic allergy. *J. Soc. Cosmet. Chem.* 10:96–97.

Hjorth, N. 1961. *Eczematous allergy to balsams*, pp. 112–123. Copenhagen: Munksgaard.

Hjorth, N. 1967. Perfume dermatitis. *Contact Dermatitis Newslett.* 1:2–5.

Hjorth, N. and Trolle-Lassen, C. 1963. Skin reactions to ointment bases. *Trans. St. John's Hosp. Dermatol. Soc.* 49:127–140.

Hjorth, N. and Fregert, S. 1972. Contact dermatitis. In *Textbook of Dermatology*, eds. A. Rook, D. S. Wilkinson, and F. J. G. Ebling, pp. 305–385. Philadelphia: Davis.

Holland, B. D., Cox, W. C. and Dehne, E. J. 1950. "Prophetic" patch test; report on results of some 14,000 completed tests performed by Army Industrial Hygiene Laboratory. *Arch. Dermatol.* 61:611–618.

Hood, D. B., Neher, R. J., Reinke, R. E. and Zapp, J. A. 1965. Experience with the guinea pig in screening primary irritants and sensitizers. *Toxicol. Appl. Pharmacol.* 7:478.

Hopf, G. 1971. Empfehlungen für Hautverträglichkeitsprüfungen von Körperpflegemitteln (kosmetischen Erzeugnissen). *Fette Seifen Anstrichm.* 73:467–469.

Hunziker, N. 1969. *Experimental studies on guinea pig's eczema.* Berlin: Springer.

Idman, M. 1976. Anticipating the effects of chemicals—an evolving concept. *Ambio* 5:175–179.

Idson, B. 1968. Topical toxicity and testing. *J. Pharm. Sci.* 57:1–11.

Idson, B. 1971. *Percutaneous absorption of topics in medicinal chemistry.* New York: Interscience.

Ischy, R., Hunziker, N., Bujard, E., and Jadassohn, W. 1969. Experimental eczema. 31st communication: Can eczema be provoked in the tongue of the guinea pig? *Dermatologica* 139:413–416.

Jadassohn, J. 1896a. Zur Kenntniss der medicamentösen Dermatosen. *Verhdlg. Deutsch. Derm. Gesellsch. 5. Congress*: 103–129.

Jadassohn, J. 1896b. A contribution to the study of dermatoses produced by drugs. *Verh. Dtsch. Dermatol. Ges.* In *Selected essays and monographs*, transl. L. Elking, 1900: 207–229. London: New Sydenham Society.

Jadassohn, W., Bujard, E. and Brun, R. 1955. The experimental eczema of the guinea pig nipple. *J. Invest. Dermatol.* 24:247–253.

Jarrett, A. 1973. *The physiology and pathophysiology of the skin*, Vol. 1. London: Academic Press.

Johnson, R. A., Baer, H., Kirkpatrick, C. H., Dawson, C. R. and Khurana, R. G. 1972. Comparison of the contact allergenicity of the four pentadecyl-catechols derived from poison ivy urushiol in human subjects. *J. Allergy* 49:27–35.

Jungermann, E. and Silberman, H. C. 1972. The absorption and desorption of cosmetic chemicals on skin. *J. Soc. Cosmet. Chem.* 23:139–152.

Justice, J. D., Travers, J. J. and Vinson, L. J. 1961. The correlation between animal tests and human tests in assessing product mildness. *Proc. Sci. Sect. Toilet Goods Assoc.* 35:12.

Kahn, G. 1971. Intensified contact sensitization to benzyl salicylate. *Arch. Dermatol.* 103:497–500.

Kastner, E. 1968. Parfüm and Allergie. *J. Soc. Cosmet. Chem.* 19:807–821.

Katz, M. and Poulsen, B. J. 1971. Absorption of drugs through the skin. In *Handbuch der experimentellen Pharmakologie, 28/1,* eds. B. Brodie and J. D. Gilette, pp. 104–174. Berlin: Springer.

Katz, M. and Poulsen, B. J. 1972. Corticoid, vehicle and skin interaction in percutaneous absorption. *J. Soc. Cosmet. Chem.* 23:565–590.

Katz, M. and Shaikh, Z. 1965. Percutaneous corticosteroid absorption correlated to partition coefficient. *J. Pharm. Sci.* 54:591–594.

Kero, M. and Hannuksela, M. 1980. Guinea pig maximization test, open epicutaneous test and chamber test in induction of delayed contact hypersensitivity. *Contact Dermatitis* 6:341–344.

Klecak, G., Geleick, H., and Frey, J. R. 1977. Screening of fragrance materials for allergenicity in the guinea pig. I. Comparison of four testing methods. *J. Soc. Cosmet. Chem.* 28:53–64.

Kligman, A. M. and Epstein, W. 1959. Some factors effecting contact sensitization in man. In *Mechanism of Hypersensitivity,* eds. J. H. Shaffer, G. A. LoGrippo, and M. W. Chase, pp. 713–722. Boston, Mass.: Little Brown.

Kligman, A. M. 1966a. The identification of contact allergens by human assay. I. A critique of standard methods. *J. Invest. Dermatol.* 47:369–374.

Kligman, A. M. 1966b. The identification of contact allergens by human assay. II. Factors influencing the induction and measurement of allergic contact dermatitis. *J. Invest. Dermatol.* 47:375–392.

Kligman, A. M. 1966c. The identification of contact allergens by human assay. III. The maximization test. A procedure for screening and rating contact sensitizers. *J. Invest. Dermatol.* 47:393–409.

Kligman, A. M. 1966d. The SLS provocative patch test. *J. Invest. Dermatol.* 46:573–589.

Kligman, A. M. and Epstein, W. 1959. Some factors effecting contact sensitization in man. In *Mechanism of hypersensitivity,* p. 713. Boston: Little, Brown.

Kligman, A. M. and Epstein, W. 1975. Updating the maximization test for identifying contact allergens. *Contact Dermatitis* 1:231–239.

Koch, G., Magnusson, B. and Nyquist, G. 1971. Contact allergy to medicaments and materials used in dentistry. II. Sensitivity to eugenol and colophony. *Odontol. Revy* 22:275–289.

Lachapelle, J. M. and Tennstedt, D. 1979. Low allergenicity of triclosan. Predictive testing in guinea pigs and in humans. *Dermatologica* 158:379–383.

La Du, B. N. 1965. Pharmacogenetics. *Toxicol. Appl. Pharmacol.* 7:27–38.

Landsdown, A. B. G. and Grasso, P. 1972. Physico-chemical factors influencing epidermal damage by surface active damage. *Br. J. Dermatol.* 86:361–373.

Landsteiner, K. and Chase, M. W. 1937. Studies on the sensitization of animals with simple chemical compounds. IV. Anaphylaxis induced by picryl chloride and 2:4 dinitrochlorobenzene. *J. Exp. Med.* 66:337–351.

Landsteiner, K. and Chase, M. W. 1941. Studies on the sensitization of animals with simple chemical compounds. IX. Skin sensitization induced by injection of conjugates. *J. Exp. Med.* 73:431–438.

Landsteiner, K. and Chase, M. W. 1942. Experiments on transfer of cutaneous sensitivity to simple chemical compounds. *Proc. Soc. Exp. Biol. Med.* 49:688.

Landsteiner, K. and DiSomma, A. A. 1938. Studies on the sensitization of animals with simple chemical compounds. V. Sensitization to diazomethane and mustard oil. *J. Exp. Med.* 68:505–512.

Landsteiner, K. and Jacobs, J. 1935. Studies on sensitization of animals with simple chemical compounds. *J. Exp. Med.* 61:643–656.

Landsteiner, K. and Jacobs, J. 1936. Studies on the sensitization of animals with simple chemical compounds, II. *J. Exp. Med.* 64:625–629.

Lane-Petter, W. and Porter, G. 1963. The guinea pig. In *Animals for research*, ed. W. Lane-Petter, pp. 287–321. New York: Academic Press.

Larsen, W. G. 1975. Cosmetic dermatitis due to a perfume. *Contact Dermatitis* 1:142–145.

Lieu, E. J. and Tong, G. L. 1973. Physicochemical properties and percutaneous absorption of drugs. *J. Soc. Cosmet. Chem.* 24:371–384.

Lippold, B. C. 1974. Auswirkungen grenzflächenaktiver Substanzen auf Löslichkeit, chemische Stabilität und Verfügbarkeit cutan applizierter Wirkstoffe. *J. Soc. Cosmet. Chem.* 25:423–435.

Lüders, G. 1976. Reaktionen und Schäden nach äusseren Einwirkungen von Arzneimitteln und Berufsnoxen auf die Haut. *Berufsdermatosen* 24:61–70.

Magnusson, B. 1975. The relevance of results obtained with the guinea pig maximization test. In *Animal models in dermatology*, ed. H. Maibach, pp. 76–83. Edinburgh: Churchill Livingstone.

Magnusson, B. and Hersle, K. 1965. Patch test methods: I. A comparative study of six different types of patch tests. *Acta Derm. Venereol. (Stockh.)* 45:123–128.

Magnusson, B. and Kligman, A. M. 1969. The identification of contact allergens by animal assay. The guinea pig maximization test. *J. Invest. Dermatol.* 52:268–276.

Magnusson, B. and Kligman, A. M. 1970. *Allergic contact dermatitis in the guinea pig. Identification of contact allergens.* Springfield, Ill.: Thomas.

Magnusson, B. and Mobacken, H. 1972. Contact allergy to a self-hardening acrylic sealer for assembling metal parts. *Berufsdermatosen* 20:198–199.

Magnusson, B. and Möller, H. 1979. Contact allergy without skin disease. *Acta Derm.-Venereol. (Stockh.)* 59(Suppl. 85):113–115.

Magnusson, B., Blohm, S. G., Fregert, S., Hjorth, S., Havding, N., Pirilä, V. and Skog, E. 1962. Standardization of routine patch testing. *Acta Derm. Venereol. (Stockh.)* 126–127.

Magnusson, B. et al. 1966. Routine patch testing. II. Proposed basic series of test substances for Scandinavian countries and general remarks on testing technique. *Acta Derm. Venereol. (Stockh.)* 46:153–158. III. Frequency of contact allergy at six Scandinavian clinics. *Acta Derm. Venereol. (Stockh.)* 46:396–400.

Maguire, H. C. 1973a. Mechanism of intensification by Freund's complete adjuvant of the acquisition of delayed hypersensitivity in the guinea pig. *Immunol. Commun.* 1:239–246.

Maguire, H. C. 1973b. The bioassay of contact allergens in the guinea pig. *J. Soc. Cosmet. Chem.* 24:151–162.

Maguire, H. C. 1974a. Alteration in the acquisition of delayed hypersensitivity with adjuvant in the guinea pig. *Monogr. Allergy* 8:13-26.

Maguire, H. C. 1974b. Induction of delayed hypersensitivity to nitrogen mustard in the guinea pig. *Br. J. Dermatol.* 91:21-26.

Maguire, H. C. 1975. Estimation of the allergenicity of prospective human contact sensitizers in the guinea pig. In *Animal models in dermatology*, ed. H. Maibach, pp. 67-75. Edinburgh: Churchill Livingstone.

Maguire, H. C. and Chase, M. W. 1967. Exaggerated delayed-type hypersensitivity to simple chemical allergens in the guinea pig. *J. Invest. Dermatol.* 49:460-468.

Maguire, H. C. and Chase, M. W. 1972. Studies on the sensitization of animals with simple chemical compounds. XIII. Sensitization of guinea pigs with picric acid. *J. Exp. Med.* 135:357-374.

Maibach, H., ed. 1975. *Animal models in dermatology.* Edinburgh: Churchill Livingstone.

Maibach, H. I. and Epstein, W. L. 1965. Predictive patch testing for allergic sensitization in man. *Toxicol. Appl. Pharmacol.* 7:39-43.

Maibach, H. I. and Mitchell, J. C. 1975. Costus absolute (Saussurea): Predictive assay for allergic contact sensitization in guinea pigs. *Conf. Dermatol.* 1:184.

Malten, K. E. 1975. Cosmetics, the consumer, the factory worker and the occupational physician. *Contact Dermatitis* 1:16-26.

Malten, K. E. 1979. Four bakers showing positive patch-tests to a number of fragrance materials, which can also be used as flavors. *Acta Derm.-Venereol. (Stockh.)* 59(Suppl. 85):117-121.

Malten, K. E. and Zielhuis, R. L. 1964. *Industrial toxicology and dermatology in the production and processing of plastic.* New York: Elsevier.

Malten, K. E., Werwilghen, L. M. E. and Seutter, E. 1966a. The sensitization capacity of a simple epoxy resin as demonstrated in the guinea pig nipple test. 1st European Congress on Allergy, Stockholm, 1965. *Acta Derm. Venreol. (Stockh.)* Suppl.

Malten, K. E., Seutter, E., Verwilghen, M. E. and Disse, G. F. 1966b. The sensitization capacity of a simple epoxy resin as demonstrated in the guinea pig nipple test. II *Proc. 15th Int. Congr. Occup. Health, Vienna.*

Malten, K., Meneghini, C. L., Pirilä, V. and Wilkinson, D. S. 1969. Epidemiology of contact dermatitis. *Bull. Johns Hopkins Hosp.* 55:17-35.

Malten, K. E. et al. 1971. Occupational dermatitis in five European dermatological departments. *Berufsdermatosen* 19:1-13.

Marcussen, P. V. 1962. Eczematous allergy to metals. *Acta Allergol. (Kbh.)* 17:311-333.

Marzulli, F. N. 1962. Barriers to skin penetration. *J. Invest. Dermatol.* 39:387-393.

Marzulli, F. N. and Maibach, H. I. 1974. The use of graded concentrations in studying skin sensitizers: Experimental contact sensitization in man. *Food Cosmet. Toxicol.* 12:219-227.

Marzulli, F. N. and Maibach, H. I. 1976. Contact allergy: Predictive testing in man. *Contact Dermatitis* 2:1-17.

Marzulli, F. N., Carson, T. R. and Maibach, H. I. 1968. Delayed contact hypersensitivity studies in man and animals. *Proc. Joint Conf. Cosmet. Sci., Washington, D.C.* 107-122.

Maurer, T. 1974. Tierexperimentelle Methoden zur prädiktiven Erfassung sensibilisierender Eigenschaften von Kontaktallergenen. Inauguraldissertation, Universität Basel.

Maurer, T., Thomann, P., Weirich, E. G., and Hess, R. 1975. The optimization test in the guinea pig. A method for the predictive evaluation of the contact allergenicity of chemicals. *Agents Actions* 5:174–179.

Maurer, T., Thomann, P., Weirich, E. G., and Hess, R. 1978. Predictive evaluation in animals of the contact allergenic potential of medically important substances. I. Comparison of different methods of inducing and measuring cutaneous sensitization. *Contact Dermatitis* 4:321–333.

Maurer, T., Thomann, P., Weirich, E. G., and Hess, R. 1979. Predictive evaluation in animals of the contact allergenic potential of medically important substances. II. Comparison of different methods of cutaneous sensitization with "weak" allergens. *Contact Dermatitis* 5:1–10.

Meneghini, C. L., Rantuccio, R. and Lomuto, M. 1971. Additives, vehicles and active drugs of topical medicaments as causes of delayed-type allergic dermatitis. *Dermatologica* 143:137–147.

Meyer, F. and Ziegenmeyer, J. 1975. Resorptionsmöglichkeiten der Haut. *J. Soc. Cosmet. Chem.* 26:93–104.

Meyer, J. C., Grundmann, H.-P., Weiss, H., and Trachsel, H. 1979. Spättyp-Ueberempfindlichkeit gegenüber Staphylokokkenantigenen bei Meerschweinchen. *Dermatologica* 159:383–385.

Middleton, J. D. 1978. Predictive animal tests for delayed dermal hypersensitivity in man. *Soap Perfum. Cosmet.* 51(5):201–205.

Miescher, G. 1962. Ekzem, Histopathologie, Morphologie, Nosologie. In *Handb. Haut-Geschl. Krankh. Erg.-Werk*, ed. J. Jadassohn, vol. 2, pt. 1, p. 1. Berlin: Springer.

Mikkelsen, T. and Trolle-Lassen, C. 1969. Viscosity of test substances in petrolatum. *Contact Dermatitis Newslett.* 6:128–129.

Mitchell, J. C. 1975. Contact hypersensitivity to some perfume materials. *Contact Dermatitis* 1:196–199.

NACDG (North American Contact Dermatitis Group). 1973. News and notes. Allergen list. *Arch. Dermatol.* 107:457.

NACDG. 1972. Epidemiology of contact dermatitis in North America: 1972. *Arch. Dermatol.* 108:537–540.

Nakayama, H. et al. 1974. *Allergen controlled system.* Tokyo: Kamhara Shuppan.

Nethercott, J. R. 1981. Allergic contact dermatitis due to an epoxy acrylate. *Br. J. Dermatol.* 104:697–703.

Newcomer, V. D. and Landau, J. W. 1964. The current role of animals in the development of topically applied preparations. In *The evaluation of therapeutic agents and cosmetics*, eds. T. H. Sternberg and V. D. Newcomer, pp. 102–124. New York: McGraw-Hill.

Nicholas, P. 1978. "Economic" safety evaluation. *Soap Perfum. Cosmet.* 51(5):197–205.

Nilzén, A. and Wikström, K. 1955. The influence of sodium lauryl sulfate on the sensitization of guinea pigs to chrome and nickel. *Acta Derm. Venereol. (Stockh.)* 35:292–299.

Nobréus, N., Magnusson, B., Leander, L. and Attström, R. 1974. Induction of dinitrochlorobenzene contact sensitivity in dogs. Transfer of sensitivity by thoracic duct lymphocytes and suppression of sensitivity by antithymocyte serum. *Monogr. Allergy* 8:100–109.

Oberste-Lehn, H. and Wiemann, F. W. 1950. Die Meerschweinchenhaut als dermatologisches Testobjekt. *Arch. Klin. Exp. Dermatol.* 209:539–550.

Opdyke, D. L. J. 1974. Monographs on fragrance raw materials. *Food Cosmet. Toxicol.* 12:807–1016.

Opdyke, D. L. J. 1975. The safety of fragrance ingredients. *Br. J. Dermatol.* 93:351.

Opdyke, D. L. J. 1976. The safety of fragrances. *Soap Perfum. Cosmet.* 49:237–241.

Osborne, R. A. et al. 1956. Dermatological evaluation of perfumes of low sensitizing index. *Proc. Sci. Sect. Toilet Goods Assoc.* 17:80–84.

Ostrenga, J. O. 1971. Significance of vehicle composition. I. Relationship between topical vehicle compositions, skin penetrability, and clinical efficacy. *J. Pharm. Sci.* 60:1175–1179.

Paschoud, J. M. 1967. Externe Kontaktallergene. Alphabetisch geordnete Uebersicht der Fachliteratur 1960 bis 1965. *Hautarzt* 18:145–149.

Paterson, J. S. 1966. The guinea pig or Cavy. In *The UFAW handbook on the care and management of laboratory animals*, 3rd ed., p. 241. Baltimore, Md.: Williams & Wilkins.

Pirilä, V. 1947. On occupational diseases of the skin among paint factory workers and painters in Finland. *Acta Derm. Venereol. (Stockh.)* 27(Suppl. 16).

Pirilä, V. 1962. On the primary irritant and sensitizing effects of organic solvents. *Excerpta Med. Int. Congr. Ser.* 55:463–466.

Pirilä, V. 1971. Patch testing technique. A new modification of the chamber test. *Excerpta Med. Int. Congr. Ser.* 235:50.

Pirilä, V. 1974. Chamber test versus lapptest. *Förh. Nord. Dermatol. Fören.* 20:43.

Polak, L. and Turk, J. L. 1968. Studies on the effect of systemic administration of sensitizers in guinea-pigs with contact sensitivity to inorganic metal compounds. *Clin. Exp. Immunol.* 3:245–254.

Polak, L., Barnes, J. M. and Turk, J. L. 1968. The genetic control of contact sensitization to inorganic metal compounds in guinea-pigs. *Immunology* 14:707–711.

Polak, L., Turk, J. L. and Frey, J. R. 1973. Studies on contact hypersensitivity to chromium compounds. *Progr. Allergy* 17:145–226.

Poole, R. L., Griffith, J. F. and Macmillan, F. S. K. 1970. Experimental contact sensitization with benzoyl peroxide. *Arch. Dermatol.* 102:635–639.

Poulsen, B. J., Young, E., Coquilla, V. and Katz, M. 1968. Effect of topical vehicle composition on the *in vitro* release of fluocinolone acetonide and its acetate ester. *J. Pharm. Sci.* 57:928–933.

Rackemann, F. H. and Simon, F. A. 1934. The sensitization of guinea pigs to poison ivy. *Science* 79:344.

Rand, M. J. 1972. Toxicological considerations and safety testing of cosmetics and toiletries. *Am. Cosmet. Perfum.* 87:39–48.

Rantuccio, F. and Meneghini, C. L. 1970. Results of patch testing with cosmetic components in consecutive eczematous patients. *Contact Dermatitis Newslett.* 7:156–158.

Ritschel, W. A. 1969. Sorptionsvermittler in der Biopharmazie. *Angew. Chem.* 81:757–796.

Ritz, H. L., Connor, D. S. and Sauter, E. D. 1975. Contact sensitization of guinea-pigs with unsaturated and halogenated sultones. *Contact Dermatitis* 1:349–358.

Rockwell, E. M. 1955. Study of several factors influencing contact irritation and sensitization. *J. Invest. Dermatol.* 24:35–49.

Rostenberg, A. 1947. Studies on the eczematous sensitization. I. The route by which the sensitization generalizes. *J. Invest. Dermatol.* 8:345–354.

Rostenberg, A. 1953. The allergic dermatoses. *J. Am. Med. Assoc.* 165:1118–1125.

Rostenberg, A. 1954. Concepts of allergic sensitization: Their role in producing occupational dermatoses. *Ind. Med.* 23:1–8.

Rostenberg, A. 1957. Primary irritant and allergic eczematous reactions. *Arch. Dermatol.* 75:547–558.

Rostenberg, A. 1959. A predictive procedure for eczematous hypersensitivity. *Arch. Ind. Health* 20:181–193.

Rostenberg, A. and Haeberlin, J. B. 1950. Studies in eczematous sensitization. III. The development in species other than man or the guinea pig. *J. Invest. Dermatol.* 15:233–247.

Rothenborg, H. W. and Hjorth, N. 1968. Allergy to perfumes from toilet soap and detergents in patients with dermatitis. *Arch. Dermatol.* 97:417–421.

Roudabush, R. L., Terhaar, C. J., Fassett, D. W. and Dzibua, S. P. 1965. Comparative acute effects of some chemicals on the skin of rabbits and guinea pigs. *Toxicol. Appl. Pharmacol.* 7:559–565.

Rowe, V. K. and Olson, K. J. 1965. Prediction of dermal toxicity in humans from studies on animals. *Toxicol. Appl. Pharmacol.* 7:86–92.

Rudner, E. J., Clendenning, W. E., Epstein, E., Fisher, A. A., Jilson, O. F., Jordan, W. P., Kanof, N., Larsen, W., Maibach, H., Mitchell, J. C., O'Quinn, S. E., Schorr, W. F. and Sulzberger, M. B. 1973. Epidemiology of contact dermatitis in North America. *Arch. Dermatol.* 108:537–540.

Rudzki, E. and Kleiniewsak, D. 1970. The epidemiology of contact dermatitis in Poland. *Br. J. Dermatol.* 83:543–545.

Sachs, L. 1971. *Statistische Auswertungsmethoden.* Stuttgart: Thieme.

Senma, M., Fujuware, N., Sasaki, S., Toxama, M., Sakaguchi, K., and Takaoka, I. 1978. Studies on the cutaneous sensitization reaction of guinea pigs to purified aromatic chemicals. *Acta Derm.-Venereol. (Stockh.)* 58:121–124.

Schaefer, H. 1974. Wechselbeziehungen zwischen Haut, Vehikel und Arzneimittel bei der Penetration in die menschliche Haut. I. Mechanismus der Penetration. *Fette Seifen Anstrichm.* 76:220–222.

Schaefer, H., Zesch, A. and Stüttgen, G. 1975. Penetration von Medikamenten in die Haut. *Hautarzt* 26:449–451.

Schäfer, U., Metz, J., Pevny, I., and Röckl, H. 1978. Sensibilisierungsversuche an Meerschweinchen mit fünf parasubstituierten Benzolderivaten. *Arch. Dermatol. Forsch.* 261:153–161.

Scheuplein, R. J. 1965. Mechanism of percutaneous absorption. I. Routes of penetration and the influence of solubility. *J. Invest. Dermatol.* 45:334–346.

Schubert, H. and Ziegler, V. 1971. Die sensibilisierende Wirkung von flüssigem Polysulfidkautschuk. *Berufsdermatosen* 19:229–239.

Schubert, H., Göring, H. D., and Gans, U. 1973. Untersuchungen zur Sensibilisierungsfähigkeit von Aethoxyquin und *p*-Pheneditin. *Dermatol. Monatsschr.* 159:791–796.

Schumacher, G. E. 1967. Some properties of dimethyl sulfoxide in man. *Drug. Intell.* 1:188–194.

Schwartz, L. 1951. The skin testing of new cosmetics. *J. Soc. Cosmet. Chem.* 2:321–324.

Schwartz, L. and Peck, S. 1935. The irritants in adhesive plaster. *Public Health Rep.* 50:811–819; cited by L. Schwartz et al. 1940. An outbreak of dermatitis from new resin fabric finishes. *J. Am. Med. Assoc.* 115:906–911.

Schwartz, L. and Peck, S. M. 1944. The patch test in contact dermatitis. *Public Health Rep.* 59:546–557.

Schwartz, L. and Peck, S. M. 1946. *Cosmetics and dermatitis.* New York: Hoeber.

Schwartz, K., Tulipan, L. and Birmingham, D. 1957. *Occupational diseases of the skin.* Philadelphia: Lea & Febiger.

Shelanski, H. A. and Shelanski, M. V. 1953. A new technique of human patch tests. *Proc. Sci. Sect. Toilet Goods Assoc.* 20:46–49.

Siegel, J. M. and Melther, L. 1948. Patch test versus usage tests with special reference to volatile ingredients. *Arch. Dermatol.* 57:660–663.

Simon, F. A. 1936. Observations on poison ivy hypersensitiveness in guinea pigs. *J. Immunol.* 30:275–286.

Simon, F. A., Simon, M. G., Rackemann, F. M. and Dienes, L. 1934. The sensitization of guinea pigs to poison ivy. *J. Immunol.* 27:113–123.

Skog, E. and Wahlberg, J. E. 1970. Sensitization and testing of guinea pigs with potassium bichromate. *Acta Derm.-Venereol. (Stockh.)* 50:103–108.

Smeenk, G. and Rijnbeek, A. M. 1969. The water-binding properties of the water-soluble substances in the horny layer. *Acta Derm. Venereol. (Stockh.)* 49:476–480.

Stampf, J.-L., Schlewer, G., Ducombs, G., Foussereau, J., and Benezra, C. 1978. Allergic contact dermatitis due to sesquiterpene lactones. A comparative study of human and animal sensitivity to alpha-methylene-beta-butyrolactone and derivatives. *Br. J. Dermatol.* 99:163–169.

Stampf, J.-L. and Benezra, C. 1982. The sensitizing capacity of helenin and of two of its main constituents, the sesquiterpene lactones alantolactone and isoalantolactone: A comparison of epicutaneous and intradermal sensitizing methods and of different strains of guinea pigs. Submitted for publication.

Steigleder, G. K. 1975. Differentialdiagnose des allergisch bedingten Kontaktekzems. *Hautarzt* 26:62–64.

Stemann, G. 1965. Die percutane Penetrationsvermittlung von Rhodamin B durch organische Flüssigkeiten unter besonderer Berücksichtigung ihrer physiko-chemischen Eigenschaften. Dissertation, Hamburg.

Stoughton, R. B. 1965. Percutaneous absorption. *Toxicol. Appl. Pharmacol.* 7(Suppl. 3):1–6.

Strauss, H. W. 1937. Studies in experimental hypersensitiveness in the rhesus monkey. I. Active sensitization with poison ivy. *J. Immunol.* 32:241–246. III. On the manner of development of the hypersensitiveness in contact dermatitis. *J. Immunol.* 33:215–225.

Stüttgen, G. 1972. Die Haut als Resorptionsorgan in pharmakokinetischer Sicht. *Arzneim. Forsch.* 22:324–329.

Stüttgen, G. 1965. *Die normale und pathologische Physiologie der Haut.* Stuttgart: Fischer.

Sulzberger, M. B. 1930. Arsphenamine hypersensitiveness in guinea pigs. *Arch. Dermatol.* 22:839–848.

Sulzberger, M. B. and Baer, R. L. 1938. Sensitization to simple chemicals. III. Relationship between chemical structure and properties, and sensitizing capacities in the production of eczematous sensitivity in man. *J. Invest. Dermatol.* 1:45–58.

Thorgeirsson, A., Fregert, S. and Magnusson, B. 1975. Allergenicity of epoxy reactive diluents in the guinea pig. *Berufsdermatosen* 23:178–193.

Traub, E. F., Tusing, T. W. and Spoor, H. J. 1954. Evaluation of dermal sensitivity. *Arch. Dermatol.* 69:399–409.

Treherne, J. E. 1956. The permeability of skin to some non-electrolytes. *J. Physiol. (Lond.)* 133:171–180.

Turk, J. L. 1966. Die Immunreaktion vom verzögerten Typ und ihre Bedeutung in der Medizin. *Triangel* 7:275–280.

Turk, J. L. 1967. *Delayed hypersensitivity.* Amsterdam: North-Holland.

Van der Walle, H. B., Klecak, G., Geleick, H., and Bensink, T. 1982. Sensitizing potentials of 14 mono(meth)acrylates in the guinea pig. Submitted for publication.

Vinson, L. J., Singer, E. J., Koehler, W. R., Lehman, M. D. and Mausrat, T. 1965. The nature of the epidermal barrier and some factors influencing skin permeability. *Toxicol. Appl. Pharmacol.* 7:7–19.

Voss, J. G. 1958. Skin sensitization by mercaptans of low molecular weight. *J. Invest. Dermatol.* 31:273–279.

Wagner, J. G. 1961. Biopharmaceutics: Absorption aspects. *J. Pharm. Sci.* 50:359–387.

Wahlberg, J. E. and Boman, A. 1978. Sensitization and testing of guinea pigs with cobalt chloride. *Contact Dermatitis* 4:128–132.

Weil, C. S. 1972. Guidelines for experiments to predict the degree of safety of a material for man. *Toxicol. Appl. Pharmacol.* 21:194–199.

Wolter, K., Schaefer, H., Frömming, K. M. and Stüttgen, G. 1970. Partikelgrösse und Penetration. *Fette Seifen Anstrichm.* 72:990–998.

Wurster, D. E. 1968. Factors influencing the design and formulation of dermatological preparations. In *Development of safer and more effective drugs,* ed. S. W. Goldstein, pp. 121–140. Washington, D.C.: American Pharmaceutical Association.

Zesch, A. 1974. Wechselbeziehungen zwischen Haut, Vehikel und Arzneimittel bei der Penetration in die menschliche Haut. II. Vehikel und Penetration. *Fette Seifen Anstrichm.* 76:312–318.

Ziegler, V. 1975. Tierexperimenteller Nachweis stark allergener Eigenschaften von Industrieprodukten. Dissertation zur Promotion B and der Karl-Marx-Universität, Leipzig, DDR.

Ziegler, V. 1977. Der tierexperimentelle Nachweis allergener Eigenschaften von Industrieprodukten. *Dermatol. Monatsschr.* 163:387–391.

Ziegler, V., Süss, E., Standau, H. and Hasert, K. 1972. Der Meerschweinchen-Maximisationstest zum Nachweis der sensibilisierenden Wirkung wichtiger Industrieprodukte. *Allerg. Immunol.* 18:203–208.

10

validation of guinea pig tests for skin hypersensitivity

F. Marzulli ■ H. C. Maguire, Jr.

INTRODUCTION

During the past two decades there has been a proliferation of federal regulatory agencies in the United States. This has led to increasing requirements for tests on animals and humans to characterize the potential toxicity of a wide variety of personal products, drugs, pesticides, and other chemicals with which humans may come into contact. Ethical considerations require that laboratory animals be used for this purpose rather than humans. Monetary, political, and time considerations would favor elimination of the use of both humans and animals and reliance instead on *in vitro* tests. In some cases the latter approach is achievable. However, in the area of skin sensitization, tests for contact allergy potential require the use of intact mammals with functioning immunologic systems.

Traditionally, the animal species of choice for skin hypersensitivity tests has been the guinea pig. The first useful test was that devised by Draize et al. (1944) on the basis of observations reported by Landsteiner and Jacobs (1935). Candidate drugs and cosmetics were administered to guinea pigs by

The statistical computations were the work of Dr. John Atkinson (Department of Mathematics, Food and Drug Administration). Dr. Atkinson's invaluable assistance is greatly appreciated. The excellent technical assistance of Deborah Cipriano in the conduct of the guinea pig tests is acknowledged.

This work was supported by Food and Drug Administration contract 223-77-2341.

intradermal (id) injection in a prescribed manner (details of which follow) to ascertain their potential for human sensitization under conditions of use.

Subsequent variations in the basic procedure have included topical application to the skin without (Hood et al., 1965; Klecak et al., 1977) and with (Buehler, 1965) occlusion of the skin test site. A significant development in prospective testing in guinea pigs occurred with the introduction of complete Freund's adjuvant (CFA) as a means of enhancing the skin sensitization potential (Landsteiner and Chase, 1940; Magnusson and Kligman, 1969).

To date, a number of prospective testing methods have been developed and widely touted as superior to the original Draize technique, and yet we have limited information about their usefulness in predicting skin sensitization potential in humans. One attempt to compare guinea pig assays was made by Prince and Prince (1977). They concluded that, in general, CFA (adjuvant) techniques were clearly superior to nonadjuvant techniques in detecting weak contact sensitizers. Magnusson and Kligman (1970) reached a similar conclusion. However, there remains the separate problem of the applicability of test results in guinea pigs to conditions of use by humans and to the results of testing in humans.

The work described in this chapter is an attempt to predict by animal testing the effects of a compound when used by humans. While recognizing that predictive tests in humans have deficiencies in forecasting the sensitization potential of a chemical "in the field," we carried out a large-scale comparison of test results obtained in guinea pigs and in humans. In the main study five guinea pig predictive test methods were used to evaluate 11 possibly allergenic substances that have been used in the cosmetic industry; the results have been compared with the findings of predictive tests in humans. In a subsidiary small study three additional test methods were evaluated, using 5 of the 11 original test materials. Experience with humans suggested that most of the 11 chemicals were weak or negligible sensitizers. In addition, the allergenicity of 10 of the 11 chemicals had been evaluated by prospective testing in humans and the resulting sensitization rates were available for comparison. In the initial and major phase of this investigation, each of the 11 chemicals was subjected simultaneously to testing by five different techniques: (1) the guinea pig Draize method, (2) the Buehler method, (3) the guinea pig maximization test (GPMT) of Magnusson and Kligman (1969), (4) a strictly epicutaneous (split adjuvant) test that we devised some years ago, and (5) a test that utilizes immunopotentiation with cyclophosphamide (Hunziker, 1968; Maguire, 1973; Maguire and Ettore, 1967).

The last three tests make use of CFA; the first two do not. The further investigation undertaken to supplement the main work involved a limited evaluation of 5 of the 11 chemicals by three nonocclusive, non-CFA techniques, having as reference the standard guinea pig Draize test and the GPMT. In all the work the basic approach was to investigate each compound simultaneously with different techniques.

The results indicate the merits and limitations of each testing technique for the evaluation of compounds of weak allergenicity, and suggest ways for improving the reliability of methods for identifying and ranking in the guinea pig weak contact allergens of humans.

EXPERIMENTAL

Materials

Guinea pigs. Female Hartley-strain guinea pigs weighing about 350 g at the time of purchase were obtained from commercial sources. The guinea pigs were housed in metal cages on wood shavings in temperature-controlled ($65 \pm 5°F$) rooms with a 12-h (7 a.m. to 7 p.m.) light cycle. They were fed fresh Purina Guinea Pig Chow and had constant access to tap water. Water delivery was by demand from tubes external to the guinea pig cages.

Chemicals. Cyclophosphamide was purchased as a powder from Sigma Chemical Co. (St. Louis, Mo.) and diluted in pyrogen-free saline immediately before use. CFA (0638-60; Difco Laboratories, Detroit, Mich.) contained 0.5 mg heat-killed tubercle bacilli (*Mycobacterium butyricum*) per milliliter in a vehicle consisting of sterile light mineral oil and Arlacel A. The compounds tested and their sources were: dimethyl sulfoxide (DMSO), Crown Zellerbach Corp., Chemical Products Division, Washington, D.C.; ethanol, Pharm Co., Publicker Industries Co., Linfield, Pa.; dimethyl citraconate (12%, v/v; lot AE 10393), Food and Drug Administration, Washington, D.C.; methyl crotonate (6%, v/v; lot J8009), Food and Drug Administration; Germall 115 (imidazolidinyl urea; 10%, v/v, Sutton Laboratories Inc., Roselle, N.J.; Formalin (aqueous formaldehyde; 37%, v/v), Baker Chemical Co., Phillipsburg, N.J.; captan (1%, w/v; Vancide no. 898E), Vanderbilt Co., Norwalk, Conn.; Dowicil 200 (quaternium-15; 5%, v/v; lot 01138005), Dow Chemical Co., Coral Gables, Fla.; hydroxycitronellal (20%, v/v), Fritzche-Dodge and Olcott, Inc., New York; vetivert acetate (20%, v/v), Givaudan Corp., Clifton, N.J.; methyl methacrylate (10%, v/v), Eastman-Kodak Co., Rochester, N.Y.

Sensitization Techniques[1]

Draize guinea pig technique. A concentration of 0.1% test compound (w/v for solids and v/v for liquids) in saline was used throughout. In each round of testing, 10 guinea pigs were clipped on the left flank and injected id with 0.05 ml of test solution as their initial sensitizing exposure. The injection site was examined 24 h later and the reactions measured and recorded. Nine subsequent id injections were made, each time with a volume of 0.1 ml; a new site on the left flank was used each time. These injections were given three times per week. Two weeks after the last (tenth) injection, the guinea pigs were challenged at a clipped site on the opposite flank with 0.05 ml of test solution given id. A similar injection was made in 10 control guinea pigs. The

---

[1] See Chapter 9.

reactions (at 24 h) of the first (induction) and final (challenge) injections in the experimental animals, as well as the 24-h reactions of the naïve control guinea pigs, were compared to determine whether a change in reactivity to test material had taken place as a result of the sensitization procedure.

Buehler guinea pig assay. The vehicle and concentration of test material are shown for each compound in Table 1. Ten guinea pigs were clipped on the left flank; 0.5 ml of test compound was applied to the area, covered by Blenderm (3M Corp., Minneapolis, Minn.), and fixed in place by an encircling

TABLE 1   Results of Three Rounds of Testing of 11 Compounds
in Five Guinea Pig Bioassays for Allergenicity

| Compound | Concentration and vehicle[a] | Test | Number of guinea pigs with reaction[b] | | | |
			Round 1	Round 2	Round 3	Cumulative
DMSO	–[c]	Draize	0	0	0	0
		Buehler	0	0	0	0
		Cy/CFA[d]	0	0	0	0
		GPMT	0	0	0	0
		Split adjuvant	0	0	0	0
Ethanol	–[c]	Draize	0	0	0	0
		Buehler	0	0	0	0
		Cy/CFA	0	0	0	0
		GPMT	0	0	0	0
		Split adjuvant	0	0	0	0
Hydroxy-citronellal	20% (w/w) in petrolatum	Draize	0	0	0	0
		Buehler	0	0	0	0
		Cy/CFA	2	0	2	4
		GPMT	2	4	2	8
		Split adjuvant	2	2	1	5
Methyl methacrylate	10% (v/v) in 100% ethanol	Draize	0	2	0	2
		Buehler	0	0	0	0
		Cy/CFA	0	0	0	0
		GPMT	0	0	0	0
		Split adjuvant	0	0	0	0
Captan	1% (w/w) in petrolatum	Draize	10	6	10	26
		Buehler	0	1	0	1
		Cy/CFA	8 (8)	10 (12)	10	28
		GPMT	9	7 (9)	8	24 (29)
		Split adjuvant	7	6	8	10

(See footnotes on p. 241.)

TABLE 1 Results of Three Rounds of Testing of 11 Compounds
in Five Guinea Pig Bioassays for Allergenicity (*Continued*)

Compound	Concentration and vehicle[a]	Test	Round 1	Round 2	Round 3	Cumulative
Formalin	5% (v/v) in saline	Draize	6	1	3	10
		Buehler	0	0	0	0
		Cy/CFA	4 (8)	0	0	4 (28)
		GPMT	2 (8)	1	2	5 (28)
		Split adjuvant	2	0	0	2
Dowicil 200	5% (w/w) in petrolatum	Draize	0	0	0	0
		Buehler	0	0	0	0
		Cy/CFA	1	3	5	9
		GPMT	9	2	5 (9)	16 (29)
		Split adjuvant	4	3	4	11
Methyl crotonate	6% (v/w) in petrolatum[e]	Draize	0	0	0	0
		Buehler	0	0	0	0
		Cy/CFA	1	1	0	2
		GPMT	2	3	1	6
		Split adjuvant	3	1	0	4
Vetivert acetate	20% (w/w) in petrolatum[e]	Draize	0	0	0	0
		Buehler	0	0	0	0
		Cy/CFA	1	2	0 (9)	3 (29)
		GPMT	2	5	4	11
		Split adjuvant	6	2	2	10
Dimethyl citraconate	12% (v/w) in petrolatum	Draize	0	0	0	0
		Buehler	0	0	0	0
		Cy/CFA	0	0	0	0
		GPMT	0	0	0	0
		Split adjuvant	1	0	1	2
Germall 115	10% (w/w) in petrolatum[e]	Draize	0	0	0	0
		Buehler	0	0	0	0
		Cy/CFA	0	3	0	3
		GPMT	0	2	1	3
		Split adjuvant	0	0	0	0

[a]For tests other than the Draize test, for which a concentration of 0.1% test compound was used throughout.

[b]Ten guinea pigs were used in each round (cumulative no. = 30) except where the numbers used are indicated in parentheses.

[c]Except for the Draize test, induction with ethanol and DMSO (50:50, v/v) and a separate challenge with either 100% ethanol or 100% DMSO.

[d]Cy/CFA, cyclophosphamide/complete Freund's adjuvant bioassay.

[e]Challenge with 25% test compound in round 2 (except in the Draize test).

bandage of Elastoplast (Beiersdorf Inc., South Norwalk, Conn.). This occlusive bandage was secured by adhesive tape at either end; it was removed after 6 h. The application was repeated 7 and 14 d later. On d 28 an area on the right flank was clipped and 0.5 ml of test compound was applied, using the same technique as for the left flank except that Scanpor tape (Norgesplaster, A.S., Oslo, Norway), which was less irritating, was substituted for regular adhesive tape. The dressing was removed after 24 h. Ten control guinea pigs were challenged in parallel. All reactions were read in experimental and control guinea pigs 24 and 48 h later and comparisons were made between groups.

Guinea-pig maximization test of Magnusson and Kligman (1969). Ten guinea pigs were clipped in the mid-dorsal region near the scapula. Three sets of two id injections (0.1 ml each) were given to each animal as follows: (1) CFA emulsified with an equal volume of sterile distilled water; (2) a 5% concentration of test compound in saline, and (3) a 10% concentration of test compound in saline emulsified with an equal volume of CFA. On d 6 the injection sites were inspected and if there was no significant irritation 5% sodium lauryl sulfate was applied; if there was significant irritation, no sodium lauryl sulfate was applied to the site. On d 7 the area of the injections was clipped and 0.5 ml of the test compound (concentrations and vehicles specified in Table 1) was applied to a 1-in square of Whatman No. 2 filter paper. The paper was positioned face-down on the induction site and sealed in place with Blenderm, Elastoplast, and adhesive tape as in the Buehler wrappings. A challenge was made on d 21 with 0.5 ml of test material at a high nonirritant concentration (see Table 1). The application was made to a clipped site on the left flank with Whatman No. 2 filter paper, and which was sealed with Blenderm, Elastoplast, and Scanpore adhesive tape. The dressing was removed 24 h later and readings were made 1 and 2 d later (i.e., 48 and 72 h after the challenge).

Split adjuvant technique. The concentration and vehicle for each test compound are shown in Table 1. Ten guinea pigs were clipped on the right anterior flank, the area was shaved to the glistening layer with a razor blade, and dry ice was applied for 10 s with firm pressure. A dressing containing a window was placed over the clipped, shaved, frozen site and 0.2 ml of test material was applied to the induction site and covered with Blenderm tape. The dressing was held in place with adhesive tape. Two days later 0.2 ml of test material was applied to the area sealed. On d 4 two injections of 0.075 ml CFA were made adjacent to the induction site, followed by application of 0.2 ml of test material on the induction site. The site was resealed and on d 7 a further 0.2 ml of test material was applied through the window. On d 9 the dressing was removed. A challenge was made on d 22 by the GPMT method.

Cyclophosphamide/CFA bioassay. The concentration and vehicle for each test compound are shown in Table 1. Three days prior to induction (i.e., on d −3) 10 guinea pigs were weighed and given by intraperitoneal (ip) injection 150 mg of cyclophosphamide per kilogram of body weight. On d 0 the animals were clipped on the right anterior flank and dry ice was applied to the induction area for 5 s. A dressing containing a window was applied as in the split adjuvant technique and 0.2 ml of test material was placed on a 1-in square of Whatman No. 2 filter paper and applied to the induction site through the window. This was sealed with Blenderm and adhesive tape. On each of d 1, 2, 3, and 4 the window was opened, 0.2 ml of the test material applied, and the window resealed. On the afternoon of d 4 the dressing was removed and two id injections (0.075 ml each) were made with CFA immediately adjacent to the induction site. On d 9 a 6-h application of allergen to the induction site was made under occlusion. The guinea pigs were challenged on d 22 by the GPMT technique.

Altered Draize technique. Preliminary tests were carried out with each chemical (in saline) to identify the highest concentration that failed to give a significant irritation reaction at 24 h when 0.1 ml was injected id on the flank. These concentrations (w/v) were: $\frac{1}{2}$% hydroxycitronellal, $\frac{1}{2}$% methyl crotonate, $\frac{1}{2}$% vetivert acetate, $\frac{1}{2}$% dimethyl citraconate, and $\frac{1}{2}$% Germall 115. For induction, 10 guinea pigs were clipped as for the standard Draize test. They were injected on d 0 and three times weekly, for a total of 10 injections, with 0.1 ml of the test solution. A fresh adjacent site was used for each successive injection. A challenge was made 2 wk after the last inducing injection with 0.1 ml of the test solution, as in the standard Draize test, using a freshly clipped site on the right flank. Control animals were challenged in parallel. The reactions were read at 24 h and comparisons were made as in the standard Draize test.

Nonocclusive topical test. Ten guinea pigs were clipped on the left flank. The test material (0.5 ml, concentration and vehicle as in Table 4) was applied to a 1-in^2 area and massaged gently into the skin for a few seconds. This was repeated daily 5 d/wk for 4 wk, for a total of 20 applications. The application site was clipped three times per week to maintain close contact between the test material and the surface epidermis. The animals were left untreated for 10 d after the last inducing application and then a challenge was made to a freshly clipped site on the opposite flank, using a fixed concentration of test materials (Table 4). Reactions were recorded after 24 and 48 h. Control animals were tested in parallel and appropriate comparisons were made. The sensitization and challenge schedule is similar to that of the open epicutaneous test (Klecak, 1977) (see Chapter 9). However, the latter makes use of a number of different concentrations for induction and challenge, whereas in this work fixed concentrations of test materials were used.

Nonocclusive topical test with DMSO. The nonocclusive topical test described above was modified by pretreating the induction site with 0.02 ml of 100% DMSO 10–15 min before application of the test material (concentration and vehicle as in Table 4). DMSO was not used at challenge (Maguire, 1974).

RESULTS

Results of three rounds (replicates) of tests (10 animals per round) with 11 compounds in five guinea pig assays for allergenicity are shown in Table 1. For comparison, Table 2 shows results obtained when 10 of these chemicals were tested on humans by the human Draize[2] predictive tests for delayed skin hypersensitivity [modified by using a high induction concentration of test material (Marzulli and Maibach, 1980)].

Two types of comparison between these results are possible, one quantitative and one qualitative. As will be seen, the quantitative approach is less useful.

Quantitative Assessment

Coefficients of correlation (R) between the response fractions obtained by each guinea pig test and the response fraction obtained by the human test were estimated.[3] The results were: Draize, 0.69; GPMT, 0.65; cyclophosphamide/CFA, 0.51; split adjuvant, 0.41; and Buehler, 0.24. A positive correlation between the results of the guinea pig and human tests was obtained in all cases except with the Buehler guinea pig technique. These positive results are only weakly supportive of a quantitative relation between guinea pig and human test results; a high sensitization index in guinea pigs does not necessarily indicate a similarly high sensitization index in humans.

---

[2] Note that there is a Draize guinea pig test and a completely different Draize human test for skin sensitization. The test species (human or guinea pig) is mentioned in connection with a Draize test.

[3] Logarithmic transformations were involved. Rates were transformed to their square foots. This gives skewed results; nevertheless, this transformation tends to stabilize variances.

TABLE 2 Results of Prospective Testing (Modified Draize Test) in Humans

| Compound | Concentration (%) | | Reactions |
	Induction	Challenge	
Ethanol	100	100	0/94
Hydroxycitronellal	20	20	1/99
Methyl methacrylate	10	10	0/184
Captan	1	1	9/205
Formalin	5	1	4/52
Dowicil 200	5	5	1/183
Methyl crotonate	12	12	1/99
Vetivert acetate	20	2	1/62
Dimethyl citraconate	12	12	0/104
Germall 115	10	10	1/184

TABLE 3 Validation of Guinea Pig Predictive Test Methods
by Comparison of Results with Those of a Human
Predictive Test Method[a]

Guinea pig test method	Results (frequency in 30 evaluations) compared with predictive test method in humans		
	Agreement	False positive	False negative
Draize	14	1	15
Buehler	10[b]	0	20[b]
Cy/CFA	23[c,d]	0	7[c,e]
GPMT	29[d]	0	1[d]
Split adjuvant	22[c,e]	2	6[c,d]

[a]The results from the guinea pig predictive tests are shown in Table 1. The results for DMSO are not included in this comparison since it was not tested in humans. Three rounds of each test were carried out on each of the 10 remaining chemicals (a total of 30 evaluations per test). Ten guinea pigs were used for each evaluation. The results of the modified Draize test in humans are shown in Table 2. If one or more human subjects showed a reaction, the chemical was considered allergenic. If one or more guinea pigs showed a reaction, an evaluation was considered to have shown a positive response.
[b]Significantly different from values from GPMT (chi-square test, $p < 0.01$).
[c]Significantly different from values from GPMT (chi-square test, $p < 0.05$).
[d]Significantly different from values from guinea pig Draize test (chi-square test, $p < 0.01$).
[e]Significantly different from values from guinea pig Draize test (chi-square test, $p < 0.05$).

Qualitative Assessment

In the qualitative assessment, a substance was considered allergenic if one or more subjects showed a positive response in any test round (guinea pigs) or group (humans). Otherwise, it was considered a negative finding for allergenicity. In this qualitative assessment a positive response rate of 1/100 has the same thrust as a rate of 9/10, both being considered an allergenic finding. Table 3 shows comparisons between guinea pig test results, including (1) the frequency with which guinea pig and human test results agree, (2) the frequency with which the guinea pig test is falsely positive, and (3) the frequency with which the guinea pig test is falsely negative.

The adjuvant techniques (GPMT, cyclophosphamide/CFA, and split adjuvant) show significantly (chi-square test) greater agreement with human predictive findings than the nonadjuvant techniques (Draize and Buehler). On comparing the adjuvant techniques with one another, however, the GPMT test emerges as superior to the other two. All five guinea pig techniques were comparable in producing false positive results (in relation to the human test results). There was no significant difference between any of the five guinea pig test methods in this regard. False negative findings (meaning that the guinea pig test failed to indicate an allergenic potential that was seen in human predictive testing) were observed with the highest frequency in the Draize and Buehler methods and the lowest frequency in the GPMT.

The overall findings of these tests support the conclusion that the GPMT best duplicates human predictive findings, as measured by the human modified Draize method.

Additional Guinea Pig Techniques

The standard Draize guinea pig test and the GPMT were used as references for evaluating the usefulness of a nonocclusive topical test and its possible enhancement with DMSO. In addition, we altered the Draize guinea pig test ("altered Draize") to find out whether a higher induction concentration would improve the Draize guinea pig test, as it does the Draize human test.

The guinea pig test results are shown in Table 4 and comparisons with human findings are shown in Table 5. The results here are not as dramatic as in the first series of tests, largely because there were fewer compounds tested (five) and fewer replicates (two). Nevertheless, these results confirm the earlier finding that the GPMT is the test of choice among the guinea pig test methods evaluated. DMSO pretreatment of the induction site prior to application of a putative sensitizer did not make that site more prone to the development of contact sensitivity. Increasing the induction and challenge concentrations of an allergen in the altered Draize test resulted in the identification of vetivert acetate as an allergen; this would have been missed in the standard guinea pig Draize test. Further alteration of the guinea pig Draize test along these lines might be worthwhile.

DISCUSSION

New cosmetics, new drugs, and other substances that come into contact with human skin, and whose allergenicity is unknown, are continually being developed. As part of an evaluation of their safety, it is necessary to measure their relative allergenic potential for contact dermatitis.

While allergic contact dermatitis can be induced in a variety of laboratory animals, such as mice, rats, hamsters, and chickens, the guinea pig remains the animal of choice for the bioassay of putative contact allergens of humans (Asherson and Ptak, 1969; Jaffee and Maguire, 1981; Maguire et al., 1976). Compounds that produce a high incidence of contact sensitivity in the human—that is, strong and moderate sensitizers—are readily identified in the guinea pig by classical techniques such as the guinea pig Draize method (Draize, 1965) or the more recently developed Buehler method (Buehler and

TABLE 4 Results of Two Rounds of Testing of Five Compounds
with Five Guinea Pig Bioassays for Allergenicity

Compound	Concentration and vehicle[a]	Test	Round 1	Round 2	Cumulative
			Number of guinea pigs with reaction[b]		
Hydroxycitronellal	20% (w/w) in petrolatum	Draize	0	0	0
		Altered Draize	0	0	0
		NTT[c]	0	0	0
		NTT-DMSO	0	0	0
		GPMT	2	4	6
Methyl crotonate	6% (w/w) in petrolatum	Draize	0	0	0
		Altered Draize	0	0	0
		NTT	0	0 (9)	0 (19)
		NTT-DMSO	0	0	0
		GPMT	0	0 (9)	0 (19)
Vetivert acetate	20% (w/w) in petrolatum	Draize	1	0	1
		Altered Draize	2	0	2
		NTT	1	0	1
		NTT-DMSO	0	1	1
		GPMT	1	0	1
Dimethyl citraconate	12% (w/w) in petrolatum	Draize	0	0	0
		Altered Draize	0	0 (9)	0 (19)
		NTT	0	0 (9)	0 (19)
		NTT-DMSO	0	0 (9)	0 (19)
		GPMT	2	2 (9)	4 (19)
Germall 115	10% (w/w) in petrolatum	Draize	0	0	0
		Altered Draize	1	2	3
		NTT	5	5	10
		NTT-DMSO	3	3	6
		GPMT	4	4 (9)	8 (19)

[a]For tests other than the Draize and altered Draize tests. A concentration of 0.1% of test compound was used for the Draize test. In the altered Draize test 0.5% was used.

[b]Ten guinea pigs were used in each round (cumulative number = 20) except where numbers used are indicated in parentheses.

[c]NTT, nonocclusive topical test.

Griffith, 1975; Ritz and Buehler, 1980). However, in the case of weak and very weak contact sensitizers, these methods are less successful; more reliable methods for the evaluation of such compounds in the guinea pig are needed (Magnusson and Kligman, 1977). While the incidence of sensitization with such compounds may be small, the population at risk often is very large so that significant numbers of individuals may be injured. For different compounds, the sensitization rates vary, the acceptable risk to a large extent being determined by the conditions of use and the purpose of the final product.

TABLE 5   Comparison of Results of Sensitization Tests in Guinea Pigs
with Those of a Predictive Test Method in Humans[a]

Guinea pig test method	Results (frequency in 10 evaluations) compared with predictive test in humans		
	Agreement	False positive	False negative
Draize	3	0	7
Altered Draize	5[b]	0	5[b]
NTT	5[b]	0	5[b]
NTT-DMSO	5[b]	0	5[b]
GPMT	9[c]	0	1[c]

[a]The results of the guinea pig predictive tests are shown in Table 4.
Two rounds of each test were carried out on each of five chemicals (a
total of 10 evaluations per test). Ten guinea pigs were used for each evaluation. The results of the modified Draize test on humans are shown in
Table 2. If one or more human subjects showed a reaction the chemical
was considered allergenic. If one or more guinea pigs showed a reaction,
an evaluation was considered to have shown a positive response.
[b]Close to significantly different from values from the GPMT
(chi-square test, $p > 0.05$ but < 0.1).
[c]Significantly different from values from the guinea pig Draize test
(chi-square test, $p < 0.01$).

Clearly, testing of allergens in laboratory animals should be preliminary
to their testing in humans, and the animal methods should be of such
sensitivity and reliability as to preclude the exposure of large numbers of
human volunteers to significant sensitizers. In product development there is a
distinct economic advantage in being able to exclude allergenic materials at a
relatively early stage of development. In specific instances it may be possible
to reduce the allergenicity of chemicals of particular usefulness (by chemical
modification or a change of vehicle). For this purpose, the need for sensitive,
reliable bioassays of allergenicity that can readily be done in laboratory
animals is obvious. Such testing in humans is inappropriate.

The efficiency of adjuvant techniques is clearly demonstrated by the
present study and has been alluded to in other investigations as well
(Magnusson and Kligman, 1969; Maurer et al., 1975). In addition, the present
work demonstrates the overall superiority of the GPMT over two other
candidate guinea pig test methods with regard to ability to duplicate human
predictive findings.

Finally, the results of this study provide a basis for further recommending that compounds about which little is known be tested first by the Draize
guinea pig technique and then by the GPMT. Positive findings in the Draize
guinea pig test would suggest that the compound is a strong skin sensitizer
and might imply that further testing with the GPMT is unnecessary. Negative
findings in both the Draize and the GPMT indicate that the chemical is not

likely to be a significant sensitizer in humans. Positive findings in the GPMT with negative results in the Draize guinea pig test suggest that the compound is likely to be a weak or moderate skin sensitizer in humans.

As part of this study, the contact allergenicity of ethanol was evaluated. In the modified human Draize test none of the 94 subjects were sensitized (Table 2). Furthermore, we failed to sensitize any of 150 guinea pigs to this substance (Table 1). Thus, a report of allergenicity of ethanol in humans (Stotts and Ely, 1977) was not confirmed.

REFERENCES

Asherson, G. L. and Ptak, W. L. 1969. Contact and delayed hypersensitivity in the mouse. I. Active sensitization and passive transfer. *Immunology* 15:405.

Buehler, E. V. 1965. Delayed contact hypersensitivity in the guinea pig. *Arch. Dermatol.* 91:171.

Buehler, E. V. and Griffith, J. F. 1975. Experimental skin sensitization in the guinea pig and man. In *Animal Models in Dermatology*, ed. H. I. Maibach, p. 56. New York: Churchill Livingstone.

Draize, J. H. 1965. Dermal toxicity. In *Appraisal of the Safety of Chemicals in Foods, Drugs and Cosmetics.* Austin, Texas: Association of Food and Drug Officials of the United States, Texas State Department of Health.

Draize, J. H., Woodard, G., and Calvery, H. O. 1944. Methods for the study of irritation and toxicity of substances applied topically to the skin and mucous membranes. *J. Pharmacol. Exp. Ther.* 82:377.

Hood, D. B., Neher, R. J., Reinke, R. E., and Zapp, J. A., Jr. 1965. Experience with the guinea pig in screening primary irritants and sensitizers. *Toxicol. Appl. Pharmacol.* 7:485 (abstract).

Hunziker, N. 1968. Effect of cyclophosphamide on the contact eczema in guinea pigs. *Dermatologica* 48:39.

Jaffee, B. D. and Maguire, H. C., Jr. 1981. Delayed-type hypersensitivity and immunological tolerance to contact allergens in the rat. *Fed. Proc.* 40:991 (abstract 4312).

Klecak, G. 1977. Identification of contact allergens: Predictive tests in animals. In *Dermatotoxicology and Pharmacology*, eds. F. N. Marzulli and H. I. Maibach, p. 305. Washington, D.C.: Hemisphere.

Klecak, G., Geleick, H., and Frey, J. R. 1977. Screening of fragrance materials for allergenicity in the guinea pig. I. Comparison of four testing methods. *J. Soc. Cosmet. Chem.* 28:53.

Landsteiner, K. and Chase, M. W. 1940. Studies on the sensitization of animals with simple chemical compounds. VII. Skin sensitization by intraperitoneal injections. *J. Exp. Med.* 71:237.

Landsteiner, K. and Jacobs, J. 1935. Studies on the sensitization of animals with simple chemical compounds. *J. Exp. Med.* 61:643.

Magnusson, B. and Kligman, A. M. 1969. The identification of contact allergens by animal assay. The guinea pig maximization test. *J. Invest. Dermatol.* 52:568.

Magnusson, B. and Kligman, A. M. 1970. Allergic contact dermatitis in the guinea pig. In *Identification of Contact Allergens.* Springfield, Ill.: Thomas.

Magnusson, B. and Kligman, A. M. 1977. Usefulness of guinea pig tests for detection of contact sensitizers. In *Dermatotoxicology and Pharmacology*, eds. F. N. Marzulli and H. I. Maibach, p. 551. Washington, D.C.: Hemisphere.

Maguire, H. C. 1973. The bioassay of contact allergens in the guinea pig. *J. Soc. Cosmet. Chem.* 24:151.

Maguire, H. C. 1974. Induction of delayed hypersensitivity to nitrogen mustard in the guinea pig. *Br. J. Dermatol.* 91:21.

Maguire, H. C., Jr. 1980. Allergic contact dermatitis in the hamster. *J. Invest. Dermatol.* 75:166.

Maguire, H. C., Jr., and Ettore, V. L. 1967. Enhancement of dinitrochlorobenzene (DNCB) contact sensitization by cyclophosphamide in guinea pigs. *J. Invest. Dermatol.* 48:39.

Maguire, H. C., Jr., Rank, R., and Weidanz, W. 1976. Allergic contact dermatitis to low molecular weight contact allergens in the chicken. *Int. Arch. Allergy Appl. Immunol.* 50:737.

Marzulli, F. and Maibach, H. 1980. Contact allergy: Predictive testing of fragrance ingredients in humans by Draize and maximization methods. *J. Environ. Pathol. Toxicol.* 3(5, 6):235.

Maurer, T., Thomann, P., Weirich, E. G., and Hess, R. 1975. The optimization test in the guinea pig. A method for the predictive evaluation of the contact allergenicity of chemicals. *Agents Actions* 5:174.

Prince, H. N. and Prince, T. G. 1977. Comparative guinea pig assays for contact hypersensitivity. *Cosmet. Toiletries* 92:53.

Ritz, H. L. and Buehler, E. V. 1980. Planning, conduct and interpretation of guinea pig sensitization patch tests. In *Current Concepts in Cutaneous Toxicity*, eds. V. A. Drill and P. Lazar, p. 25. New York: Academic.

Stotts, J. and Ely, W. J. 1977. Induction of human skin sensitization to ethanol. *J. Invest. Dermatol.* 69:219.

11

factors influencing allergic contact sensitization

Bertil Magnusson ■ Albert M. Kligman

INTRODUCTION

Many factors influence the contact sensitization process. These include dose of allergen, number of exposures, scheduling and route of exposures, and so on. The elicitation of the reaction in sensitized animals is also influenced by many factors. Additionally, genetic background, age, pregnancy, and the general state of health of the test animals are important variables.

More than in most types of bioassay, the experimenter is a critical factor. The induction of sensitization and challenge testing require scrupulous attention to details. An important source of error is inadvertent bias by the person reading the challenge reactions. This trouble can be avoided by blind reading of animals selected at random by an assistant.

In this presentation we have concerned ourselves mainly with variables that pertain to practical matters. The most complete study to date is the monograph on contact dermatitis in the guinea pig (Magnusson and Kligman, 1970).

The procedures used by Magnusson and Kligman were as follows. The guinea pigs were white females of the Hartley strain weighing between 250 and 550 g. Groups of 25 animals each were used. Three allergens were intensively studied: 2,4-dinitrochlorobenzene (DNCB), *p*-nitrodimethylaniline

(NDMA), and *p*-phenylenediamine (PPDA). DNCB and NDMA are fat soluble and PPDA both fat and water soluble. Attempts were made to select a dose that would sensitize about 50% of the animals. This increased the likelihood that a promoting or inhibiting effect would attain a level of statistical significance.

Sensitization. Animals were sensitized by injection or by topical application. The former is more convenient and dosage more precisely controllable. A single intradermal injection was made into the skin over the sacrum. The hair was first removed with an electric clipper. The routine dose of the three allergens was 0.1 ml of a 0.005 or 0.01% concentration in propylene glycol. The higher concentration was used when the mean weight of the animals was 500 g or more. One-half to two-thirds of the animals become sensitized with these doses.

Topical application utilized both the open and the closed patch techniques. An area on the flank was first clipped free of hair and then shaved clean with an electric razor.

With the open technique, a circular area of 380 mm^2 was defined with a metal stamp lightly moistened with ink. A volume of 0.1 ml of allergen was applied uniformly with a micropipette.

Closed patch induction consisted of a single application of 0.04 ml allergen via ready-made test patches. The latter consisted of 80 mm^2 circles of filter paper holding up to 0.05 ml. The paper disk was centered on a larger circle of water-repellent paper (380 mm^2). The patch was covered with an overlapping impermeable plastic tape firmly held in place for 24 hr by elastic adhesive bandage encircling the trunk.

The standard allergen concentration for topical induction was 0.05 or 0.1% in 70% ethanol. The higher concentration was used in animals with a mean weight of 500 g or more. This usually sensitized one-half to two-thirds of the animals.

Challenge. The animals were challenged topically on the flank 9 or 10 days after the sensitizing dose. The area was clipped free of hair and shaved clean with an electric razor. Three different concentrations of the allergen were used. DNCB and NDMA were employed in 0.1, 0.05, and 0.025% and PPDA in 5, 1, and 0.5% concentrations. Ethanol (95%) was the vehicle. These concentrations were determined to be below the threshold level of irritation.

For open patch testing, three circular areas (22 mm in diameter, 380 mm^2) were marked off with a metal stamp lightly moistened with ink. Fresh areas were always chosen for challenge. A volume of 0.015 ml of the allergen solution was uniformly applied with a micropipette.

For closed patch challenge, three of the aforementioned cellulose patches were spaced out on impermeable tape mounted on the elastic bandage. Volumes of 0.04 ml of the allergen were pipetted on the patches, with the most concentrated one in the most caudal position. The patches were applied in the same manner as for closed patch induction and held in place for 24 hr.

Evaluation of challenge reactions. With open testing the reactions were evaluated at 24 hr. With closed patches 48 hr readings—that is, 24 hr after removal of the patch—proved best. The reactions were evaluated blind.

The intensity of the reactions was evaluated according to the following scale: no visible change = 0; slight or discrete erythema = 1; moderate and confluent erythema = 2; and intense erythema and swelling = 3.

The results were expressed in two ways; (1) the proportion of animals sensitized and (2) the intensity of the reaction. These data were reduced to one integrated figure, the mean response. The latter was calculated by summing the numerical reading for all three challenge concentrations and dividing this by the total number of readings, including the negative ones. Analysis of variance was used for testing statistical significance.

THE EXPERIMENTAL ANIMAL

Genetic Factors

Heredity plays a strong role in all immunologic processes, including contact allergy. By inbreeding, Chase (1959) established a strain of guinea pigs with very high susceptibility to DNCB. Polak et al. (1968) studied genetic control with three metallic sensitizers, potassium dichromate, beryllium fluoride, and mercuric chloride, using an outbred Hartley strain of guinea pigs and two inbred ones, strain 2 and strain 13. It was difficult to sensitize the outbred strain with these three allergens. Strain 2 guinea pigs could be sensitized to dichromate and beryllium but not to mercury. Strain 13 could be sensitized to mercury but not to the other metals. Crossbreeding experiments indicated that the ability to become sensitized to a particular metal was inherited as a simple Mendelian dominant trait.

More recently Polak et al. (1974) found that strains 2 and 13 sensitized either with dinitrofluorobenzene (DNFB) or a homologous DNP skin protein conjugate differed in their response to the DNP skin protein conjugate. It was concluded that sensitization with hapten leads to the formation of a set of autologous hapten-protein conjugates and that genetic factors control the response to individual haptens.

In our studies (Magnusson and Kligman, 1970) white outbred Hartley guinea pigs from a Danish breeder did not differ in sensitizability to DNCB from animals obtained from the Rockefeller Institute, New York. The latter were known to be readily sensitized to this allergen.

With strong allergens healthiness is of greater significance than genotype. Mycotic and bacterial infections and stress of various kinds are important sources of inconsistent results.

Age

Contact sensitization can be induced in the newborn. All of the 2-day-old animals exposed to DNCB by Hunziker and Schinas (1962) became sensitized. On the other hand, Salvin et al. (1962) sensitized only 57% of 1-day-old guinea pigs as compared to 100% of adult animals injected with 1-fluoro-2,4-dinitrochlorobenzene in Freund's complete adjuvant (FCA). Baer and Bowser (1963) showed that animals 6 months to 2 yr old were less readily sensitized to pentadecylcatechol than guinea pigs 2 months old.

These findings were confirmed in our studies (Magnusson and Kligman, 1970). With DNCB, NDMA, and PPDA we found mature animals, 11-13 months old (900-1,000 g), much less sensitizable than younger guinea pigs 1-3 months old (300-500 g). Infant animals, 1-2 wk old (150-200 g) were somewhat less sensitizable than adult animals.

Guinea pigs 1-3 months old are most suitable when one is trying to detect weak allergens.

Sex

Chase (1941) thought there might be a sex-linked difference in susceptibility to contact sensitization, females being more sensitizable. The contrary opinion was expressed by Fasett (1963). Most authors have found no differences in the sensitizability of male and female guinea pigs to various contact sensitizers (Nilzén, 1952; Magnusson and Kligman, 1970; Ziegler, 1975).

We prefer nonetheless to use groups of female guinea pigs. The aggressive social behavior of males may result in considerable skin damage, interferring with the interpretation of challenge reactions.

Pregnancy

A markedly decreased reactivity to an irritant, croton oil, has been observed in pregnant guinea pigs just prior to delivery (Rockwell, 1955). Fasett (1963) did state that female guinea pigs "should not be used because of their lower reactivity especially if pregnant."

We induced sensitization to DNCB at the time of conception and found that allergic reactivity to DNCB progressively declined as pregnancy progressed (Magnusson and Kligman, 1970). Animals exposed once to PPDA in late pregnancy showed a strikingly lower rate of sensitization than age-matched nonpregnant females. The effect is probably on cutaneous expression and not on the sensitization process; that is to say, the phenomenon is related to the capacity of skin to mount an inflammatory reaction and is accordingly nonimmunologic. Our findings parallel those in which female sex hormones have been found to decrease the tuberculin reaction (Lurie et al., 1949; Seeberg, 1950; Pepys, 1955).

Dietary Factors

Vitamin C. Interest in the effect of vitamin C on contact allergy was aroused when Mayer and Sulzberger (1931) observed greater sensitization of guinea pigs on a winter rather than summer diet. Subsequently it was claimed that scorbutic animals were more easily sensitized (Sulzberger and Oser, 1935) and that adding vitamin C to the diet decreased sensitization (Streitmann and Wiedmann, 1937). Frey et al. (1966) observed that a diet poor in vitamin C (but also poor in vitamins A and E) favored sensitization. Other investigators have found just the opposite—that is, that a diet deficient in vitamin C inhibited contact sensitization (Chapman and Morell, 1935; Kile and Pepple, 1938) or that neither hypervitaminosis C nor a scorbutic diet influences the process (Storck, 1939). We too could not show that a scorbutic diet had any effect on sensitization of guinea pigs (Magnusson and Kligman, 1970). The animals showed clinical signs of scurvy at the time of sensitization to DNCB. Neither was the allergic contact reaction affected by placing guinea pigs on a scorbutic diet immediately or 2 wk after sensitization to DNCB and maintaining the diet for 2, 3, or 5 wk.

Thus, vitamin C deficiency probably does not influence either the process of contact sensitization or its elicitation.

Vitamin A. Hypervitaminosis A has been noted to suppress the tuberculin reaction in guinea pigs (Uhr et al., 1963; Jansz et al., 1967). The effect of hypervitaminosis A on allergic contact reactions has been studied by Knop and Rupec (1972). Oral administration of vitamin A acid at toxic levels was found to suppress earlier allergic reactions in DNCB-sensitized guinea pigs. Whether this has anything to do with the labilizing effect of vitamin A on lysosomes (Uhr et al., 1963; Knop and Rupec, 1972) is completely unknown.

Ambient Conditions

Temperature. In a small series Rockwell (1955) found that cold (40°F and 60% RH) enhanced sensitization to DNCB in guinea pigs; however, she could not repeat this result.

Conflicting results have been reported on the effect of low temperature on the allergic reaction itself. Rockwell (1955) and Suskind and Ishihara (1965) observed an increased skin reactivity to DNCB with low temperature while Nilzén and Wikström (1955b) found an suppressive effect.

We have studied the effect of low temperature during induction and of low and high temperature during challenge of sensitized guinea pigs (Magnusson and Kligman, 1970). In two experiments low ambient temperature (below the freezing point in one of the experiments) during the induction phase did not influence sensitization to DNCB and PPDA. In three crossover experiments neither elevation of the temperature to 32°C nor lowering to around the freezing point influenced the allergic reactions in animals sensitized to DNCB, NDMA, and PPDA.

Season. Mayer and Sulzberger (1931) reported that guinea pigs were more easily sensitized to neoarsphenamine and Ursol in the winter than in the summer. This finding has been confirmed by de Weck and Brun (1956) using DNCB and picryl chloride, by Godfrey (1975) using dinitrophenyl thiocyanate in FCA, and by Baer and Hooton (1976) using pentadecylcatechol and DNFB. However, no seasonal differences were found by Magnusson and Kligman (1970) regarding sensitization to DNCB, NDMA, and PPDA. Ziegler's (1975) results were similar to ours in chromate-sensitive animals. According to Parker et al. (1975) there is a tendency for seasonal variation to be more evident with weaker sensitizers, such as oxazolone, than with the stronger agents, such as DNFB.

Variations in diet, ambient temperature, humidity, and duration of daylight are some of the factors that might help to explain seasonal effects. Guinea pigs living under more or less constant conditions the year round do not clearly show seasonal rhythms in either the induction or the challenge phase.

INDUCTION OF HYPERSENSITIVITY

Site of Allergen Exposure

For both intradermal and topical induction, most workers prefer the back or nuchal area. The footpads are used for inducing sensitization by injection of adjuvant (Arnason and Waksman, 1964).

We have compared different regions in regard to induction of sensitivity (Magnusson and Kligman, 1970). The guinea pigs were sensitized by a single intradermal injection of DNCB, NDMA, or PPDA. Injection over the scapula yielded higher rates than over the sacrum. In turn, the sacrum was clearly superior to the footpad and to the sternum. The sacrum and parietal region of the head were equivalent. The site of allergen deposition is thus of some importance and might become decisive with weak allergens.

Route of Allergen Exposure

According to Ginsberg et al. (1939) and Seeberg (1951) intradermal and topical application of allergen are equivalently sensitizing, while subcutaneous injection is decidedly inferior (Seeberg, 1951; Frey and Geleick, 1962). Schnitzer (1942) was able to sensitize a small proportion of guinea pigs to DNCB by intramuscular injection. Occasionally, with the aid of adjuvant, contact sensitization may be established even by intraperitoneal injection (Landsteiner and Chase, 1940). By intravenous and intraperitoneal injections of DNCB a few weak sensitizations were induced by Frey and Geleick (1962).

We were particularly concerned to compare intracutaneous with open and occluded applications (Magnusson and Kligman, 1970). Intradermal injection of DNCB, NDMA, and PPDA was clearly more effective than occluded (24 hr) topical exposure. Occlusion markedly enhanced the efficacy of the topical route. The subcutaneous and intramuscular routes gave low sensitization rates. Intraperitoneal injection did not sensitize.

Dose

With weak allergens the dose becomes a critical factor. The objective of enhancing the immunologic response by manipulating the dose was studied by increasing (1) the concentration of the sensitizer, (2) the number of exposures, (3) the exposure area, and (4) the volume of sensitizer (Magnusson and Kligman, 1970).

Concentration. With topical exposure the sensitization rates to DNCB, NDMA, and PPDA increased as the surface concentration increased (quantity per square centimeter). Similarly, by intradermal injection, higher concentrations were more sensitizing.

Number of exposures. A course of ten injections was recommended by Draize et al. (1944) for testing the allergenicity of new substances in guinea pigs. We found that increasing the number of intradermal exposures from one to five or from five to ten significantly increased the sensitization rates. However 15 exposures were no more effective.

Area. When the surface concentration was kept constant, the sensitization rates were not affected by the size of the area of topical application. With DNCB and NDMA an area difference of 100 times made no difference in mean response. These results verify earlier observations by Schnitzer (1942).

These studies clearly indicate the overriding importance of the concentration per unit area of surface and not the size of the area exposed. The total quantity of allergen is not an influential factor. For every substance there is a threshold concentration; this may be quite low for potent allergens and proportionately higher for weak ones.

Volume. Increasing the volume of injection of an allergen solution of constant concentration from 0.1 to 0.5 ml enhanced the sensitization achieved by a single injection of DNCB, NDMA, and PPDA. A larger volume, 1.0 ml, reversed the trend.

Enlarging the volume fivefold necessarily increases the quantity of allergen by the same factor. However, 0.5 ml would appear to be the upper limit. When a sensitizing course consists of repeated injections, there is probably little to be gained by giving more than the usual 0.1 ml.

Interval between Exposures

Strong allergens can produce high sensitization rates by a single exposure. Repeated exposures are required for weaker allergens. It has become customary with new compounds to use a modified Landsteiner technique, giving ten doses at intervals of 2–3 days (Draize et al., 1944).

We sought to find the interval between allergen injections that would give maximal sensitization rates (Magnusson and Kligman, 1970). Four intradermal injections in the sacral skin of DNCB, NDMA, and PPDA, one injection every third day, were more effective than the same total dose given once. Four injections at an interval of 3 days between exposures was much superior to daily administration, and 6-day intervals were no better than 3. With PPDA we found lower sensitization rates with exposures every sixth compared to every third day.

Our results validate the common practice of applying allergen every 2 or 3 days.

Repeated Exposures to the Same versus Different Regions

In humans Epstein et al. (1963) found that four repeated allergen applications to one extremity were far more sensitizing than exposure of each extremity once in succession. Repeated stimulation of the same draining lymph nodes was held responsible for increased effectiveness.

We have made the same observation in the guinea pig (Magnusson and Kligman, 1970). Four successive applications, one every other day, of various allergens to one extremity, by injection or topically, gave sharply higher sensitization rates than the same number of exposures at the same intervals, each time at a different extremity. Limiting the allergen exposures to the same region or same site is thus a simple tactic for greatly enhancing contact sensitization.

Vehicle

The influence of the vehicle on the induction and elicitation of contact allergy has received little attention (Hjorth and Thomsen, 1968; Marzulli and Maibach, 1976). Usually the investigator rather arbitrarily chooses a solvent suitable to his purpose. DNCB, the most commonly used experimental allergen, is usually dissolved in ethanol, acetone, or olive oil for topical application (Landsteiner and Chase, 1939; Nilzén, 1952; Chase, 1954; Frey and Wenk, 1957). Often the same vehicle is used for both induction and elicitation.

The vehicles used for sensitization to DNCB by injection have been ethanol (Frey and Geleick, 1962), acetone (Frey and Geleick, 1962), and propylene glycol (Maguire and Maibach, 1961). In the Landsteiner-Draize procedure the substance is injected in a 0.1% solution or suspension in physiological saline (Draize, 1959).

Stevens (1967) compared the effect of vehicles on sensitization to DNCB using the open technique for both induction and challenge. In declining order of effectiveness were dimethyl formamide, olive oil, paraffin oil, acetone, propylene glycol, glycerine, and ethanol. These findings are difficult to interpret. Vakilzadeh (1973) has shown that by using 90% dimethyl-sulfoxide (DMSO) as a solvent for DNCB the minimum exposure time was reduced from 12 to 6 hr with both topical and intradermal induction compared to acetone and ethanol as solvents.

In a limited study we found that for topical sensitization to DNCB, NDMA, and PPDA, 70% ethanol was superior to petrolatum, propylene glycol, and acetone (Magnusson and Kligman, 1970). For intradermal sensitization propylene glycol and peanut oil were equally effective with DNCB, but with NDMA and PPDA peanut oil was superior. Propylene glycol was markedly more effective than 70% ethanol with all three allergens. In the case of PPDA, equivalent results were obtained with water and propylene glycol. It would thus appear that generalizations are hazardous.

Surface Active Agents

The hope of achieving greater contact and penetration through wetting action has probably been the reason for the intensive study of surfactants as promoters of sensitization. According to Nilzén and Wikström (1955a), guinea pigs became sensitized to chromate and nickel when 1% sodium lauryl sulfate (SLS) was added to the solutions. Without SLS, sensitization did not occur. Analogous studies in guinea pigs have been carried out by others with SLS and other anionic surfactants. All these damage the "barrier" and can provoke irritation. Some authors have achieved sensitization to nickel and chromate; others have not.

Investigators have reached conflicting conclusions with nonionic surfactants as well. Levine (1960), for instance, sensitized animals to penicillin with the aid of Tween 80. Wikström (1962) secured sensitization to chromate using a nonionic surfactant; other experiments have been unsuccessful.

These divergent results are probably attributable to different methods. Technique becomes decisive with weaker allergens.

We have found that anionic surfactants (dodecyl benzene sulfonate and sodium lauryl sulfate) added to the sensitizer (DNCB, NDMA, PPDA, tetrachlorosalicylanilide) in irritating concentrations (1 or 5%) promoted sensitization (Magnusson and Kligman, 1970). The higher concentration was more damaging to the skin and more sensitizing. In subtoxic concentration (0.1%), no enhancement occurred. Nonirritating, nonionic surfactant (1 and 10% Tween 80) did not promote sensitization.

Our results indicate that the promoting effects of the surfactants are very likely attributable to their capacity to promote penetration and produce inflammation and not to their surface-tension lowering or wetting effects.

Chemical and Physical Insults

It has been proved many times that sensitization is promoted by applying the allergen to damaged skin. By mixing the allergen with equal parts of soft soap, Burckhard (1939) obtained increased sensitization to turpentine. Landsteiner and Di Somma (1940) achieved higher sensitization rates to picric acid when the skin was pretreated with cantharidin. Rockwell (1955) enhanced the sensitization to dinitrochlorobenzene by sandpapering or by irritating the skin with croton oil.

We have compared the effects of pretreatment of the exposure site with croton oil, stripping with Scotch tape, and moderate abrasion with a fine-grain sandpaper (Magnusson and Kligman, 1970). The three modes of insults were adjusted to give moderate and similar degrees of inflammation.

All three of the skin-damaging methods enhanced sensitization. The order of increasing effectiveness was sandpapering, stripping, and croton oil. Thus the chemical insult was more effective than the physical ones. This corresponds to experience in humans, in whom chemical irritation with sodium lauryl sulfate and dimethylsulfoxide enhanced sensitization more than physical trauma such as ultraviolet radiation, freezing, or Scotch tape stripping (Kligman, 1966). Chemicals produce an inflammation that evolves more slowly, is more intense at peak, and regresses more slowly.

Among the several factors that might contribute to the enhancing effect of inflammation is that it brings immunocompetent cells to the skin, increasing the possibility of peripheral sensitization.

Occlusion

Rather little attention has been paid to the possible advantage of tightly sealing the application site when attempting to sensitize topically. Occlusion is one of the most effective means for increasing penetration; it also prevents loss of the allergen.

Burckhardt (1939) successfully used occlusion to promote sensitization to turpentine. Vinson and Choman (1960) exploited the occlusive technique to study the influence of surfactants on sensitization to nickel sulfate. Occlusion has been successfully used for both sensitizing and challenging by Buehler (1965). Ziegler (1975) has modified the sensitization technique of Polak and Turk (1968) by using occlusion during topical induction.

We have compared the effects of open exposure, partial occlusion (elastic bandage), and complete occlusion (3 *M* Blenderm) firmly secured by elastic bandage on sensitization to DNCB, NDMA, and PPDA (Magnusson and Kligman, 1970). The effect of maintaining complete occlusion for 1, 3, and 6 days, respectively, was also studied.

A striking promoting effect was obtained by sealing the exposure area. With PPDA, for instance, 24 of 26 animals became sensitized under complete occlusion, in comparison to only 7 of 23 when the area was left open. Partial occlusion was superior to open application but uniformly less effective than complete sealing. Prolonging the duration of occlusion from 1 to 3 days further increased the enhancement. Six days of occlusion, however, were no more effective than three.

The traditional open technique may be effective enough with potent allergens. The occlusion technique, although somewhat more troublesome, has great potential usefulness in promoting sensitization to weak allergens.

Potentiation of Hypersensitivity by Adjuvant

Both immediate and delayed types of allergic states may be potentiated by suspending the antigen in Freund's complete adjuvant (FCA) (Freund, 1956; Finger, 1964).

Landsteiner and Chase (1941) were the first to use a form of adjuvant to promote allergic contact dermatitis (picryl chloride). Others who have employed FCA to promote contact sensitization include Mayer (1955) with picryl chloride, Voss (1958) with mercaptans, Hunziker (1960), Gross et al. (1968), and Polak et al. (1973) with dichromate, and Epstein and Wenzel (1962) with neomycin.

Whether Freund's adjuvant is indispensable or even superior to other methods of inducing contact sensitization has not been thoroughly established. We have quantitatively studied the effect of FCA in relation to other variables (Magnusson and Kligman, 1970). In addition to DNCB, NDMA, and PPDA, the sensitizers used were potassium dichromate, nickel sulfate, Marfanil, neomycin, tetrachlorosalicylanilide, formaldehyde, epoxy resin, and di-*t*-butylphenyldisulfide.

Our findings may be summarized as follows:

Emulsification of contact allergen in FCA generally enhances sensitization greatly. This promoting effect is especially marked in the case of weaker allergens, which may fail to sensitize at all without adjuvant.

Sensitization is dose-dependent. Multiple simultaneous injections of the allergen in adjuvant are more potentiating than multiple single injections. Sensitization tends to increase with repeated injections up to a definite maximum. Beyond this number, the effect is lessened. When single injections were given on alternative days, ten injections were far superior to five, but 15 were considerably less effective than ten, though better than five.

Intradermal administration of allergen in FCA was far more effective than the subcutaneous, intramuscular, or intraperitoneal routes.

Injecting the allergen and adjuvant separately into nearby sites may be as effective, or even more effective, than combining the allergen and adjuvant in a single mixture. For only three of the eight sensitizers studied did the allergen-adjuvant mix give significantly higher sensitization responses than injecting the allergen and adjuvant separately. Effectiveness varies inversely with distance between the injection sites of allergen and FCA. Complete separation into different extremities totally deprives the adjuvant of its potentiating effect.

A greater promoting effect is obtained when the adjuvant is injected simultaneously with, or within a few days after, the allergen than when the adjuvant is injected before the allergen. In the latter case, the adjuvant effect is greatly weakened.

ELICITATION OF HYPERSENSITIVITY

Site of Challenge

There are few reports on regional variations in reactivity to allergens in sensitized guinea pigs. Mu (1931) found that neoarsphenamine reactions were stronger on the flank than on the abdomen. Storck (1955) observed that the reactions appeared earlier on areas close to the head than they did caudally. The flank is the specified challenge site in the Landsteiner-Draize technique (Draize, 1959).

The skin is not the same everywhere, and different regions have different capacities to express inflammation. If marginal states of sensitivity are to be detected, it is important to select sites of maximal reactivity.

In guinea pigs sensitized to DNCB, NDMA, and PPDA we have compared the challenge responses on the flank with those on the back and the abdomen; the back was compared with the scapula and sacrum (Magnusson and Kligman, 1970). No significant differences were observed, except for reactions over the scapula, which were stronger than over the sacrum.

Interval between Induction and Challenge

The minimum time that allergic contact sensitization can be demonstrated in guinea pigs is 5-7 days, according to most authors (Simon, 1936; Landsteiner and Chase, 1939; Schnitzer, 1942; Frey and Wenk, 1957). However, little is known concerning the waxing and waning of the intensity of sensitization with time. Since it is customary practice to challenge animals about 2 wk after the inductive stimulus, it is a matter of consequence to find out whether this time falls within the period of peak sensitivity.

The animals in each of our studies were sensitized on the same day by a single intradermal injection of DNCB, NDMA, or PPDA (Magnusson and Kligman, 1970). Each group of 25 animals was challenged once at times varying from 5 days to 8 wk after the inductive injection. This scheme eliminated the possibility of booster or inhibiting effects from repeated challenge.

Sensitization was detectable at 5 days; by 9 days it reached a maximum, which was maintained up to the 14th day, and then the level began to decline. By 3 wk the incidence and intensity of sensitization had weakened considerably. The convention of challenging 2 wk after the last induction, as specified by Draize et al. (1944), is probably appropriate.

Interval between Challenge and Reading

Customarily intradermal or topical challenge tests are read at 24 hr and sometimes again at 48 hr. With DNCB-sensitized animals, Nilzén (1952) observed that 70% of the animals were already positive within 4 hr. The time pattern of the challenge response has not been systemically studied.

In groups of animals sensitized to DNCB, NDMA, or PPDA or to one of three weaker allergens (tetrachlorosalicylanilide, malathion, and streptomycin) we have rated the challenge responses at 24, 48, 72, and 94 hr after elicitation (Magnusson and Kligman, 1970). Maximum responses with open testing were generally attained at 48-72 hr. Closed patches (left on for 24 hr), however, gave maximal readings 48-72 hr after the patch was removed. It is quite clear that one should never limit the reading of challenge responses to 24 hr. Closed patches should not be read earlier than 24 hr after removal because of the irritation induced by the adhesive.

Occlusion

With potent sensitizers, open testing usually gives sufficiently clear-cut responses. With weaker allergens, however, the hypersensitivity may be so marginal as to remain undetected unless the challenge conditions are optimal. Greater sensitivity is to be expected from closed-patch testing because of enhanced penetration and prevention of loss of the test substance. As early as 1931 Mayer and Sulzberger effectively utilized closed patches in PPDA-sensitized guinea pigs. By restraining the guinea pigs during induction and challenge, Buehler (1965) used occlusive patches and secured superior results.

We have compared the effectiveness of open and occluded testing in animals sensitized to DNCB, NDMA, or PPDA. Occlusion was performed with impermeable plastic tape (Blenderm) secured with elastic bandage and left on for 24 hr. Each animal was challenged with two concentrations of the allergen by both the open and the closed technique. Occlusion of the test areas for 24 hr significantly increased the allergic reactions compared to those observed with uncovered sites. With PPDA, for instance, 19 out of 25 of the animals were positive with the occluded patch and only 11 were positive with open testing.

REFERENCES

Arnason, B. G. and Waksman, B. H. 1964. Tuberculin sensitivity. Immunologic considerations. *Fortschr. Tuberk. Forsch.* 13:1.

Baer, H. and Bowser, R. T. 1963. Antibody production and development of contact skin sensitivity in guinea pigs of various ages. *Science* 140:1211.

Baer, H. and Hooton, M. 1976. Effect of season of immunization on the induction of delayed contact sensitivity in the guinea pig. *Int. Arch. Allergy Appl. Immunol.* 51:140.

Buehler, E. V. 1965. Delayed contact hypersensitivity in the guinea pig. *Arch. Dermatol.* 91:171.

Burckhardt, W. 1939. Experimentelle Sensibilisierung des Meerschweinchens gegen Terpentinöl (Pinen). *Acta Derm. Venereol. (Stockh.)* 19:359.

Chapman, C. W. and Morrell, C. A. 1935. Influence of vitamin C on development of skin sensitivity to neoarsphenamine in the guinea pig. *Proc. Soc. Exp. Biol.* 32:813.

Chase, M. W. 1941. Inheritance in guinea pigs of the susceptibility to skin sensitization with simple compound. *J. Exp. Med.* 73:711.

Chase, M. W. 1954. Experimental sensitization with particular reference to picryl chloride. *Int. Arch. Allergy* 5:163.

Chase, M. W. 1959. Models for hypersensitivity studies. In *Cellular and humoral aspects of the hypersensitive states*, ed. H. S. Lawrence, p. 251. New York: Hoeber-Harper.

De Weck, A. and Brun, R. 1956. De l'eczéma expérimental. 2ème communication. La sensibilisation du cobaye au dinitrochlorobenzène et au chlorure de picryle. *Dermatologica* 113:335.

Draize, J. H. 1959. Dermal toxicity. In *Appraisal of the safety of chemicals in foods, drugs and cosmetics*, p. 46. Austin, Texas: Association of Food and Drug Officials of the United States, Texas State Department of Health.

Draize, J. H., Woodard, G. and Calvery, H. O. 1944. Methods for the study of irritation and toxicity of substances applied topically to the skin and mucous membranes. *J. Pharmacol. Exp. Ther.* 82:377.

Epstein, S. and Wenzel, F. J. 1962. Cross-sensitivity to various "mycins." *Arch. Dermatol.* 86:183.

Epstein, W. L., Kligman, A. M. and Senecal, I. P. 1963. Role of regional lymph nodes in contact sensitization. *Arch. Dermatol.* 88:789.

Fasett, D. W. 1963. Dermatitis and skin tests with textile materials. *Am. Dyest. Rep.*, August 19.

Finger, H. 1964. *Das Freundsche Adjuvans. Wesen und Bedeutung.* Stuttgart: Gustav Fischer.

Freund, J. 1956. The mode of action of immunologic adjuvants. *Fortschr. Tuberk. Forsch.* 7:130.

Frey, J. R. and Geleick, H. 1962. Sensibilisierungsweg und Sensibilisierungserfolg beim Kontaktekzem des Meerschweinchens durch Dinitrochlorbenzol. *Dermatologica* 124:389.

Frey, J. R. and Wenk, P. 1957. Experimental studies on the pathogenesis of contact eczema in the guinea-pig. *Int. Arch. Allergy* 11:81.

Frey, J. R., De Weck, A. L. and Geleick, H. 1966. Sensitization, immunological tolerance and desensitization of guinea pigs to neoarsphenamine.—II. Influence of various factors on sensitization to NEO. *Int. Arch. Allergy* 30:385.

Ginsberg, J. E., Stewart, C. and Baker, S. 1939. Cutaneous sensitization studies. II. Gross and microscopic changes in ragweed and 2-4 dinitrochlorobenzene sensitization of guinea pigs, and in poison ivy sensitization of human beings. *J. Invest. Dermatol.* 2:113.

Godfrey, H. P. 1975. Seasonal variation of induction of contact sensitivity and of lymph node T lymphocytes in guinea pigs. *Int. Arch. Allergy Appl. Immunol.* 49:411.

Gross, P. R., Katz, S. A. and Samitz, M. H. 1968. Sensitization of guinea pigs to chromium salts. *J. Invest. Dermatol.* 50:424.

Hjorth, N. and Thomsen, K. 1968. Difference in the sensitizing capacity of neomycin in creams and in ointments. *Br. J. Dermatol.* 80:163.

Hunziker, N. 1960. De l'eczéma expérimental. 8ème communication. À propos de l'hypersensibilité au bichromate de potassium chez le cobaye. *Dermatologica* 121:93.

Hunziker, N. and Schinas, G. 1962. Experiences sur cobayes nouveaunes. Eczema au dinitrochlorobenzene. *Dermatologica* 124:235.

Jansz, A., Flad, H.-D., Koffler, D. and Miescher, P. A. 1967. The effect of vitamin A on experimental immune thyroiditis. *Int. Arch. Allergy* 31:69.

Kile, R. L. and Pepple, A. W. 1938. Further investigations of poison ivy hypersensitiveness in guinea pigs. *J. Invest. Dermatol.* 1:59.

Kligman, A. M. 1966. The identification of contact allergens by human assay. II. Factors influencing the induction and measurement of allergic contact dermatitis. *J. Invest. Dermatol.* 47:375.

Knop, G. and Rupec, M. 1972. Die Beeinflussung des experimentellen Ekzems durch Vitamin A. *Z. Haut. Geschlechtskr.* 47:579.

Landsteiner, K. and Chase, M. W. 1939. Studies on the sensitization of animals with simple chemical compounds. *J. Exp. Med.* 69:767.

Landsteiner, K. and Chase, M. W. 1940. Studies on the sensitization of animals with simple chemical compounds. VII. Skin sensitization by intraperitoneal injections. *J. Exp. Med.* 71:237.

Landsteiner, K. and Chase, M. W. 1941. Studies on the sensitization of animals with simple chemical compounds. IX. Skin sensitization induced by injection of conjugates. *J. Exp. Med.* 73:431.

Landsteiner, K. and Di Somma, A. A. 1940. Studies on the sensitization of animals with simple chemical compounds. *J. Exp. Med.* 72:361.

Levine, B. B. 1960. Studies on the mechanism of the formation of the penicillin antigen. I. Delayed allergic cross-reactions among penicillin G and its degradation products. *J. Exp. Med.* 112:1131.

Lurie, M. B., Harris, T. N., Abramson, S. and Allison, J. M. 1949. Constitutional factors in resistance to infection. II. The effect of estrogen on tuberculin skin sensitivity and on the allergy of the internal tissues. *Am. Rev. Tuberc.* 59:186.

Magnusson, B. and Kligman, A. M. 1970. *Allergic contact dermatitis in the guinea pig. Identifications of contact allergens.* Springfield, Ill.: Thomas.

Maguire, H. C., Jr. and Maibach, H. I. 1961. Effect of cyclophosphoramide, 6-mercaptopurine, actinomycin D and vincaleukoblastine on the acquisition of delayed hypersensitivity (DNCB contact dermatitis) in the guinea pig. *J. Invest. Dermatol.* 37:427.

Marzulli, F. N. and Maibach, H. I. 1976. Effects of vehicles and elicitation concentration in contact dermatitis testing. I. Experimental contact sensitization in humans. *Contact Dermatitis* 2:325.

Mayer, R. L. 1955. Tubercle bacilli as immunological adjuvants. In *Experimental tuberculosis*, Ciba Foundation Symposium, eds. G. E. W. Wolstenholme and M. P. Cameron, p. 188. London: Churchill.

Mayer, R. L. and Sulzberger, M. D. 1931. Zur Frage der jahreszeitlichen Schwankungen der Krankheiten. Der Einfluss der Kost auf Experimentelle Sensibilisierung. *Arch. Dermatol. Syph.* 163:245.

Mu, J. W. 1931. Regional variability of skin hypersensitiveness to neoarsphenamine in guinea pigs and rabbits. *Proc. Soc. Exp. Biol.* 29:783.

Nilzén, Å. 1952. Some aspects of epidermal testing of guinea-pigs sensitized and not sensitized to 2,4-dinitrochlorobenzene. *Acta Derm. Venereol. (Stockh.)* 32(Suppl. 29):231.

Nilzén, Å. and Wikström, K. 1955a. The influence of lauryl sulphate on the sensitization of guinea pigs to chrome and nickel. *Acta Derm. Venereol. (Stockh.)* 35:292.

Nilzén, Å. and Wikström, K. 1955b. Factors influencing the skin reaction in guinea pigs sensitized with 2,4-dinitrochlorobenzene. *Acta Derm. Venereol. (Stockh.)* 35:415.

Parker, D., Sommer, G. and Turk, J. L. 1975. Variation in guinea pig responsiveness. *Cell. Immunol.* 18:233.

Pepys, J. 1955. The relationship of nonspecific and specific factors in the tuberculin reaction. A review. *Am. Rev. Tuberc.* 71:49.

Polak, L. and Turk, J. L. 1968. Studies on the effect of systemic administration of sensitizers in guinea-pigs with contact sensitivity to inorganic metal compounds. *Clin. Exp. Immunol.* 3:245.

Polak, L., Barnes, J. M. and Turk, J. L. 1968. The genetic control of contact sensitization to inorganic metal compounds in guinea-pigs. *Immunology* 14:707.

Polak, L., Turk, J. L. and Frey, J. R. 1973. Studies on contact hypersensitivity to chromium compounds. *Progr. Allergy* 17:145.

Polak, L., Polak-Wyss, A. and Frey, J. R. 1974. Development of contact sensitivity to DNFB in guinea pigs genetically differing in their response to DNP skin protein conjugates. *Int. Arch. Allergy* 46:417.

Rockwell, E. M. 1955. Study of several factors influencing contact irritation and sensitization. *J. Invest. Dermatol.* 24:35.

Salvin, S. B., Gregg, M. B. and Smith, R. F. 1962. Hypersensitivity in newborn guinea pigs. *J. Exp. Med.* 115:707.

Schnitzer, A. 1942. Beitrag zur Frage des Mechanismus der Sensibilisierung. *Dermatologica* 85:339.

Seeberg, G. 1950. Cutaneous absorption during the menstrual cycle and its influence on intradermal reactions of the delayed type. *Acta Derm. Venereol. (Stockh.)* 30:231.

Seeberg, G. 1951. Eczematogenous sensitization via the lymphatic glands as compared with other routes. *Acta Derm. Venereol. (Stockh.)* 31:592.

Simon, F. A. 1936. Observations on poison ivy hypersensitiveness in guinea pigs. *J. Immunol.* 30:275.

Stevens, M. A. 1967. Use of the albino guinea-pig to detect the skin-sensitizing ability of chemicals. *Br. J. Ind. Med.* 24:189.

Storck, H. 1939. Tierexperimentelle Untersuchungen über den Einfluss von Vitamin C auf allergische Vorgänge. *Schweiz. Z. Allg. Pathol.* II:338.

Storck, H. 1955. Tierexperimentelle Untersuchungen zur Frage der ekzematösen Sensibilisierung. *Arch Dermatol. Syph.* 191:430.

Streitmann, B. and Wiedmann, A. 1937. Vergleichende Untersuchungen über die Sensibilisierungsfähigkeit einzelner Aresnobenzolderivate. *Arch. Dermatol. Syph.* 175:696.

Sulzberger, M. B. and Oser, B. L. 1935. Influence of ascorbic acid in diet on sensitization of guinea pigs to neoarsphenamine. *Proc. Soc. Exp. Biol.* 32:716.

Suskind, R. R. and Ishihara, M. 1965. The effects of wetting on cutaneous vulnerability. *Arch. Environ. Health* 11:529.

Uhr, J. W., Weissman, G. and Thomas, L. 1963. Acute hypervitaminosis A in guinea pigs. II. Effects on delayed-type hypersensitivity. *Proc. Soc. Exp. Biol.* 112:287.

Vakilzadeh, F. 1973. Die Beeinflussung des experimentellen Kontaktekzems durch Dimethylsulfoxyd (DMSO). Verkürzung der Minimalkontaktdauer bei intracutaner Sensibilisierung. *Z. Haut. Geschlechtskr.* 48:271.

Vinson, L. J. and Choman, B. R. 1960. Percutaneous absorption and surface active agents. *J. Soc. Cosmet. Chem.* 11:127.

Voss, J. G. 1958. Skin sensitization by mercaptans of low molecular weight. *J. Invest. Dermatol.* 31:273.

Wikström, K. 1962. Epidermal treatment of guinea pigs with potassium bichromate. *Acta Derm. Venereol. (Stockh.)* 42(Suppl. 49).

Ziegler, V. 1975. Tierexperimenteller Nachweis stark allergener Eigenschaften von Industrieprodukten. Dissertation zur Promotion B an der Karl-Marx-Universität Leipzig (DDR).

12

diagnostic patch testing

■ Niels Hjorth ■

INTRODUCTION

Although great progress has been made within the field of experimental and clinical immunology, no useful *in vitro* tests have been devised to demonstrate lymphocyte-mediated contact allergy in humans. Instead, the sensitivity must be looked for and proved by a reproduction of the acute lesions after contact with a suspected substance under an occlusive patch.

Like any other clinical or laboratory examination it is subject to sources of error. However, with standardized methods and meticulous attention to detail, patch testing represents a sound and reasonably reliable method for identifying allergens responsible for contact dermatitis.

INDICATIONS FOR PATCH TESTING

Previously, patch testing was performed only if allergic contact dermatitis was suspected. More extensive use of a standard series of diagnostic test substances has, however, revealed that clinical suspicions are most unreliable (Cronin, 1972; Magnusson et al., 1969; Rudner et al., 1975; Wilkinson, 1972) and that, in fact, many cases with nonspecific patterns of dermatitis did suffer from contact dermatitis (Fregert et al., 1969). Recent studies showed that about 40% of patients with contact dermatitis of the hands have one or several contact sensitivities, of which two-thirds are relevant to the dermatitis (Wilkinson et al., 1970a). This justifies a more extensive use of patch testing. Patients with dermatitis of the hands of more than 1 month's duration and all patients with occupational dermatitis causing absence from work must be tested. Possibly the eczema is caused by an allergen that can be avoided—for example, by use of rubber gloves—or whose impact can be diminished by minor changes in the process of work. In chronic dermatitis of the legs, especially stasis dermatitis, the majority of patients are sensitive to one or

267

several medicaments used for topical treatment (Bandmann et al., 1972). Pompholyx or dyshidrotic eczema can develop in sensitive persons after ingestion of traces of their allergens in the daily food, such as nickel (Christensen and Möller, 1975) or chromate (Fisher, 1973).

Any chronic eczema of the anogenital area can be complicated by contact sensitivity.

The observations above justify a more extensive use of patch testing.

PATCH TESTING TECHNIQUE

A standardized procedure for patch testing was developed in the 1960s by a Scandinavian group (Magnusson and Hersle, 1965; Magnusson et al., 1969) and brought into widespread usage by two more recent study groups, the North American Contact Dermatitis Group (Rudner et al., 1975) and the International Contact Dermatitis Research Group (Fregert et al., 1969). Test results can be compared only provided the same techniques are followed.

Basically a patch test implies the application to the skin of a certain amount of the suspected allergen in a suitable concentration and a suitable vehicle. The concentration and the vehicle are usually chosen on the assumption that penetration through the skin is promoted by airtight occlusion.

In practice, the substance is applied to a test unit placed on adhesive tape, which is then fixed onto the skin. The test unit must be left on for at least 24 hr, but because many reactions develop later than that, the units are usually removed after 2 or 3 days.

TEST UNITS

It is common practice to use ready-made test materials. The North American Contact Dermatitis Group at present prefers Al-Test IMECO. This is a unit of circular 10-mm-diameter filter paper disks, welded to polythene foil, which is stiffened by a paper-backed aluminum foil. The Al-Test is supplied in rolls of 1,000 units, convenient for serial patch testing. Aluminum foil affords good occlusion of the centrally placed test material. Many other test units are currently available. One of them, the Finn Chamber Test, is a flat cup of aluminum 10 mm in diameter (Pirilä, 1975). This has the advantage of a stiff brim, which provides sufficient occlusion to allow the use of porous, nonocclusive, less irritant tapes. Reactions to adhesive tape are common, but most are of a nonallergic nature, and the major concern is interference with the reading of patch test reactions. For that reason many dermatologists prefer Dermicel (Johnson & Johnson), which has, however, less adhesive power than conventional adhesive tape, a drawback of most acrylic tapes. Scanpore (Norgesplaster, Oslo) has better adhesive properties than most other acrylic tapes by virtue of a thicker coat of adhesive and has been recommended for use with the Finn Chamber Test.

VEHICLES

Textiles, leather, and so on can be applied to the skin as they are and covered by adhesive tape. Most chemicals, however, are dissolved in some vehicle in a suitable concentration for testing. Petrolatum is the most suitable, since it does not evaporate, protects against oxidation, and increases the shelf stability of the test substance (Trolle-Lassen and Hjorth, 1966). Petrolatum is therefore used for most diagnostic test substances included in standard series.

Substances brought in by the patients can be diluted in an adequate solvent such as water, alcohol, or methyl ethyl ketone. Irritant solvents such as benzene, chloroform, and kerosene are obviously unsuitable.

CONCENTRATION

The concentration of the test substance is highly important since the choice of too low a concentration causes false negative patch test reactions, and concentrations that are too high cause irritant reactions and a risk of patch test sensitization.

Often a suitable concentration can be found in handbooks on patch testing (Bandmann and Dohn, 1967; Bandmann and Fregert, 1975; Fisher, 1973; Malten et al., 1976; Rook et al., 1968). The concentrations given in these will usually not cause irritant reactions or sensitizations, but they may, in fact, be too low because they have not been tried out on a sufficient number of sensitive patients. Difficulties arise when patients bring their own materials, such as industrial chemicals, for testing. Open patch tests with various dilutions are advisable for a start. If these give no reactions, occlusive patch tests with lower concentrations can be performed.

It should be realized that the concentration chosen for routine testing will cause false negative reactions in some cases and irritant reactions in others.

Some standard test substances such as formaldehyde, cobalt, and tars cause false positives in children. Presumably the concentrations chosen for routine testing should be selected with regard to the age of the patients tested. No systematic studies of this problem have been performed.

AMOUNT OF TEST MATERIAL

The dose of test substance applied from a syringe is usually adequate if the string of ointment is 5 mm long. If the test substance is a fluid, the filter paper should be saturated.

Scrapings from solid materials must cover the filter paper and they should be wetted with some solvent.

TEST SITES

Most dermatologists apply the tests on the upper or lower back, but the lateral side of the upper arm can also be chosen. The inner surface of the upper arm, the thighs, and the legs may be unsuitable test sites because of inadequate absorption (Bandmann and Rohrbach, 1964; Bandmann and Fregert, 1975; Magnusson and Hersle, 1965).

TIME OF READING

With most allergens a sufficient amount is usually absorbed within 24 hr to provoke a positive response, which may not develop for one or more further days. Conventionally the tests are left in place for 2 days and then removed. If the patient can come only once, it is advisable to let the patient remove the test 2 days after application and appear for reading the next day. This assumes that all test sites were marked for future identification at the time of application.

Positive reactions usually itch, are red, and are to a varying extent infiltrated and studded with papulovesicles. Such a reaction persists for several days or even weeks.

A positive reaction that develops 6 days or more after the application of a patch test is called a late reaction or a flare-up reaction (Wilkinson et al., 1970b).

Some reactions are of an irritant nature but difficult to distinguish from true allergic responses. But most irritant reactions are sharply demarcated with a brownish eroded or glistening surface. Sometimes they are bullous. Compression of the test site between the fingers may reveal a finely wrinkled surface called a "soap effect." Irritant reactions rarely itch but may burn and be painful.

Sweat retention may develop from patch testing. Such papular non-specific reactions are particularly common in a hot summer. At all times of the year nonspecific pustular sweat gland reactions can be found in atopic individuals after testing with metal salts.

TEST SUBSTANCES

Common test substances are available from a number of pharmaceutical firms, which supply them in suitable concentrations and in suitable vehicles.[1] The substances available include a standard series of 20–30 substances, known to be the most common allergens (Table 1). There are slight differences

[1] Patch test substances are supplied by (1) Hollister-Stier Laboratories, Spokane, Washington 94577; (2) Trolab, laboratory for dermatological tests, A. N. Hansensvej 6, DK-2900 Hellerup, Denmark; and (3) Allergopharma, Bahnhofstrasse 4, D-2057 Reinbek, Germany.

TABLE 1   Example of a Patch Test Series Comprising 20 Substances

Substance	Number of tests
Metals (chromium, nickel, cobalt)	3
Mixtures of rubber chemicals	5
Topical medicaments (neomycin, Vioform, local anesthetics, parabens)	5
Balsams (balsam of Peru, rosin, turpentine, wood tars)	4
Miscellaneous agents (formaldehyde, paraphenylenediamine, epoxy resin)	3

between the North American (Rudner et al., 1975) and European (Fregert et al., 1969) recommended series. These substances give a clue to 60–80% of cases of allergic contact dermatitis. The rest are caused by huge numbers of environmental allergens. These derive from several spheres of a patient.

In the personal environment, cosmetics, textiles, and leather are the important allergens. Hair dyes may cause patch test sensitization; permanent wave lotions and mascara and other eye cosmetics may cause irritant reactions. Creams and lipsticks, on the other hand, commonly give false negative reactions.

Textiles should be moistened in water or alcohol in order to wash out the allergen. But even so, up to half of those tested show false negative reactions. Extracts must then be prepared; for example, by means of ether, hot ethanol, or other solvents.

To obtain material from a shoe a mastoid curette must be employed. With proper technique, false positives are rare. In the home and kitchen rubber gloves and indoor plants are reasonably common allergens. It should be noted that not all causes of rubber sensitivity can be revealed by patch testing and that, on the other hand, not all reactions to rubber mixes are indicative of rubber glove sensitivity. Sensitivity to Black Rubber Mix and Naphthyl Mix does not usually coincide with rubber glove sensitivity.

Some plants can be tested as they are, but since the allergen may be largely confined to one organ, several parts of the plant should be employed in the test. Most cases can probably be detected by testing with suitable extracts and mixtures thereof. Extracts of the Compositae (supplied by Hollister-Stier) are used in the detection of weed allergy in hand eczema and in dermatitis on exposed surfaces, especially in farmers. Primin, the sensitizer in *Primula*, is commercially available for patch testing (supplied by Trolab).

Hobbies involve manifold chemical contacts with substances such as glues, dyes, exotic woods, and so forth, and if they involve amateur gardening, exposures to sensitizing plants—apart from the obvious *Rhus*—are unavoidable.

Industrial allergens are commonly detected by standard testing, which includes nickel, chromate, cobalt, and epoxy resin, but obviously there must be a wealth of different materials not included. They must be selected according to the history of the individual patient. Protective gloves and protective creams and cleansers should not be forgotten.

SIGNIFICANCE OF PATCH TEST REACTIONS

A positive reaction to a patch test properly performed indicates that the patient is sensitive to the substance tested and that the allergen may be involved in the causation of dermatitis.

Corroboration of the history determines whether exposure to the substance in question is relevant to the development of dermatitis. Establishment of sensitivity to rubber can explain a nonspecific dermatitis of the leg as being caused by a rubber boot. This is a typical example of an unexpected sensitivity that could only be detected by patch testing and is most easily detected by inclusion of rubber chemicals in a series of standard tests.

Positive reactions can be (1) relevant to the actual dermatitis, (2) of past relevance, (3) of questionable relevance, and (4) of unknown relevance (Wilkinson et al., 1970b).

A reaction of past relevance could be a positive reaction to nickel in the standard series, associated with a history of previous dermatitis from a zip fastener. The finding of a positive reaction to neomycin associated with a clear-cut history of dermatitis from an unknown applied medicament would be of questionable relevance.

Some patients are sensitive to substances that are not known to occur in their environment. Such reactions of unknown relevance should challenge the clinician to trace the origin of the sensitization. The positive reaction indicates that the patient has been sensitized by contact either with the test substance or with a chemically related allergen. Reactions of unknown relevance at the time of reading may later prove highly important as a clue to dermatitis. More and more reactions to chromate have proved to be relevant (Table 2). Nonspecific patterns of dermatitis of the body were common in the 1950s in patients sensitive to formaldehyde. These reactions were of unknown relevance until it was established that formaldehyde resins were used as fixatives for

TABLE 2   Year of Detection of New
Sources of Chromate Contact

Source	Year
Dichromate	1923
Eau de Javelle (cleansing agent)	1930
Leather	1938
Cement	1950
Matches	1962
Game-table felt	1970
Sodium sulfate	1972

textiles. Similarly, reactions to balsam of Peru may indicate a perfume sensitivity. Questionably relevant would apply to a reaction to a common perfume chemical in a patient with dermatitis of the hands. The perfume chemical may or may not occur in the toilet soap used, and the reaction is therefore of questionable relevance.

Obviously, the relevance of a positive patch test can only be established provided the clinician has an adequate knowledge of the occurrence of the allergen in the patient's environment. The occurrences of the common allergens are listed in many handbooks (Bandmann and Fregert, 1975; Fisher, 1973; Malten et al., 1976; Rudner et al., 1975), and at least one should be consulted before a positive reaction is discarded as being of questionable or unknown relevance.

FALSE POSITIVE REACTIONS

False positive reactions are of irritant and of nonimmunological character. Many substances are irritant if applied in a sufficiently high concentration under occlusion on normal skin. Even substances included in the standard patch test series cause irritant reactions in a small number of susceptible individuals.

Materials brought in by the patients pose the greatest problems. Many industrial chemicals are irritant under the condition of a patch test. Some, such as gasoline, kerosene, and detergents, should never be tested. Patients may be sensitive to organic dyes used for motor oils or gasoline, but the vehicle is so irritant that it is impossible to verify the sensitivity by testing with dilutions of the material. Other solvents are also irritant. This applies to benzene and chloroform, which should not be used for testing, even if they are the only solvents suitable for a particular test substance.

Recent dermatitis in the test area, and even an active dermatitis elsewhere, may decrease the threshold for irritant reactions (Björnberg, 1968). If reading of the reaction is performed immediately after removal of the adhesive tape, reactions may be read as positive although the local erythema will disappear after 20-30 min. Rubbing or fingering of the test area will prolong this type of irritant erythema. The adhesive tape employed for fixation of the test units may provoke irritant or allergic reactions or miliaria. Any of these complicates the reading so that nonallergic reactions are read as positives.

Strong positive reactions in the neighborhood of the test site may lower the threshold for both allergic and irritant patch test reactions.

FALSE NEGATIVE REACTIONS

A patch test may give a negative reaction, even if the patient has a clinical (i.e., relevant) sensitivity to the substance tested. Such false negative reactions are generally due to insufficient penetration through the skin. The most common cause of error is loosening of the adhesive tape. This results in inadequate occlusion and therefore inadequate penetration of test material. Open patch tests require ten times the concentration recommended for occlusive patch tests.

The laboratory technician may apply too little test material to the patch. This is particularly obvious if the filter paper patch is not saturated with a testing solution. An unfortunate choice of vehicle may prevent release and thus penetration of the test substance into the skin. A powdered test substance may be too crude, and for that reason unable to penetrate.

The concentration of the allergen may be too low. Neomycin dermatitis is usually caused by ointment with 0.5% neomycin. However, penetration of neomycin through normal skin is so slow that only half of those who are clinically sensitive will develop a positive patch test reaction to 0.5% neomycin. Testing with an excessive concentration of 20% is required to prove the sensitivity.

If only a small fraction of a composite test mixture is allergenic, the very bulk of inert material may preclude an adequate concentration on normal skin. With eosin in lipstick contact dermatitis could develop when sufficient amounts of an impurity of eosin had accumulated in the skin of the vermilion border. This could not be verified with a 48 hr patch test with the lipstick but only with the excessive concentration of 50% eosin in a lipstick base. Similarly, lanolin sensitivity is best demonstrated by patch testing with wool alcohols, which contain a concentrate of the allergens.

Some irritants must be diluted to avoid irritant reactions, but this may prevent testing in search of allergy to a component of the mixture. Perfumes in toilet soaps and detergents cannot be expected to give positive reactions in persons sensitive to them. To avoid the irritant effect of the alkaline soap or detergent, the product must be diluted to such an extent that testing is no longer meaningful (Sulzberger and Baer, 1945).

Very sensitive individuals react to patch tests applied in nearly all body regions. On average, however, half of the positive reactions obtained by testing on the back will be missed if the tests are applied on the front of the thighs (Magnusson and Hersle, 1965).

Negative reactions may be recorded if only one reading is performed, and this is done after 2 days (Fregert et al., 1969). The time of reaction is commonly longer. Local steroid therapy of the test area can reduce the reactivity of the skin, and so can systemic steroid therapy provided the daily dosage exceeds 20 mg prednisone or equivalent. Exhaustion of the immunological reactivity after a widespread acute dermatitis has been reported but is very rare.

SIDE EFFECTS OF PATCH TESTING

Most patients find it a nuisance to carry strips of adhesive tape on their backs for 2 days, partly because it prevents them from having a bath and partly because some itching is unavoidable, especially in summer. Occlusive tapes may cause miliaria rubra. In a pigmented Caucasian temporary hypopigmentation can follow the removal of the adhesive tape. Some test substances can cause a hypopigmentation from pigment incontinence (Osmundsen, 1970). Sun exposure of the test sites leaves hyperpigmented spots from tar and other photosensitizers. Scarring is very rare.

Positive reactions itch, and if they are strong, they may provoke a flare-up of distant sites of dermatitis, dyshidrotic eruptions and id-like dissemination. Such spread can be stopped by a short course of prednisone (40–60 mg/day).

Patch testing may in some cases sensitize to the substance tested. This is rare with substances included in the standard series, whose concentrations and vehicles have been chosen after mass testing. Materials of unknown composition brought in by the patients bring more problems. Sensitization sometimes becomes apparent as a late reaction develops 7 days or more after testing, but some cases can be established only by repeated testing. For unknown reasons patch test sensitizations are often transient and impossible to verify by repeated testing 1 yr later (White and Baer, 1950).

Contact sensitivity tends to decline with the years, especially with avoidance of contact with the allergen. Repeated patch tests may provoke the sensitivity, and even in such cases a late reaction may develop. The clinical significance of this is probably limited since such a patient will easily be resensitized by clinical contact with the allergen.

New important environmental allergens must be introduced in standard patch test series. A suitable test concentration cannot be predicted. With alantolactone, an allergen in the Compositae plant family, a cautious choice of 1% in petrolatum was found to cause patch test sensitization. Consequently, the concentration was adjusted to a safe 0.1%. Patch test sensitizations may also occur if the test substances undergo chemical changes during storage. This happens with turpentine, whose allergen content initially increases and then declines during storage.

Such phenomena are unpredictable and therefore unavoidable. Systemic symptoms may follow occlusive patch tests with Apresoline (Kligman, 1966). Insecticides and some war gases may similarly cause systemic pharmacological effects after absorption.

Fainting, malaise, and fever have been observed after epicutaneous tests with lauryl ether sulfate containing an allergenic sultone impurity (Magnusson and Gilje, 1973). Such symptoms occurred only in patients with a delayed-type hypersensitivity to the test substance and must have an immunological basis, as does contact urticaria from the insect repellent Deet (Maibach and Johnson, 1975). The general reactions described are rare.

WHY PATCH TEST?

Contact sensitivities are very often missed, even at clinics that are specially focused on contact dermatitis (Agrup et al., 1970; Cronin, 1972).

This can have far-reaching clinical consequences. If a worker develops occupational hand eczema, contact substances specific for the place of work will be suspected. A change of job may be recommended. This would be unlikely to help if the hand eczema were due to protective rubber gloves. Unless patch tests are performed, rubber gloves may not come into focus, and only patch testing could reveal that sensitivities to specific materials were nonexistent. This worker should change his gloves and not his job.

Several studies have assessed the accuracy of clinical estimates of contact sensitivities. The clinical diagnosis of a primary nickel sensitization is usually obvious, but secondary dyshidrotic eruptions of the hands may not be ascribed to a nickel sensitivity (Agrup et al., 1970; Cronin, 1972; Wilkinson, 1972). Chromate, cobalt and rubber sensitivities are often unexpected findings at standard patch testing (Agrup et al., 1970), and so are sensitivities to individual components of local therapeutics. A bullous streaky dermatitis from a weekend outing is assumed to be diagnostic of *Rhus* dermatitis. Only recently has the phototoxic *Heracleum* dermatitis, which in Europe is the usual cause of streaky plant dermatitis, been recognized in the United States (Camm et al., 1976). Standard patch tests with *Primula obconica* reveal that many cases of dermatitis from it are missed by dermatologists.

Many dermatologists trust their clinical acumen in the diagnosis of allergic contact dermatitis and feel, as a consequence, that the benefits of patch testing do not outweigh the risks of the procedure. Systematic investigation has, however, failed to support this complacency and has, on the contrary, shown that half of all contact sensitivities were relevant and unexpected by the clinician.

REFERENCES

Agrup, G., Dahlquist, J., Fregert, S. and Rorsman, H. 1970. Value of history and testing in suspected contact dermatitis. *Arch. Dermatol.* 101:212–215.

Bandmann, H.-J. and Dohn, W. 1967. *Die Epicutantestung.* Munich: Bergmann.

Bandmann, H.-J. and Fregert, S. 1975. *Patch testing.* New York: Springer Verlag.

Bandmann, H.-J. and Rohrbach, W. 1964. Die epicutane Testreaktion und ihre Abhängigkeit von dem Auflageort der Läppchenprobe. *Arch. Klin. Exp. Dermatol.* 220:155.

Bandmann, H.-J., Calnan, C. D., Cronin, E., Fregert, S., Hjorth, N., Magnusson, B., Maibach, H. J., Malten, K. E., Meneghini, C. P., Pirilä, V. and Wilkinson, D. S. 1972. Dermatitis from applied medicaments. *Arch. Dermatol.* 106:335–337.

Björnberg, A. 1968. *Skin reactions to primary irritants in patients with hand eczema*, p. 117. Göteborg, Sweden: Isacson.

Camm, E., Buck, H. W. L. and Mitchell, J. C. 1976. Phytophotodermatitis from Heracleum mantegazzianum. *Contact Dermatitis* 2:68–72.

Christensen, O. B. and Möller, H. 1975. External and internal exposure of the antigen in the hand eczema of nickel allergy. *Contact Dermatitis* 1:136–141.

Cronin, E. 1972. Clinical prediction of patch test results. *Trans. St. John's Hosp. Dermatol. Soc.* 58:153–162.

Fisher, A. A. 1973. *Contact dermatitis.* Philadelphia: Lea & Febiger.

Fregert, S., Hjorth, N., Magnusson, B., Bandmann, H.-J., Calnan, C. D., Cronin, E., Malten, K., Menghini, C. L., Pirilä, V. and Wilkinson, D. S. 1969. Epidemiology of contact dermatitis. *Trans. St. John's Hosp. Dermatol. Soc.* 55:17–35.

Kligman, A. M. 1966. The identification of contact allergens by human assay. III. The maximization test: A procedure for screening and rating contact sensitizers. *J. Invest. Dermatol.* 47:393.

Magnusson, B. and Gilje, O. 1973. Allergic contact dermatitis from a dishwashing liquid containing lauryl ether sulphate. *Acta Derm. Venereol. (Stockh.)* 53:136–140.

Magnusson, B. and Hersle, K. 1965. Patch test methods. 2. Regional variations of patch test responses. *Acta Derm. Venereol. (Stockh.)* 45:257.

Magnusson, B., Fregert, S., Hjorth, N., Høvding, G., Pirilä, V. and Skog, E. 1969. Routine patch testing V. *Acta Derm. Venereol. (Stockh.)* 49:556–563.

Maibach, H. J. and Johnson, H. L. 1975. Contact urticaria syndrome. *Arch. Dermatol.* 111:726–730.

Malten, K. E., Nater, J. P. and van Ketel, W. G. 1976. Patch testing guidelines. Nijmegen: Dekker & van de Vegt.

Osmundsen, P. E. 1970. Pigmented contact dermatitis. *Br. J. Dermatol.* 83:296–301.

Pirilä, V. 1975. Chamber test versus patch test for epicutaneous testing. *Contact Dermatitis* 1:48–52.

Rook, A., Wilkinson, D. S. and Elling, F. J. G. 1968. *Textbook of dermatology*, vol. 1. Oxford: Blackwell.

Rudner, E. J., Clendenning, W. E., Epstein, E., Fisher, A. A., Jillson, O. F., Jordan, W. P., Kanoj, N., Larsen, W., Maibach, H. J., Mitchell, J. C., O'Quinn, S. E., Schorr, W. and Sulzberger, M. B. 1975. The frequency of contact sensitivity in North America 1972–1974. *Contact Dermatitis* 1:277–280.

Sulzberger, M. B. and Baer, R. L. 1945. Unusual or abnormal effects of soap on the "abnormal skin." In *Medical uses of soap*, ed. M. Fishbein, pp. 51–59. London: Lippincott.

Trolle-Lassen, C. and Hjorth, N. 1966. Deterioration of substances used for patch testing. *Berufsdermatosen* 14:176–188.

White, W. A. and Baer, R. L. 1950. Failure to prevent experimental sensitization. Observations on the "spontaneous" flare-up phenomenon. *J. Allergy* 21:344–348.

Wilkinson, D. S. 1972. Contact dermatitis of the hands. *Trans. St. John's Hosp. Dermatol. Soc.* 58:163–171.

Wilkinson, D. S., Bandmann, H.-J., Calnan, C. D., Cronin, E., Fregert, S., Hjorth, N., Magnusson, B., Maibach, H. J., Malten, K. E., Menghini, C. L. and Pirilä, V. 1970a. The role of contact allergy in hand eczema. *Trans. St. John's Hosp. Dermatol. Soc.* 56:19–25.

Wilkinson, D. S., Fregert, S., Magnusson, B., Bandmann, H.-J., Calnan, C. D., Cronin, E., Hjorth, N., Maibach, H. J., Malten, K. E., Menghini, C. L. and Pirilä, V. 1970b. Terminology of contact dermatitis. *Acta Derm. Venereol. (Stockh.)* 50:287–292.

13

contact allergy: predictive testing in humans

Francis N. Marzulli ■ Howard I. Maibach

INTRODUCTION

Investigative dermatologists employ basically similar patch test procedures to forecast the allergenic potential of topical skin preparations in subjects without skin disease and to diagnose contact allergy in clinical patients (that is, those who have presented themselves to the physician for treatment).

In diagnostic tests, a preparation is applied to a clinical patient's skin under an occlusive patch for 48 hr and the skin is evaluated for evidence of erythema, edema, or more severe skin changes occurring 24, 48, and 72 hr after removal of the patch. Allergenic materials are thereby identified by reproducing skin disease on a small scale with offending chemicals. Diagnostic test results obtained in this manner are finding their way into the scientific literature with increasing frequency. Two groups of dermatologists, the North American Contact Dermatitis Group[1] (NACDG) and the International Contact Dermatitis Research Group (ICDRG) (Fregert et al., 1969), which had its origin in the Northern Dermatologic Society of Scandinavia (Magnusson et al., 1962), have been especially active in this regard.

The authors thank John Atkinson, Division of Mathematics, Food and Drug Administration, Washington, D.C., for statistical analyses.

[1] Established in December 1970 by 13 dermatologists. W. G. Larsen, M.D., secretary-treasurer, 2250 N.W. Flanders St., Portland, Oregon 97210.

In this setting, clinical patients from a wide geographic area are tested with a standard screening series tray. Substances, concentrations, and methods are agreed on at the start. Results are centrally reported, analyzed, and evaluated in terms of a sensitization index (percentage of positive skin reactions).

The more recently formed NACDG has lately reported a study of 1,200 clinical patients tested with 16 materials (Rudner et al., 1973). A high incidence of skin reactions was disclosed with nickel sulfate, p-phenylene-diamine, potassium dichromate, thimerosal, ethylenediamine, neomycin sulfate, and ammoniated mercury. This suggests the possibility that these, or chemically related substances, might be responsible for skin disease in these patients. A mathematical evaluation of the data of Table 1, reported by the NACDG (Rudner et al., 1973), shows a number of interesting findings. Nickel

TABLE 1   Skin Reactions Reported by Two Research Groups on Clinical Patients Evaluated with a Diagnostic Test Kit[a]

Compound[b]	North American Contact Dermatitis Group Concentration (%)	North American Contact Dermatitis Group Reactors No. (1,200 tested)[c]	North American Contact Dermatitis Group Reactors %	International Contact Dermatitis Research Group Concentration (%)	International Contact Dermatitis Research Group Reactors No. (4,824 tested)[d]	International Contact Dermatitis Research Group Reactors %	North American vs. International[e]
Nickel sulfate	2.5	131	11	5	321	6.7	S
Potassium dichromate	0.5	91	8	5.0	318	6.6	NS
Thimerosal	0.1	91	8				
p-Phenylenediamine	1	98	8	1	237	4.7	S
Ethylenediamine	1	85	7				
Neomycin sulfate	20	71	6	20	176	3.7	S
Benzocaine	5	54	5	5	192	4.0	NS
Ammoniated mercury	1	65	5				
Mercaptobenzothiazole	2	58	5	2	99	2.0	S
Formalin, aqueous	2	43	4	2	169	3.5	NS
Thiram	2	50	4	2	97	2.0	S
Woolwax alcohol	30	37	3	30	127	2.6	NS
Paraben mixture[f]	15	38	3	15	91	1.9	S
Dibucaine HCl	1	32	3				
Cyclomethycaine sulfate	1	23	2				

[a]Data from Rudner et al. (1973).
[b]All prepared in petrolatum, except formalin.
[c]Male and female, black and white subjects.
[d]Male and female, white subjects.
[e]S = significant at 95% level; NS = not significant.
[f]Methyl, ethyl, propyl in equal amounts.

sulfate, *p*-phenylenediamine, neomycin sulfate, mercaptothiobenzothiazole, thiram, and paraben show significantly higher sensitization indices (95% confidence) when tested on 1,200 patients by the NACDG than when tested by the ICDRG on 4,825 patients. These results could be interpreted as signifying that climatic or genetic differences might have influenced the outcome or, more likely, greater frequency of exposure of U.S. and Canadian citizens to a wider array of chemicals may be responsible for the higher index in those countries. Marzulli and Maibach (1974b) showed that greater exposure could also occur in the form of a higher concentration of a sensitizing ingredient. This, in turn, could result in elicitation of a higher reaction frequency from chemicals with a proclivity to sensitize.

The type of patient referred for testing must also be considered in evaluating the significance of the results. For instance, in some clinics (such as that of Fregert et al. in Sweden) many referrals are for alleged occupational exposure; other clinics, because of their location, have few occupationally afflicted patients. Some centers test patients who are referred mainly for intractable eczema, whereas others investigate more acute problems.

A further evaluation of the data of Table 1 is given in Table 2. The table shows that nickel sulfate produces a significantly greater number (95% confidence) of skin reactions in clinical patients than any other material tested by the NACDG. This analysis (Table 2) also suggests that reactions to these 15 compounds can be placed in ten different categories, each of which is significantly different (95% confidence) from the others.

Nickel sulfate, with a reaction rate of 11% the most frequently encountered sensitizer in U.S. and Canadian dermatologic patients, is arbitrarily assigned to category 1. *p*-Phenylenediamine, potassium dichromate, and thimerosal with an 8% reaction rate and ethylene diamine with a 7% rate represent a significantly lower reaction rate and are classified as category 2. Neomycin with a 6% reaction rate represents category 3. Ammoniated mercury with a 5.4% reaction rate is in category 4 and so on to cyclomethycaine, with a reaction rate of 2%, which is category 10.

PREDICTIVE METHODS

Systematic predictive test procedures (as contrasted with diagnostic) for skin sensitization have evolved over a period of about 30 yr (Draize et al., 1944; Rostenberg and Sulzberger, 1937; Schwartz, 1941, 1951, 1960; Shelanski, 1951). Currently they generally require multiple occlusive patches for induction of sensitization (ten patches, 48 hr each, same site) followed by a 2 wk rest period and then challenge (48 hr) with a patch at a new skin site (Marzulli and Maibach, 1973). There are a number of variations in these procedures, including the use of provocative chemical agents such as sodium lauryl sulfate (SLS) (Kligman, 1966b), special skin preparation such as stripping (Spier and Sixt, 1955) or freezing (Epstein et al., 1963), special

TABLE 2   Reactors Observed by North American Contact Dermatitis Group among 1,200 Patients Tested Diagnostically for Skin Sensitization with 15 Compounds[a]

Compound	No. reactors	1 (131)	2 (98)	3 (91)	4 (91)	5 (85)	6 (71)	7 (65)	8 (58)	9 (54)	10 (50)	11 (43)	12 (38)	13 (37)	14 (32)	15 (23)	Category[b]
1. Nickel sulfate	131		+	+	+	+	+	+	+	+	+	+	+	+	+	+	1
2. p-Phenylenediamine	98			0	0	0	+	+	+	+	+	+	+	+	+	+	2
3. Potassium dichromate	91				0	0	0	+	+	+	+	+	+	+	+	+	2
4. Thimerosal	91					0	0	+	+	+	+	+	+	+	+	+	2
5. Ethylenediamine	85						0	0	+	+	+	+	+	+	+	+	2
6. Neomycin sulfate	71							0	0	0	+	+	+	+	+	+	3
7. Ammoniated mercury	65								0	0	0	+	+	+	+	+	4
8. Mercaptobenzothiazole	58									0	0	0	+	+	+	+	5
9. Benzocaine	54										0	0	0	0	+	+	5
10. Thiram	50											0	0	0	+	+	6
11. Formalin	43												0	0	0	+	7
12. Paraben mixture	38													0	0	0	8
13. Woolwax alcohol	37														0	0	8
14. Dibucaine HCl	32															0	9
15. Cyclomethycaine sulfate	23																10

[a]Items to the right of heavy line are significantly different (95% confidence) from others on that line.
[b]See text.

patches (Magnusson and Hersle, 1965), high concentrations at induction (Marzulli and Maibach, 1974b), and 25-200 test subjects (Draize et al., 1944; Kligman, 1966a). Other background information and references to studies on predictive methods are contained in review papers by Giovacchini (1972) and Hardy (1973). Methods of historic and current interest are summarized in Table 3.

It is apparent from the cited variations in proposed test procedures that methodologies have proliferated. It is not entirely clear, however, how useful these variations are and what limitations obtain under use conditions, as validation has not kept pace with the announcement of each new departure. Furthermore, predictive tests are often performed on a single chemical entity, whereas ultimate use may occur as part of a multicomponent formulation in a marketed product, where the vehicle and associated ingredients may influence the outcome.

If indeed one has an adequate laboratory test for identifying allergenic potential, two important considerations obtain in employing it for successfully marketing a cosmetic or topical drug.

TABLE 3 Predictive Tests for Skin Sensitization of Humans

Test	No. subjects	Test substance amount or concentration	Vehicle	Skin site	Type patch	Induction No. patches	Duration	Rest	Challenge	Reference
Schwartz	200	Fabric			Fabric	1	5 days	10 days	48 hr patch; observe 10 days	Schwartz, 1941
Schwartz	200	1 in. fabric liquid or powder		Arm, thigh, or back	Cellophane covered with 2 × 2 in. Elastoplast	1	72 hr	7–10 days	72 hr; same site; observe 3 days	Schwartz, 1960
"Prophetic" Schwartz-Peck	200	¼ in. square 4-ply gauze, liquid saturated[a]	Petrolatum or corn oil	Arm or back	1 in. square nonwaterproof cellophane covered with 2 in. square adhesive plaster	1	24 hr or 3 or 4 days	10–14 days	48 hr; any site especially thin keratin; observe 3 days; compare new and old formulas	Schwartz and Peck, 1944; Schwartz, 1951
"Repeated insult" Shelanski	200	Proportional to area of ultimate use	Mineral oil		Occlusion; follows Schwartz test	10–15	24 hr every other day; same site	2–3 wk	48 hr patch	Shelanski, 1951; Shelanski and Shelanski, 1953
"Repeated insult" Draize	100 males 100 females	0.5 ml or 0.5 gram		Arm or back	1 in. square	10	24 hr alternate days	10–14 days	Repeat patch on new site	Draize et al., 1944; Shelanski, 1951; Draize, 1959
Modified Draize	200	0.5 ml or 0.5 gram (high concentration)	Petrolatum	Arm	Square BandAid, no perforations	10	48 hr	2 wk	Patch on new site 72 hr with nonirritant concentration	Marzulli and Maibach, 1973, 1974
"Maximization" Kligman	25	1 ml 5% SLS[b] followed by 1 ml 25% test material	Petrolatum	Forearm or calf	1.5 in. square Webril occluded with Blenderm; held in place with perforated plastic tape	5 (same site)	24 hr SLS followed by 48 hr test material for each of five inducing applications	10 days	1 in. square patch on lower back or forearm; 0.4 ml of 10% SLS for 1 hr followed in 24 hr by 0.4 ml of 10% test material for 48 hr	Kligman, 1966
Modified "maximization"	25	Same as maximization				7	24 hr SLS followed by 48 hr test material for each of seven inducing applications; no patch for 24 hr between each of seven inducing applications	10 days	2% SLS for ½ hr followed by 48 hr patch with test material	Kligman and Epstein, 1974

[a] Modified for solids, powders, ointments, and cosmetics. Concentration, amount, area, and site of application are considered important in evaluating results. Authors recommended that cosmetics be tested uncovered.
[b] Sodium lauryl sulfate (SLS) pretreatment is used to produce moderate inflammation of the skin. SLS is mixed with test material when compatible. SLS is eliminated when the test material is a strong irritant.

283

1. The sample size of test subjects must be large enough so that results are valid for the population at large, yet small enough to permit logistic feasibility in the laboratory.
2. The laboratory test must have the capacity to predict likelihood of occurrence under use conditions.

Henderson and Riley (1945) in their classic paper discussed some of the complexities and mathematical considerations involved in extrapolating from a small test population to large numbers of users. Briefly stated, there may be no skin reactions in a test population of 200 random subjects, yet as many as 15 of every 1,000 of the general population may react (95% confidence), and up to 22 of every 1,000 may react (99% confidence). If the test population is reduced to 100 subjects, up to 30 of every 1,000 of the general population may react (95% confidence). Conversely, when 1 of 200 subjects in a test population becomes sensitized, a test population of 10,000 subjects might show from 1 to 275 sensitized, with 95% confidence.

The possibility that the laboratory test may not predict what is likely to happen in the field stems from a large number of variables that may affect the outcome of the test. These include the skin site, climatic conditions, area and frequency of application, and others.

Validation of a laboratory test procedure for predicting skin sensitization in the field can be undertaken in a variety of ways, none of which is completely satisfactory.

One approach is to evaluate the test system by comparing predictive test results with those obtained from other sources, such as:

1. Limited use tests on a final formulation prior to marketing.
2. Industry and Food and Drug Administration (FDA) consumer complaint data.
3. Retrospective epidemiologic data.
4. Monitoring programs such as the Department of Health, Education, and Welfare (HEW)-sponsored investigation of consumer's perceptions of adverse reactions to cosmetic products (HEW, 1975).
5. Diagnostic test results in dermatologic clinics.

All of the above items can be important; however, item 5 represents our major source of precise information at present. When the incidence of sensitization predicted by the prophetic test methods exceeds the incidence observed in the diagnostic clinic, or in other words, when an ingredient is predicted to be a strong sensitizer, yet marketed products containing the ingredient appear to be well tolerated (as evidenced by a lack of sensitized dermatologic patients), it may mean that the concentration used in the marketed product may be exceedingly low or the product may provide limited (time) skin contact (see the section on formaldehyde below). On the other hand, when the sensitization frequency observed in diagnostic tests exceeds that suggested by predictive tests, it may mean that individuals who cannot tolerate a widely used product are being systematically identified by clinical dermatologists (see parabens below). When both diagnostic and predictive tests show a high frequency of sensitization, a substance with strong sensitization potential is suggested (*p*-phenylenediamine), and when both diagnostic and predictive tests show a low frequency of sensitization, it is apparent that the predictive test is accurately forecasting a low allergenic potential and is not revealing false positives.

One can add the art of successful marketing of safe preparations to the aforementioned mathematic and scientific approaches to predicting the safe use of an ingredient. In some cases, despite a careful evaluation of conditions that appear to be of importance, one may not be aware of certain hidden factors that may play a role in the outcome. This aspect is best regulated by comparing a new product with an old one that has stood the test of time in the market place. Studies of this kind may occasionally provide a more meaningful interpretation of the likelihood of success (safety) in the marketplace than a carefully obtained sensitization index on a panel of 200 laboratory subjects.

EVALUATION OF SOME COMMON CONTACT SENSITIZERS

Formaldehyde

Formaldehyde (aqueous solution) is a strong sensitizer. In predictive tests conducted on 331 normal subjects with 1-10% formalin (formalin is 37% formaldehyde) at induction, 1% at challenge, 4.5-7.8% of the test population showed evidence of skin sensitization (Marzulli and Maibach, 1974b). Diagnostic tests on clinical patients reported by the NACDG (Rudner et al., 1973) showed a sensitization index of 4%. Earlier reports by other investigators indicate that in earlier times, formaldehyde sensitivity in clinical patients reached as high as 24%. The possibility that some of these reactions were irritant responses (false positives) due to the use of too high a concentration of formaldehyde at challenge has been postulated (Epstein and Maibach, 1966). On the other hand, the general recognition that formaldehyde is a potent sensitizer by both industry and many of those likely to be exposed to it professionally may also have contributed to this decreased incidence in recent years. The Cosmetic Product Registry of the FDA shows that formaldehyde is used in about 5% of 8,000 preparations in the registry (FDA, 1972). Despite this rather extensive use of formaldehyde in cosmetic products, the prediction rate is roughly the same as the incidence seen in diagnostic tests. One explanation for the fact that it has not sensitized a greater number of patients who use cosmetics is that formaldehyde is largely confined to use at low concentrations as a preservative in shampoos. These preparations do not remain in continuous contact with skin, as they are rinsed off. The use of formaldehyde as a nail hardener, on the other hand, is accompanied by a significant number of serious injuries to sensitive nail and adnexal tissues. This type of exposure may contribute substantially to that portion of the 4% sensitization index seen in clinical patients which is cosmetic-related.

Parabens

Methyl and propyl paraben are abundantly used as preservatives in foods, drugs, and cosmetics, providing many opportunities for exposure. Methyl and propyl paraben appear in 36 and 31%, respectively, of cosmetic products registered with the FDA (FDA, 1972). Predictive tests for skin sensitization (Marzulli and Maibach, 1973) show a sensitization index of 0.3% (397 subjects). Diagnostic tests for skin sensitization show a reaction rate of 3% by the NACDG, 1.9% by the ICDRG, and 0.7% when tested in 1968 on 273 chronic dermatitis patients by Schorr (1968) (note correction from 0.8 to 0.7% in the original article). The diagnostic test results show a significantly higher reaction rate in patients than was observed in predictive tests on normal people. This in itself is, of course, not surprising. The fact that each of the diagnostic test results is significantly different from the others is interesting. It may be due to differences in exposure in different geographic areas as well as in different time frames; that is, greater susceptibility as exposure time increases. The widespread use of parabens may account for the tenfold difference between diagnostic and predictive test results obtained with certain test populations. The status of topical parabens with special reference to skin hypersensitivity is discussed in greater detail in a recent review paper (Marzulli and Maibach, 1974a). It was concluded that "allergic contact dermatitis (from parabens) exists. Fortunately, the number of cases is relatively small. It is hoped that alternatives to the parabens will be carefully studied so that they do not surprise us and prove to be a greater topical or systemic hazard."

p-Phenylenediamine

p-Phenylenediamine (PPDA) is well known as a skin irritant and skin sensitizer. Its principal use in cosmetics is as a hair dye ingredient. In preditive tests at 1% concentration it produced sensitization reactions in 53% of a normal test population (Marzulli and Maibach, 1974b). Other "para" substances are encountered which are immunologically related to p-phenylenediamine. These include p-aminobenzoic acid, a sunscreen; sulfonamide, an antibacterial agent; procaine, a local anesthetic; and p-aminosalicylic acid, an antitubercular agent. In diagnostic tests, 8% of clinical patients showed skin reactions when tested with PPDA (Rudner et al., 1973). An FDA complaint file for 1974 (Cosmetic Injury Reports, 1974) showed that 1.9% of consumer compalints (639) involved oxidative hair dyes containing PPDA or PPDA-like materials. These predictive, diagnostic, and consumer complaint data tend to support the high allergenic potential of PPDA. The fact that a cautionary statement warns the hair dye user to test behind the ear prior to each use may be responsible for reducing the expected reaction rate under use conditions. In addition, hair dyes are applied primarily to the hair, mainly by trained cosmeticians, after admixture with peroxide. These circumstances could also contribute substantially to reducing the reaction rate under use conditions. Nevertheless, PPDA remains in the second highest category (category 2) of diagnostic test reactions seen by investigative clinical dermatologists.

Peru Balsam

Peru balsam (or balsam of Peru) is an oleoresin obtained from *Myroxylon pereirae*, a tree that grows mainly in Central America. Peru balsam is a dark brown, viscous liquid which contains 50–60% cinnamein, an ester of cinnamic and benzoic acid, and about 28% resin, styracine, and vanillin. It has had considerable past use in perfumes, flavors, toilet waters, hair lotions, and at one time in topical antiscabic and disinfectant drugs. Peru balsam oil is prepared from Peru balsam by extraction with volatile solvents or by distillation. The oil contains large amounts of benzyl benzoate and benzyl cinnamate. The sensitization potentials of the oil and the parent material are decidedly different (Opdyke, 1974), as are their compositions.

In predictive tests, Shelanski and Shelanski (1953) reported that Peru balsam produced no evidence of skin sensitization when tested at 8% concentration on 50 subjects with a repeated insult method. Failure to elicit sensitization may have resulted from the low concentration of Peru balsam that was used. Hjorth (1961), in a classic and extensive study of Peru balsam, recommended that 25% concentration be used to avoid false negative responses, the same concentration recommended earlier by Bonnevie. Kligman (1966), using a maximization procedure obtained a 28% sensitization rate (Opdyke, 1974) when Peru balsam was tested on 25 human volunteers at 8% concentration. The possibility that the irritant effects of SLS were super-imposed on those of Peru balsam cannot be excluded.

In one diagnostic series of tests conducted on 5,558 patients in Scandinavia, a reaction rate of 6.9% to Peru balsam was obtained (Magnusson et al., 1968). In another diagnostic series conducted in 1970 on a selected group of 281 female patients with contact allergy of the hands, 27% of those who reacted to a diagnostic series of allergens showed a reaction to Peru balsam (Calnan et al., 1931). Hjorth (1961) states that 0.4–7% of patients in European clinics react positively to Peru balsam. At the Finsen Institute in Denmark, Hjorth's data, collected from February 1, 1954 to October 31, 1958, show an incidence of 3.2% (239 of 7,500 patients). Records of the NACDG for the period July 1, 1972 to June 30, 1973 show a 4.5% incidence of skin reactions when tested on 177 male and female patients with 25% Peru balsam.

It would appear from the total findings that results for both diagnostic and predictive testing with Peru balsam are complicated as well as variable. On close inspection, some of the factors involved in the variability emerge. Peru balsam is not one substance but several. Benzyl benzoate, benzyl cinnamate, benzoic acid, cinnamic acid, and vanillin are not considered important allergens in Peru balsam (Hjorth, 1961). According to Hjorth (1961), "only resin A (esters of coniferyl alcohol) of which Peru balsam contains 1 to 3% is sensitizing to some patients." The 8% test concentration of Peru balsam used by Shelanski and Shelanski (1953) in predictive tests may therefore be too low. On the other hand, maximization test results of Kligman (1966) may be high if irritant effects of Peru balsam and SLS are additive.

With regard to diagnostic testing, a sensitization rate from about 3.2% (Hjorth, 1961) to 4.5% (NACDG) appears to be representative of the actual reaction rate expected in ordinary clinical patients, whereas higher rates may be observed in selected patients with hand dermatitis of unknown etiology.

Because ingredients of Peru balsam are found in perfumes, spices, and fruits, the allergenic effects of the primary allergen may therefore extend to secondary allergens. Hence, as Hjorth puts it, "sensitization to balsam of Peru results in complicated patterns of multiple sensitivities. The number and kind may vary from subject to subject." In some cases, then, diagnostic reactions are to the primary allergen, in other cases, to related materials (cross-sensitization).

Of interest to the perfume industry is the fact that fractions of Peru balsam that can be eluted with petroleum esters and benzene are rarely allergenic in patients sensitized to Peru balsam (Hjorth, 1961). Thus, highly purified Peru balsam which does not contain resin A, and is available for perfumery, is not expected to be a problem when used in cosmetics. As cosmetic injury reports received by the FDA for the fiscal year 1974 suggest that 3.1% (2.4% for 1970-1973) of the total (639) are due to fragrance preparations, some of which may contain Peru balsam and other potentially allergenic fragrance substances, it would appear that the cosmetic industry may be aware of the requirements for selecting safe perfume ingredients.

Nickel and Chromium

Two metallic substances, nickel and chromium, and compounds containing these metals are responsible for skin irritation, contact dermatitis, and cancer (Sunderman et al., 1973; Baetjer et al., 1974) in industrial workers. They are also among the most frequently encountered contact allergens for the population at large. Nickel offers opportunities for contact in the form of coins, inexpensive jewelry, and metal fastenings on clothing. It is a frequent sensitizer of women, ostensibly because of their greater contact with the metal in the home and in their dress. Sweating skin enhances solubilization of the metal, favoring skin penetration and ultimately sensitization. Hexavalent chromium in the form of dichromate is encountered by contact with tanned leather such as is used for gloves.

A selected population (skewed) of normal human volunteers known to be nonreactive to nickel was exposed experimentally by Vandenberg and Epstein (1963) to a "triple freeze" procedure (irritation, occlusion, freezing, repeated exposure) for inducing sensitization with 25% $NiCl_2$ and 0.1% SLS. On challenge with 5% $NiCl_2$ (nonoccluded), 9% (16 of 172) of the subjects were sensitized. As the latent period in nickel sensitivity appears to be quite long, it was decided to reexpose some of the nonreactors to the triple freeze induction procedure. When the procedure was carried out a second time, 26% (5 of 19) of this group were sensitized. The authors concluded that nickel is slow to sensitize; the rate of sensitization can be raised by prolonged exposure. It is of interest, however, that nickel hypersensitivity induced by this technique did not result in clinical disease in these subjects in skin sites making contact with identification bracelets or watch bands.

Kligman (1966) used his "maximization" procedure to test for the skin sensitization potential of nickel sulfate on healthy subjects, 90% of whom were black. Here, SLS was used both at induction and at challenge, posing greater opportunities for absorption of nickel at the test site. Ten percent nickel sulfate was used at induction and 2.5% at challenge (Kligman, 1966a). Kligman reported that 48% (12 of 25) of the subjects were sensitized, and classified nickel as a "grade 3" sensitizer. (By this technique grade 1 is called a weak sensitizer and is applied to sensitization rates of 0–8%, whereas grade 5 is an extreme sensitizer and is characterized by sensitization rates of 84% or more.)

The results of diagnostic tests (Table 1) show that nickel sulfate is the most frequently encountered sensitizer when tested with tray substances used by the NACDG or the ICDRG on clinical patients. Although the reaction rate is significantly higher in the NACDG subjects (11 vs. 6.7%), the diagnostic test findings of both these groups appear to be more closely related to the original predictive findings of Vandenberg and Epstein (1963), namely, a 9% sensitization rate. Vandenberg and Epstein were able to increase the sensitization rate to 26% by repeating the provocative procedure, and Kligman was able to further increase it to 48% by using SLS at challenge. This fact suggests that although nickel is slow to sensitize, the reaction rate first observed may be increased by further contact with the metal.

It has been reported by several groups that subjects may also lose their hypersensitivity to nickel (probably following a prolonged period of avoidance) (Morgan, 1953; TeLintum and Nater, 1973). In one such study, a persistent positive patch test to nickel sulfate was retained in only 39 of 57 nickel-positive patients after an interval of 2–15 yr (TeLintum and Nater, 1973).

Chromium eczema is one of the most frequently encountered occupational dermatoses; it involves workers in a wide variety of trades. These include industries in which there is frequent contact with chemicals, leather, metal, paint, cement, paper pulp, timber, building materials, and various household articles such as detergents and glue.

A review of our present knowledge of skin hypersensitivity to chromium and its compounds is given in an article by Polak et al. (1973).

Although chromium has been much studied clinically and in basic human and animal experiments, there is little published information regarding its capacity to sensitize normal human subjects. Using the maximization procedure, Kligman (1966a) obtained sensitization rates of 48% (11 of 23) with chromium sulfate and 56% (13 of 23) with chromium trioxide, in predictive tests on healthy subjects. These rates are significantly higher than the 8% incidence of skin reactions reported for clinical patients diagnostically tested by the NACDG (Table 1). These diagnostic findings, as related to the predictive findings, may be at variance with one another for the same reasons as those given for nickel.

Mercury

Mercurials are widely used in inorganic form (mercuric salts and ammoniated mercury) for the topical treatment of skin diseases, disinfection, and a variety of industrial uses. Organic forms of mercurials (phenylmercuric salts and thimerosal, also called Merthiolate, which is sodium ethylmercurithiosalicylate) are used as antiseptics and preservatives.

Many complicating factors may contribute to a proper interpretation of mercury sensitivity. When mercuric chloride is used for elicitation, skin irritation is a strong possibility; when thimerosal is used, the possibility arises that some component (thiosalicylic acid) other than mercury may be responsible (Ellis, 1947; Ellis and Robinson, 1942; Gaul, 1958). Hansson and Moller (1970) suggest that young skin may react differently from old skin to thimerosal; in addition, this compound may have a peculiar predilection to produce false positive responses. Epstein (1974) recommends that in equivocal situations, one must repeat testing, employ various dilutions and usage tests, and use ammoniated mercury for elicitation in order to establish sensitivity to mercury.

Phenylmercuric acetate (PMA) was tested in healthy subjects for skin sensitization potential by Marzulli and Maibach (1973). There was a 2% incidence (1 of 56) of sensitization reactions in a small test panel using 0.125% PMA for induction and 0.01% for challenge (modified Draize test). A 0.01% concentration of PMA was considered to be nonirritating, whereas a 0.05% concentration was irritating to skin.

Anti-infective skin preparations of ammoniated mercury normally do not exceed 5% concentration. In tests by Kligman (1966) using the maximization procedure (25% ammoniated mercury at induction and 10% at challenge) a 59% incidence (44 of 74) of skin reaction was obtained in healthy subjects.

By this technique, ammoniated mercury would be characterized as a moderate (grade 3) sensitizer. In diagnostic testing of dermatologic patients, using 1% ammoniated mercury, the NACDG obtained a sensitization index of 5% (Table 1).

Clearly, additional predictive work is needed to provide a more precise interpretation of the sensitization potential of various mercurials in healthy subjects. One cannot overstress the importance of avoiding skin irritation effects with mercurials of any type in such studies.

Neomycin

Neomycin sulfate is a well-known broad-spectrum topical antibiotic of the aminoglycoside family produced from cultures of *Streptomyces fradiae*. It is used for superficial skin infections due to staphylococci and many gram-negative bacteria. When first introduced for these purposes, it produced only rare skin reactions. Widespread, continued use in both prescription and nonprescription ointments in many European communities and the United States resulted in a dramatic rise in the rate of neomycin-related skin reactions (Pirilä and Rouhunkoski, 1959). Sensitivity to neomycin is often accompanied by sensitivity to related compounds (kanamycin, paromomycin, and framycetin) and to unrelated compounds (bacitracin) (Pirilä and Rouhunkoski, 1959, 1962). Whether these are cross-reactions or concomitant sensitization is not entirely clear (Schorr et al., 1973). Neomycin represents a type of substance whose proclivity to sensitize is easily missed. This may be chiefly because it is a poor penetrant of intact skin. Sensitized individuals may show a skin reaction when tested by intradermal injection while at the same time they are patch test negative (Schorr et al., 1973).

Repeated use, especially on broken skin, may be required to produce skin hypersensitivity. Calnan and Sarkany (1958) recognized this early, yet did not recommend the use of SLS and other substances which might enhance absorption for patch testing because of the possibility of producing false positive reactions.

Marzulli et al. (1968) reported provocative patch tests with neomycin on healthy subjects. Results showed a relatively low incidence of skin sensitization (1.6% or 3 of 186) when 5% concentration was used *at both induction and challenge*. No sensitization was induced in similar tests using 0.5% (0 of 54) and 20% (0 of 42) concentrations of neomycin. In further tests, the use of SLS at induction and at challenge increased the incidence of skin reactions. The rates of sensitization appeared to be 5.5% (3 of 54) when tested at 0.5% concentration, 2.6% (5 of 186) at 5% concentration, and 48% (12 of 25) at 20% concentration.

Kligman (1966a) reported a skin reaction incidence of 28% (7 of 25) using the maximization provocative procedure. He used 25% neomycin at induction and 10% at challenge.

The use of SLS in provocative tests with neomycin clearly increases the apparent incidence of skin sensitization reactions. In view of Calnan's warning, however, one must consider the possibility that some of these may have been false positive reactions.

Diagnostic test results on clinical patients evaluated by the NACDG show a 6% incidence of skin reactions to neomycin sulfate (Table 1), using 20% for elicitation.

The overall findings with neomycin suggest that provocative patch tests may fail to detect the proclivity of neomycin to sensitize in some instances and may overstate the incidence when SLS is used.

Thiram

Thiram (tetramethylthiuram disulfide), the methyl analogue of disulfiram, is used as an agricultural fungicide and insecticide for turf and seed treatment. Thiram and disulfiram (tetraethylthiuram disulfide) are also used as accelerators in the rubber industry. Disulfiram has also had limited use as a drug (Antabuse).

Workers in the rubber industry sometimes become sensitized to thiram. In addition, dermatitis has been reported from rubber in wearing apparel and in shoes (Blank and Miller, 1952; Gaul, 1957).

Predictive tests with guinea pigs show that thiram has the capacity to produce skin sensitization in this species (D. Hood, personal communication). Kligman (1966a) found that 16% of a normal test population (4 of 25) became sensitized to thiram when subjected to standard predictive procedures using 25% concentration at induction and 10% at challenge.

Around 1952, thiram was incorporated at about 0.5% concentration in a germicidal soap. Blank (1956) patch-tested six subjects known to be sensitive to thiram with an 8% solution of this soap. As all six reacted to the soap preparation, he notified the manufacturers that persons with rubber-related thiram allergy might develop dermatitis from using this soap. He suggested that the manufacturers monitor this carefully. They did and later reported that consumer complaints from thiram antiseptic soap (1 in 2,000,000 bars sold) were no different in numbers from those received when their more traditional antiseptic soap (cresylic acid) was previously marketed. The manufacturers claimed that they eventually withdrew thiram soap from the market for reasons unrelated to skin sensitization reactions.

These conclusions regarding the lack of adverse effects of thiram when incorporated into soap appear to be somewhat at variance with findings reported by Baer and Rosenthal (1954). These investigators found that 1 in 309 dermatologic patients who used soap containing 1% thiram developed a skin hypersensitivity to the product. Seven other subjects had to discontinue using it because of other adverse effects. The concentration of thiram in these soap studies was higher than that reported above.

Diagnostic tests conducted on dermatologic patients by the NACDG (Rudner et al., 1973), using 2% concentration for elicitation, showed that 4% of the test population reacted to thiram. The rather high incidence of skin reactions to thiram by dermatologic patients in the NACDG test indicates both the ubiquitous nature of this substance and its capacity to produce skin sensitization in significant numbers of persons who come into contact with it.

On the basis of the overall findings, one must conclude that predictive tests accurately foretell the fact that thiram is a contact sensitizer.

Benzocaine

Benzocaine (ethyl aminobenzoate), the ethyl ester of *p*-aminobenzoic acid, is a procaine-like surface anesthetic with only slight water solubility. It is often used at 2–5% concentration in topical antipruritic dermatologic ointments and creams, for superficial burns, and at 20% concentration for sunburn. Its use for these conditions is questionable in view of the risk of producing dermatitis from this and a host of related materials such as hair dyes with *p*-phenylenediamine, fabrics treated with azo dyes, sulfonamide-type drugs, and *p*-aminobenzoic acid-type sunscreens (Wilson, 1966).

In predictive tests on healthy subjects, using the modified Draize procedure, Marzulli and Maibach (1974b) reported that benzocaine produced a 6% incidence (6 of 99), in skin sensitization, using 20% concentration at induction and 10% at challenge. Kligman obtained a 22% incidence (5 of 23) in tests on normal subjects with the SLS maximization procedure. He used 25% at induction and 10% at challenge.

Bandmann et al. (1972) called attention to the possibility of producing iatrogenic allergic contact dermatitis when dermatologists prescribe benzo-caine-containing preparations for their patients. In a study of 4,000 eczema patients in five European clinics they concluded that 14% (560 of 4,000) suffered dermatitis from applied medicaments. Benzocaine and neomycin each made up the largest share—4% in each case. Elicitation was accomplished with 5% benzocaine and 20% neomycin sulfate.

Diagnostic tests performed by the NACDG show a reaction rate of 5% (Table 1) when dermatologic patients were patch-tested with benzocaine.

Although benzocaine is known to be a significant skin sensitizer, clinical experience suggests that this potential is not likely to exceed the rate observed in dermatologic test patients.

Ethylenediamine

Ethylenediamine is a strongly alkaline solvent and emulsifier substance. It has been used in an antibiotic anti-inflammatory topical preparation (Mycolog[2]) where, although not an active ingredient, it, like benzocaine, has produced iatrogenic allergic contact dermatitis (Fisher et al., 1971). Cross reactions to chemically related substances used such as topical antihistamines may also occur (Fisher et al., 1971).

Maibach (1975) conducted predictive tests on healthy subjects, using the

---

[2] Nystatin; neomycin sulfate; gramicidintriamcinolone acetonide.

modified Draize procedure. He obtained a sensitization index of 8% (5 of 61) using 5% ethylenediamine dihydrochloride at induction and 1% at challenge.

Fisher et al. (1971), in a study of 100 patients suspected of allergic contact dermatitis from topical medications, found 18% (18 of 100) sensitive to ethylenediamine dihydrochloride (1%). Six patients who were patch test negative to Mycolog cream containing triamcinolone acetonide, neomycin sulfate, gramicidin nystatin, ethylenediamine hydrochloride, and other minor ingredients showed significant skin reactions when tested with ethylenediamine hydrochloride alone in petrolatum.

In diagnostic tests with dermatologic patients, the NACDG found that 7% of the subjects showed positive reactions. The subjects' responses were elicited with 1% ethylenediamine.

The overall findings with ethylenediamine show that this is a potent sensitizer and suggest that predictive tests by the modified Draize procedure accurately foretell this potential.

SUMMARY AND CONCLUSION

Essentially three types of tests are needed to evaluate skin sensitization potential. The predictive test is needed to identify allergenic substances; the diagnostic test is used to find out what substances may actually be producing dermatologic problems; and the use test provides information regarding safety of ingredients in a particular combination for a specific use before they enter the marketplace. Inclusion of a known sensitizer or new ingredient in a marketed product will, of course, require more frequent and more careful monitoring than is needed when commonly used substances of known sensitization potential are used.

We have reviewed in some detail skin sensitization predictive and diagnostic data on 11 compounds. These are among the most frequently encountered sensitizers to which large numbers of humans in Western Europe, the United States, and Canada are exposed in normal living. They include drugs (benzocaine and neomycin), cosmetic ingredients (*p*-phenylenediamine and Peru balsam), preservatives (formaldehyde, ethylenediamine, parabens, and mercurials), and ingredients of wearing apparel (nickel, chromium, and thiram).

Eight of these substances have been studied in dermatologic patients by the ICDRG and all 11 have been studied by the NACDG. Use of this type of subject was expected to reveal the (diagnostic) incidence of sensitization in a select population whose skin was seriously enough affected that medical assistance was sought. These individuals would therefore be expected to comprise a dermatologically vulnerable population.

The reported scientific literature contains a paucity of systematic predictive studies of skin sensitization in which a sensitization index is reported on a significant population. For the most part, reported predictive studies have been done by two methodologies, namely, the modified Draize procedure and the maximization procedure. Both methods offer some assistance in forecasting skin sensitization in humans.

The modified Draize procedure showed essentially the same incidence of sensitization potential in predictive tests conducted on a normal test population as was observed by diagnostic tests on clinical patients with four compounds, namely, benzocaine, formaldehyde, ethylenediamine, and paraben. It may have overstated the potential of *p*-phenylenediamine; nevertheless, this is indeed a potent sensitizer. On the other hand, it tended to understate the potential of neomycin.

The maximization procedure is a harsher methodology, whose main usefulness may be in providing a measure of the uppermost limits of sensitization. With a poor skin penetrant such as neomycin, it was useful.

The data for the maximization test must be viewed, like those for all other tests, with judgment. When first promulgated, a high concentration of compound (such as 25% of a single compound) and a high concentration of SLS were suggested (Kligman, 1966). Subsequently the test has frequently been used with final formulations (usually lower concentrations) and lower SLS concentrations instead (Kligman and Epstein, 1975). Data developed with the technique will be required to make an adequate comparison with the more frequently employed modified Draize techniques.

A comparison of results obtained on 21 fragrance ingredients by both the modified Draize and maximization methods was reported recently (Marzulli and Maibach, 1980). The results showed good agreement for 10 of 21 test substances. These included alantroot oil, diethyl malleate, dihydro-coumarin, balsam peru, cinnamon bark oil, ethyl acrylate, and benzilidine acetone, all potent sensitizers by both predictive methods (Table 4). Vetiver acetate appeared intermediate and methyl crotonate a low grade sensitizer by

TABLE 4   Predictive Test Results with 21 Fragrance Ingredients Tested by Both Draize and Maximization Methods

Both positive	Both negative	Positive maximization only	Positive Draize only
Alantroot oil	Bitter fennel	Dimethyl citraconate	Jasmine
Diethyl maleate			Coumarin
Dihydrocoumarin			Citronellal
Balsam peru			Geraniol
Cinnamon bark oil			Eugenol
Ethyl acrylate			Isoeugenol
Benzilidine acetone			α-amyl cinnamic
Vetiver acetate			alcohol
Methyl crotonate			Hydroxycitronellal
Costus oil			
Cinnamic aldehyde			

both methods. Bitter fennel was not considered a skin sensitizer by Draize or by recent maximization tests.

Costus oil and cinnamic aldehyde appeared significantly more potent by the maximization test. Dimethyl citraconate was a suspected low grade sensitizer by the maximization method and negative by the Draize procedure.

On the other hand, jasmine, coumarin, citronellal, geraniol, eugenol, isoeugenol, α-amyl cinnamic alcohol, and hydroxycitronellal possessed a sensitization potential by the Draize procedure, yet showed no such proclivity by the maximization test. In this series, the vehicle, test concentration, or size of test population may have been responsible for failure of the maximization procedure to detect a sensitization potential seen by the Draize method. The use of sodium lauryl sulfate (SLS) may have been required to elicit a sensitization potential in some of those cases where its absence was accompanied by a negative outcome.

REFERENCES

Baer, R. L. and Rosenthal, S. A. 1954. The germicidal action in human skin of soap containing tetramethylthiruam disulfide. *J. Invest. Dermatol.* 23:193–211.

Baetjer, A. M., Birmingham, D. J., Enterline, P. E., Mertz, W. and Pierce, J. O., II 1974. *Chromium*, pp. 1–155. Washington, D.C.: Commitee on Biological Effects of Atmospheric Pollutants, National Research Council–National Academy of Sciences.

Bandmann, H. J., Calnan, C. D., Cronin, E., Fregert, S., Hjorth, N., Magnusson, B., Maibach, H., Malten, K. E., Meneghini, C. L., Pirilä, V. and Wilkinson, D. S. 1972. Dermatitis from applied medicaments. *Arch. Dermatol.* 106:335–337.

Blank, I. H. 1956. Allergic hypersensitivity to an antiseptic soap. *J. Am. Med. Assoc.* 160:1225–1226.

Blank, I. H. and Miller, O. G. 1952. A study of rubber adhesives in shoes as the cause of dermatitis of the feet. *J. Am. Med. Assoc.* 109:1371–1374.

Calnan, C. D. and Sarkany, I. 1958. Contact dermatitis from neomycin. *Br. J. Dermatol.* 70:435–445.

Calnan, C. D., Bandmann, H. J., Cronin, E., Fregert, S., Hjorth, N., Magnusson, B., Malten, K., Meneghini, C. L., Pirilä, V. and Wilkinson, D. S. 1970. Hand dermatitis in housewives. *Br. J. Dermatol.* 82:543–548.

Cosmetic Injury Reports. FY 1974. Filed in Division of Cosmetics Technology, Bureau of Foods, Food and Drug Administration, Washington, D.C.

Draize, J. H. 1959. Dermal toxicity. In *Appraisal of the safety of chemicals in foods, drugs and cosmetics*. Austin, Texas: Association of Food and Drug Officials of the United States, Texas State Department of Health.

Draize, J. H., Woodard, G. and Calvery, H. D. 1944. Methods for the study of irritation and toxicity of substances applied topically to the skin and mucous membranes. *J. Pharmacol. Exp. Ther.* 83:377–390.

Ellis, F. A. 1947. The sensitizing factor in merthiolate. *J. Allergy* 18:212–213.

Ellis, F. A. and Robinson, H. M. 1942. Cutaneous sensitivity to merthiolate and other mercurial compounds. *Arch. Dermatol.* 46:425–430.

Epstein, E. 1974. Mercury allergy and patch testing. *Arch. Dermatol.* 109:98–99.

Epstein, E. and Maibach, H. I. 1966. Formaldehyde allergy. *Arch. Dermatol.* 94:186–190.

Epstein, W. L., Kligman, A. M. and Senecal, I. P. 1963. Role of regional lymph nodes in contact sensitization. *Arch. Dermatol.* 88:789–792.

FDA (Food and Drug Administration), Division of Cosmetics Technology/ Product Experience Branch, April 11, 1972. Subchapter D—Cosmetics, Part 170, Voluntary registration of cosmetic product establishments, part 171, voluntary filing of cosmetic product ingredients and cosmetic raw material composition statements. *Fed. Regist.* 37(70).

Fisher, A. A., Pascher, F. and Kanof, N. B. 1971. Allergic contact dermatitis due to ingredients of vehicles. *Arch. Dermatol.* 104:186–190.

Fregert, S., Hjorth, N., Magnusson, B., Bandmann, H. J., Calnan, C. D., Cronin, E., Malten, K., Meneghini, C. L., Pirilä, V. and Wilkinson, D. S. 1969. Epidemiology of contact dermatitis. *Trans. St. John's Hosp. Dermatol. Soc.* 55:17–35.

Gaul, L. E. 1957. Results of patch testing with rubber anti-oxidants and accelerators. *J. Invest. Dermatol.* 29:105–110.

Gaul, L. E. 1958. Sensitizing component in thiosalicylic acid. *J. Invest. Dermatol.* 31:91–92.

Giovacchini, R. P. October 1972. Old and new issues in the safety evaluation of cosmetics and toiletries. *CRC Crit. Rev. Toxicol.* 361–378.

Hansson, H. and Moller, H. 1970. Patch test reactions to merthiolate in healthy young subjects. *Br. J. Dermatol.* 83:349–356.

Hardy, J. 1973. Allergy, hypersensitivity and cosmetics. *J. Soc. Cosmet. Chem.* 24:423–468.

Henderson, C. R. and Riley, E. C. 1945. Certain statistical considerations in patch testing. *J. Invest. Dermatol.* 6:227–232.

HEW (Department of Health, Education, and Welfare) June 1975. Investigation of consumer's perceptions of adverse reactions to consumer products. Contracted to Westat, Inc., Rockville, Maryland. Contract No. 223738052. Rockville, Maryland: Consumer Safety Statistics Staff, Office of Planning and Evaluation, Office of the Commissioner, Food and Drug Administration.

Hjorth, N. 1961. Eczematous allergy to balsam, allied perfumes and flavoring agents, with special reference to Balsam of Peru. *Acta Derm. Venereol. (Stockh.)* 41(Suppl. 46):6–216.

Kligman, A. M. 1966a. The identification of contact allergens by human assay. III. The maximization test. A procedure for screening and rating contact sensitizers. *J. Invest. Dermatol.* 47:393–409.

Kligman, A. M. 1966b. The SLS provocative patch test in allergic contact sensitization. *J. Invest. Dermatol.* 46:573–585.

Kligman, A. M. and Epstein, W. 1975. Updating the maximization test for identifying contact allergens. *Contact Dermatitis* 1:231–239.

Magnusson, B. and Hersle, K. 1965. Patch test methods. *Acta Derm. Venereol. (Stockh.)* 45:123–128.

Magnusson, B., Blohm, S., Fregert, S., Hjorth, N., Havding, G., Pirilä, V. and Skog, E. 1962. Standardization of routine patch testing. Proceedings of the Northern Dermatologic Society of Gothenburg, *Acta Derm. Venereol. (Stockh.)* 126–127.

Magnusson, B., Blohm, S. G., Fregert, S., Hjorth, N., Havding, G., Pirilä, V.

and Skog, E. 1968. Routine patch testing. IV. *Acta Derm. Venereol. (Stockh.)* 48:110–114.

Maibach, H. I. 1975. Report 105 under Contract FDA 223-75-2340. *Skin sensitization.*

Marzulli, F. N. and Maibach, H. I. 1973. Antimicrobials: Experimental contact sensitization in man. *J. Soc. Cosmet. Chem.* 24:399–421.

Marzulli, F. N. and Maibach, H. I. 1974a. Status of topical parabens: Skin hypersensitivity. *Int. J. Dermatol.* 13:397–399.

Marzulli, F. N. and Maibach, H. I. 1974b. The use of graded concentrations in studying skin sensitizers: Experimental contact sensitization in man. *Food Cosmet. Toxicol.* 12:219–227.

Marzulli, F. N. and Maibach, H. I. 1980. Contact allergy: Predictive testing of fragrance ingredients in humans by Draize and maximization methods. *J. Environ. Path. Toxicol.* 3:235–245.

Marzulli, F., Carson, T. and Maibach, H. 1968. Delayed contact hypersensitivity studies in man and animals. *Proceedings of a joint conference on cosmetic sciences.* Washington, D.C., April 21–23, pp. 107–122.

Morgan, J. K. 1953. Observations on the persistance of skin sensitivity with reference to nickel eczema. *Br. J. Dermatol.* 65:84–94.

Opdyke, D. L. J. 1974. Monographs on fragrance raw materials. *Food Cosmet. Toxicol.* 12:807–1016.

Pirilä, V. and Rouhunkoski, S. 1959. On sensitivity to neomycin and bacitracin. *Acta Derm. Venereol. (Stockh.)* 39:470–476.

Pirilä, V. and Rouhunkoski, S. 1962. The patterns of cross-sensitivity to neomycin. *Dermatologica* 125:273–278.

Polak, L., Turk, J. L. and Frey, J. R. 1973. Studies on contact hypersensitivity to chromium compounds. *Progr. Allergy* 17:145–226.

Rostenberg, A., Jr. and Sulzberger, M. B. 1937. Some results of patch tests. *Arch. Dermatol. Syphilol.* 35:433–455.

Rudner, E. J., Clendenning, W. E., Epstein, E., Fisher, A. A., Jillson, O. F., Jordan, W. P., Kanof, N., Larsen, W., Maibach, H., Mitchell, J. C., O'Quinn, S. E., Schorr, W. F. and Sulzberger, M. B. 1973. Epidemiology of contact dermatitis in North America. *Arch. Dermatol.* 108:537–540.

Schwartz, L. 1941. Dermatitis from new synthetic resin fabric finishes. *J. Invest. Dermatol.* 4:459–470.

Schwartz, L. 1951. The skin testing of new cosmetics. *J. Soc. Cosmet. Chem.* 2:321–324.

Schwartz, L. 1960. Twenty-two years experience in the performance of 200,000 prophetic-patch tests. *South. Med. J.* 53:478–483.

Schwartz, L. and Peck, S. M. 1944. The patch test in contact dermatitis. *Publ. Health Rep.* 59:546–557.

Shelanski, H. A. 1951. Experience with and considerations of the human patch test method. *J. Soc. Cosmet. Chem.* 2:324–331.

Shelanski, H. A. and Shelanski, M. V. 1953. A new technique of human patch tests. *Proc. Sci. Sect. Toilet Goods Assoc.* 19:46–49.

Schorr, W. F. 1968. Paraben allergy: A cause of intractable dermatitis. *J. Am. Med. Assoc.* 204:107–110.

Schorr, W. F., Wenzel, F. J. and Hegedus, S. I. 1973. Cross-sensitivity and aminoglycoside antibiotics. *Arch. Dermatol.* 107:533–539.

Spier, H. W. and Sixt, I. 1955. Untersuchungen über die Abhängigkeit des Ausfalles der Ekzem Lappchenpraben von der Hornschichtdicke. *Hautarzt* 6:152–159.

Sunderman, F. W., Jr. 1973. The current status of nickel carcinogenesis. *Ann. Clin. Lab. Sci.* 3:156–180.

TeLintum, J. C. A. and Nater, J. P. 1973. On the persistence of positive patch test reactions to Balsam of Peru, turpentine and nickel. *Br. J. Dermatol.* 89:629–634.

Vandenberg, J. J. and Epstein, W. L. 1963. Experimental nickel contact sensitization in man. *J. Invest. Dermatol.* 41:413–418.

Wilson, H. 1966. Dermatitis from anesthetic ointments. *Practitioner* 197:673–677.

14

the contact urticaria
syndrome

Geo von Krogh ■ Howard I. Maibach

INTRODUCTION

Contact urticaria describes a wheal-and-flare response elicited within 30 to 60 min after cutaneous exposure to certain agents. Delayed-onset contact urticaria (up to 4–6 h) (Calnan, 1982) is of unknown frequency and should be sought; the mechanism for the delay may be slower percutaneous penetration.

The number of recent publications on verified contact urticaria indicates a higher incidence than was previously suggested and justifies the term "contact urticaria syndrome" for a disease entity with a broad spectrum of clinical manifestations (Maibach and Johnson, 1975). The diagnosis may easily be missed; this chapter summarizes current clinical experience and presents a rational approach to diagnostic and pathogenetic evaluation when suspected cases are encountered.

In reproducing contact urticaria in the laboratory (i.e., the equivalent of the patch test for delayed hypersensitivity), observation of the wheal and flare is greatly simplified by application to normal (or only slightly damaged) skin. Moderately or markedly inflamed skin does not permit observation or quantification of additional erythema, unless it is extreme. Patients applying contact urticants to already damaged skin note the equivalent of subjective irritation (burning, stinging, and itching) but not a marked visible change.

Certain types of physical urticaria, strictly representing subgroups of contact urticaria, are not included in this review.

Reprinted with permission from the *Journal of the American Academy of Dermatology.*

ETIOLOGY

Table 1 is an updated list of agents that elicit contact urticaria. It includes an impressive number of chemicals in medicaments, industrial contactants, cosmetic products, foods, and drinks, and many chemically undefined environmental agents. While the role of ingested food in exacerbating

TABLE 1   Agents Producing Contact Urticaria[a]

Agent	Reference
	Chemically defined agents
Acrylic monomer	Key, 1961
Aliphatic polyamines	Key, 1961
Aminophenazone	Camarasa et al., 1978
Aminothiazole	Key, 1961
Ammonia	Key, 1961
Ammonium persulfate	Calnan and Shuster, 1963; Brubaker, 1972; Fisher and Dooms-Goossens, 1976; Widstrøm, 1977
Bacitracin	Comaish and Cunliffe, 1967
Balsam of Peru	Friis and Hjorth, 1973; Rudzki and Grzywa, 1976; Forsbeck and Skog, 1977; Von Temesvári et al., 1978, 1979
Benzaldehyde	Forsbeck and Skog, 1977
Benzoic acid	Forsbeck and Skog, 1977; Von Temesvári et al., 1978; Kirton, 1978
Benzophenone	Ramsey et al., 1972
Camphor	Von Temesvári et al., 1978
CaOCl$_2$	Neering, 1977
Cassia oil	Rudzki and Grzywa, 1976; Rietschel, 1978
Cephalosporin	Tuft, 1975
Chloramphenicol	Kosáková, 1977
Chlorpromazin	Odom and Maibach, 1976
Cetyl alcohol	Gaul, 1969
Cinnamic acid	Forsbeck and Skog, 1977
Cinnamic aldehyde	Rudski and Grzywa, 1976; Forsbeck and Skog, 1977; Kirton, 1978; Nater et al., 1977
Clioquinol	Von Liebe et al., 1979
Cobalt chloride	Smith et al., 1975
Diethyl toluamide	Maibach and Johnson, 1975
Dimethyl sulfoxide	Odom and Maibach, 1976
Epoxy resin	Woyton et al., 1974
Ethylaminobenzoate	Ryan et al., 1980
Formaldehyde	Key, 1961; Helander, 1977; McDaniel and Marks, 1979
Lanolin	Von Liebe et al., 1979
Lindane	Key, 1961
Mechlorethamine	Daughters et al., 1973
Monoamylamine	Tharp, 1973
NaOCl	Neering, 1977
p-Aminodiphenylamine	Von Liebe et al., 1979
Paraben (ethyl, methyl)	Henry et al., 1979

(See footnote on p. 303.)

TABLE 1 Agents Producing Contact Urticaria[a] (*Continued*)

Agent	Reference
Penicillin	Maucher, 1972
Phenylmercuric proprionate	Mathews, 1968
Platinum salts	Key, 1961
Polyethylene glycol 3–400	Fisher, 1978
Polysorbate	Maibach and Conant, 1977
Salicylic acid	Odom and Maibach, 1976
Sodium sulfide	Key, 1961
Sorbic acid	Rietschel, 1978
Stearyl alcohol	Gaul, 1969
Streptomycin	Odom and Maibach, 1976
Sulfur dioxide	Key, 1961
Vanillin	Von Temesvári et al., 1978

Chemically undefined agents

Agent	Reference
Animals:	
Arthropods	Odom and Maibach, 1976; Zschunke, 1978
Danders	Odom and Maibach, 1976
Hair (rat-tail)	Rudzki and Grzywa, 1976
Marine animals	Odom and Maibach, 1976
Serum (horse, tetanus)	Odom and Maibach, 1976
Saliva (cat, dog)	Odom and Maibach, 1976
Cosmetics:	
Nail polish	Odom and Maibach, 1976
Hair spray	Odom and Maibach, 1976
Perfumes	Odom and Maibach, 1976; Rothenborg et al., 1977
Foods:	
Chicken	Hjorth and Roed-Petersen, 1976
Egg	Von Temesvári et al., 1979
Flour	Maibach, 1976
Fruits	Andersen and Løwenstein, 1978; Hannuksela and Lahti, 1977
Lamb	Maibach, 1976
Lettuce/endive	Krook, 1977
Seafood	Hjorth and Roed-Petersen, 1976
Spices	Von Temesvári et al., 1978; Hjorth and Roed-Petersen, 1976
Turkey	Maibach, 1976
Vegetables	Hjorth and Roed-Petersen, 1976
Plants:	Odom and Maibach, 1976
Cactus	
Nettles	
Marine plants	
Rhus	
Textiles:	
Wool	Rudzki and Grzywa, 1976
Silk	Rudzki and Grzywa, 1976
Rubber	Nutter, 1979
Wood:	
Exotic woods	Key, 1961; Schmidt, 1978

[a]Modified from Odom and Maibach (1976) and updated according to Table 2.

eczema is often questioned by dermatologists, it is of interest to note the increasing evidence that ingredients of barley, meat, eggs, vegetables, and spices may penetrate intact skin, evoking urticarial responses. As will be further discussed, externally applied food components may also maintain a status eczematicus.

CLASSIFICATION/PATHOGENESIS

On the basis of pathogenetic mechanisms, contact urticaria is divided into three major groups (Maibach and Johnson, 1975; Odom and Maibach, 1976).

Type A: Nonimmunologic Mechanisms

A wide variety of chemical compounds release histamine and other vasoactive substances to the skin without involving immunologic processes (Monroe and Jones, 1977). These include biogenic polymers released from certain plants (nettles) and animals (caterpillars, jellyfish) and some medications—for example, cinnamic aldehyde (Mathias et al., 1980), thurfyl nicotinate (Trafuril), compound 48/80, and dimethyl sulfoxide (DMSO) (Odom and Maibach, 1976).

Type B: Immunologic Mechanisms

Contact urticaria due to hypersensitivity was long considered a rare phenomenon. From available publications and unpublished cases reported by colleagues, Maibach and Johnson (1975) collected a diverse list of possible etiologic agents strongly suspected of eliciting contact urticaria of an immediate hypersensitivity type. To shed further light on this subject, suggestions for future evaluation of pathogenetic mechanisms were given (Odom and Maibach, 1976).

Unfortunately, in many subsequent reports the evaluation is incomplete. Table 2 lists 86 patients who were previously not comprehensively reviewed. Indications of immunologic mechanisms exist in 10 of these cases (12%). However, when the remaining 76 patients were exposed to the provoking agent(s), symptoms with a possible allergic background were evoked in other organs in 17 (22%) by history and 7 (9%) by the skin test(s). It is likely that if detailed methods for pathogenetic evaluation are followed, future studies will disclose an increasing number of chemicals responsible for immunologic contact urticaria.

Type C: Uncertain Mechanism

This classification is reserved for contact urticaria elicited by chemicals for which neither an immune nor a direct action can be proved. Ammonium persulfate, used in hair bleaches, is the classic example. It has been responsible for wheal-and-flare reactions at the site of application, generalized urticaria,

TABLE 2 Investigative Information on 86 Patients with Contact Urticaria Previously Not Comprehensively Reviewed[a]

Reference	Substance	Pure chemical	No. of cases	History Dermal	History Extra-dermal	Test response Immediate Open	Test response Immediate Patch	Test response Immediate ID	Test response Delayed	Test response Control	Classification
Camarasa et al., 1978	Cibalgine	Aminophenazone	1	GU			Pos			–	ND
Fisher, 1978	Lotrimin Tinactin	Polyethylene glycol 400	1	D		Pos			Neg	Neg	ND
	Americaine Otic	Polyethylene glycol 300	1	D		Pos			Neg	Neg	ND
Forsbeck and Skog, 1977	Balsam of Peru	Cinnamic acid/aldehyde	16	GU			Pos		Neg	Neg	Uncertain
		Benzoic acid	9	D							
		Benzaldehyde									
Fisher and Dooms-Goossens, 1976	Hair bleach	Ammonium persulfate	1	GU		Pos			Neg	Neg	ND
Helander, 1977	Leather	Formaldehyde	1	LU			Pos + GU		Neg	–	ND
Henry et al., 1979	Cosmetic products	Ethyl- or methyl paraben	1	LU		Pos			Neg	–	Immunol
Hjorth and Roed-Petersen, 1976	Seafood, chicken, vegetables, spices	?	9	D		Pos 3/9	Pos 6/9	Pos 9/9	Pos 6/9	–	Immunol
Kosáková, 1977	Chloramphenicol ointment	Chloramphenicol?	1	D			Pos + GU/AR			–	ND
Kirton, 1978	Cinnamon cake	Cinnamic aldehyde	1	GU			Pos		Pos	–	ND
	Cosmetic products	Cinnamic aldehyde + benzoic acid	1	*			Pos		Neg	–	ND
Krook, 1977	Lettuce/endive	?	2	D	OL	Pos	Pos	Pos 1/2	Pos	Neg	ND

(See footnote on p. 307.)

305

TABLE 2 Investigative Information on 86 Patients with Contact Urticaria Previously Not Comprehensively Reviewed[a] (Continued)

Reference	Substance	Pure chemical	No. of cases	History Dermal	History Extra-dermal	Immediate Open	Immediate Patch	Immediate ID	Delayed	Control	Classification
Von Liebe et al., 1979	Permanent hair products	p-Aminodiphenylamine Lanolin Clioquinol	1	GU		Pos			Pos / Neg	Neg	ND
Maibach, 1976	Lamb, turkey, flour	?	1	D		Pos		Pos	Neg	Neg	ND
Maibach and Conant, 1977	Cream	Polysorbate	1	D		Pos			Neg	–	ND
Mathias et al., 1980	Mouthwash	Cinnamic aldehyde	1	*		Pos			–	Pos	Nonimmunol
McDaniel and Marks, 1979	Starch	Formaldehyde Terpinyl acetate	1	GU		Pos			Neg	Neg	ND
Nater et al., 1977	No data	Cinnamic aldehyde	1	D		Pos			Neg	Neg	ND
Neering, 1977	Chlorinated water Cleansing powder	NaOCl CaOCl₂	1	GU		Neg	Pos + GU		Neg	Neg	ND
Nutter, 1979	Rubber	Hevea braziliensis latex	1	*		Pos		Pos	Pos	Neg	ND
Rietschel, 1978	Toothpaste, detergent	Cassia oil + sorbic acid	1	LU		Pos	Pos		Neg	Neg	ND
Rothenborg et al., 1977	Detergent	Terpenes de limette, de citron, et d'oranges; Citrufix	12	D		Pos	Pos		Pos	–	ND
Rudzki and Grzywa, 1976	Rat-tail hair	?	1	LU		Pos					
	Silk		1	GU		Pos					
	Knit fibers		1	LU		Pos					
	Egg white		2	GU	GI	Pos					
	Chocolate	Balsam of Peru	1	D	BA	Pos	Pos		Neg		
		Cinnamic aldehyde	1	D		Pos	Pos		Neg		
	Shaving cream	Cinnamic aldehyde	1	D		Pos			Pos		
Ryan et al., 1980	Benzocaine gel	Ethyl aminobenzoate	1	LU		Pos			Pos	–	Nonimmunol

306

Reference	Source	Allergen	n						
Schmidt, 1978	Teak	?	1	*	GI	Pos + GU/GI	Pos	–	ND
Von Temesvári et al., 1978	Foods	Balsam of Peru	1	GU		Pos			
	Drinks	Balsam of Peru	1	GU		Pos			
	Detergents	Balsam of Peru + cinnamon oil	1	GU	GI	Pos			
	Cosmetics	Balsam of Peru + cinnamon oil + vanillin + benzoic acid	1	GU + D	AR	Pos + OL/GI		Neg for Balsam of Peru	ND
		Balsam of Peru + cinnamon oil + camphor			GI	Pos			
		Balsam of Peru	1	LU	GI	Pos + GU/GI			
		Capsicum	1	GU	AR/GI	Pos + GU/GI			
		Vanillin							
Von Temesvári et al., 1979	Eggs	?	1	GU	BA/GI	Pos + GU/BA/AR	Pos + GU/BA/AR	Neg	ND
	Cosmetics	Balsam of Peru							
Rietschel, 1978	Cephalosporins		1	LU	BA + RC	Pos + RC		–	ND
Widstrom, 1977	Hair bleach	Ammonium persulfate	1	D	RC	Pos + GU	Pos	–	ND
Woyton et al., 1974	Epoxy resin	Epidian 1-5, Araldit, Epoxide 201, ERL 4221	1	D		Pos + GU/BA	Pos	–	ND
Zschunke, 1978	Cockroaches	?	4	GU + D	BA + RC	Pos		Neg	ND
Total			86			25	80	33	

[a] Abbreviations: LU, localized urticaria; GU, generalized urticaria; D, dermatitis/dermatosis; (*), uncharacteristic cutaneous symptoms (itching, tingling, burning, "intolerance," etc.); BA, bronchial asthma; RC, rhinoconjunctivitis; OL, orolaryngeal dysfunction; GI, gastrointestinal dysfunction; AR, anaphylactoid reaction; Pos, positive immediate test response; Neg, negative cutaneous test response; ND, not determined; Immunol, immunologic; and Nonimmunol, nonimmunologic.

and even vascular collapse. Although this chemical probably acts through histamine release, it is not known whether liberation is effectuated immunologically or through direct action on the mast cells. The fact that some individuals react on the first exposure and the negative outcome of passive transfer attempts favor a nonimmunologic mechanism, while the negative results obtained in tests with controls disagree with the concept of direct histamine release (Calnan and Shuster, 1963; Brubaker, 1972).

STAGING THROUGH SYMPTOMATOLOGY

Clinical Heterogeneity

Previous reviews (Maibach and Johnson, 1975; Odom and Maibach, 1976) emphasized the heterogeneity of clinical manifestations in contact urticaria, varying from localized or generalized urticaria to concurrent involvement of other organs. This allowed a tentative staging of the syndrome: stage 1, wheal-and-flare response restricted to the area of contact (localized urticaria, LU); stage 2, generalized urticaria (GU) including angioedema; stage 3, urticaria combined with bronchial asthma (BA); and stage 4, urticaria combined with anaphylactoid reactions (AR). Subsequent experience indicates that an even broader spectrum of symptomatology exists.

Extracutaneous Manifestations

As shown in Table 2, extracutaneous symptoms may include rhino-conjunctivitis (RC) and orolaryngeal (OL) or gastrointestinal (GI) dysfunctions. The convenient four-step staging remains rational, but should be updated according to the list of clinical phenomena in Table 3; this summarizes the distribution of symptoms presented historically or evoked by diagnostic skin tests in the patients reviewed in Table 2.

TABLE 3 Contact Urticaria Syndrome: Distribution of Symptoms in 86 Patients

Stage	Description	History	Skin test
	Cutaneous reactions only		
1	Localized urticaria (LU)	8	80
	Dermatitis/dermatosis (D)	48	0
	Nonspecific symptoms (itching, tingling, burning, etc.)	4	0
2	Generalized urticaria (GU)	35	8
	Extracutaneous reactions		
3	Bronchial asthma (BA)	7	2
	Rhinoconjunctivitis (RC)	6	1
	Orolaryngeal (OL)	2	1
	Gastrointestinal (GI)	7	3
4	Anaphylactoid reactions (AR)	2	2

Fifteen percent had a history indicating simultaneously occurring non-dermatologic symptoms when they were exposed to the suspected agent. Rhinoconjunctivitis and GI dysfunctions were as frequent as respiratory effects. Historically, anaphylactoid reactions were triggered in one case by dermal contact with paprika (*Capsicum*) and in another by ingestion of vanilla, cinnamon, and benzoic acid (Temesvári et al., 1978).

Cutaneous Manifestations

Only 9% of the patients in Table 2 reported a history of typical localized wheal-and-flare reactions. Generalized urticaria was considerably more frequent, being reported in one-third of the cases. Dermal manifestations also included nonurticarial phenomena; half of the patients presented with dermatitis. Nonspecific sensations such as itching, tingling, and burning also occurred. In three cases described by Forsbeck and Skog (1977), contact urticaria was unexpectedly diagnosed in individuals with psoriasis, erysipelas, or drug reaction, respectively.

We do not imply that tabulations based on the literature provide a realistic assessment of the epidemiology. Undoubtedly, the mundane non-immunologic forms ("nettle rash," reactions to certain insects, DMSO, and thurfyl nicotinate) must be common, yet not often the subject of derma-tology or allergy publications. Obscure chemical causes will probably pre-dominate in future publications. In spite of their current obscurity, any of the three mechanisms may be involved.

SKIN TESTING

Epidermal Tests

When diagnostically tested, 10% of 86 patients reacted with widespread urticaria and 9% with extradermal symptoms (Tables 2 and 3). The incidence of systemic reactions triggered by the tests was lower than indicated his-torically, presumably because a smaller quantity was used in the test situation. Thus, 12 of 82 patients (15%) who reacted exclusively cutaneously when challenged had a positive history of reactions in other organs as well.

Anaphylactoid responses. Anaphylactoid responses to the small amount of material used in skin testing have been documented in at least nine instances (Table 4). Note that such a response may occur even with open testing on normal skin (Daughters et al., 1973). A risk of unpredictable test reactions must always be kept in mind, as a highly sensitized individual may react fatally when antigens are rapidly absorbed.

Diagnostic tests should therefore be performed where resuscitation equipment and personnel are available for immediate response to anaphy-lactoid reactions. Even if most patients who react with extradermal symptoms after epidermal diagnostic tests had a positive history of similar

TABLE 4   Documented Cases of Anaphylactoid Reactions to Cutaneously Tested Agents

Reference	Agent	Testing method
Comaish and Cunliffe, 1967	Bacitracin	Intradermal injection
Levene and Withers, 1969	Streptomycin	Intradermal injection
Maucher, 1972	Penicillin	Epidermal occlusive
Daughters et al., 1973	Mechlorethamine	Epidermal open
Woyton et al., 1974	Epoxy resin	Epidermal occlusive
Maibach, 1982	Neomycin	Epidermal occlusive
Kosáková, 1977	Chloramphenicol	Epidermal occlusive
Camarasa et al., 1978	Aminophenazone	Epidermal occlusive
Von Temesvári et al., 1979	Egg	Intradermal scarification
	Peru balsam	Epidermal occlusive

reactions, it is deluding oneself to believe that historical data are reliable predictors of test responses. In Table 5 the cutaneous and systemic test responses evoked in the 86 patients in Table 2 are correlated with test procedures. From a diagnostic viewpoint, the occlusive patch test is apparently reliable and was used most frequently by the investigators. The open challenge was negative in 7 of 35 cases (20%). While the latter procedure seldom evokes extracutaneous reactions, occlusive patch testing was followed by such responses in 7 of 69 cases (10%). Open application is apparently safer and is therefore recommended for the first test.

INTRADERMAL TESTS: RELEVANCE

Although the apparent risk associated with intradermal tests, as presently known, may not be greater than that with closed epidermal tests (Table 5), we remain concerned about anaphylactoid responses. Penicillin skin

TABLE 5   Contact Urticaria Syndrome: Test Response Correlated
to Test Procedure in 86 Patients

			Test response		
			Positive (115)		
			Cutaneous		
Test procedure	n	Negative (11)	Test site only	Generalized	Systemic
Epidermal					
Open	35	7	28	0	0
Occlusive	69	3	56	8	7
Intradermal	16	1	14	1	1
Total	120	11	98	9	8

testing is not necessarily directly analogous to the contact urticaria syndrome; penicillin allergy represents a complex syndrome in itself. Nevertheless, anaphylactic responses are far more common with the intradermal injection method than with the prick test. We believe great care is indicated when using intradermal tests in the contact urticaria syndrome, until extensive clinical experience indicates the contrary.

Even if the results from topical and intradermal test procedures frequently agree, a positive intradermal test by itself is not diagnostic of contact urticaria. Recent publications show numerous cases where contact urticaria syndrome is probably the correct diagnosis, but it is not proved because intradermal exposure to the suspected agent was the only cutaneous diagnostic approach (Grunnet, 1976; Cronin, 1979; Powell and Smith, 1978; Noyes et al., 1979; Praehl and Roed-Petersen, 1979).

The reasons for this are twofold: presumably most cases are elicited naturally by topical contact rather than by injection, and many chemicals intradermally injected in normal individuals produce a nonspecific wheal-and-flare. On the other hand, we emphasize that there are clinical situations where intradermal introduction of the suspected agent may be the only way to demonstrate a cutaneous hyperreactivity mediated by immediate mechanisms. This seems to be a frequent phenomenon when the sensitivity is due to high-molecular-weight food proteins. How, then, do we discriminate between a relevant and a nonrelevant response? In the immunologic type this may be settled when the patient responds vigorously to the intradermal test and a large control population does not. In the nonimmunologic type the discrimination is more difficult.

Protein contact dermatitis. The term "protein contact dermatitis" was introduced by Hjorth and Roed-Petersen (1976) in relation to patients with recurrent eczema who demonstrate immediate reactions when affected skin is exposed to certain types of food. Often these individuals repeatedly encounter certain types of animal or plant proteins for a protracted time, for example, through occupational handling. Within 10–30 min after the proteins come in contact with affected skin, usually the hands, the patients frequently experience aggravation of symptoms with a broad range of severity: from itching of various degrees of intensity to erythema, urticarial swelling, and in some cases prompt development of dyshidrotic vesicles.

Only 6 of 33 food handlers with recurrent hand dermatitis, reported by Hjorth and Roed-Petersen (1976), exhibited delayed hypersensitivity. Contact urticaria elicited by food proteins was demonstrated in 9 cases, 3 of which reacted exclusively when the suspected food was applied to eczematous skin. When the food proteins that induced positive immediate patch tests on normal skin in 6 of the patients were introduced in scratch tests, 15 of the food handlers exhibited a positive reaction. A total of 25 reacted with a positive scratch test to incriminated food such as chicken, seafood, vegetables, and spices. In 10 of these the test revealed the only explanation for the cause of the dermatitis. Of patients tested with dialyzed extract of fish, positive reactions usually occurred only when relatively high-molecular-weight protein fractions were used. Five of eight with a positive scratch test to fish also had specific circulating immunoglobulin E (IgE) against fish protein. Other common allergens were garlic, onion, chives, cucumber, horseradish, leek, parsley, and tomato.

Other hand eczemas. Immediate reactions aggravating chronic hand dermatitis have been reported after protracted contact with lettuce and endive (Krook, 1977), wheat flour, turkey, and lamb (Maibach, 1976), and apple and potato (Andersen and Lowenstein, 1978). Two of Krook's patients revealed a contact urticaria on normal skin, while a third reacted only to food introduced by scratch test.

Occupational contact dermatitis caused by obstetric work and/or contact with cows is common among veterinarians (Praehl and Roed-Petersen, 1979). Seven of nine with a positive prick test to cow hair and dander gave a history of itching and flare-up of hand eczema after contact with cows and/or giving obstetric aid to cows. Three had a positive prick test to amnion and allantoic fluids. Four also had a positive radioallergosorbent test (RAST) to cow hair or dander; specific IgE against bovine amnion or allantoic fluids could not be demonstrated. An identical case was reported by Schmidt (1978). So far, the allergen(s) that causes symptoms in those assisting with cows' delivery remains unidentified.

Orolaryngeal and other phenomena associated with food proteins. The orolaryngeal area is another site where similar reactions may be provoked by food contact. One of the patients described by Krook (1977) nearly suffocated from a throat edema that developed quickly when the patient was eating endive. Maibach (1975) described a patient with delayed hypersensitivity to Merthiolate who received a throat spray containing this chemical; the application was followed within minutes by edema requiring tracheotomy. This is also likely to be a form of contact urticaria rather than only delayed sensitivity.

In a selected group of individuals with a positive scratch chamber test to birch pollen, 112 of 152 (74%) said that they experienced itching, tingling, and/or edema of lips, mouth, and tongue, or irritation of the throat such as hoarseness, when eating raw apple, potato, carrot, or tomato (Hannuksela and Lahti, 1977). Abdominal disturbances, rhinitis, angioedema, and aggravation of hand dermatitis were recorded in some patients. When scratch-tested with extracts from the incriminated products, an 80–90% correlation existed between positive reactions and the presence of symptoms, although there were some false positive and negative reactions. Positive reactions were rare in patients who did not react to birch pollen. Cooking destroyed the allergenic properties of the tested products. Similar reactions when handling or ingesting apples or potatoes have been reported in patients allergic to either birch pollen or hazelnut. While immunochemical similarities between extracts from birch pollen and hazelnut were demonstrated, their antigenic relation to apples, potatoes, and possibly other vegetable products remained obscure (Andersen and Løwenstein, 1978).

Development of anaphylactic reactions was reported after ingestion of celery (Hannuksela and Lahti, 1977; Forsbeck and Ros, 1979) and sunflower seed (Noyes et al., 1979) in cases where the reaction was correlated with a positive scratch test to the respective products.

COEXISTENCE OF CONTACT URTICARIA AND ATOPIC DERMATITIS?

Allergists have scratch-tested atopics for years, recommending elimination diets and exposures, while dermatologists emphasize caution in the interpretation of a positive intradermal test as the only tool in evaluating food allergy (Maibach, 1976). The situation remains controversial and has resulted in an unfortunate paucity of communication between allergy and dermatology. We believe that many reports of food hypersensitivity of the immediate type may include patients troubled by a true contact urticaria. This possibility has not been systematically evaluated.

The potential existence of the contact urticaria syndrome was overlooked in a recent study of possible food allergy in 119 patients suffering from asthma, rhinitis, eczema, urticaria or episodic mouth irritation, or vomiting, in combination with asthma. Based on total IgE levels, 88% of these individuals had an atopic background. Their sera were tested for specific IgE antibodies against egg, cow's milk, fish, cereal flours, and various types of nuts, and patients were investigated subsequently with elimination and challenge with the corresponding food.

A 79% correlation was found between symptoms and occurrence of specific IgE antibodies. Of 27 patients with one or more positive RAST tests to food allergens, 20 (74%) reacted within one hour after challenge with either nuts, egg, fish, or wheat, complaining of swelling or irritation of the mouth or tongue, and a 100% correlation existed between such symptoms and identification of specific IgE against the incriminated food (Wraith et al., 1979).

In our view, the value of including epidermal diagnostic and provocative test procedures in analogous future studies is unquestionable in evaluating to what extent hypersensitivity reactions from oral or gastrointestinal mucous membranes correspond to a true contact urticarial phenomenon on eczematous or previously affected skin sites as well as on nondiseased skin in atopic individuals. The skin may be an important, but so far disregarded, route of allergen introduction in highly protein allergic patients with atopic dermatitis.

SPECIAL FACTORS INFLUENCING THE INCIDENCE
OF POSITIVE DIAGNOSTIC TESTS

Previously Affected or Slightly Affected Skin

In investigations of the incidence of contact urticaria, diagnostic tests should include application of suspected products to affected or previously affected skin whenever tests on normal skin give a negative result. Eczematous skin, with its impaired barrier to penetration, may be more susceptible to contact urticaria than healthy skin. Relatively large molecules, such as the proteinaceous ones, presumably can pass through damaged epidermis better than through undamaged epidermis. However, even after apparent cure of an eczema, previously affected areas may remain more responsive than unaffected skin, reacting with pathological responses of an immediate type when again encountering the etiologic stimulus. Maibach (1976) reported a patient who was allergic to turkey, lamb, and flour, according to the history and positive scratch tests, and who was given an open test on intact, normal skin with negative results; after application of the pertinent foods to chronically slightly inflamed skin of the arms and back, a wheal-and-flare response occurred.

Of food handlers with recurrent hand dermatitis and positive scratch tests to suspected food, six were given open tests on unaffected and previously affected skin (Hjorth and Roed-Petersen, 1976). A positive reaction occurred in four cases when pertinent food was applied to previously dermatitic but now healthy skin, but in only one case when the test was performed on previously nondiseased skin.

A cold-buffet manager with relapsing hand-dermatitis gave a positive scratch test but a negative immediate open test on normal skin. When the open test was repeated on previously eczematous but now normal fingers, symptoms developed within 10 min (Krook, 1977).

In several of these cases the response consisted of prompt itching followed by urticarial responses either alone or in combination with an eruption of vesicles and all macroscopic features of a dermatitis (Hjorth and Roed-Petersen, 1976; Krook, 1977). We emphasize that skin testing on grossly eczematous skin is hardly productive; the wheal-and-flare response presumably is not recognized in this grossly damaged skin. However, recently healed or slightly involved skin, whose major abnormality is scaling, dramatically shows the wheal and flare.

Anatomic Site Specificity

There is a range of skin permeability on different anatomic sites (Maibach et al., 1971). The importance of acknowledging this fact when diagnosing contact urticaria has been convincingly demonstrated.

A man who experienced recurrent episodes of erythema when applying polysorbate-containing cream to his forehead revealed immediate urticarial reactions to polysorbate only when the substance was applied to the forehead, not to the arm or the back (Maibach and Conant, 1977).

In 16 healthy individuals who were openly tested with various concentrations of cinnamic aldehyde, the strength and number of positive reactions were significantly greater on the antecubital fossa than on the volar part of the forearm (Mathias et al., 1980).

Vehicle Dependence

The incidence of positive reactions in the latter study was vehicle dependent and increased with observation time and number of readings. Reactions to cinnamic aldehyde in ethanol usually appeared within 15 min and frequently faded within $\frac{1}{2}$ h. With petrolatum as the vehicle, positive reactions often occurred somewhat later, but always within 46–60 min. The study indicates that a single reading at 30 min could miss a substantial number of positive reactions.

Temperature Dependence

In an outbreak of hand eczema among cleaning personnel after the introduction of a lemon-scented detergent, it was noted that the patients complained of a burning, stinging sensation when their hands were submerged in hot detergent solution. Identical closed-patch tests were placed on both forearms for 20 min, one arm being exposed to $43°C$ and the other to $23-25°C$. Minimal or no reactions were seen on the "cold" arm, whereas one of the lemon perfume components evoked wheal-and-flare-like responses on the heated forearm in 9 of 12 cases (Rothenborg et al., 1977).

OCCURRENCE OF COMBINED IMMEDIATE AND DELAYED IMMUNE RESPONSES

Biopsies were obtained from two patients who exhibited promptly developing vesicles when the juice from lettuce or endive was applied to previously affected skin. The microscopic picture revealed subcorneal vesiculation, spongiosis, and infiltration of lymphocytes in the lower epidermis and in the corium—that is, a histological appearance in accord with that of contact dermatitis of the delayed type (Krook, 1977). An almost healed, still weakly erythematous patch site, which had been provoked by lettuce and endive juice 2 wk previously and read as positive after 72 h, was rechallenged with the same allergens and biopsied after 30 min. The macro- and microscopic pictures demonstrated identical features, as accounted for above.

Similar histological pictures were evident in two cases with immediate reactions to lemon perfume when biopsies were taken immediately after removal of the 20-min test (Rothenborg et al., 1977).

In guinea pigs sensitized to citraconic anhydride, epidermal challenge with the substance provoked an urticarial response, commencing within 30 min and reaching a peak after about 2 h. Seven to eight hours later this response underwent a progressive transformation into a delayed eczematous response.

Histologically, the initial response consisted of dilated dermal vessels surrounded by edema and mononuclear and eosinophilic cells. Later, invasion of basophils occurred (Hunziker and Brun, 1978). The final microscopic picture was similar to that in contact dermatitis of the delayed type induced by dinitrochlorobenzene (DNCB) sensitization (Jansa, 1977).

These reports indicate that immediate and delayed hypersensitivity to a substance may occur simultaneously in the same individual. While this phenomenon was previously considered most unusual (Ramsey et al., 1972), such cases have been increasingly recognized and add a new dimension to the field of contact dermatitis. Of the 67 patients in Table 2 who were tested for both types of response, 22 (33%) developed a positive delayed test response after the initial wheal-and-flare reaction. This type of combined reaction occurred with food products and such diverse substances as teak, rubber latex, cinnamic aldehyde, p-aminodiphenylamine, ethylaminobenzoate, ammonium persulfate, epoxy resin, and lemon perfume. Seventeen presented with a history of eczema, and the remainder with urticarial responses or uncharacteristic immediate sensations. We suggest that the term "contact dermatitis of the immediate and delayed type" be used for patients who exhibit combined reactions in the test situation, whether the initial reaction is uncharacteristic, urticarial, or vesicular.

IDENTIFICATION OF SPECIFIC ANTIBODIES

The factors involved in the interplay between immediate and delayed hypersensitivity are not understood. The patients probably reflect diverse mechanisms, where the identified hypersensitivity is either primarily responsible for a toxic or allergic dermatitis, or contributes secondarily to a flare-up of a preexisting toxic, allergic, or atopic eczema.

The most appropriate method for determining whether an antibody-antigen response is involved in contact urticaria is the use of passive serum transfer in vivo (the Prausnitz-Küstner test) (Odom and Maibach, 1976). Detection of specific circulating antibodies is desirable in future investigations. As yet, efforts have been limited to tracing the specific IgE (Hjorth and Roed-Petersen, 1976; Praehl and Roed-Petersen, 1979). This is reasonable when the syndrome occurs in atopic individuals. However, among those exhibiting contact urticaria, whether as an isolated phenomenon or associated with simultaneously occurring delayed hypersensitivity, atopics do not seem to be overrepresented.

In 46 of the patients listed in Table 2, specification of atopic manifestations and/or heredity was given. Atopic association was demonstrated in only 7 (15%). Food allergy may be more frequent among atopics, as investigations of selected materials seem to indicate (Hannuksela and Lahti, 1977; Wraith et al., 1979), but "protein contact dermatitis" does develop in other individuals. Only 6 of the 25 food handlers accounted for by Hjorth and Roed-Petersen

(1976) had a personal and/or family history of atopy. Specific IgE may be predominantly responsible for simultaneous reactions of the immediate type from extradermal organs in the contact urticaria syndrome through liberation of histamine from mast cells and basophils. However, IgG and IgM may also contribute through activation of the complement cascade by the classical pathway. Interestingly, through passive transfer experiments *in vivo*, it is known that specific IgG may contribute to some of the delayed hypersensitivity reactions (Askenase et al., 1975).

The immunopathogenetic circumstances may in this respect be analogous to tumor situations, when target cells may become increasingly susceptible to lytic destruction by mononuclear effector cells that have been exposed to tumor-specific IgG. *In vitro* assays show that such effector cells have Fc receptors on their membranes with affinity for the activated Fc regions of the IgG. Due to extreme economy in the use of immunoglobulins, the reaction may synergistically contribute to a cell-mediated immune response (Currie, 1974).

PRACTICAL EVALUATION

History

Because of the diversity of clinical manifestations of the contact urticaria syndrome, patients may be encountered not only in dermatology but in allergy and gastroenterology as well. The syndrome is an important differential diagnosis in patients with bronchial asthma, rhinoconjunctivitis, and orolaryngeal or gastrointestinal dysfunctions, and it should be kept in mind when evaluating unexplained vascular collapse.

From a dermatologic viewpoint, only a few of these individuals will present a typical story of an immediate, localized wheal-and-flare response; the majority will give a history of recurring dermatitis or generalized urticarial attacks. Some report only noncharacteristic sensations such as itching, burning, and tingling, symptoms likely to be disregarded by a physician who is not alert to the possibility of contact urticaria. As there is no standard test battery for routine evaluation of this diagnosis, diagnostic clues must be obtained from a careful history including any occurrence of immediate reactions, whether confined to the skin or not, and their correlation to preceding types of activity. These data should also include any personal and family history of atopic diseases.

Diagnostic Tests

Immediate readings of all epidermal tests are not routinely possible in dermatologic practice, but should—with guidance from the history—be performed liberally for selected substances. As the contact urticaria syndrome represents a scientifically relatively unexplored area, efforts should be initiated

at larger centers to evaluate the prevalence of the syndrome due to various substances in selected populations. These should include patients with occupational
dermatitis, atopic eczema, chronic "toxic" dermatitis, and urticaria recidivans.

Tests should be performed on normal and involved skin as well; this is
of particular interest in a disease such as atopic dermatitis, where the reason
for chronic occurrence on certain sites is obscure.

We do not intend to present a fixed scheme for evaluation of all
suspected cases. Development of the diagnostic patch test for delayed
hypersensitivity has taken decades; in spite of the fact that Jadassohn's work
was done at the beginning of the century, standardization of the techniques
continues and much new information has become available very recently.

Table 6 is an outline of the course that we advocate for cutaneous
evaluation of a suspected case of contact urticaria. Choice of the anatomic
test site must be guided by common sense and depends on the distribution of
affected versus normal skin in the individual patient. Both immediate and
delayed responses should be noted.

The advantages of open testing are obvious: ready observation and low

TABLE 6   Test Procedures for Evaluation of Immediate-Type Responses,
in Recommended Order[a]

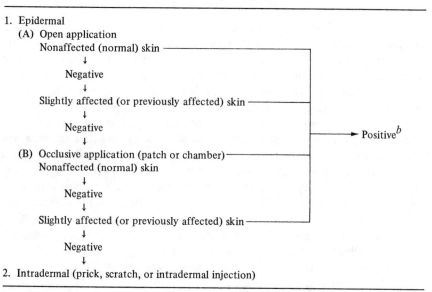

1. Epidermal
   (A) Open application
       Nonaffected (normal) skin
           ↓
       Negative
           ↓
       Slightly affected (or previously affected) skin
           ↓
       Negative
           ↓   → Positive[b]
   (B) Occlusive application (patch or chamber)
       Nonaffected (normal) skin
           ↓
       Negative
           ↓
       Slightly affected (or previously affected) skin
           ↓
       Negative
           ↓
2. Intradermal (prick, scratch, or intradermal injection)

[a]The goals are twofold: rational standardization of diagnostic and pathogenetic
evaluation, and minimization of hazardous extracutaneous reactions. An environment with
equipment to handle anaphylactoid reactions is required whenever evaluation of possible
contact urticaria is initiated. Choice of anatomic test site requires common sense and is
dependent on current skin status of individual patients; when testing diseased skin, only
slightly affected sites should be selected so that interpretations will be clear.
[b]If positive reactions are obtained, discontinue further evaluation.

risk of extracutaneous reactions; the advantage of closed testing is the possibility that enhanced penetration will lead to a positive response that is not noted in the open testing. For the open test, approximately 0.1 ml of the suspected substance is spread with a glass rod. The observation period must be at least 30 min, but should preferably be 1 h with three or four readings to avoid missing any positive reactions. A positive response consists of a follicular erythema evolving into a wheal or wheal-and-flare response.

If the response is negative on normal skin, the test should be repeated on previously affected or still involved skin. Only when this produces a negative result should a closed patch test be tried. The patch is removed after 15-20 min.

As a routine, the ventral forearm is practical for testing immediate responses if the patient is simultaneously tested on the back for delayed hypersensitivity. Alternatively, duplicate applications in parallel rows may be made to the back; one is left open and observed for immediate reactions, and the other is covered and read after 48-96 h.

Intradermal Tests

As already noted, intradermal tests combined with clinical and historical data are apparently relevant in some cases of protein contact dermatitis. As the tests are not diagnostic, we do not recommend intradermal application of incriminated substances in routine screening for contact urticaria. Intradermal tests are research-type procedures; when they are positive, extensive controls are mandatory for proper interpretation of specificity.

Immunoglobulin Determinations

Total IgE and occurrence of specific IgE antibodies (RAST) should be evaluated in atopic individuals, and in some of these cases RAST may give additional clues to which antigen(s) should be further tested topically. Determination of specific antibodies of other globulin classes should be an important aim of future research.

Passive Transfer

Passive transfer is accomplished by injecting 0.1 ml of freshly obtained serum from the patient into the forearm of a human volunteer or into a monkey. After 24 h 0.1 ml of the eliciting agent is applied topically to the injection site and to a contralateral saline control site. A positive result, indicated by a wheal-and-flare response only at the site of injection of the donor serum, is considered indirect proof that a reaction is mediated by an IgE mediated immediate allergic reaction. Caution must be used in performing the test in humans because of the possibility of hepatitis.

Compound 48/80

Compound 48/80 is diluted to 0.05 mg/ml, and 0.01 ml is injected id into the patient's forearm. Because of the histamine-liberating effect of the drug, a wheal-and-flare response is noted. Injection is repeated at the same site two or three times at 8-h intervals. Usually no response can be elicited by the third injection. Twenty-four hours after the initial injection, 0.1 ml of the test substance is applied to the site pretreated with compound 48/80 and to a control site. If a typical urticarial response occurs at the control site but not at the prepared site, the response may be partly mediated by histamine. Component 48/80 is available on an experimental basis (Sigma Chemical Co., St. Louis, Mo.).

In conclusion, the experience available to date indicates a broad syndrome complex. It it likely that increasing awareness of this syndrome will lead to the discovery of even broader clinical involvements. We hope that the testing scheme presented here will help document the etiology in a scientifically useful and acceptable manner.

REFERENCES

Andersen, K. E. and Løwenstein, H. 1978. An investigation of the possible immunological relationship between allergen extracts from birch pollen, hazelnut, potato and apple. *Contact Dermatitis* 4:73–79.

Askenase, P. W., Haynes, H. D., Tauber, D., et al. 1975. Specific basophil hypersensitivity induced by skin testing and transferred using immune serum. *Nature (Lond.)* 256:52–54.

Brubaker, M. M. 1972. Urticarial reaction to ammonium persulfate. *Arch. Dermatol.* 106:413–414.

Calnan, C. 1982. Delayed onset contact urticaria. *Contact Dermatitis,* in press.

Calnan, C. and Shuster, S. 1963. Reactions to ammonium persulfate. *Arch. Dermatol.* 88:812–815.

Camarasa, J. M. G., Alomar, A., and Perez, M. 1978. Contact urticaria and anaphylaxis from aminophenazone. *Contact Dermatitis* 4:243–244.

Comaish, J. S. and Cunliffe, W. J. 1967. Absorption of drugs from varicose ulcers. A cause of anaphylaxis. *Br. J. Clin. Pract.* 21:97–98

Cronin, E. 1979. Immediate-type hypersensitivity to henna. *Contact Dermatitis* 5:198–199.

Currie, G. A. 1974. Cancer and the immune response. In *Current Topics in Immunology,* ed. J. Turk, No. 2, Ch. 5, pp. 36–53. Edinburgh: Arnold.

Daughters, D., Zackheim, H., and Maibach, H. I. 1973. Urticaria and anaphylactoid reactions after topical application of mechlorethamine. *Arch. Dermatol.* 107:429–430.

Fisher, A. A. and Dooms-Goossens, A. 1976. Persulfate hair bleach reactions. Cutaneous and respiratory manifestations. *Arch. Dermatol.* 112:1407–1409.

Fisher, A. A. 1978. Immediate and delayed allergic contact reactions to polyethylene glycol. *Contact Dermatitis* 4:135–138.

Forsbeck, M. and Ros, A.-M. 1979. Anaphylactoid reaction to celery. *Contact Dermatitis* 5:191.

Forsbeck, M. and Skog, E. 1977. Immediate reactions to patch tests with balsam of Peru. *Contact Dermatitis* 3:201–205.

Friis, B. and Hjorth, N. 1973. Immediate reactions to patch tests with balsam of Peru. *Contact Dermatitis Newslett.* 13:389.

Gaul, L. E. 1969. Dermatitis from cetyl and stearyl alcohols. *Arch. Dermatol.* 99:593.

Grunnet, E. 1976. Contact urticaria and anaphylactoid reaction induced by topical application of nitrogen mustard. *Br. J. Dermatol.* 94:101–103.

Hannuksela, M. and Lahti, A. 1977. Immediate reactions to fruits and vegetables. *Contact Dermatitis* 3:79–84.

Helander, I. 1977. Contact urticaria from leather containing formaldehyde. *Arch. Dermatol.* 113:1443.

Henry, J. C., Tschen, E. H., and Becker, L. E. 1979. Contact urticaria to parabens. *Arch. Dermatol.* 115:1231–1232.

Hjorth, N. and Roed-Petersen, J. 1976. Occupational protein contact dermatitis in food handlers. *Contact Dermatitis* 2:28–42.

Hunziker, N. and Brun, R. 1978. Contact urticaria and dermatitis to citraconic anhydride in guinea pigs. *Contact Dermatitis* 4:236–238.

Jansa, P. 1977. Cellular evaluation of hypersensitivity to 2,4-dinitrochlorobenzene. *Neoplasma* 24:529–532.

Key, M. M. 1961. Some unusual allergic reactions in industry. *Arch. Dermatol.* 83:3–6.

Kirton, V. 1978. Contact urticaria and cinnamic aldehyde. *Contact Dermatitis* 4:374–375.

Kosáková, M. 1977. Sub-Schock bei der Epikutanprobe mit Chloramphenicol. *Berufs-Dermatosen* 25:134–135.

Krook, G. 1977. Occupational dermatitis from *Lactuca sativa* (lettuce) and *Cichorium* (endive). Simultaneous occurrence of immediate and delayed allergy as a cause of contact dermatitis. *Contact Dermatitis* 3:27–36.

Levene, G. and Withers, A. 1969. Anaphylaxis to streptomycin and hyposensitization. *Trans. St. John's Hosp. Dermatol. Soc.* 55:184–188.

McDaniel, R. and Marks, M. J. 1979. Contact urticaria due to sensitivity to spray starch. *Arch. Dermatol.* 115:628.

Maibach, H. I. 1975. Acute laryngeal obstruction presumed secondary to thiomersal (Merthiolate) hypersensitivity. *Contact Dermatitis* 1:221–222.

Maibach, H. I. 1976. Immediate hype⸱ ⸱ensitivity in hand dermatitis. Role of food-contact dermatitis. *Arch. Dermatol.* 112:1289–1291.

Maibach, H. I. 1982. Immediate sensitivity to neomycin. Personal observation.

Maibach, H. I. and Conant, M. 1977. Contact urticaria to a corticosteroid cream: Polysorbate 60. *Contact Dermatitis* 3:350–351.

Maibach, H. I. and Johnson, H. L. Contact urticaria syndrome. Contact urticaria to diethyltoluamide. *Arch. Dermatol.* 111:726–730.

Maibach, H. I., Feldman, R., Milby, T., et al. 1971. Regional variation in percutaneous penetration in man. *Arch. Environ. Health* 23:208–211.

Mathews, K. P. 1968. Immediate type hypersensitivity to phenylmercuric compounds. *Am. J. Med.* 44:310.

Mathias, T., Chappler, R. R., and Maibach, H. I. 1980. Contact urticaria from cinnamic aldehyde. *Arch. Dermatol.* 116:74–76.

Maucher, O. M. 1972. Anaphylaktische Reaktionen beim Epicutantest. *Hautarzt* 23:139–140.

Monroe, E. W. and Jones, H. E. 1977. Urticaria. An updated review. *Arch. Dermatol.* 113:80–90.

Nater, J. P., de John, J. M., Baar, A. J. M., et al. 1977. Contact urticarial skin responses to cinnamaldehyde. *Contact Dermatitis* 3:151–154.

Neering, H. 1977. Contact urticaria from chlorinated swimming pool water. *Contact Dermatitis* 3:279.

Noyes, J. H., Boyd, G. K., and Settipane, G. A. 1979. Anaphylaxis to sunflower seed. *J. Allergy Clin. Immunol.* 63:242–244.

Nutter, A. F. 1979. Contact urticaria to rubber. *Br. J. Dermatol.* 101:597–598.

Odom, R. B. and Maibach, H. I. 1976. Contact urticaria: A different contact dermatitis. *Cutis* 18:672–676.

Powell, R. F. and Smith, E. B. 1978. Tumbleweed dermatitis. *Arch. Dermatol.* 114:751–754.

Praehl, P. and Roed-Petersen, J. 1979. Type I allergy from cows in veterinary surgeons. *Contact Dermatitis* 5:33–38.

Ramsey, D. L., Cotten, H. J., and Baer, R. L. 1972. Allergic reaction to benzophenone; simultaneous occurrence of urticarial and contact sensitivities. *Arch. Dermatol.* 105:906–908.

Rietschel, R. L. 1978. Contact urticaria from synthetic cassia oil and sorbic acid limited to the face. *Contact Dermatitis* 4:347–349.

Rothenborg, H. W., Menné, T., and Sjølin, K.-E. 1977. Temperature dependent primary irritant dermatitis from lemon perfume. *Contact Dermatitis* 3:37–48.

Rudzki, E. and Grzywa, Z. 1976. Immediate reactions to balsam of Peru, cassia oil and ethyl vanillin. *Contact Dermatitis* 2:360–361.

Ryan, M. E., Davis, B. M., and Marks, J. G. 1982. Contact urticaria and allergic contact dermatitis to benzocaine gel. *J. Am. Acad. Dermatol.*, in press.

Schmidt, H. 1978. Contact urticaria to teak with systemic effects. *Contact Dermatitis* 4:176–177.

Schmidt, H. Contact urticaria. *Contact Dermatitis* 4:230–232.

Smith, J. D., Odom, R. B., and Maibach, H. I. 1975. Contact urticaria to cobalt chloride. *Arch. Dermatol.* 111:1610–1611.

Tharp, C. K. 1973. Contact urticaria. *Arch. Dermatol.* 108:135.

Tuft, L. 1975. Contact urticaria from cephalosporins. *Arch. Dermatol.* 111:1609.

von Liebe, V., Karge, H.-J., Burg, G. 1979. Kontakturtikaria. *Hautarzt* 30:544–546.

von Temesvári, E., Podányi, B., Kovács, I., et al. 1978. Contact urticaria provoked by balsam of Peru. *Contact Dermatitis* 4:65–68.

von Temesvári, E., Albonczy, É., and Somlai, B. 1979. Kontakturtikaria durch Ei. *Dermatosen* 27:69–71.

Widstrøm, L. 1977. Allergic reactions to ammonium persulfate in hair bleach. *Contact Dermatitis* 3:343.

Woyton, A., Wasik, F., and Blizanowska, A. 1974. From "Summary." *Przegl. Dermatol.* 61:303–308.

Wraith, D. G., Merrett, J., Roth, A., et al. 1979. Recognition of food-allergic patients and their allergens by the RAST technique and clinical investigation. *Clin. Allergy* 9:25–36.

Zschunke, E. 1978. Contact urticaria, dermatitis and asthma from cockroaches. *Contact Dermatitis* 4:313–314.

15

light-induced dermal toxicity: effects on the cellular and molecular level

Andrija Kornhauser ▪ Wayne Wamer ▪ Albert Giles, Jr.

INTRODUCTION

Die Sonne ist auch da wenn die Wolken schwarz und undurch-dringlich scheinen.—Ernst Jucker[1]

Toxicology has evolved as a multidisciplinary field of study and is still in rapid evolutionary development. As such, toxicology overlaps many other basic biomedical disciplines, including biochemistry, pharmacology, and physiology. A recent event in this development has been the intersection of toxicology with photobiology, opening the field of phototoxicology.

Sunlight is the most potent environmental agent influencing life on the earth. Historically, exposure to the sun has been believed to be healthful and beneficial. It has only recently become apparent that many of the effects of solar radiation are detrimental. In a broad sense, therefore, the evolution of life can be regarded as a continuous adaptation to light by simultaneously utilizing solar energy and protecting against its detrimental effects.

Modern civilization presents a challenge for basic phototoxicologic research. This challenge arises from alterations in the life-styles of a large portion of the population, including holiday trips, clothing styles, and particularly the fashion of suntanning among Caucasians. It is also possible that environmental factors may change the quality of light reaching the earth's

[1] From *Ein gutes Wort zur rechten Zeit*, Verlag Paul Haupt, Bern, 1957.

323

surface. Many of these factors lead to an essentially increased exposure to light for a large segment of the population (Fitzpatrick et al., 1974). In the past decade, phototoxic reactions to drugs, cosmetics, and many industrial and environmental chemicals have become a major health problem.

Definitions of phototoxicity are numerous and frequently inconsistent. In the broadest sense, photosensitivity is any toxicity induced by photons. Phototoxicity is used to describe all nonimmunologic light-induced toxic skin reactions. Sunburn is the most frequently occurring phototoxic reaction, requiring only the interaction of ultraviolet (UV) light with skin. In most cases of phototoxicity, however, we deal with an endogenous or exogenous chemical (chromophore) that absorbs light and transfers the energy to, or reacts in the excited state with, cellular components. Such toxic reactions would most properly be termed chemical phototoxicity.

Chronic phototoxic exposure can lead to neoplastic changes. It is established that the consequence of lifelong enhanced exposure to light is a significant increase in skin tumors (Urbach et al., 1974), including basal and squamous cell carcinomas and, to a certain extent, malignant melanomas. This is confirmed by the pronounced increase in frequency of skin cancers in that part of the population, particularly those Celts and Teutons, which in the course of history settled in regions with higher solar irradiation (Africa, Australia, and North America).

Phototoxicity studies, particularly those related to human disorders, have so far been based predominately on gross anatomic or histological procedures. Although our knowledge of the molecular events that occur during these processes is rapidly growing, much basic research remains to be done. In this chapter we discuss some molecular and cellular events that take place on exposure to light.

LIGHT CHARACTERISTICS

Aside from artificial light sources, solar radiation is the primary source of light that elicits biological effects. A portion of the solar spectrum containing the biologically most active region (290–700 nm) is shown in Fig. 1.

The UV part of the spectrum includes wavelengths from 200 to 400 nm. Portions of the UV spectrum have distinctive features from both the physical and medical points of view. The accepted designations for the biologically important parts of the UV spectrum are UVA, 400–315 nm; UVB, 315–280 nm; and UVC, 280–220 nm (Fig. 2). Wavelengths less than 290 nm (UVC) do not occur at the earth's surface, since they are absorbed, predominantly by ozone, in the stratosphere. The most thoroughly studied photobiological reactions that occur in skin are induced by UVB. Although UVB wavelengths represent only approximately 1.5% of the solar energy received at the earth's surface (WHO, 1979), they elicit most of the known biological effects. Light

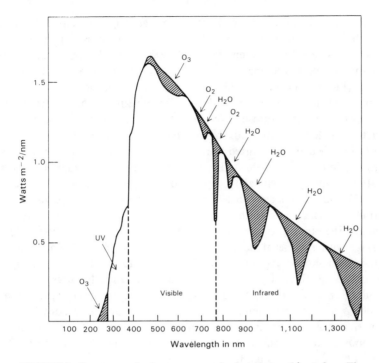

FIGURE 1 Spectrum of solar energy received at the earth's surface. The absorption bands of atmospheric O_2, O_3, and H_2O are shown.

distributed over these wavelengths inhibits cell mitosis, makes vitamin D, and induces sunburn and skin cancer. The UVA wavelengths elicit most of the known chemical phototoxic and photoallergic reactions. The visible portion of the spectrum, representing about 50% of the sun's energy received at sea level, includes wavelengths from 400 to 700 nm. Visible light is necessary for such biological events as photosynthesis, circadian cycles, vision, and pigment darkening. Furthermore, visible light in conjunction with certain chromophores (e.g., dyes, drugs, and endogenous compounds) and molecular oxygen induces photodynamic effects.

Understanding the toxic effects of light impinging on the skin requires knowledge of the skin's optical properties. Skin may be viewed as an optically inhomogeneous medium, composed of three layers that have characteristic

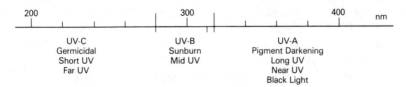

FIGURE 2 Biologically important regions of the UV spectrum.

refractive indices, chromophore distributions, and light-scattering properties. Light entering the outermost layer, the stratum corneum, is in part reflected— 4–7% for wavelengths between 250 and 3000 nm (Anderson and Parrish, 1981)—due to the difference in refractive index between air and stratum corneum (Fresnel reflection). Absorption by urocanic acid (a deamination product of histidine), melanin, and proteins containing the aromatic amino acids tryptophan and tyrosine in the stratum corneum produces further attenuation of light, particularly at shorter UV wavelengths. Approximately 40% of the UVB is transmitted through the stratum corneum to the viable epidermis (Everett et al., 1966). The light entering the epidermis is attenuated by scattering and, predominately, absorption. Epidermal chromophores consist of proteins, urocanic acid, nucleic acids, and melanin. Passage through the epidermis results in appreciable attenuation of UVA and particularly UVB radiation. The transmission properties of the dermis are largely due to scattering, with significant absorption of visible light by melanin, β-carotene, and the blood-borne pigments bilirubin, hemoglobin, and oxyhemoglobin. Light traversing these layers of the skin is extensively attenuated, most drastically for wavelengths less than 400 nm. Longer wavelengths are more penetrating. It has been noted that there is an "optical window"—that is, greater transmission—for light at wavelengths of 600–1300 nm, which may have important biological consequences (Anderson and Parrish, 1981). These features are presented in Fig. 3.

Normal variations in the skin's optical properties frequently occur. The degree of pigmentation, or skin melanin content, may result in variations in the attenuation of light, particularly between 300 and 400 nm, by as much as 1.5 times more in Negroes than in Caucasians (Pathak, 1967). Alterations in the amount or distribution of other natural chromophores account for further variations in skin optical properties. Urocanic acid, deposited on the skin's surface during perspiration (Anderson and Parrish, 1981), and UV-absorbing lipids, excreted in sebum (Beadle and Burton, 1981), may significantly reduce UV transmission through the skin. Epidermal thickness, which varies over regions of the body and increases after exposure to UVB radiation, may significantly modify UV transmission (Soffen and Blum, 1961; Parrish and Jaenicke, 1981).

Certain disease states also produce alterations in the skin's optical properties. Alterations of the skin's surface, such as by psoriatic plaques, decrease transmitted light. This effect may be lessened by application of oils whose refractive index is similar to that of skin (Anderson and Parrish, 1981). Disorders such as hyperbilirubinemia, porphyrias, and blue skin nevi result in increased absorption of visible light due to accumulation or altered distribution of chromophoric endogenous compounds.

The penetration of light into and through dermal tissues has important consequences. Skin, as the primary organ responsible for thermal regulation, is overperfused relative to its metabolic requirements (Anderson and Parrish,

Wavelength in Nanometers

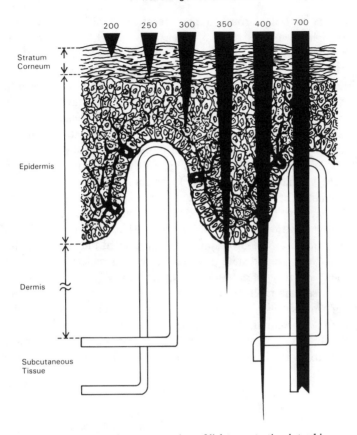

FIGURE 3   Schematic representation of light penetration into skin.

1981). It is estimated that the average cutaneous blood flow is 20–30 times that necessary to support the skin's metabolic needs. The papillary boundaries between epidermis and dermis allow capillary vessels to lie close to the skin's surface, permitting the blood and important components of the immune system to be exposed to light. The equivalent of the entire blood volume of an adult may pass through the skin, and potentially be irradiated, in 20 min. This corresponds to the time required to receive 1–2 MEDs.[2] The accessibility of incident radiation to blood has been exploited in such regimens as phototherapy of hyperbilirubinemia in neonates, where light is used as a therapeutic agent. However, in general there is a potential for light-induced toxicity due to irradiation of blood-borne drugs and metabolites.

[2] The MED is defined as the minimal dose of UV irradiation that produces definite, but minimally perceptible, redness 24 h after exposure.

FUNDAMENTAL CONCEPTS IN PHOTOCHEMISTRY

Damage to cells through a photoreaction is initiated at the site where the chromophore absorbs specific wavelengths of light. Absorption of UV or visible photons results in electronically excited molecules; dissipation of this energy may result in an adverse phototoxic effect on the cell.

The sequence of events initiated by light absorption is shown in Fig. 4. The transition of a ground-state molecule to a excited singlet electronic state accompanies absorption of a visible or UV photon. Molecules in their singlet excited states exist for only about 10^{-8}-10^{-9} s before either returning to the ground state or converting (intersystem crossing) to a longer lived (10^{-4}-10^1 s) metastable triplet state. Both excited singlet and populated triplet states relax to the ground state through (1) transfer of energy to another molecule and (2) emission of light (fluorescence or phosphoresence) or release of heat.

Alternatively, the excited molecule may undergo photochemistry such as *cis-trans* isomerization, fragmentation, ionization, rearrangement, and intermolecular reactions. The probability that an excited molecule will choose any given path to the ground state depends on both its molecular structure and its environment and may be determined experimentally (Turro, 1965).

All these factors—light absorption, the nature of the excited states, the extent of intersystem crossing, and photochemical reactions—will finally determine the phototoxic potential of a endogenous or exogenous compound. However, we are not yet able to predict the phototoxic potential of a compound from its molecular structure alone. Reliable predictive tests are

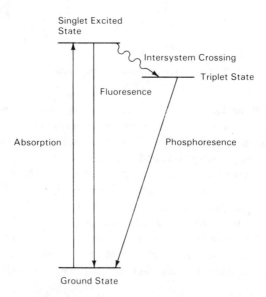

FIGURE 4 Electronic energy diagram of physical events accompanying the absorption of a photon.

still required to evaluate suspected compounds. Several lists of compounds that are phototoxic in humans have appeared (e.g., Parrish et al., 1979). Classes of compounds known to be phototoxic in humans are:

Psoralens
Sulfonamides
Sulfonylureas
Phenothiazine
Tetracyclines
Coal tar
Anthracene
Acridine
Phenanthrene

The mechanisms through which absorption of light causes a chemical alteration in the chromophore, eventually resulting in a phototoxic response, are shown in Fig. 5. Compounds such as psoralens may react directly in their excited states with a biological target. Because of the short lifetimes of most excited states, direct reaction requires close association, or complex formation, between the chromophore and the target before light absorption. Alternatively, a stable toxic photoproduct may be formed after absorption of light. Chlorpromazine and protriptyline are examples of this mechanism (Kochevar, 1981). The phototoxicity of these compounds is in large part the result of the toxicity of their photoproducts.

The other mechanisms shown in Fig. 5 are frequently categorized as photodynamic mechanisms. Photodynamic reactions usually involve compounds that absorb UVA or visible light. In type I photodynamic reactions the chromophore, in an excited triplet state, is reduced either by an electron or by hydrogen transfer from a compound in the environment. This reduction results in the generation of highly reactive free radicals, whose subsequent attack on biological substrates may result in toxicity. In type II photodynamic reactions the chromophore transfers its energy to O_2 generating singlet oxygen ($^1O_2$), an active oxidizing agent. Although $^1O_2$ has not been directly detected in photodynamic actions so far investigated *in vivo*, a large body of evidence supports its involvement.

CELLULAR TARGETS AND MECHANISMS OF PHOTOTOXICITY

A vigorous effort is under way to discover the biological targets in phototoxicity. Cellular injury by photons may be studied on either the histological or the molecular level. The characteristic histological change induced by photons is the appearance of the so-called sunburn cell (SBC) (Daniels et al., 1961), a dyskeratotic cell with bright eosinophilic cytoplasm

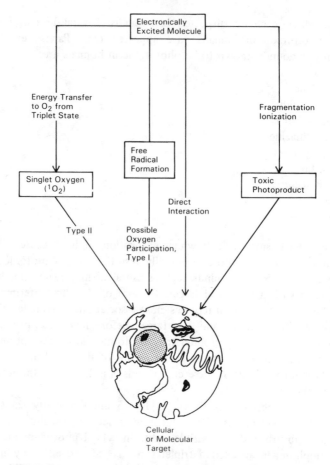

FIGURE 5 Diagram of basic phototoxicity mechanisms. The electronically excited molecule, located within or near a cell, may elicit a phototoxic response through several mechanisms.

and a pyknotic nucleus. SBCs appear 24–48 h after UVB irradiation (Woodcock and Magnus, 1976) and may persist 1 wk or longer (Parrish et al., 1979). The mechanisms of SBC formation are still obscure, although its morphological and biochemical characteristics have been investigated (Danno and Horio, 1980; Olson et al., 1974). The primary chromophore for sunburn cell production is not known; however, Young and Magnus (1981) found evidence that DNA may be an important chromophore. They detected SBCs in mouse epidermis after administration of 8-methoxypsoralen (8-MOP) and UVA irradiation (PUVA conditions). They speculated that since the primary molecular lesion in PUVA treatment is in DNA, the fact that PUVA can promote SBC formation supports the view that DNA may be a significant chromophore in SBC induction.

The mechanisms by which photosensitized cells are damaged are in most cases poorly understood. On the subcellular level, the primary targets in a phototoxic reaction include nucleic acids, proteins, and plasma and organelle membranes. Subcellular effects may differ depending on the photosensitizer's structure and intracellular localization. Sensitizers such as rose bengal, porphyrin, and anthracene accumulate selectively in cell plasma membranes (Ito, 1978). Acridine orange and psoralens are localized in the cell nucleus (Van de Vorst and Lion, 1976; Pathak et al., 1974; Bredberg et al., 1977). Some photosensitizers may become concentrated in lysosomes and on irradiation may induce lysosomal rupture (Allison et al., 1966). Table 1 shows results from some studies of the mechanisms of action for several important classes of phototoxic compounds. It includes two endogenous photosensitizers, porphyrins and kynurenic acid. As reflected in Table 1, most compounds that evoke chemical phototoxicity are thought to act through a photodynamic mechanism. Further, it appears that a compound may elicit a phototoxic response through several modes. Studies are needed to correlate specific molecular alterations (such as DNA cross-linking and photooxidation of enzymes and of DNA) with cell toxicity and mutagenesis. To date, only the mechanism of psoralen phototoxicity is relatively well understood. Much more remains to be learned about the mode of action for other groups of photosensitizers.

SPECIFIC MOLECULAR ALTERATIONS IN CELLS

On the molecular level, DNA is the most sensitive target in a cell exposed to UV light. As previously discussed, other cellular constituents may also be affected, generally with less severe consequences for the cell.

Thymine Dimers

Cyclobutane-type pyrimidine dimers in DNA are the most important and best-studied lesions induced in cells by UV, predominately at wavelengths less than 300 nm (Rothman and Setlow, 1979; Rosenstein and Setlow, 1980; Kantor et al., 1980). They result from the formation of covalent bonds between adjacent pyrimidines of the same DNA strand and interfere with normal DNA function. Beukers and Berends (1960) first demonstrated the formation of these dimers *in vitro*, and Wacker et al. (1960) found them in DNA from UV-irradiated bacteria *in vivo*. These findings marked the beginning of a new era in molecular biology. Thymine dimers (TT) (Fig. 6) were later shown to occur in a number of higher systems and, more recently, in mammalian and human skin after UV irradiation (Pathak et al., 1972). Studies initiated by Cleaver and Trosko (1970) demonstrated the involvement of TT in xeroderma pigmentosum (XP). This finding represents one of the rare cases in which a specific molecular lesion can be correlated with a malignant process. In another approach, Hart et al. (1977) used cell extracts from

TABLE 1 Mechanisms and Targets of Selected Groups of Phototoxic Compounds

Compound	Structure	Mechanism of phototoxicity	Cellular target	Reference
Psoralens		Direct addition	DNA	Pathak et al., 1974
		Photodynamic	DNA, proteins, ribosomes, membranes	de Mot et al., 1981 Poppe and Grossweiner, 1975 Singh and Vadasz, 1978 Pathak, 1982
Phenothiazines, e.g., chlorpromazine	S, Cl, CH₂CH₂N(CH₃)₂	Stable (toxic) photoproduct	DNA	Kochevar, 1981
		Photodynamic	DNA, membranes	Kochevar, 1981 Copeland et al., 1976
Porphyrins	HO₂C, CO₂H, NH, HN	Photodynamic	Membranes, DNA, proteins	Spikes, 1975 Verweij et al., 1981 Jori and Spikes, 1981
Dyes, e.g., acridine orange	(CH₃)₂N, N(CH₃)₂	Photodynamic	Proteins, membranes, DNA	Hass and Webb, 1981 Ito, 1978 Wacker et al., 1964 Wagner et al., 1980
Kynurenic acid	OH, CO₂H	Photodynamic	Membranes	Wennersten and Brunk, 1977, 1978 Pileni and Santus, 1978
Anthracene		Photodynamic	Membranes, DNA	Allison et al., 1966 Blackburn and Taussig, 1975

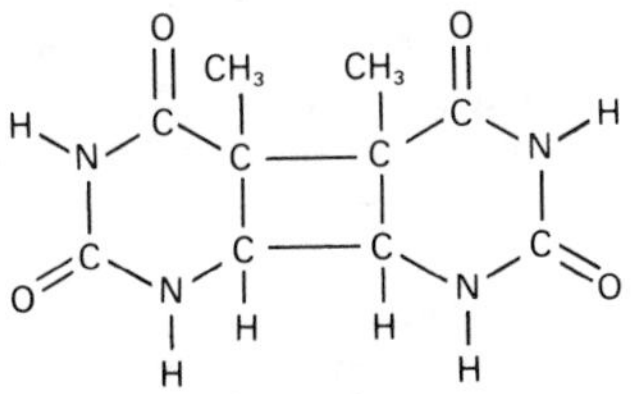

FIGURE 6 Structure of the thymine dimer (*cis, syn*).

UV-irradiated Amazon mollies (small fish) and reported evidence that pyrimidine dimers in DNA gave rise to tumors.

Until recently, sensitive assays for TT required use of radiolabeled thymidine. However, very sensitive techniques have now been developed for measuring TT. These methods, including radioimmunoassays (Mitchell and Clarkson, 1981) and endonuclease digestion followed by determination of DNA chain length (D'Ambrosio et al., 1981), have made quantitation of TT in human biopsies feasible.

Several possible reaction mechanisms for the sensitized photodimerization of pyrimidines have been suggested, including population of the triplet state of a suitable sensitizer (Lamola, 1968). Our previous work showed that a Schenck type of mechanism (Schenck, 1960) involving a complex-forming reaction is highly favored in photosensitized thymine dimer formation (Kornhauser and Pathak, 1972; Kornhauser et al., 1974). Also, we found that only a few of the potential sensitizers caused measurable thymine dimerization. A small amount (1–2%) of thymine dimer was detected after UV irradiation, even in the absence of a sensitizer. Acetone, ethyl acetoacetate, and dihydroxyacetone were more potent sensitizers than acetophenone and benzophenone (Table 2).

The following conclusions can be derived from our results:

1. The sensitized energy transfer taking place during thymine dimerization most likely does not occur through a simple physical mechanism. The ability of the sensitizer in its excited state to form a complex with the pyrimidine molecule appears to be a prerequisite for this type of photosensitization.
2. Ethyl acetoacetate and dihydroxyacetone, molecules that are commonly present in any viable cell and were not previously known to be photosensitizers, proved as effective as acetone or acetophenone. On the other hand, urocanic acid, a major UV-absorbing compound in mammalian skin, did not show sensitizing ability in inducing thymine dimerization. The UV energy absorbed by urocanic acid is believed to induce its *cis-trans* isomerization (Baden and Pathak, 1967).

TABLE 2   Formation of Thymine Dimers (TT)
after Irradiation of [2-^{14}C] Thymine
in the Presence of Different Sensitizers[a]

No.	Sensitizer	TT formed (%)
1	None	1–2
2	Acetone	30–40
3	Dihydroxyacetone	25–30
4	Acetophenone	5–10
5	Benzophenone	5–8
6	4-Methoxyacetophenone	2–4
7	Ethyl acetoacetate	35–45
8	Phenyl cyanide	1–3
9	Carbazole	3–6
10	Fluorene	2–3
11	Naphthalene	1–3
12	Xanthene-9-one	1–3
13	Urocanic acid	1–3

[a]Solutions of [2-^{14}C] thymine (2×10^{-3} M) and sensitizer (10^{-4}–10^{-1} M) were irradiated with a total UV ($\leqslant 300$ nm) dose of 1.2 J/cm^2. Irradiations were carried out in water (1, 2, 3, 13), water and ethanol (3:1) (4, 6–12), and water and dioxane (3:1) (5, 12).

3. Topical preparations containing acetone, dihydroxyacetone, or other acetone derivatives should be used cautiously, since they might damage the epidermal DNA when skin is exposed to UV radiation. Interestingly, one of these compounds, dihydroxyacetone, has been used in cosmetics, notably as the active component in "sunless" tanning lotions (Maibach and Kligman, 1960).

The studies discussed above have practical applications for correlating the structure of a potential phototoxic agent with its ability to induce pyrimidine dimerization or other molecular lesions in cells.

DNA-Protein Cross-Links

The previous discussion focused on the reaction between bases, specifically thymine, within a strand of DNA to form a homoadduct. However, DNA in the cell has a complex and richly varied environment, making possible additional light-induced reactions.

Heteroadducts of DNA—that is, adducts formed by covalent attachment of a large number of different types of compounds (both normal cellular constituents, such as proteins, and exogenous compounds such as drugs, food additives, and cosmetics—have profound effects on cells. Artificially produced covalent linkages like DNA-protein cross-links, of the type not observed in normal viable cells, may result in a phototoxic response or be expressed as mutagenic or carcinogenic events.

The chemical nature of the DNA-protein cross-links is not yet known. An *in vitro* photochemical reaction between thymine and cysteine has been observed (Schott and Shetlar, 1974) and may be one of the mechanisms for covalent linking of DNA to protein *in vivo* (Smith, 1974). Similarly, it has been reported that irradiation of thymine-labeled DNA and lysine in aqueous solvent produces a photoproduct that behaves like a thymine-lysine adduct (Shetlar et al., 1975). Furthermore, 11 of the common amino acids combine photochemically with uracil in different model systems (Smith, 1974). These pyrimidine-amino acid adducts are regarded as models for the coupling sites between proteins and DNA. In addition to reactions directly induced by UV, model systems provide evidence that acetone and acetophenone are effective photosensitizers for the covalent addition of amino acids to pyrimidine bases (Fisher et al., 1974). It is reasonable to assume that suitable chromophores present in drugs, cosmetics, and so on, will also be able to photosensitize the cross-linking of proteins and nucleic acids *in vitro* and *in vivo*.

The cross-linking of DNA and protein in bacteria was the first *in vivo* photochemical heteroadduct reaction reported (Smith, 1962). Several studies of UV-induced DNA and protein cross-links in mammalian cells *in vitro* have been based mainly on reduced DNA extractability after UV irradiation (Todd and Han, 1976). Evidence that this lesion plays a significant role in killing UV-irradiated cells has been obtained under several experimental conditions.

Mammalian (eukaryotic) cells, in general, represent a suitable model for the cross-linking reaction. Within the nuclei of eukaryotic cells, DNA is in intimate contact with proteins responsible for structurally organizing DNA and controlling macromolecular synthesis. Such a DNA-protein complex is commonly referred to as chromatin. The proximity of nuclear proteins to DNA should facilitate the formation of UV-induced DNA-protein covalent bonds. Todd and Han (1976) studied the general features of UV-induced (254 nm) DNA-protein cross-links in asynchronous and synchronous HeLa cells. Cross-linking was demonstrated by the detection of unextractable DNA in irradiated cells. Fornace and Kohn (1976), using a sensitive alkaline elution assay, measured UV-induced DNA-protein cross-links in both normal and xeroderma pigmentosum human fibroblasts. They noted that normal cells exhibit a repair phase lacking in XP cells.

No *in vivo* data on DNA-protein cross-linking in mammalian skin, other than our preliminary work, have been reported. To study the possible role of the DNA-protein cross-links in epidermis, we focused on the isolation of chromatin from irradiated and nonirradiated guinea pig skin (Kornhauser et al., 1976; Kornhauser, 1976). The backs of guinea pigs were irradiated with a moderate physiological dose (80 mJ/cm^2; 290–350 nm) that corresponds to approximately four times the minimal erythema dose in an average fair-skinned Caucasian. Epidermis was obtained from both the irradiated and the control (nonirradiated) sites and was homogenized. Chromatin was isolated from the homogenates by using Sepharose B-4 and DEAE cellulose chromatography and density gradient centrifugation; its biological activity was determined by chemical methods and biological tests (Kornhauser et al., 1976).

A comparison of the sucrose gradient centrifugation profiles of the UV-irradiated epidermal chromatin and the nonirradiated epidermal DNA, including calf thymus DNA (molecular weight 1.3×10^6) as an internal standard, showed (1) a significant breakdown of the high-molecular-weight DNA fraction and the presence of low-molecular-weight DNA fragments on top of the sucrose gradient after UV-irradiation, and (2) an increment in the high-molecular-weight DNA 60 min after irradiation (the regeneration or repair phase).

We were able to obtain 4–5 mg extractable DNA free of protein from 1 g wet epidermal tissue. Immediately after UV irradiation, the yield of extractable DNA was reduced by 20–30%, presumably as a result of DNA-protein cross-linking and possibly of DNA strand breakage. The latter molecular lesion is consistent with previous findings (Zierenberg et al., 1971).

The results discussed above can be summarized as follows:

1. UV irradiation, at physiological doses (5 MED) of 290–350 nm, decreased the actual amount of dissociable chromosomal DNA by 20–30% as a result of cross-linking of DNA to protein and DNA strand breakage.
2. A comparison of corresponding elution profiles from Sepharose columns of dissociable DNA isolated from UV-irradiated and non-irradiated epidermal specimens indicated cross-linking of protein to DNA.
3. UV irradiation caused significant breakdown of the high-molecular-weight DNA that was isolated after irradiation.
4. In the regeneration phase, an active repair process was operating in the viable cells of the epidermis.

So far, no other evidence for the cellular repair of DNA-protein heteroadducts has been found *in vivo*. It is conceivable that cells exposed to light have evolved a repair system for eliminating this type of heteroadduct; this system is different from photoreactivation, which is specific for pyrimidine dimers (Setlow and Setlow, 1963).

All these findings suggest that UV radiation, even in moderate doses, can induce measurable alterations of the chromosomal material chromatin in mammalian skin. At present, it is not known what biochemical changes accompany light-induced lesions in chromatin. It is possible that damage by photons may alter such important chromatin functions as regulation of gene expression and/or steroid hormone receptor regulation. Thus further studies of lesions in chromatin are indispensable for a complete understanding of light-induced effects on cells.

Psoralen Phototoxicity

In addition to DNA-protein cross-linking, cross-links between DNA strands are possible. Because of the distance between bases in the DNA double helix, light-induced cross-linking without a bridging molecule (a drug, component of a cosmetic, etc.) is not observed. A very important class of cross-linking agents is the furocoumarins, whose derivatives are commonly called psoralens. The furocoumarins are a group of naturally occurring and synthetic substances that, when added to any of several biological systems and irradiated with UVA, produce various biological effects. These effects are not observed with either psoralens or light alone.

The photobiological reactions of furocoumarins with DNA have received widespread attention in recent years. On the molecular level, the following facts are known:

1. Psoralens intercalate into DNA—that is, slip in between adjacent base pairs—by forming molecular complexes involving weak chemical interactions ("dark reaction").

2. On UVA irradiation of such a system, *in vitro* or *in vivo*, covalent bond formation between a pyrimidine base and the furocoumarin molecule takes place (C_4 cycloaddition). Because of their structure, psoralens in this reaction can react either at their 3,4 double bond or at their corresponding 4′,5′ site, yielding monoadducts (in the former case the product is not fluorescent, and in the latter case it is).

3. On absorption of an additional photon, a further chemical reaction yielding a "cross-linked DNA" may take place. Thus psoralens can behave as photoreactive bifunctional agents, one molecule reacting with two pyrimidines in opposite strands of DNA. The structures of psoralen mono- and di-adducts with thymine are shown in Fig. 7. Figure 8 schematically shows DNA cross-linked by a psoralen molecule. The result is a cross-linked DNA in which the individual strands cannot be separated by standard denaturation conditions. Both types of lesions, the monofunctional adduct and the cross-linked product, can be repaired *in vivo* (Pathak and Kramer, 1969; Baden et al., 1972).

Dall'Acqua (1977) showed that the photoaddition of furocoumarins to DNA is not a random process. Specific sites exist in DNA for the photochemical interaction with psoralens; the sites that can be considered specific receptors for the photobiological activity of psoralens are represented by alternating sequences of adenine and thymine in each complementary strand

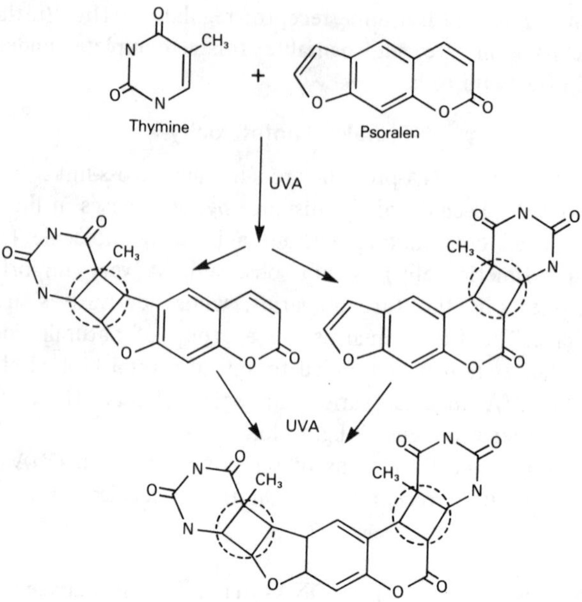

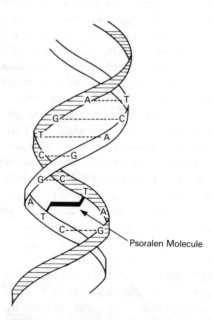

FIGURE 7 Photoaddition products of psoralen with thymine
after UV irradiation *in vitro*.

FIGURE 8 Schematic representation of
DNA cross-linked by a psoralen molecule.

of the polynucleotide. Psoralen has a greater photoreactivity toward thymine than it has toward cytosine. The receptor sites have a high capacity for intercalation and subsequent photoreaction with psoralens (Dall'Acqua, 1977).

The covalent addition of furocoumarins to DNA, particularly the cross-linking reaction, is usually believed to be responsible for the major effects of psoralen photosensitization. These include mutation and lethality in prokaryotic and eukaryotic systems, inhibition of DNA synthesis, sister chromatid exchange, and carcinogenesis. However, the relation between psoralen photoaddition to DNA and the appearance of erythema remains to be elucidated. Some very recent observations suggest a relation between erythema production and the ability of a compound to form $^1O_2$ (Pathak, 1982).

Structures of some furocoumarins and coumarins are shown in Fig. 9. The cutaneous photobiological activity of psoralens is highly dependent on structure. The ability to sensitize cutaneous tissue appears to be a unique characteristic of the psoralen ring system; for instance, pyranocoumarins, which have a similar linear tricyclic ring system, lack photosensitizing activity (Pathak, 1967). Furthermore, cutaneous phototoxicity is expressed only with linear derivatives; angular furocoumarins, such as angelicins, do not photo-sensitize mammalian skin (Dall'Acqua et al., 1981). The ability of linear furocoumarins to evoke phototoxicity appears to be concomitant with their ability to photosensitize the formation of $^1O_2$. Angular furocoumarins like angelicins, on the other hand, do not sensitize the formation of $^1O_2$ (de Mol, 1981) and are not phototoxic. This correlation between $^1O_2$ production and appearance of erythema suggests that $^1O_2$ may be a mediator in erythema produced by psoralens (Pathak, 1982). Unsubstituted psoralen exhibits the

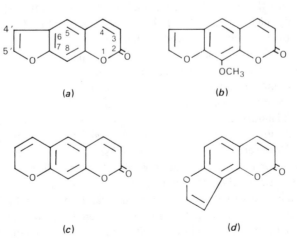

(a) (b)

(c) (d)

FIGURE 9 Structures of some furocoumarins and pyrano-coumarin: (*a*) psoralen; (*b*) 8-methoxypsoralen (8-MOP); (*c*) pyranocoumarin; (*d*) angelicin.

most severe phototoxicity. This photobiological activity is reduced by adding methyl (on carbon 3) or halogen substituents (Pathak, 1967).

Skin photosensitization is one of the most widely studied properties of furocoumarins. Several types of photodermatoses occur when skin comes into contact with plants or vegetable products and is later exposed to sunlight. Much less is known about potential adverse cutaneous effects after chronic ingestion of foods that contain furocoumarins, such as figs, limes, parsnips, and cloves (Pathak et al., 1974).

Although furocoumarins are potent phototoxic compounds, they are also used as therapeutic agents. Psoralen derivatives have been applied clinically to treat vitiligo (leukoderma) and increase the tolerance of human skin to solar radiation. A new clinical discipline, photochemotherapy (PCT), is increasingly being introduced to treat psoriasis and other skin disorders (Parrish et al., 1974; Wolff et al., 1976; Gilchrest et al., 1976).

PCT involves the interaction of light and orally administered drug in order to produce a beneficial effect. Psoralen PCT has entered medical terminology as PUVA (psoralen plus UVA). The PUVA regimen is effective, clean, and acceptable to patients. Some problems, however, persist; these include possible induction of cataracts (Cloud et al., 1960), hematologic effects (Friedmann and Rogers, 1980), alteration of the immune response (Strauss et al., 1980), skin aging (Bergfeld, 1977), and a possible increase of cutaneous cancers (Stern et al., 1979; Honigsmann et al., 1980).

The use of psoralens in PCT has raised some additional questions concerning their phototoxicity. The structurally similar psoralens 8-MOP, 5-MOP, and 4,5',8-trimethylpsoralen (TMP) have similar topical phototoxicity. However, when they are orally administered, the phototoxicity of TMP and 5-MOP is greatly diminished compared to that of 8-MOP (Mandula et al., 1976; Honigsmann et al., 1979). Recently, this has been exploited by two European teams, who introduced 5-MOP as an alternative to 8-MOP in the PCT of psoriasis (Honigsmann et al., 1979; Grupper and Berretti, 1981). While the clearing of psoriatic lesions was comparable with 5-MOP and 8-MOP, acute side effects (including phototoxicity) were significantly reduced in the 5-MOP regimen. As more has been learned about the biotransformations of psoralens (Mandula et al., 1976), it appears that metabolism may play a central role in determining the relative oral phototoxicity of substituted psoralens. However, it has not been established that reduced delivery of the phototoxic psoralen to the epidermis, due to metabolism or lack of absorption, is the basis for the observed differences in oral phototoxicity.

We have reported serum and epidermal levels of 5-MOP and 8-MOP (Giles et al., 1981). Determinations of psoralen levels in the epidermis, the primary target organ for phototoxicity, have not been reported for either humans or an animal model. For this study we chose a guinea pig model system that has been found by us and others (Harber, 1969) to be reliable for predicting phototoxicity in humans. Our results indicated that, after equivalent oral doses, metabolism and/or absorption constrain 5-MOP to lower epidermis levels than 8-MOP. Therefore, by orally administering 5-MOP it should be possible to maintain epidermal drug concentrations at lower levels than in an 8-MOP regimen.

Because psoralens, as used in PCT, react covalently with DNA, there is a potential risk of mutagenicity and oncogenicity. Indeed, in an *in vitro* study, 8-MOP and 5-MOP exhibited essentially the same activity in inducing chromosome damage in human cells (Natarajan et al., 1981). Furthermore, it was reported that topical 5-MOP combined with UVA induced carcinogenesis in mice comparable to that observed with 8-MOP (Zajdela and Bisagni, 1981). These two studies suggest that 5-MOP and 8-MOP have a similar oncogenic potential when topically administered.

Extrapolating our findings with orally dosed guinea pigs to clinical applications, we can say that a 5-MOP therapeutic regimen may minimize damage to epidermal DNA, reducing the risk of carcinogenesis which is suspected in 8-MOP PCT. For this reason, and because of the reduced acute side effects in a 5-MOP regimen, we feel that 5-MOP should be tested further, along with other psoralen derivatives, as an alternative to 8-MOP in PCT.

Photosensitized Oxidations

Many phototoxic compounds, such as porphyrins and dyes, affect biological substrates through photosensitized oxidations. These substances absorb light (long-wavelength UV and particularly visible) and sensitize photooxidization from their triplet excited states. Following excitation there are two distinct mechanisms (type I and type II) that result in photooxidation (Fig. 10).

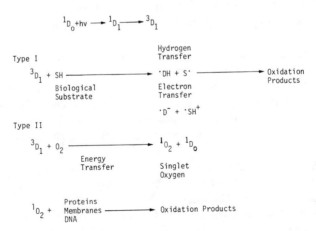

FIGURE 10 Mechanisms of photosensitized oxidation. The ground state sensitizer ($^1D_0$) is excited to the lowest excited singlet state ($^1D_1$) and undergoes intersystem crossing to the lowest excited triplet state ($^3D_1$).

Although opinion is divided, type II is probably the more common mechanism producing $^1O_2$, a highly reactive oxidizing agent. A unique feature of $^1O_2$ involvement in photodynamic action is the fact that the generation and reaction sites may be different, the diffusion range of $^1O_2$ in cytoplasm being on the order of 0.1 μm (Moan et al., 1979). In contrast, in the type I (radical) mechanism the sensitizer and substrate must be closer at the time of photon absorption. The major processes involving $^1O_2$ are photooxidative loss of histidine, methionine, tryptophan, tyrosine, and cysteine in proteins; photooxidation of guanine base in DNA; and formation of hydroperoxides with unsaturated lipids.

It has been recognized for decades that membrane damage plays a role in the photoinactivation of cells, especially in the presence of photodynamic sensitizers (Raab, 1900; Blum, 1941). The mechanism of cell membrane damage and disruption has been extensively studied for several photodynamic sensitizers. Photohemolysis of red blood cells sensitized by protoporphyrin (metal-free porphyrin) has been studied most extensively because in several porphyrias—diseases of abnormal porphyrin metabolism—the red cells contain unusually high levels of photosensitizing porphyrins. Oxygen is required for protoporphyrin-photosensitized red cell lysis. On the molecular level, it is known that $^1O_2$, formed by energy transfer from protoporphyrin triplet in red blood cell membranes, oxidizes unsaturated lipids (Lamola et al., 1973; Goldstein and Harber, 1972). Incorporation of cholesterol hydroperoxides, such as those formed in cholesterol photooxidation by protoporphyrin, leads to increased osmotic fragility and hemolysis of red blood cells (Lamola et al., 1973). Protoporphyrin has also been shown to photosensitize protein cross-linking in membranes (Verweij et al., 1981). It has been suggested that additional, more subtle, membrane functions, such as active transport of small molecules, are altered by membrane protein cross-linking (Kessel, 1977; Lamola and Doleiden, 1980).

Photooxidation of cell membrane components and proteins is not the only mode of photodynamic damage. Various photodynamic sensitizers were found to be mutagenic in bacterial (Gutter et al., 1977), yeast (Kobayashi and Ito, 1976), and mammalian cells (Gruener and Lockwood, 1979). Thus direct photodynamic damage to DNA is suspected, although alternative mechanisms for photodynamic mutagenesis have been proposed (Mukai and Goldstein, 1976).

There is evidence from *in vitro* studies that the bases in DNA, particularly guanosine, are oxidized by photodynamic dyes (Wacker et al., 1964). Photooxidation products of guanosine have been isolated and characterized (Cadet and Teoule, 1978). Further, photooxidation of guanosine has been found in bacteria (Wacker et al., 1964). The detailed mechanism of photooxidation of bases in DNA is not fully understood. When cells are in an environment containing a photodynamic active dye, such as porphyrins or toluidine blue, damage to DNA from $^1O_2$ might be expected to result from extracellular as well as intracellular dye. However, it has been found that toluidine blue, which is not taken up by cells, does not damage DNA (Ito and Kobayashi, 1977). Porphyrins, on the other hand, accumulate in cells and the efficiency of inducing DNA lesions follows the cellular uptake curve (Moan and Christensen, 1981). It is generally felt that accessibility of the sensitizing dye to DNA is a major factor determining photomutagenic potential.

Both type I and type II mechanisms have been proposed for the photooxidation of DNA. The major pathway will be determined by the structure of the photosensitizing compound, the extent and type of binding to DNA, the oxygen concentration, and the polarity of the cellular environment (Kochevar, 1981; Ito, 1978).

CELLULAR MEDIATORS INDUCED BY LIGHT

We have reviewed various sensitized and unsensitized light-induced reactions, such as pyrimidine dimer formation, DNA-protein cross-linking, and various photooxidations. It is still not known how these molecular events are involved in the complex physiological processes that give rise to erythema in sunburn or phototoxic reactions. Generally, a UV-induced effect in tissue may be a direct photon effect or may be mediated by diffusible substances induced by photons. Such substances include prostaglandins (PGs), histamines, kinins, lysosomal enzymes, activated oxygen species (e.g., $^1O_2$, superoxide radical).

PGs have dominated research in this area and have been implicated in many physiological processes. The almost ubiquitous occurrence of the PG synthetase enzyme system and the presence of its substrate fatty acids in membrane phospholipids of mammalian cells suggest that PGs can be formed in most types of cells, where they can act as intracellular messengers (Silver and Smith, 1975).

The role of PGs in cutaneous pathology and inflammation is well established (Goldyne, 1975). PGs were found in whole rat skin homogenates; when the epidermis was separated from the dermis, most of the PG activity was located in the epidermis. The realization that PGs are important in cellular control mechanisms has motivated a great deal of research on their possible role in the etiology of cancer (Snyder and Eaglstein, 1974).

A tentative pathway of PG formation and its interrelation with the adenylate cyclase system in cutaneous tissue after UV irradiation is shown in Fig. 11. Tissue (specifically membrane) damage, induced by light makes membrane phospholipids "accessible" to the enzyme phospholipase. This is the first step in inducing the arachidonic acid cascade, which results in PG production.

Prostaglandins E_2 (PGE_2) and F_2 (PGF_2) are produced in skin irradiated with UVB. PGE_2 is believed to play a part in the pathogenesis of UVB-induced tissue injury. This is supported by the observation that inhibitors of PG synthetase such as indomethacin and aspirin can suppress UVB-

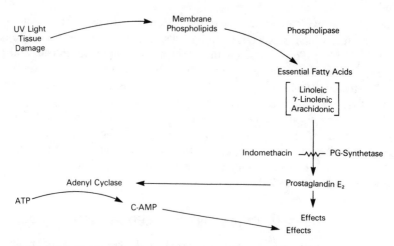

FIGURE 11 Tentative pathway of prostaglandin formation and its interrelation with the adenylate cyclase system in cutaneous tissue following UV irradiation.

induced erythema (Snyder and Eaglstein, 1974). On the other hand, erythema due to psoralen phototoxicity (PUVA) cannot be suppressed with indomethacin (Morison et al., 1977) and no increase in PG activity is found in exudate from PUVA-inflamed skin (Greaves, 1978). For these reasons, mediators other than PG are likely to be involved in the pathogenesis of PUVA-induced inflammation.

PGs are rapidly metabolized near the site of their synthesis, which increases the difficulty of studying their role in inflammation. A metabolite of PGE_2, 13,14-dehydro-15-keto-PGE_2 (PGE_2-M), is much more stable and accumulates in plasma, where it can be measured (Tashjian et al., 1977). The introduction of a specific assay for the measurement of PGE_2-M provides an opportunity to examine, in a relatively noninvasive manner, the systemic levels of PGE_2 after a single acute UV injury.

The systemic effect of UVB and PUVA on PGE_2 plasma levels has been investigated in a preliminary study of eight fair-skinned Caucasians. The subjects were divided into two groups. Four were exposed to whole-body UVB irradiation and four to whole-body PUVA irradiation. The aim was to produce the equivalent of a moderate sunburn over most of the body surface. For the PUVA subjects, a less aggressive approach was adopted. It was necessary to monitor the radiant exposure very carefully, since the dose-response curve for PUVA is steep and phototoxic burns are more painful and persistent than sunburns. Plasma samples were obtained from each subject at appropriate time intervals. Plasma PGE_2-M concentrations, including a pre-irradiation baseline for each subject, were determined by radioimmunoassay (Tashijian et al., 1977; White et al., 1982, personal communication).

It was found that plasma concentrations of PGE_2-M were increased significantly in the four subjects treated with UVB but not in any of the PUVA-treated subjects. This is consistent with data on the effects of indomethacin on PUVA-induced erythema (Morison et al., 1977). Animal studies with an increased dose of UVA could confirm these findings and give valuable information about the proposed different mechanisms of UVB and PUVA phototoxicity.

PHOTOIMMUNOLOGY

In a broad sense, immunology is the study of how and why the body reacts against anything that is foreign and how an organism can recognize the difference between self and nonself. That UV light can significantly influence the immune system is a very recent discovery.

The discipline of photoimmunology began with two important observations: (1) UVB induces suppression of contact dermatitis (hypersensitivity) in mice evoked by dinitrochlorobenzene or similar compounds, and (2) UV-induced alterations in immune functions are involved in the pathogenesis of photocarcinogenesis in mice (Kripke, 1980). UVB-induced tumors in mice are highly antigenic; they are immunologically rejected when transplanted into normal syngeneic recipients, but grow progressively in immunosuppressed animals. Subtumorigenic doses of UVB produce specific systemic alterations, which permit progressive growth of these highly antigenic tumors after transplantation.

The mechanism(s) of these reactions is far from understood. The available evidence suggests that both processes involve suppressor T lymphocytes that inhibit normal immunologic reaction (hypersensitivity, tumor rejection). UVB-mediated alteration of antigen processing cells (macrophages) has also been suggested (Kripke, 1980). The primary chromophore responsible for initiating events leading to alterations in the immune system is not known. A correlation of the action spectrum for UV-induced suppression of contact sensitivity with the absorption spectrum of components in the skin suggests that urocanic acid may play this role (DeFabo et al., 1981).

Evidence for the involvement of the immune system in the etiology of photocarcinogenesis in humans is not complete. It is possible that chronic exposure to UV causes nonspecific immunosuppression and thus leads to the development of light-induced skin tumors. Long-term clinical treatment with PUVA also induces immunosuppression (Morison et al., 1979), and this may be one of the mechanisms of PUVA-mediated carcinogenesis.

The immune system involves complex molecular and cellular interactions that are still poorly understood. However, even these fragmentary observations dramatically demonstrate the relevance of photobiology to dermatology and carcinogenesis. Furthermore, the studies also show that immunologic approaches will be important in extending basic knowledge and clinical treatments of various forms of cancer.

PHOTOTOXICITY TESTING

Because of the proliferation of topically applied compounds in use today, as both drugs and cosmetics, the need has arisen for a rapid and meaningful test for phototoxicity. To date, a uniform test method has not been established. Tests with human subjects are of unique value since they directly predict the clinical behavior of a compound, and several test protocols with human subjects are in use (Kligman and Breit, 1968; Harber et al., 1974). However, since total reliance on human testing is not practical, we briefly mention some alternative test methods.

Over the past 15 yr, the use of microbiological phototoxicity tests has increased. The Daniels test, employing the pathogenic yeast *Candida albicans*, is perhaps the best known example (Daniels, 1965). Although simple to perform, this test does not reliably predict the clinical phototoxicity of compounds such as sulfanilamide and demeclocycline (demethylchlortetra-cycline) (Daniels, 1965). A nonpathogenic yeast, *Candida utilis*, has been suggested as an alternative test organism (Kagen and Gabriel, 1980). Bacterial systems have also been studied (Ashwood-Smith et al., 1980; Harter et al., 1976).

Phototoxicity tests with animal model systems are potentially more predictive than those with simpler organisms. Several test systems are in use, mostly employing hairless mice (Forbes et al., 1976) and guinea pigs (Harber, 1969).

Table 3 shows the results of several comparative phototoxicity tests. We have also included results from the guinea pig model for phototoxicity in use in our laboratory (Giles et al., 1979). For a number of psoralens, the guinea pig model appears to accurately predict human phototoxicity. 5,7-Dimethoxy-coumarin (entry 8 in Table 3), which was reported to be lethal in a bacterial system (Harter et al., 1976), was found to be inactive in humans and guinea pigs (Giles et al., 1979). Carbethoxypsoralen (entry 3), a compound of potential therapeutic importance, was found to be weakly phototoxic in humans (Dubertret et al., 1978) and inactive in guinea pigs (Pathak et al., 1967). The sterically hindered psoralen derivatives (entries 3 and 4) and pyranocoumarins (entry 5) are new and their phototoxicity has not been completely tested.

5-Methylangelicin (entry 9) is an example of the angelicins being developed for potential use in photochemotherapy (Dall'Acqua et al., 1981). These compounds show strong photobiological activity, yet they do not provoke skin phototoxicity.

EPILOG

Since its beginning around the turn of the century, the science of photobiology has had various stages of development. At a very early stage, through the classical experiments by O. Raab and others, it was shown that

TABLE 3 Comparison of Phototoxicity of Selected Compounds in Different Organisms; Topical Phototoxicity Is Reported for Guinea Pigs and Humans

Compound	Human	Guinea pig	Bacteria
8-Methoxypsoralen	+	+	+
5-Methoxypsoralen	+	+	+
3-Carbethoxypsoralen	±	−	ND* Petite mutations in yeast
3-(α,α-Dimethylallyl) psoralen	ND	−	ND
Pyranocoumarins	ND	−	+ (*E. coli*)
Anthracene	+	+	+
6-Methycoumarin	(Photoallergic) −	−	ND
5,7-Dimethoxycoumarin	−	−	+ (*B. subtilis*)
5-Methylangelicin	−	−	+

*ND, not done.

many dyes and pigments can sensitize various cells and organisms to visible light. The introduction of phototherapy by Niels R. Finsen dates from the same period. These developments extended the boundaries of photobiology to physicists, biologists, and clinicians.

The past three decades marked the beginning of molecular photobiology;

an early milestone was the isolation of thymine dimers from living systems exposed to UV. The molecular basis of a genetic disease was established. The rapid expansion of molecular photobiology significantly contributed to the development of molecular biology and related disciplines and enabled the advent of a new clinical discipline, photochemotherapy.

One of the objectives of photobiology will be to shed more light on the relation between phototoxicity and photocarcinogenesis, which has been poorly established so far. It is still believed that chronic phototoxicity can lead to carcinogenesis. In at least a few cases, however, such as chronic phototoxicity evoked by anthracene or prophyrins, no carcinogenic developments were observed. A possible explanation for this phenomenon is that the primary targets of anthracene and other photodynamic sensitizers are molecules not directly involved in the transmission of genetic information.

One of the major conceptual advances in the field in the past few years is the perception that photon toxicity is not limited to skin; it can, and often does, induce significant systemic alterations. Therefore, the significance of photobiology greatly exceeds that of dermatology. Basic photobiology should become common knowledge in all branches of basic and clinical medicine.

In all civilizations humans have worshiped the sun. They have recognized that the sun is the most important of the factors that sustain life on the earth, and that many of our daily rhythms are dependent on the cycles of sunlight. We know today that sunlight is also one of the most potent carcinogens present in the environment. To survive the insult of photons, humans have evolved a group of defense mechanisms. These include keratinization (thickening of the stratum corneum), production of melanin (the most important protective pigment in skin), and synthesis of urocanic acid (an absorber of UV). The dietary pigment carotenoids also provide some protection by absorbing in the visible region and quenching singlet oxygen and various active radical species.

The protective mechanisms evolved against the detrimental effects of the sun are, in a growing number of cases, inadequate due to our modern life-styles. We must therefore increase our understanding of light-induced toxic reactions and judiciously use this knowledge to protect the public health.

REFERENCES

Allison, A. C., Magnus, I. A., and Young, M. R. 1966. Role of lysosomes and of cell membranes in photosensitization. *Nature (Lond.)* 209:874–878.
Anderson, R. R. and Parrish, J. A. 1981. The optics of skin. *J. Invest. Dermatol.* 77:13–19.
Ashwood-Smith, M. J., Poulton, G. A., Barker, M., and Midenberger, M. 1980. 5-Methoxypsoralen, an ingredient in several suntan preparations, has lethal mutagenic and clastogenic properties. *Nature (Lond.)* 285:407–409.
Baden, H. P. and Pathak, N. A. 1967. The metabolism and function of urocanic acid in skin. *J. Invest. Dermatol.* 48:11–17.

Baden, H. P., Parrington, J. M., Delhanty, J. D. A., and Pathak, M. A. 1972. DNA synthesis in normal and xeroderma pigmentosum fibroblasts following treatment with 8-methoxypsoralen and long wave ultraviolet light. *Biochim. Biophys. Acta* 262:247–255.

Beadle, P. C. and Burton, J. L. 1981. Absorption of ultraviolet radiation by skin surface lipid. *Br. J. Dermatol.* 104:549–551.

Bergfeld, W. F. 1977. Histopathologic changes in skin after photochemotherapy. *Cutis* 20:504–507.

Beukers, R. and Berends, W. 1960. Isolation and identification of the irradiation product of thymine. *Biochim. Biophys. Acta* 41:550–551.

Blackburn, G. M. and Taussig, P. E. 1975. The photocarcinogenicity of anthracene: Photochemical binding to deoxyribonucleic acid in tissue culture. *Biochem. J.* 149:289–291.

Blum, H. F. 1941. *Photodynamic Action and Diseases Caused by Light.* New York: Reinhold.

Bredberg, A., Lambert, B., Swanbeck, G., and Thyresson-Hok, M. 1977. The binding of 8-methoxypsoralen to nuclear DNA of UVA irradiated human fibroblasts *in vitro*. *Acta Derm. Venereol.* 57:389–391.

Cadet, J. and Teoule, R. 1978. Comparative study of oxidation of nucleic acid components by hydroxyl radicals, singlet oxygen and superoxide anion radicals. *Photochem. Photobiol.* 28:661–667.

Cleaver, J. E. and Trosko, J. E. 1970. Absence of excision of ultraviolet-induced cyclobutane dimers in xeroderma pigmentosum. *Photochem. Photobiol.* 11:547–550.

Cloud, T. M., Hakim, R., and Griffin, A. C. 1960. Photosensitization of the eye with methoxsalen. I. Chronic effects. *Arch. Ophthalmol.* 64:364–351.

Copeland, E. S., Alving, C. R., and Grenan, M. M. 1976. Light-induced leakage of spin label marker from liposomes in the presence of phototoxic phenothiazines. *Photochem. Photobiol.* 24:41–48.

Dall'Acqua, F. 1977. New chemical aspects of the photoreaction between psoralen and DNA. In *Research in Photobiology,* ed. A. Castellani, pp. 245–255. New York: Plenum.

Dall'Acqua, F., Vedaldi, D., Caffieri, S., Guiotto, A., Rodighiero, P., Baccichetti, F., Carlassare, F., and Bordin, F. 1981. New monofunctional reagents for DNA as possible agents for the photochemotherapy of psoriasis: Derivatives of 4,5'-dimethylangelicin. *J. Med. Chem.* 24:178–184.

D'Ambrosio, S. M., Whetstone, J. W., Slazinski, L., and Lowney, E. 1981. Photorepair of pyrimidine dimers in human skin *in vivo*. *Photochem. Photobiol.* 34:461–464.

Daniels, F. 1965. A simple microbiological method for demonstrating phototoxic compounds. *J. Invest. Dermatol.* 44:259–263.

Daniels, F., Jr., Brophy, D., and Lobitz, W. C., Jr. 1961. Histochemical responses of human skin following ultraviolet irradiation. *J. Invest. Dermatol.* 37:351–357.

Danno, K. and Horio, T. 1980. Histochemical staining of cells for sulphhydryl and disulphide groups: A time course study. *Br. J. Dermatol.* 102:535–539.

DeFabo, E. C., Noonan, F. P., and Kripke, M. L. 1981. An *in vivo* action spectrum for ultraviolet radiation-induced suppression of contact sensitivity in BALB/c mice. *9th Annu. Meet. Am. Soc. Photobiol. Program Abstr.* 185.

De Mol, N. J. and Beijersbergen van Henegouwen, G. M. J. 1981. Relation between some photobiological properties of furocoumarins and their extent of singlet oxygen production. *Photochem. Photobiol.* 33:815–819.

Dubertret, L., Averbeck, D., Zajdela, F., Bisagni, E., Moustacchi, E., Touraine, R., and Latarjet, R. 1978. Photochemotherapy (PUVA) of psoriasis using 3-carbethoxypsoralen, a noncarcinogenic compound in mice. *Br. J. Dermatol.* 101:379–389.

Everett, M. A., Yeargers, E., Sayre, R. M., and Olson, R. L. 1966. Penetration of epidermis by ultraviolet rays. *Photochem. Photobiol.* 5:533–542.

Fisher, G. J., Varghese, A. J., and John, H. E. 1974. Ultraviolet induced reactions of thymine and uracil in the presence of cysteine. *Photochem. Photobiol.* 20:109–120.

Fitzpatrick, T. B., Pathak, M. A., Harber, L. C., Seiji, M., and Kukita, A. 1974. An introduction to the problem of normal and abnormal responses of man's skin to solar radiation. In *Sunlight and Man*, eds. M. A. Pathak, L. C. Harber, M. Seiji, and A. Kukita, pp. 3–14. Tokyo: Univ. of Tokyo Press.

Forbes, P. D., Davies, R. E., and Urbach, F. 1976. Phototoxicity and photocarcinogenesis: Comparative effects of anthracene and 8-methoxypsoralen in the skin of mice. *Food Cosmet. Toxicol.* 14:303–306.

Fornace, A. J. and Kohn, K. W. 1976. DNA-protein cross-linking by ultraviolet radiation in normal human and xeroderma pigmentosum fibroblasts. *Biochim. Biophys. Acta* 435:95–103.

Friedman, P. S. and Rogers, S. 1980. Photochemotherapy of psoriasis: DNA damage in lymphocytes. *J. Invest. Dermatol.* 74:440–443.

Gilchrest, B., Parrish, J. A., Tannenbaum, L., Haynes, H., and Fitzpatrick, T. B. 1976. Oral methoxsalen photochemotherapy of mycosis fungoides. *Cancer (Philadelphia)* 38:683–689.

Giles, A., Tobin, P., and Kornhauser, A. 1979. 8-MOP and 5,7-dimethoxycoumarin (DMC) phototoxicity, oral vs. topical. *7th Annu. Meet. Am. Soc. Photobiol. Program Abstr.* 146.

Giles, A., Wamer, W., and Kornhauser, A. 1981. Comparison of 5-MOP and 8-MOP phototoxicity to their epidermal and blood levels in the guinea pig. *9th Annu. Meet. Am. Soc. Photobiol. Program Abstr.* 110.

Goldstein, B. D. and Harber, L. C. 1972. Erthropoietic protoporphyria: Lipid oxidation and red cell membrane damage associated with photochemolysis. *J. Clin. Invest.* 51:892–902.

Goldyne, M. E. 1975. Prostaglandins and cutaneous inflammation. *J. Invest. Dermatol.* 64:377–385.

Greaves, M. W. 1978. Does ultraviolet-evoked prostaglandin formation protect skin from actinic cancer? *Lancet* i:189.

Gruener, N. and Lockwood, M. P. 1979. Photodynamic mutagenicity in mammalian cells. *Biochem. Biophys. Res. Commun.* 90:460–465.

Grupper, C. and Berretti, B. 1981. 5-MOP in PUVA and RE-PUVA—a monocentric study: 250 patients with a follow-up of three years. Presented at the 3d International Symposium on Psoriasis, Stanford, Calif.

Gutter, B., Speck, W. T., and Rosenkranz, H. S. 1977. A study of the photoinduced mutagenicity of methylene blue. *Mutat. Res.* 44:177–182.

Harber, L. C. 1969. Use of guinea-pigs in photobiologic studies. In *The Biologic Effects of Ultraviolet Radiation*, ed. F. Urbach, pp. 291–295. New York: Pergamon.

Harber, L. C., Baer, R. L., and Bickers, D. R. 1974. Technique of evaluation of phototoxicity and photoallergy in biologic systems, including man, with particular emphasis on immunologic aspects. In *Sunlight and Man*, eds. M. A. Pathak, L. C. Harber, M. Seiji, and A. Kukita, pp. 515–528. Tokyo: Univ. of Tokyo Press.

Hart, R. W., Setlow, R. B., and Woodhead, A. D. 1977. Evidence that pyrimidine dimers in DNA can give rise to tumors. *Proc. Natl. Acad. Sci. U.S.A.* 74:5574–5578.

Harter, M. L., Felkner, I. C., and Song, P. S. 1976. Near-UV effects of 5,7-dimethoxycoumarin in *Bacillus subtilis. Photochem. Photobiol.* 24:491–493.

Hass, B. S. and Webb, R. B. 1981. Photodynamic effects of dyes on bacteria. *Mutat. Res.* 81:277–285.

Honigsmann, H., Jaschke, E., Gschnait, W. B., Fritsch, P., and Wolff, K. 1979. 5-Methoxypsoralen (Bergapten) in photochemotherapy of psoriasis. *Br. J. Dermatol.* 101:369–378.

Honigsmann, H., Wolf, K., Gschnait, F., Brenner, W., and Jaschke, E. 1980. Keratoses and nonmelanoma skin tumors in long-term photochemotherapy (PUVA). *J. Am. Acad. Dermatol.* 3:406–414.

Ito, T. 1978. Cellular and subcellular mechanisms of photodynamic action: The $^1O_2$ hypothesis as a driving force in recent research. *Photochem. Photobiol.* 28:493–508.

Ito, T. and Kobayashi, K. 1977. A survey of *in vivo* photodynamic activity of xanthenes, thiazines, and acridine in yeast cells. *Photochem. Photobiol.* 26:581–587.

Jori, G. and Spikes, J. D. 1982. Photosensitized oxidations in complex biological structures. In *Oxygen and Oxy-Radicals in Chemistry and Biology*, eds. M. A. J. Rodgers and E. L. Powers, pp. 441–457. New York: Academic.

Kagan, J. and Gabriel, R. 1980. *Candida utilis* as a convenient and safe substitute for the pathogenic yeast *C. albicans* in Daniel's phototoxicity test. *Experientia* 36:587–588.

Kantor, G. J., Sutherland, J. C., and Setlow, R. B. 1980. Action spectra for killing non-dividing normal human and xeroderma pigmentosum cells. *Photochem. Photobiol.* 31:459–464.

Kessel, D. 1977. Effects of photoactivated porphyrins at the cell surface of leukemia L1210 cells. *Biochemistry* 16:3443–3449.

Kligman, A. M. and Breit, R. 1968. The identification of phototoxic drugs by human assay. *J. Invest. Dermatol.* 51:90–99.

Kobayashi, K. and Ito, T. 1976. Further *in vivo* studies on the participation of singlet oxygen in the photodynamic inactivation and induction of genetic changes in *Saccharomyces cerevisiae. Photochem. Photobiol.* 23:21–28.

Kochevar, I. 1981. Phototoxicity mechanisms: Chlorpromazine photosensitized damage to DNA and cell membranes. *J. Invest. Dermatol.* 77:59–64.

Kornhauser, A. 1976. UV-induced DNA-protein cross-links *in vivo* and *in vitro. Photochem. Photobiol.* 23:457–460.

Kornhauser, A. and Pathak, M. A. 1972. Studies on the mechanism of the photosensitized dimerization of pyrimidines. *Z. Naturforsch. Teil B* 27:550–553.

Kornhauser, A., Burnett, J. B., and Szabo, G. 1974. Isotope effects in the photosensitized dimerization of pyrimidines. *Croat. Chem. Acta* 46:193–197.

Kornhauser, A. M., Pathak, M. A., Zimmermann, E., and Szabo, G. 1976. The *in vivo* effect of ultraviolet irradiation (290–350 nm) on epidermal chromatin. *Croat. Chem. Acta* 48:385–390.

Kripke, M. L. 1980. Immunologic effects of UV radiation and their role in photocarcinogenesis. *Photochem. Photobiol. Rev.* 5:257–292.

Lamola, A. A. 1968. Excited state precursors of thymine photodimers. *Photochem. Photobiol.* 7:619–632.

Lamola, A. A. and Doleiden, F. H. 1980. Cross linking of membrane proteins and protoporphyrin-sensitized photohemolysis. *Photochem. Photobiol.* 31:597–601.

Lamola, A. A., Yamane, T., and Trozzalo, A. M. 1973. Cholesterol hydroperoxide formation in red cell membranes and photochemolysis in erythropoietic protoporphyria. *Science* 179:1131–1133.

Maibach, H. I. and Kligman, A. M. 1960. Dihydroxyacetone: A suntan-simulating agent. *Arch. Dermatol.* 82:505–507.

Mandula, B. B., Pathak, M. A., and Dudek, G. 1976. Photochemotherapy: Identification of a metabolite of 4,5′,8-trimethylpsoralen. *Science* 193:1131–1134.

Mitchell, D. L. and Clarkson, J. M. 1981. The development of a radio-immunoassay for the detection of photoproducts in mammalian cell DNA. *Biochim. Biophys. Acta* 655:40–54.

Moan, J. and Christensen, T. 1981. Photodynamic effects on human cells exposed to light in the presence of hematoporphyrin. Localization of the active dye. *Cancer Lett.* 11:209–214.

Moan, J., Pettersen, E. O., and Christensen, T. 1979. The mechanism of photodynamic inactivation of human cells *in vitro* in the presence of haematoporphyrin. *Br. J. Cancer* 39:398–407.

Morison, W. L., Paul, B. S., and Parrish, J. A. 1977. The effects of indomethacin on long-wave ultraviolet-induced delayed erythema. *J. Invest. Dermatol.* 68:120–133.

Morison, W. L., Parrish, J. A., Block, K. J., and Krugler, J. I. 1979. Transient impairment of peripheral blood lymphocyte function during PUVA therapy. *Br. J. Dermatol.* 101:391–397.

Mukai, F. and Goldstein, B. 1976. Mutagenicity of malonaldehyde, a decomposition product of peroxidized polyunsaturated fatty acids. *Science* 191:868–869.

Natarajan, A. T., Verdegaal-Immerzeel, E. A. M., Elly, A. M., Ashwood-Smith, M. J., and Poulton, G. A. 1981. Chromosomal damage induced by furocoumarins and UVA in hamster and human cells including cells from patients with ataxia telangiectasia and xeroderma pigmentosum. *Mutat. Res.* 84:113–124.

Olson, R. L., Gaylor, J., and Everett, M. A. 1974. Ultraviolet-induced individual cell keratinization. *J. Cutan. Pathol.* 1:120–125.

Parrish, J. A. and Jaenicke, K. F. 1981. Action spectrum for phototherapy of psoriasis. *J. Invest. Dermatol.* 76:359–362.

Parrish, J. A., Fitzpatrick, T. B., Tannenbaum, L., and Pathak, M. 1974. Photochemotherapy of psoriasis with oral methoxsalen and long-wave ultraviolet light. *N. Engl. J. Med.* 291:1207–1122.

Parrish, J. A., White, H. A. D., and Pathak, M. A. 1979. Photomedicine. In *Dermatology in General Medicine*, eds. T. B. Fitzpatrick, A. Z. Eisen, K. Wolff, I. M. Freedberg, and K. F. Austen, pp. 942–994. New York: McGraw-Hill.

Pathak, M. A. 1967. Photobiology of melanogenesis: Biophysical aspects. In *Advances in Biology of Skin*, vol. 8, *The Pigmentary System*, eds. W. Montagna and F. Hu, pp. 400–419. New York: Pergamon.

Pathak, M. A. 1982. Molecular aspects of drug photosensitivity with special emphasis on psoralen photosensitization reaction. *J. Natl. Cancer Inst.*, in press.

Pathak, M. A. and Kramer, D. M. 1969. Photosensitization of skin *in vivo* by furocoumarins (psoralens). *Biochim. Biophys. Acta* 195:197–206.

Pathak, M. A., Worden, L. R., and Kaufman, K. D. 1967. Effect of structural alterations on the potency of furocoumarins (psoralens) and related compounds. *J. Invest. Dermatol.* 48:103–118.

Pathak, M. A., Kramer, D. M., and Gungerich, U. 1972. Formation of thymine dimers in mammalian skin by ultraviolet radiation *in vivo*. *Photochem. Photobiol.* 15:177–185.

Pathak, M. A., Kramer, D. M., and Fitzpatrick, T. B. 1974. Photobiology and photochemistry of furocoumarins (psoralens). In *Sunlight and Man*, eds. M. A. Pathak, L. C. Harber, M. Seiji, and A. Kukita, pp. 335–368. Tokyo: Univ. of Tokyo Press.

Pileni, M. and Santus, R. 1978. On the photosensitizing properties of *N*-formyl kynurenine and related compounds. *Photochem. Photobiol.* 28:525–529.

Poppe, W. and Grossweiner, L. I. 1975. Photodynamic sensitization by 8-methoxypsoralen via the singlet oxygen mechanism. *Photochem. Photobiol.* 22:217–219.

Raab, O. 1900. Uber die Wirkung Fluorescierender Stoffe auf Infusoriera. *Z. Biol.* 39:525–535.

Rosenstein, B. S. and Setlow, R. B. 1980. Photoreactivation of ICR 2A frog cells after exposure to monochromatic ultraviolet radiation in the 252–313 nm range. *Photochem. Photobiol.* 32:361–366.

Rothman, R. H. and Setlow, R. B. 1979. An action spectrum for cell killing and pyrimidine dimer formation in hamster V-79 cells. *Photochem. Photobiol.* 29:57–61.

Schenck, G. O. 1960. Selektivitat und typische Reaktions-mechanismen in der Stranlenchemie. *Z. Electrochem.* 64:997–1011.

Schott, H. N. and Shetlar, M. D. 1974. Photoaddition of amino acids to thymine. *Biochem. Biophys. Res. Commun.* 59:1112–1116.

Setlow, J. K. and Setlow, R. B. 1963. Nature of the photoreactivable ultra-violet lesion in deoxyribonucleic acid. *Nature (Lond.)* 197:560–562.

Shetlar, M. D., Schott, H. N., Martinson, H. G., and Lin, E. T. 1975. Formation of thymine-lysine adducts in irradiated DNA-lysine systems. *Biochem. Biophys. Res. Commun.* 66:88–93.

Silver, M. J. and Smith, J. B. 1975. Prostaglandins as intracellular messengers. *Life Sci.* 16:1635–1648.

Singh, H. and Vadasz, J. A. 1978. Singlet oxygen: A major reactive species in the furocoumarin photosensitized inactivation of *E. coli* ribosomes. *Photochem. Photobiol.* 28:539–546.

Smith, K. C. 1962. Dose-dependent decrease in extractability of DNA from bacteria following irradiation with ultraviolet light or with visible light plus dye. *Biochem. Biophys. Res. Commun.* 8:157–163.

Smith, K. C. 1974. Molecular changes in nucleic acids produced by ultraviolet and visible radiation. In *Sunlight and Man*, eds. M. A. Pathak, L. C.

Harber, M. Seiji, and A. Kukita, pp. 57–66. Tokyo: Univ. of Tokyo Press.

Snyder, D. S. and Eaglstein, W. H. 1974. Intradermal antiprostaglandin agents and sunburn. *J. Invest. Dermatol.* 62:47–50.

Soffen, G. A. and Blum, H. F. 1961. Quantitative measurements of cell changes following a single dose of ultraviolet light. *J. Cell. Comp. Physiol.* 58:81–96.

Spikes, J. D. 1975. Porphyrins and related compounds as photodynamic sensitizers. *Ann. N.Y. Acad. Sci.* 44:496–508.

Stern, R. S., Thibodeu, L. A., Kleinerman, R. A., Parrish, J. A., Fitzpatrick, T. B., and 22 Participating Investigators. 1979. Risk of cutaneous carcinoma in patients treated with oral methoxsalen photochemotherapy for psoriasis. *N. Engl. J. Med.* 300:809–813.

Strauss, G. H., Greaves, M., Price, M., Bridges, B. A., Hall-Smith, P., and Vella-Briffa, D. 1980. Inhibition of delayed hypersensitivity reaction in skin (DNCB test) by 8-methoxypsoralen photochemotherapy. *Lancet* ii:556–559.

Tashjian, A. H., Jr., Voelkel, E. F., and Levine, L. 1977. Plasma concentrations of 13,14-dihydro-15-keto-prostaglandin E_2 in rabbits bearing the VX_2 carcinoma: Effects of hydrocortisone and indomethacin. *Prostaglandins* 14:309–317.

Todd, P. and Han, A. 1976. UV-induced DNA to protein cross-linking in mammalian cells. In *Aging, Carcinogenesis, and Radiation Biology*, ed. K. C. Smith, pp. 83–104. New York: Plenum.

Turro, N. J. 1965. *Molecular Photochemistry.* Reading, Mass.: Benjamin.

Urbach, F, Epstein, J. H., and Forbes, P. D. 1974. Ultraviolet carcinogenesis: Experimental, global and genetic aspects. In *Sunlight and Man*, eds. M. A. Pathak, L. C. Harber, M. Seiji, and A. Kukita, pp. 259–283. Tokyo: Univ. of Tokyo Press.

Van de Vorst, A. and Lion, Y. 1976. Indirect EPR evidence for the production of singlet oxygen in the photosensitization of nucleic acid constituents by proflavine. *Z. Naturforsch.* 31C:203–204.

Verweij, H., Dubbelman, T., and Van Steveninck, J. 1981. Photodynamic protein cross-linking. *Biochim. Biophys. Acta* 647:87–84.

Wacker, A., Dellweg, H., and Weinblum, D. 1960. Strahlenchemische Veranderung der bakterien-Deoxyribonucleinsaure *in vivo. Naturwissenschaften* 47:477.

Wacker, A., Dellweg, H., Trager, L., Kornhauser, A., Lodenmann, E., Turk, G., Selzer, R., Chandra, P., and Ishimoto, M. 1964. Organic photochemistry of nucleic acids. *Photochem. Photobiol.* 3:369–395.

Wagner, S., Taylor, W. D., Keith, A., and Snipes, W. 1980. Effects of acridine plus near ultraviolet light on *Escherichia coli* membranes and DNA *in vivo. Photochem. Photobiol.* 32:771–780.

Wennersten, G. and Brunk, U. 1977. Cellular aspects of phototoxic reactions induced by kynurenic acid I. *Acta Derm. Venereol.* 57:201–209.

Wennersten, G. and Brunk, U. 1978. Cellular aspects of phototoxic reactions induced by kynurenic acid II. *Acta Derm. Venereol.* 58:297–305.

WHO. 1979. *Ultraviolet Radiation, Environmental Health Criteria 14,* p. 18. Geneva: World Health Organization.

Wolff, K., Fitzpatrick, T. B., Parrish, J. A., Gschnait, F., Gilchrest, B., Honigsmann, H., Pathak, M. A., and Tannenbaum, L. 1976. Photochemotherapy for psoriasis with orally administered methoxsalen. *Arch. Dermatol.* 112:943–950.

Woodcock, A. and Magnus, J. A. 1976. The sunburn cell in mouse skin: Preliminary quantitative studies on its production. *Br. J. Dermatol.* 95:459–468.

Young, A. R. and Magnus, I. A. 1981. An action spectrum for 8-MOP induced sunburn cells in mammalian epidermis. *Br. J. Dermatol.* 104:541–547.

Zajdela, F. and Bisagni, E. 1981. 5-Methoxypsoralen, the melanogenic additive in sun-tan preparations, is tumorigenic in mice exposed to 365 nm. UV radiation. *Carcinogenesis* 2:121–127.

Zierenberg, B. E., Kramer, D. M., Geisert, M. G., and Kirste, R. G. 1971. Effects of sensitized and unsensitized longwave UV-irradiation on the solution properties of DNA. *Photochem. Photobiol.* 14:515–520.

16

immunologically mediated contact photosensitivity in guinea pigs

Leonard C. Harber ■ Alan R. Shalita ■ Robert B. Armstrong

INTRODUCTION

Immunologically mediated contact photosensitivity reactions to simple chemicals used as drugs, cosmetics, and soaps and for other purposes have become an increasingly important medical and socioeconomic problem (J. H. Epstein, 1971). Their incidence has significantly increased during the last two decades. Not infrequently, the photodermatitis they produce may result in severe and disabling skin disease (Pathak and Epstein, 1971). An obligatory component of the photosensitivity reaction is that appropriate light exposure follows contact with the chemical.

Research in several laboratories in Europe and the United States has led to the development of the guinea pig as a reliable animal model for the study of immunologic reactions of the delayed hypersensitivity type in contact photosensitivity dermatitis (Harber and Shalita, 1975). To the best of our knowledge, no other animal species have been demonstrated to be suitable experimental models for the study of this process.

Contact photosensitivity reactions in both humans and guinea pigs are

This study was supported in part by grant ES01041-03 from the National Institute of Environmental Health Sciences.

mediated by at least one additional mechanism, called a phototoxic reaction. The similarities and differences between phototoxic and photoimmunologic mechanisms are summarized in Table 1 (Harber and Baer, 1972).

The phototoxic reaction can, in many respects, be considered analogous to a primary irritant reaction and may occur on first exposure. It requires no incubation period and is dependent on the concentration of the potential photosensitizer and the number of exciting photons (Harber and Baer, 1972). Phototoxic reactions are usually initiated by wavelengths corresponding to the absorption spectrum of the excited molecule and need not have immunologic properties. The existence of the phototoxic reaction was first demonstrated in paramecia (Raab, 1900), and since that time similar reactions have been documented in viruses, bacteria, fungi, erythrocytes, mice, rats, and rabbits (Spikes, 1968). The term "phototoxic" was first used in 1939 to describe the photosensitivity reaction to sulfanilamide in humans (S. Epstein, 1939). Later it was expanded to include other chemicals (S. Epstein, 1941). The term "phototoxicity," as presently used in contact photosensitivity, refers to all known photosensitivity reactions that do not involve an immunologic

TABLE 1 Comparison of Phototoxic and Photoimmunologic Reactions[a]

Reaction	Phototoxic	Photoimmunologic
Reaction possible on first exposure	Yes	No
Incubation period necessary first exposure	No	Yes
Chemical alteration of photosensitizer	No	Yes
Covalent binding with carrier	No	Yes
Clinical changes	Usually like sunburn	Varied morphology
Flares at distant previously involved sites possible	No	Yes
Persistent light reaction can develop	No	Yes
Cross-reactions to structurally related agents	Infrequent	Frequent
Broadening of cross-reactions following repeated photopatch testing	No	Possible
Concentration of drug necessary for reaction	High	Low
Incidence	Usually relatively high (theoretically 100%)	Usually very low (but theoretically could reach 100%)
Action spectrum	Usually similar to absorption	Usually higher wavelength than absorption spectrum
Passive transfer	No	Possible
Lymphocyte stimulation test	No	Possible
Macrophage migration inhibition test	No	Possible

[a]Harber and Baer, 1972.

mechanism. According to this definition, "photodynamic sensitization," used in numerous nonmammalian photosensitivity studies, is a subdivision of phototoxicity. Photodynamic reactions can be considered a type of photo-toxic reaction in which oxygen is required for occurrence of the reaction (Harber and Baer, 1972). However, it has been shown that not all phototoxic reactions require oxygen. For example, Matthews (1963) induced a phototoxic reaction to 8-methoxypsoralen in bacteria of the *Sacrina lutea* variety using a 100% nitrogen environment. To date, it has not been determined whether or not some photoimmunologic reactions may also occur in the absence of oxygen.

PHOTOTOXIC AND PHOTOIMMUNOLOGIC COMPOUNDS

Phototoxic and photoimmunologic compounds have several biochemical features in common. They both include, for the most part, di- and tricyclic resonating compounds that fluoresce. Their absorption spectrum is usually in the ultraviolet range, but may extend well into the visible light region. This is particularly true of organic dyes. To the best of our knowledge, all of the known reactions to topical phototoxic agents reported in humans can be reproduced in guinea pigs. There are, however, numerous other laboratory animals equally well suited for phototoxicity studies (Harber et al., 1974; Morikawa et al., 1974). The most commonly reported phototoxic agents noted in humans (Harber and Bickers, 1981) are the following:

Aminobenzoic acid derivatives
Anthraquinone dyes
Chlorothiazides
Chlorpromazine
Coal tar derivatives
    Anthracene
    Acidine
    Phenanthrene
    Pyrene
Nalidixic acid
Phenothiazine
Protriptyline
Psoralens
Sulfanilamide
Tetracyclines

The guinea pig is well suited for use in assaying these compounds.

The photoimmunologic chemicals most commonly noted in human (Harber and Bickers, 1981) are:

Aminobenzoic acids
Bithionol
Chlorpromazine (Thorazine)
Chlorpropamide (Diabinase)
Fentichlor
Halogenated salicylanilides
Jadit
6-Methylcoumarin
Musk ambrette
Promethazine (Phenergan)
Sulfanilamide
Thiazides

Most clinical and laboratory studies related to allergic contact photo-sensitivity have been based on Wilkinson's original observation that 3,3',4',5-tetrachlorosalicylanilide (TCSA), which was used as an antibacterial agent in soap, had a high photosensitizing potential in humans (Wilkinson, 1961). Other major contact photoimmunologic agents in humans include the di- and trihalogenated salicylanilides (Harber et al., 1967) and chemically related compounds such as bithionol (Jillson and Baughman, 1963), hexa-chlorophene, and trichlorocarbonalide (Harber et al., 1968). In Europe, Jadit (4-chloro-2-hydroxybenzoic acid N-n-butylamide), a topical antifungal agent, has also been associated with a high index of contact photosensitization (Fregert and Möller, 1964; Jung et al., 1968).

Guinea pigs have been an excellent model for studying the induction of photosensitivity to the halogenated salicylanilides with TCSA being the most extensively studied agent (Harber and Shalita, 1975; Herman and Sams, 1972). The major advantages of TCSA include its solubility, low cost, and high index of photosensitization.

Selected clinical studies in humans and guinea pigs appear to indicate that many compounds can be both phototoxic and photoallergic. Indeed most, if not all, of the agents reported as photoallergenic in humans can be shown to be phototoxic in guinea pigs if tested in sufficiently high concentration with appropriate wavelengths of exciting light. However, relatively few of the phototoxic compounds have induced photoallergy in humans (Harber and Baer, 1969).

CONTACT PHOTOSENSITIVITY TECHNIQUE

Guinea Pig Models of Photoallergic Contact Dermatitis

General. The major advantages of an animal model as compared to a human one for predicting photosensitivity include the ability to control more variables in a humane fashion. However, it is fully appreciated that the final phase of testing must occur in humans under actual usage conditions. When animals are used in the early test phases, it is possible to minimize the risk of engendering harmful reactions in humans such as persistent light reactors. While a variety of laboratory animals might be considered candidates (Harber et al., 1974; Morikawa et al., 1974), the guinea pig has been the most popular in the study of photoallergic contact dermatitis (Vinson and Borselli, 1966; Harber et al., 1981).[1]

The Hartley strain albino guinea pig is the one most commonly used for photobiologic studies. These animals are exceedingly well suited for investigating contact photosensitivity reactions of both the phototoxic and the photoimmunologic type, but one must also be aware of their limitations (Harber, 1969). To our knowledge, the term "Hartley" does not represent an inbred monitored genetic strain of albino guinea pigs, but is a name used by vendors who deliver mixed "pools" of animals from various breeders. It has been our impression that animals in the weight range 375–450 g are best suited for contact photosensitivity studies. The guinea pig, compared to other animals, is generally remarkably resistant to common cutaneous bacterial infections; however, it is highly susceptible to gastrointestinal disturbances.

Induction Technique

The general overall procedures described for inducing photoallergic contact dermatitis are similar. The nuchal hair is removed, an appropriate concentration of the substance to be evaluated is applied, and the nuchal area is then irradiated. Various modifications, noted in Table 2, may be attempted to increase the index of photosensitization of weakly antigenic compounds or to decrease the potential variability in the assay.

Studies indicate that the nuchal region of the guinea pig has a relatively lower threshold for erythema than the thoracic and lumbar areas (Morison et al., 1981). Accordingly, this site is usually avoided for elicitation but preferred for induction procedures.

Most of the nuchal hair is routinely shortened with ordinary hair clippers. The residual stubble can be removed with commercial depilatories. Unscented ones are desirable, since some fragrances are phototoxic (e.g., psoralens) and others may be photoallergens (e.g., musk ambrette). The possibility of such extraneous reactions should be excluded by use of appropriate control animals. Once the hair has been removed, photosensitization may be enhanced by further altering the nuchal induction site before applying the test compound and irradiation. Several options have been reported, as noted in Table 2. Sodium lauryl sulfate (20%) has been applied as a substitute for UVB irradiation (Horio, 1976). Cellophane tape stripping was

[1] Recent studies by M. Takagawa and Y. Myochi (University of Kyoto) indicate the feasibility of using inbred strains of mice (BALB/C, DCA/2, C3H, C57BL) for the induction of photoallergic contact dermatitis to TCSA, TBS, and bithionol.

TABLE 2 Modifications of the Induction Technique

Nuchal technique[a] (added factors)	Example of photosensitizer	Reference
Ultraviolet radiation (type B)	Halogenated salicylanilides	Morikawa et al., 1974; Harber et al., 1967; Herman and Sams, 1971; Griffith and Carter, 1968; Cripps and Etna, 1970
Sodium lauryl sulfate	Halogenated salicylanilides	Horio, 1976
Skin "stripping" with cellophane tape	Musk ambrette	Kochevar et al., 1979
Stripping plus id injection of Freund's adjuvant	Musk ambrette Methyl coumarin	Ichikawa et al., 1981 Harber et al., 1981

[a]These procedures precede irradiation of topically applied chemical with ultraviolet (type A) radiation (Harber, 1981).

shown to enhance the index of photosensitivity of animals being tested with both musk ambrette and 6-methylcoumarin (Kochevar, 1979). A postulated mechanism increased percutaneous penetration of the compound. Similarly, the index of photosensitization of these weaker photoallergens has been increased by id injection of Freund's complete adjuvant (0.1 ml in 4 sites at the perimeter of the nuchal induction site) with cellophane tape stripping (Ichikawa et al., 1981).

After the induction site has been prepared as described above, the compound to be tested is applied. It has proved convenient to use 0.1 to 0.5 ml of compound in concentrations of 1–10%. Acetone, ethanol, and water are commonly used vehicles. In general, there is little data about the time required for compounds to penetrate to a depth at which photosensitization can occur. Experimental evidence indicates that TCSA, one of the halogenated salicylanilides, penetrates throughout the epidermis within minutes and persists there for several days (Horio and Ofuji, 1974). Prior treatment by cellophane tape stripping would be expected to remove or substantially reduce any permeability barrier. Neither is there much data about the length of time most compounds will persist in adequate amounts before being removed or metabolically altered. Empirically, a 20- to 30-min wait before irradiation has proved adequate for the induction models cited here.

Ultraviolet radiation, the final step in the induction procedure, is routinely delivered by fluorescent tubes. This type of light source offers substantial advantages in convenience, reliability, and cost. Since compounds that have been used with animal models absorb in the range 320–400 nm (UVA), tubes with this spectral emission are used. If shorter wavelengths are to be excluded, a window glass or equivalent filter must be interposed to cut off the small quantities of UVB emitted by these tubes. The irradiance of the bank of fluorescent tubes should be measured with a photometer (International Light IL 600A research photometer) and the exposure time to deliver 10–30 J/cm^2 should be determined. In addition to the UVA, some procedures have employed UVB exposure during the induction phase. The doses used, ~6 J/cm^2, are sufficient to cause an intense erythematous reaction. The precise nature of the mechanism by which UVB facilitates an increased index of photosensitization is not known.

Three to five repetitions of the induction sequence are performed within 1–2 wk. A period of 2–3 wk is allowed for the photoimmune reaction to develop before attempting to elicit photosensitivity.

Elicitation procedure. The procedure for testing each animal for photoreactivity involves many of the same steps as the induction procedure. The hair is removed with clippers with or without depilatory; the test chemical is applied, in this case in duplicate to symmetrical sites. One of these test areas is then exposed to UVA radiation.

The nuchal area is avoided to minimize the possibility of false positive reactions, as this region, being more sensitive, might react nonspecifically. Instead, the thoracic and lumbar areas of the back are used for elicitation, as shown in Fig. 1. Preliminary studies must first be done in other animals to

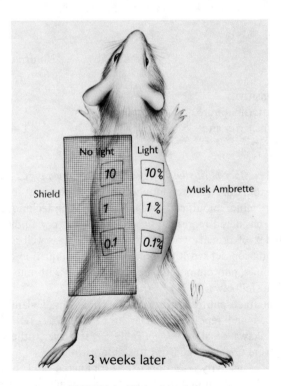

FIGURE 1 Elicitation phase.

ensure that at the concentration to be applied during the elicitation phase the compound is not a primary irritant or phototoxic agent. (Usually, 10 control animals giving negative results in the presence and absence of light at twice the highest test concentration provide a reasonable standard.) For example, phototoxic reactions have been noted in some animals treated with 2-4% TCSA before irradiation; accordingly, lower concentrations (e.g., 0.1-1.0%) should be used. The compound to be tested is always applied in duplicate to symmetrical sites. Volumes on the order of 0.2 ml are applied for each concentration tested. One site is irradiated to test for the photoallergic reaction. The other site is not irradiated and is covered with light opaque material. It serves as a control to test for contact allergic reactions. At 20-30 min after application of the potential photosensitizer, half the elicitation sites are exposed to 10 J/cm^2 UVA radiation. This light should be filtered to avoid the possibility of a misleading erythematous reaction to UVB. Experience with control animals indicates that guinea pigs do not have any detectable reaction following exposure to this dose of UVA radiation.

Scoring and interpretation of erythema. All test sites, both irradiated and nonirradiated, are scored and interpreted 24 h later. Scoring of data; 0, no erythema; 1, minimal but definite erythema; 2, moderate erythema; 3, considerable erythema; and 4, maximal erythema.

Interpretation of data:

	Irradiated		Nonirradiated
Normal	0		0
Contact photosensitivity	1-4		0
Contact sensitivity (nonphoto)	1-4	=	1-4
Contact photosensitivity and contact sensitivity	1-4	>	1-4

Results of contact photosensitivity studies in guinea pigs. Primary contact photosensitivity to TCSA has been induced in guinea pigs in at least six different laboratories with minor modifications of the preceding technique. Our data in Table 3 can be considered representative of the laboratory findings of others in terms of the index of primary contact photosensitivity as well as the percentage of animals showing contact sensitization alone or a combination of the two.

Table 4 shows photoimmunologic data elicited with musk ambrette and methyl coumarin (Ichikawa, 1981).

Primary contact photosensitization to tribromosalicylanilide (TBS) has also been induced and reported by Harber et al. (1967), Herman and Sams (1972) and Morikawa et al. (1974) (Table 5). However, others (Vinson and Borselli, 1966) were unable to confirm this observation.

Cross photosensitivity reactions to brominated and chlorinated sali-cylanilides have also been noted in studies by various investigators. Table 6 is a representative example. For reasons which remain unclear, it has been difficult

TABLE 3 Induction of Contact Photosensitivity
to TCSA in 65 Guinea Pigs[a]

Type of sensitivity	No. of animals sensitized
CS[b]	4
CPS[c]	20
CS and CPS	12

[a]Harber et al., 1967.
[b]CS, contact sensitivity.
[c]CPS, contact photosensitivity.

to induce primary photosensitivity with bithionol. The data in guinea pigs related to the contact photosensitivity of hexachlorophene is consistent in that although Harber et al. (1968) have found it to be a weak photosensitizer in selected guinea pig experiments, Morikawa et al. (1974), were unable to demonstrate contact or photocontact sensitization. Trichlorocarbanilide has also been reported to be non-photosensitizing in guinea pigs (Harber et al., 1968).

EVIDENCE FOR AN ALLERGIC MECHANISM

While the experimental induction of photoallergy in humans and in guinea pigs has shown all the clinical attributes of an allergic sensitization, it was necessary to obtain immunologic proof for an allergic mechanism as well. Our laboratory has presented data indicating a cell-mediated hypersensitivity by demonstrating passive transfer of contact photoallergy from actively

TABLE 4 Induction of Contact Photosensitivity
to Musk Ambrette and 6-Methyl Coumarin in Guinea Pigs

Concentration (%)	Percent with reaction after UVA[a] (10.2 J/cm²)				No UVA
	NR[b]	1+[c]	2+	3+	
Musk ambrette					
10.0	0	0	20	80	100
1.0	0	10	30	60	100
0.1	0	60	30	10	100
6-Methyl coumarin					
10.0	15	85	0	0	100
1.0	55	45	0	0	100
0.1	100	0	0	0	100

[a]UVA, ultraviolet light at 320–400 nm.
[b]NR, no reaction.
[c]North American Contact Dermatitis Group classification.

TABLE 5 Sensitization with Brominated Salicylanilides and Related Compounds[a,b]

	Contact sensitization				Photocontact sensitization			
Compound	No. of reactions	CS	PCS	CS and PCS	No. of reactions	CS	PCS	CS and PCS
3,4′,5-Tribromosalicylanilide (3,4′,5-TBS)	4/28	0	4	0	8/30	0	8	0
3,5-Dibromosalicylanilide (3,5-DBS)	4/18	0	4	0	14/19	0	14	0
4′,5-Dibromosalicylanilide (4′,5-DBS)	12/34	0	8	4	18/36	2	15	1
3-Monobromosalicylanilide (3-MBS)	0/10	0	0	0	7/10	0	4	3
5-Monobromosalicylanilide (5-MBS)	0/20	0	0	0	5/20	0	5	0
4′-Monobromosalicylanilide	10/30	2	8	0	14/30	1	11	2
Salicylanilide	0/10	0	0	0	0/10	0	0	0

[a]Morikawa et al., 1974.

[b]All materials were tested in 0.1% concentration in acetone. Reactions were scored as follows: PCS = photocontact sensitivity only, CS = contact sensitivity only, CS and PCS = contact and photocontact sensitivity but with photocontact sensitivity being the greater.

sensitized to nonsensitized guinea pigs, using a modification of the technique described by Landsteiner and Chase (1942). Passive transfer was successful in three out of five experiments (Harber and Baer, 1969). The procedure involved the collection of mononuclear peritoneal exudate cells from guinea pigs with contact photosensitization to TCSA. These cells were then injected intraperitoneally into nonsensitive guinea pigs. The passively sensitized guinea pigs were demonstrated to be photoallergic to TCSA when challenged with TCSA and light 24 h later. Exposure to TCSA or light alone evoked no response.

Additional experimental evidence in support of a conventional delayed hypersensitivity mechanism includes the *in vitro* demonstration by Jung et al. (1968) of lymphocyte transformation of cells from patients sensitive to Jadit (buclosamide). This could be achieved with a light-induced buclosamide-albumin complex, but not with buclosamide alone. These findings have received further support from an *in vitro* experiment of Herman and Sams (1970), who investigated the problem of carrier specificity in TCSA photoallergy. They showed a positive macrophage inhibition response; that is, the migration in tissue culture of sensitized cells from contact photoallergic guinea pigs was 90% inhibited by an *in vitro*-prepared TCSA-albumin conjugate, as compared to 17% inhibition with TCSA alone and 20% inhibition with albumin alone. These findings suggest an important role for the protein carrier in contact photoallergy.

An excellent comprehensive review of photoimmunologic studies in both laboratory animals and humans has been published by Herman and Sams (1972). The major thrust of their own basic science studies as well as those summarized by Harber and Baer (1972) is that contact photosensitivity is a cell-mediated type of hypersensitivity. As in other types of delayed hypersensitivity, the following can be demonstrated: (1) induction in guinea pigs, (2) passive transfer of hypersensitivity, (3) macrophage inhibition, (4) lymphocyte stimulation, and (5) induction in humans (Willis and Kligman, 1968).

The hapten-carrier protein binding sites have not yet been biochemically determined for either the photocontact allergens or the contact allergens under discussion here. We speculated previously (Harber et al., 1966), on the basis of studies by Coxon et al. (1965), that in the photoimmunologic reaction to TCSA, the complete photoantigen is formed by union of the carrier protein with the available site at the 3-carbon position of the benzoic acid nucleus of the halogenated salicylanilide. This hypothesis (Fig. 2) seems

TABLE 6 Cross Photosensitivity of Related Compounds in Guinea Pigs Photosensitized to TCSA[a]

Compound[b]	No. of reactions to challenge
3',4',5'-Trichlorosalicylanilide	12/30
3,5-Dichlorosalicylanilide	2/10
3',4'-Dichlorosalicylanilide	8/35
3-Monochlorosalicylanilide	Not done
5-Monochlorosalicylanilide	2/10
3'-Monochlorosalicylanilide	2/15
4'-Monochlorosalicylanilide	1/10
3,4',5-Tribromosalicylanilide	8/14
3,5-Dibromosalicylanilide	2/14
4'5-Dibromosalicylanilide	4/14
3-Monobromosalicylanilide	Not done
5-Monobromosalicylanilide	1/10
4'-Monobromosalicylanilide	3/10
Salicylanilide	3/10
Bithionol	0/13
Fenticlor	0/18
Hexachlorophene	0/13
Dichlorophene	0/8
Irgasan CF3	0/8
Irgasan DP-300	0/10
TCC	0/10

[a]Morikawa et al., 1974.
[b]All materials were tested in 0.1% concentration in acetone.

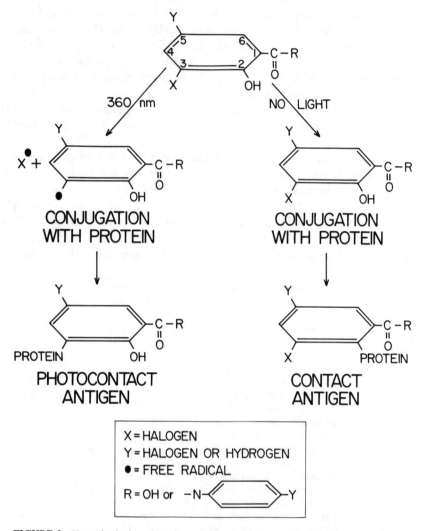

FIGURE 2 Hypothetical explanation of the mechanism involved in the production of photocontact and contact dermatitis with halogenated salicylanilides (Harber and Shalita, 1975).

attractive since a highly reactive free radical site in this position has been demonstrated to occur following the homolytic cleavage of the carbon-halogen bond after excitation with 360 nm radiation (Coxon et al., 1965).

In contrast, one would postulate, on a biochemical basis, that in the absence of light the most likely union between the halogenated salicylanilide and the carrier protein would occur at the OH group on the 2-carbon or, less likely, at the carbonyl group bridging the two aromatic rings. Other possibilities include a stable photooxidation product (Schwartz, 1969) or increased hapten-carrier protein binding (Sulzer, 1962).

FACTORS INFLUENCING CONTACT PHOTOSENSITIZATION

Among the many other factors that influence the occurrence of contact photosensitization are the clinical conditions prevailing in the skin at each particular site and particular time. These include: (1) the quantity and location of photosensitizer present in or on the skin; (2) the capacity of the photosensitizer to normally penetrate the skin through percutaneous absorption, as well as under conditions contributing to trauma, such as maceration and sunburn; (3) the pH, enzymes (such as hydrolytic peptidases and catalases), and solubility conditions at the site of exposure; (4) the quantity of activating radiation to which the skin is exposed; (5) the capacity of the spectral range that activated the photosensitizer to penetrate the skin; (6) the ambient temperature and humidity; (7) the thickness of the horny layer; (8) the degree of melanin pigmentation; and (9) the immunologic state of the affected laboratory animal or person.

With respect to the activating radiation, the action spectra of all known contact photosensitivity reactions of the immunologic type occur with wavelengths greater than 320 nm. It must be remembered that the stratum corneum permits more long UV (320–400 nm) than short UV (285–320 nm) to pass through. In addition, the vast majority of solar radiation in the UV is composed of wavelengths greater than 320 nm. Thus, the prickle cell layers are reached by relatively little short UV, in contrast to long UV and visible light, and the dermis is affected similarly.

SUMMARY

Morikawa (1972) has attempted to summarize the correlation between immunologic data obtained from patch tests in humans and data noted in various animal models. He listed numerous variables, which are summarized below:

1. Biological factors
   (a) Species
   (b) Strain
   (c) Age
   (d) Sex
   (e) Site
   (f) Hair cycle
2. Physicochemical factors
   (a) Purity

    (b) Dose
    (c) Concentration
    (d) Vehicle and solvent
    (e) pH
    (f) pK_a value
    (g) Partition coefficient
    (h) Viscosity
    (i) Polarity
    (j) Chemical structure
    (k) Light source
    (l) Energy (dose, intensity)
   (m) Wavelength

3. Environmental factors
    (a) Climatic environment, season, temperature, humidity, sunshine
    (b) Geographical environment
    (c) Sociological environment
    (d) Biological environment
    (e) Nutritional environment
    (f) Chemical environment

4. Application
    (a) Route
    (b) Area
    (c) Number
    (d) Duration
    (e) Observation time
    (f) Treatment
    (g) Closed or open, abrasion removal

5. Immunological factors

Under varied conditions with different agents each of these may have to be considered in assessing contact photosensitivity responses. Although this may seem a formidable task, it does appear that there are sufficient data available to make the following generalizations:

1. The guinea pig is at present the laboratory animal of choice for studying delayed hypersensitivity reactions mediating contact photosensitivity dermatitis.

2. In general, there is a correlation between the ability to induce contact photosensitivity of the phototoxic and photoimmunologic types in both humans and guinea pigs.

3. Use of laboratory animals as a predictive model for contact

photosensitization in humans appears to be warranted as a rapid screening procedure before studies in humans are initiated.

REFERENCES

Coxon, J. A., Jenkins, F. P. and Welti, D. 1965. The effect of light on halogenated salicylanilide ions. *Photochem. Photobiol.* 4:713.

Cripps, D. J. and Enta, T. 1970. Absorption and action spectra studies on bithionol and halogenated salicylanilide photosensitivity. *Br. J. Dermatol.* 82:230–242.

Epstein, J. H. 1971. Adverse cutaneous reactions to the sun. In *Year book of dermatology*, eds. F. D. Malkinson and R. W. Pearson, pp. 5–43. Chicago: Year Book Medical Publishers.

Epstein, S. 1939. Photoallergy and primary phototoxicity to sulfanilamide. *J. Invest. Dermatol.* 2:243.

Epstein, S. 1941. Photoallergy and primary photosensitivity to sulfanilamide. *Dermatologica* 83:63.

Fregert, S. and Möller, H. 1964. Photo cross-sensitization amongst halogen-hydroxybenzoic acid derivatives. *J. Invest. Dermatol.* 43:271.

Griffith, J. and Carter, R. O. 1968. Patterns of photoreactivity and cross reactivity in persons sensitive to TCSA. *Toxicol. Appl. Pharmacol.* 12:304–309.

Harber, L. C. 1969. Use of guinea pigs in photobiologic studies. In *The biologic effects of ultraviolet radiation*, ed. F. Urbach, pp. 291–299. Oxford: Pergamon.

Harber, L. C. and Baer, R. L. 1969. Mechanisms of drug photosensitivity reactions. *Toxicol. Appl. Pharmacol.* 3:58.

Harber, L. C. and Baer, R. L. 1972. Pathogenic mechanisms of drug-induced photosensitivity. *J. Invest. Dermatol.* 58:327.

Harber, L. C. and Bickers, D. R. 1981. *Photosensitivities: Principles of Diagnosis and Treatment*. Philadelphia: Saunders.

Harber, L. C. and Shalita, A. R. 1975. The guinea pig as an effective model for the demonstration of immunologically mediated contact photosensitivity. In *Animal models in dermatology*, ed. H. Maibach, pp. 90–102. New York: Churchill Livingstone.

Harber, L. C., Harris, H. and Baer, R. L. 1966. Photoallergic contact dermatitis. *Arch. Dermatol.* 94:255.

Harber, L. C. Targovnik, S. E. and Baer, R. L. 1967. Contact photosensitivity patterns to halogenated salicylanilides in man and guinea pigs. *Arch. Dermatol.* 96:646.

Harber, L. C., Targovnik, S. E. and Baer, R. L. 1968. Studies on contact photosensitivity to hexachlorophene and trichlorocarbanilide in guinea pigs and man. *J. Invest. Dermatol.* 51:373.

Harber, L. C., Baer, R. L. and Bickers, D. R. 1974. Techniques of evaluation of phototoxicity and photoallergy in biologic systems, including man, with particular emphasis on immunologic aspects. In *Sunlight and man*, ed. T. B. Fitzpatrick, pp. 515–528. Tokyo: Univ. of Tokyo Press.

Harber, L. C., Armstrong, R. B., Walther, R. R., and Ichikawa, H. 1982. Current status of predictive animals for drug photoallergy and their correlation with humans. In *Assessment of Safety and Efficacy of Topical Drugs and Cosmetics,* eds. A. Kligman and J. Leyden. New York: Grune & Stratton.

Herman, P. S. and Sams, W. M., Jr. 1970. Carrier protein specificity in salicylanilide sensitivity. *J. Invest. Dermatol.* 54:438.

Herman, P. S. and Sams, W. M., Jr. 1971. Requirement for carrier protein in salicylanilide sensitivity: The migration-inhibition test in contact photoallergy. *J. Lab. Clin. Med.* 77:572–579.

Herman, P. S. and Sams, W. M., Jr., 1972. *Soap photodermatitis.* Springfield, Ill.: Thomas.

Horio, T. 1976. The induction of photocontact sensitivity in guinea pigs without UVB radiation. *J. Invest. Dermatol.* 67:591–593.

Horio, T. and Ofuji, S. 1974. Distribution of fluorescent halogenated salicylanilides in guinea pig skin following topical application. *J. Invest. Dermatol.* 63:415–418.

Ichikawa, H., Armstrong, R. B., and Harber, L. C. 1981. Photoallergic contact dermatitis in guinea pigs: Improved induction technique using Freund's complete adjuvant. *J. Invest. Dermatol.* 76:498–501.

Jillson, O. F. and Baughman, R. D. 1963. Contact photodermatitis from bithionol. *Arch. Dermatol.* 88:409.

Jung, E. G., Hornke, J. and Hajou, P. 1968. Photoallergie durch 4-Chlor-2-hydroxy-benzoesauer-N-butylamid. *Arch. Klin. Exp. Dermatol.* 233:287.

Kochevar, I. E., Zalar, G. L., Einbinder, J., and Harber, L. C. 1979. Assay of contact photosensitivity to musk ambrette in guinea pigs. *J. Invest. Dermatol.* 73:144–146.

Landsteiner, K. and Chase, M. W. 1942. Experiments on transfer of cutaneous sensitivity to simple compounds. *Proc. Soc. Exp. Biol. Med.* 49:688.

Matthews, M. M. 1963. Comparative study of lethal photosensitization of *Sarcina lutea* by 8-methoxypsoralen and by toluidine blue. *J. Bacteriol.* 85:322.

Morikawa, F. 1972. Correlation between contact photosensitivity data obtained from man and laboratory animals. *Jap. J. Dermatol. Ser. A* 82:794.

Morikawa, F., Nakayama, Y., Fukada, M., Hamano, M., Yokoyama, Y., Nagura, T., Ishihara, M. and Toda, K. 1974. Techniques for evaluation of phototoxicity and photoallergy in laboratory animals and man. In *Sunlight and man*, ed. T. B. Fitzpatrick, pp. 529–557. Tokyo: Univ. of Tokyo Press.

Morison, W. L., Parrish, J. A., Anderson, R. R., and Harris, T. J. 1981. Variations in the erythemal response of guinea pig skin. *Photochem. Photobiol.* 33:283.

Pathak, M. A. and Epstein, J. H. 1971. Normal and abnormal reactions of man to light. In *Dermatology in general medicine*, eds. T. Fitzpatrick et al., p. 1020. New York: McGraw-Hill.

Raab, O. 1900. Ueber die Wirkung fluorescinder Stoffe auf Infusorien. *Z. Biol.* 39:524.

Schwartz, J. J. 1969. Experimentelle Untersuchung zur Photoallergie gegen Sulfanilamid und Chlorpromazine. *Dermatologica Suppl.* 1:139.

Spikes, J. D. 1968. Photodynamic action. In *Photophysiology*, vol. 3, ed. E. Giese. New York: Academic Press.

Sulzer, H. 1962. Photochemische Keysplung des Sulfanilamides und aromatische Amine an Eiweiss und andere hachmolekulare Verbindungen. *Arch. Klin. Exp. Dermatol.* 215:266.

Vinson, L. and Borselli, V. F. 1966. A guinea pig assay of the photosensitizing potential of topical germicides. *J. Soc. Cosmet. Chem.* 17:123.

Wilkinson, D. S. 1961. Photodermatitis due to tetrachlorosalicylanilide. *Br. J. Dermatol.* 73:213.

Willis, I. and Kligman, A. M. 1968. The mechanism of photoallergic contact dermatitis. *J. Invest. Dermatol.* 51:378.

17

phototoxicity (photoirritation) of topical and systemic agents

Howard I. Maibach ▪ Francis N. Marzulli

INTRODUCTION

Photosensitivity encompasses both allergic (photoallergy) and nonallergic (phototoxicity) light-related skin responses. Photoallergy is the light-induced counterpart of contact allergy, whereas phototoxicity is the light-induced counterpart of irritation (primary irritation). The phototoxic skin response is likened to an exaggerated sunburn and is characterized by its nonimmunologic nature; the causative photochemical is usually activated by wavelengths longer than 320 nm; the absorption spectrum and the action spectrum of the photoactive chemical are in the same general range.

The photoactive chemical may reach the skin by external application or indirectly via the blood stream after ingestion or parenteral administration. When administered either way—topically or systemically—the chemical may require chemical transformation before it becomes photoactive. Little information is available as to how often metabolic or other chemical transformation is required.

Any discussion of experimental data on phototoxicity must take into consideration the criteria required for making the diagnosis or statement. Until recently there was some confusion as to the selection of suitable methods for producing phototoxicity in animals or humans. Even now, there is a lack of uniformity in testing. Certain criteria appear a necessary minimum in such testing. The first is that adequate controls must be used to ascertain that the response noted is due to the light-activated chemical and not to the light source itself or to an unrelated toxic effect of the chemical. This is especially relevant in obtaining the minimal erythema dose (MED) with and without drug. The minimal erythema dose between subjects may vary considerably depending on recent ultraviolet light exposure, skin color, and other factors. Caution must be exercised, therefore, when stating that a chemical did or did not alter the minimal erythema dose. A second major criterion consists in discerning that the light source is of suitable spectral output to activate the chemical tested (usually > 320 nm) and at least 3,000 $\mu W/cm^2$ at a distance of 10 cm from the source. One must consider whether the demonstration of the potential for phototoxicity itself—in any experimental system—means that phototoxicity will occur in humans under the intended conditions of use. The last point in the work-up is needed to understand why phototoxic reactions occur in some but not all people. It is this situation that led investigators to falsely consider certain phototoxic reactions allergic rather than toxic. Control over factors such as skin penetration and skin contact time prior to light exposure may be involved in these response differences.

PHOTOTOXIC AGENTS

Psoralens such as xanthotoxin (8-methoxypsoralen or 8-MOP) and bergapten (5-methoxypsoralen) are among the more commonly encountered phototoxic agents. They are the furocoumarin components of plants long used for their pharmacologic or perfume properties.

Although most purified psoralens are currently produced from plant sources, it is likely that synthetic materials will become available in the future to meet the growing needs of those involved in the treatment of dermatologic disease (psoriasis and vitiligo).

Bergapten is the active component of bergamot oil, a well-known perfume ingredient, whose phototoxic skin effects have been accorded the name berlock dermatitis. Phototoxic dermatitis from this chemical was studied in considerable detail by Marzulli and Maibach (1970). On the basis of these studies, it was suggested that perfumes should contain no more than 0.3% bergamot, which is equivalent to about 0.001% bergapten, to avoid phototoxicity. This study also established that bergapten alone was responsible for phototoxic effects of the parent material in either animals or humans. Another component of bergamot, limettin (5,7-dimethoxycoumarin), although more intensely fluorescent than bergapten, did not prove to be phototoxic.

Not long ago, certain members of the cosmetics industry in the United States advised that bergapten be reduced or removed from fragrances and cosmetics (RIFM). This recommendation, which was based on the fact that bergapten is phototoxic in low concentrations in animals and humans (Marzulli and Maibach, 1970), appears to have been adopted.

This raises an important practical and philosophical issue. Should a cosmetic ingredient demonstrating a significant toxic potential such as bergamot be considered unacceptable, or can we in fact consider that there may be a suitable concentration for safe use? This is a complex issue requiring resolution. It may be imprudent to make premature dogmatic decisions in such areas, because this leads to precedents that may be difficult to deal with in the future. It is likely that some concentration of bergapten is indeed tolerated by all individuals and that there are conditions of use that may indeed be acceptable. The safety record of bergamot with and without bergapten will have to be observed over a period of time to clarify this point. As bergapten is not used in perfumes marketed in the United States and is used in other parts of the world, it might now be possible to answer this question.

Xanthotoxin (8-MOP) is the active ingredient of a drug marketed for the treatment of vitiligo. It produces skin effects, both by topical application and by oral ingestion following skin exposure to ultraviolet (UV) light irradiation. Psoralens have been used orally in crude form in Egypt since ancient times (El Mofty, 1948). Impetus for their use in this country in the treatment of vitiligo was provided in large part by the work of Lerner et al. (1953). Studies of Parrish et al. (1974) suggested that xanthotoxin is efficacious in the treatment of psoriasis. It is given orally or topically followed by ultraviolet light at large doses of UV-A (320-400 nm irradiation). What remains to be determined is the long-term human toxicity, in terms of years to a lifetime, as the drug is given for maintenance as well as initial clearing.

For some time now, investigators in this country and abroad have been applying the known capacity of psoralens to inhibit epidermal DNA synthesis in the presence of UV (Bay et al., 1970; Breza et al., 1975) to the treatment of psoriasis. A systematic evaluation under the leadership of T. Fitzpatrick, Harvard University Department of Dermatology, has involved a study of oral methoxsalen phototherapy (PUVA) at 16 selected dermatologic centers in the United States with FDA approval. Very early, PUVA was shown to be effective; however, short- and long-term concerns and different dosage regimens delayed approval by the FDA. Burning from overexposure, nausea from oral methoxsalen, and more serious consequences from the photo-carcinogenic potential of this therapy were prominent concerns. On September 21, 1981, the FDA Dermatology Advisory Committee recommended approval, with labeling for patient and physician. A commitment for follow-up human studies was also required.

Briefly stated, the photochemotherapy program is as follows. Oral methoxsalen plus UV is used on selected patients with serious psoriasis (plaquelike, pustular, or erythrodermic) covering 30% or more of the body surface. A 70 kg subject is treated two or three times each week. He receives 40 mg capsules at each treatment for up to 30 treatments, and is exposed to UV in a special cylindrical chamber 2-3 hr after taking the capsule. The intensity of UV-A (320-400 nm) is constant and duration is adjusted according to the patient's capacity for burn; that is, sufficient to produce and maintain moderate edema. Goggles are worn and eyes closed for cataract protection during treatment. Side effects may include nausea, pruritus, and severe erythema. Other reported side effects include gastric irritation, nervousness, insomnia, and depression (Emmett, 1974). Patients may use sunscreens and wear sunglasses during treatment days. An eye examination is conducted prior to therapy and at 3 months and 1 yr after the study. Maintenance therapy follows (up to one treatment per week). Pregnant patients and those with aphakia, as well as patients on systemic cytotoxic agents or topical medications, are excluded.

Coal tar derivatives constitute another important group of phototoxic agents. They occasionally produce occupational allergic contact dermatitis in exposed industrial employees and road workers.

In England an anthraquinone-based dye, disperse blue 35, was responsible for phototoxic skin reactions in dye process workers. The effects are unique in that they were produced by radiation in the visible spectrum (Gardiner et al., 1974). Hjorth and Moller (1976) demonstrated a dermatitis in young women wearing bikinis. The phototoxic agent was demonstrated to be the same disperse dye used in the bathing suit.

Chemicals known to produce phototoxic reactions and the appropriate references are listed in Tables 1*a* and 1*b*.

SOURCES OF EXPOSURE FOR HUMANS

The usual manner of topical exposure to bergapten is from perfumes, colognes, creams, ointments, and lotions containing fragrances. What we do not know is how many other minimal phototoxic agents exist that produce dermatitis of which we are unaware. With bergapten the problem was fairly straightforward. The patients that were involved developed an acute dermatitis with long-lasting pigmentation that served to remind both patient and physician that something was wrong. There are many other patients who have unexplained dermatitides in light-exposed areas. Careful investigation and systematic screening of chemicals may reveal whether some of these are phototoxic under use conditions. The forewarned mind may then be capable of making a diagnosis not otherwise made.

In this connection, it is worthwhile to point out that bergapten (5-MOP) is currently used in certain skin preparations to enhance pigmentation, employing its phototoxic and melanocyte-stimulating effect for this purpose. One such marketed European preparation contains up to 24 ppm 5-MOP (which is activated by UV-A) and a sunscreen (which absorbs UV-B). The fact that chronic skin application of 5-MOP with concomitant UV-A irradiation is tumorigenic in mice (Zajdela and Bisagni, 1981) requires that this preparation be evaluated further.

The pigmentary response was reinvestigated by Zaynoun et al. (1977). This group reported berloque pigmentation in eight Lebanese patients who used perfumes containing bergapten at concentrations as low as 12 ppm (Zaynoun et al., 1981).

TABLE 1a Phototoxicity of Topical and Systemic Agents:
Documented Phototoxic Findings in Humans

Compound	Route	Reference
Tetracyclines	Oral	Harber et al., 1961; Tromovich and Jacobs, 1953; Cullen et al., 1966; Frost et al., 1972; Maibach et al., 1967
Coal tar (multicomponent)	Topical	Tannenbaum, 1975; Bartle, 1972
Nalidixic acid	Oral	Birkett et al., 1969
Disperse blue 35 (anthraquinone base dye)	Topical	Gardiner et al., 1974; Hjorth and Moller, 1976
Cadmium sulfide	Tattoo	Bjoernber, 1963
Anthracene-acridine	Topical	Crow et al., 1961
Bergapten (5-methoxypsoralen)	Topical	Marzulli and Maibach, 1970
Xanthotoxin (8-methoxypsoralen)	Topical	Marzulli and Maibach, 1970
	Oral	Parrish et al., 1974
Sulfanilamide	id	Epstein, 1939
Dacarbazine	Infusion	Yung et al., 1981
Amyl dimethylamino benzoate, mixed *ortho* and *para* isomers	Topical	Emmett et al., 1977
Padimate A or Escalol 506 (amyl *p*-dimethylamino benzoate)	Topical	Kaidbey and Kligman, 1978

TABLE 1b Phototoxicity of Topical and Systemic Agents:
Documented Phototoxic Findings in Animals

Compound	Route	Reference
Tetracyclines	ip	Sams and Epstein, 1967; Ison and Davis, 1966
	Topical	Stott et al., 1970
Bergapten (5-methoxypsoralen)	Topical	Marzulli and Maibach, 1970
Xanthotoxin (8-methoxypsoralen)	Oral, ip, im	Bay et al., 1970
	ip	Hakim et al., 1961
Chlorpromazine	Topical	Stott et al., 1970
	ip	Sams and Epstein, 1967; Sams, 1966; Ison and Davis, 1966; Akin et al., 1979; Ljunggren and Moller, 1976
Chlorothiazide	ip	Sams and Epstein, 1967
	Topical	Stott et al., 1970
Prochlorperazine	ip	Ison and Davis, 1966
Quinoline methanols	ip	Ison and Davis, 1966
Bithionol	Topical	Kobayashi et al., 1974
Tetrachlorosalicylanilide (TCSA)	Topical	Kobayashi et al., 1974
Demeclocycline	ip	Akin et al., 1979
Griseofulvin	ip	Ljunggren and Moller, 1978
Nalidixic acid	Oral	Ljunggren and Moller, 1978
Amiodarone	Oral	Ljunggren and Moller, 1978
Kynuremic acid	Oral	Ljunggren and Moller, 1978
Chlordiazepoxide	ip	Ljunggren and Moller, 1978

The aforementioned unusual source of phototoxic agents in clothing (Hjorth and Moller, 1976) was documented in two young women having a bizarre postinflammatory hyperpigmentation on the skin beneath their bikinis. The investigators extracted the dye from the bathing suits and applied it to the skin of volunteers. After challenge with appropriate irradiation, they produced a typical phototoxic eruption.

ANIMAL TEST METHODS

By definition, phototoxicity is a form of light-related irritation that would occur in (almost) everyone following skin exposure to light of sufficient intensity and wavelength along with a light-activated chemical in adequate amount. In practice this rarely occurs. Bergamot could not have been used for the last century if it had produced ubiquitous and universal dermatitis. What happened instead was that relatively few people developed dermatitis; hence there was not sufficient impetus to track down details of the mechanism involved.

The development of suitable animal models followed the development of a satisfactory human testing model (Marzulli and Maibach, 1970). The basic requisites are nonerythrogenic light (> 320 nm) and percutaneous penetration of the phototoxic agent.

It is convenient that most phototoxic agents produce dermatitis under irradiation conditions (wavelengths > 320 nm) that do not ordinarily yield erythema. For this reason, with light sources such as the Woods light, whose principal emission is at 365 nm, the light-irradiated negative control site is expected to be free of dermatitis. This advantage makes for an all-or-none skin reaction, which simplifies evaluation.

This does not mean that the Woods light is a perfect light source. Although ideal for the study of bergapten, it may not be convenient for other chemicals. It is likely that cheap, currently marketed broader-spectrum light sources such as the (Westinghouse) BL F40W may prove more useful for screening the phototoxic potential of new chemicals. Testing is simplified when erythema rays (280–320 nm) are not involved, as this eliminates the need for estimating minimal erythema dose, a more difficult procedure for evaluating the response.

We cannot predict how often there will be topical phototoxic agents that are activated at wavelengths that produce erythema. The first example of this type is one whose general clinical relevance is not fully understood. Recently, Breza et al. (1975) from Miami showed that vinblastine produced a dermatitis in the light-exposed area following intravenous administration. Their testing suggests that light in the erythema range was required to elicit the response. They experimentally produced a similar skin response in subjects in whom the injection was given intradermally. As the drug is widely used in the treatment of malignancy, it is not clear why most patients receiving intravenous vinblastine do not develop a phototoxic dermatitis. Is it solely that they do not receive sufficient sun exposure, or are the dynamics of delivery to the skin and metabolism in these patients different from those in the ordinary patient? This issue remains *sub judice*.

An interesting example of photoallergy (not phototoxicity) has been demonstrated recently with diphenhydramine (Emmett, 1974), in which photoallergic contact dermatitis was produced with erythrogenic rays at 310 nm.

Among the newer animal test methods for phototoxicity is that of Ljunggren and Moller (1976), involving a measurement of increasing tissue fluid content of the albino mouse tail.

Forbes et al. (1977) have begun a series of phototoxicity tests on fragrance materials, using topical application of the test material to the skins of hairless mice and miniature swine (and in some cases humans) followed by exposure of the skin to either simulated sunlight or near ultraviolet (UV-A). In the first test, 21 of 160 fragrance raw materials proved to be phototoxic. Twenty of these were members of *Rutaceae* or *Umbelliferae*. The clinical significance of this list of identified chemicals was not indicated. It is not known whether they do, in fact, produce phototoxicity in humans at amounts employed in marketed products. However, human skin and pig skin appear to react similarly in phototoxicity studies, and the hairless mouse provides a more sensitive screening system.

A demonstration of variations in the erythemal response of guinea pig skin by Morison et al. (1981) provides a clear warning that photobiological studies with this species "should be confined to one area of the back, unless accompanied by appropriate controls, in order to provide meaningful comparisons."

Harber (1981) reviewed the status of mammalian and human models for predicting drug phototoxicity, citing advantages and disadvantages of various animal species.

A biochemical approach to screening for photoactivity (using glutathione as a biomolecule) before animal testing is discussed by Schothorst et al. (1979). The method appears promising but exploratory, as 8-MOP is barely positive.

EXPERIMENTAL TEST ANIMALS

Under appropriate test conditions several species have been utilized successfully to reproduce bergapten phototoxicity (Marzulli and Maibach, 1970). The hairless mouse and the rabbit appeared somewhat more sensitive to bergapten than the guinea pig. The pig (swine) was less reactive but "stripping" of the skin with cellophane tape enhanced responsiveness; the squirrel monkey appeared resistant. The hamster showed histologic changes of phototoxicity that were not apparent on gross examination.

Other anatomic test sites and different treatment schedules might alter these relative rankings. The practical point is that one can select from a variety of test species. Unfortunately, the list of chemicals of known relevance to humans is limited. Until validation is more complete and until some of the variables are better understood, it is prudent that new chemicals intended for wide human use be examined on human skin, following exploratory work on animals.

With animal models judgment is needed in defining the test parameters. For example, both the time after application to the skin and the duration of light exposure should be carefully controlled. With bergapten, maximal human responses are obtained when the skin is irradiated about 1 hr after applying the phototoxic chemical, whereas little or no response results if a 24 hr interval intervenes between chemical application and light exposure. This does coincide with what we know about percutaneous penetration in humans. In animals a 5-10 min exposure to the chemical (prior to light) is usually sufficient; in humans 1 hr is optimum.

HUMAN TESTING FOR PHOTOTOXICITY

Human bioassays can be safely performed because only small test areas are exposed. As we know of no examples in which the arm or back can not be used, cosmetic sites such as the face can be avoided. The greatest hazard to the experimental subject is the possible development of a small area of dermatitis, which heals promptly. In addition there may be a long period of hyperpigmentation (weeks to months). This is rarely a serious consideration to the informed subject. Because the dermatitis can be produced in almost every subject, it is not necessary to employ a large test panel (Burdick, 1966; Marzulli and Maibach, 1970). With sufficient light exposure and percutaneous penetration, dermatitis will occur. Obtaining high-energy light sources should present no problem; examples are furnished in Tables 2 and 3. Penetration may be enhanced in several ways. Testing a highly permeable anatomic site such as the scrotum (Feldmann and Maibach, 1967) is one method. Decreasing the barriers to penetration by removing the stratum corneum with cellophane tape is another. Increasing the concentration of the test agent manyfold over what would ordinarily be used will concomitantly increase penetration and the likelihood of detecting or identifying a phototoxic agent. It is understood that study of phototoxic agents in this experimental fashion does not duplicate human use conditions. Such tests may disclose a phototoxic potential unrelated to what will occur under use conditions. The dermatotoxicologist must use judgment in establishing the test concentration, frequency, time, and duration of chemical and light exposure, and other factors.

It is not entirely clear why stripping the skin with cellophane tape enhances the phototoxic potential of bergapten. Increased skin penetration is one obvious effect, but other factors may be involved. It is sometimes stated that stripping the skin of the stratum corneum produces *complete* percu-

TABLE 2 Some Special Units for Investigating UV Effects on Humans

Product name	Manufacturer	Product type
Blak-Ray B-100A high-intensity black light	Ultraviolet Products, Inc., 5100 Walnut Grove Ave., San Gabriel, Calif. 91778	High-intensity reflector,[a] mainly 366 nm
Blak-Ray XX-40A fixture, for use with two 40-W tubes: 48 X 6 X 4 in.	Same as above	Can be used with fluorescence-type bulbs available at electric store
Blak-Ray XX-15 fixture, 18 in. long	Same as above	Can be used with commercially available black light
Xenon Solar Simulator 70% of output < 400 nm	Solar Light Co., 6655 Lawnton Ave., Philadelphia, Pa. 19126	150-W xenon arc lamp; details in *J. Invest. Dermatol.* (1969)
Filter to cut out < 320 nm	Same as above	$\frac{1}{8}$ in. window glass (see Sams, 1966)

[a]Disadvantage is heat and small area covered.

TABLE 3 Some Characteristics of Marketed Irradiation Sources[a]

Source	Approximate irradiance at 15 in.
Fluorescent lamps with principal spectral range at 320–400 (UV-A)	
1. Sylvania FR 40 T12 PUVA (psoriasis lamp)	317 (Bare-base bulb without reflector)
2. F 40 W BL (black light); has some visible	125
3. F 40 W BLB (black light with black glass); has no visible	
Mercury vapor lamps (require ballast) with principal spectral range at 320–400 nm (UV-A)	
1. GE H 400 A33-1	1,115
2. Sylvania H 33AR 400	925
Fluorescent lamps with principal spectral range in visible (400–500 nm)	
1. Westinghouse F20T12 BB (special blue)	300

[a]Additional information: For point sources, the inverse square law applies (double distance $= \frac{1}{4}$ intensity). For extended sources (fluorescent bulbs) the inverse square law does not apply for short distances used in exposing animals or humans. By adding a reflector, one can increase intensity about fivefold; by using multiple lamps (two plus a reflector, increase may be up to tenfold. By moving closer (i.e., $7\frac{1}{2}$ in. rather than 15 in.) one doubles the irradiance.

taneous absorption, but this is not so. With hydrocortisone, stripping produces approximately a threefold increase in skin penetration (Feldmann and Maibach, 1967). With several pesticides similarly studied (H. I. Maibach and R. Feldmann, unpublished observation) a severalfold increase in penetration occurred, but it was never complete.

CHEMICAL-SKIN CONTACT TIME BEFORE LIGHT EXPOSURE

With many chemicals there is considerable lag time before significant amounts of percutaneous penetration occur (Feldmann and Maibach, 1970). Bioassays on skin must take this delay factor into consideration; for example, reading the vasoconstrictor corticoid assay at 18-24 hr after application. One might expect that light exposure could or should be delayed for many hours after application to skin. This does not appear to be the case, at least with bergamot. Animals are exposed within minutes after application; humans 1-2 hr later. By 4 hr animals are less reactive; at 24 hr light exposure will often produce no response in humans or animals. This time factor must be taken into account for predictive assays; it is of considerable interest in terms of the relationship of pharmacokinetics and site of action in skin. Future experience will determine if the time relationship found optimal for bergamot will hold for other phototoxic chemicals or require alteration.

VEHICLES

Vehicles may alter percutaneous penetration. A considerable literature defines chemical and vehicle properties that increase or decrease chemical release and penetration. Much of this work has been done with *in vitro* or other model test systems; the experience with vehicles in animal or human *in vitro* test systems is limited. Marzulli and Maibach (1970) showed that reactions to bergamot were greater in the rabbit with 70% alcohol than with 95% alcohol. K. Johnson and Y. Gressel (personal communication) noted that in the guinea pig 8-methoxypsoralen produced greater reactions in 70% alcohol than in absolute alcohol; in the rabbit the reverse response occurred. They demonstrated that mineral oil gave a similar response to 70% alcohol, but reactivity in castor oil and olive oil was greatly decreased.

Kaidbey and Kligman (1974), in studying the phototoxic properties of coal tar, methoxsalen, and chlorpromazine, found the result strongly influenced by the vehicle chosen. No single base produced optimal effects for the three chemicals; emulsion-type creams were generally more active than petrolatum. Polyethylene glycol was a uniformly poor vehicle.

The intensity of phototoxic reactions produced by topically applied methoxsalen and coal tar was investigated by Suhonen (1976) in relation to three test variables. Petrolatum proved to be a suitable vehicle for testing methoxsalen; carbowax appeared useful in testing coal tar. The optimum concentration was 5% for coal tar, 0.03–0.05% for methoxsalen. Optimum occlusion time was 1–2 hr for methoxsalen, 24 hr for coal tar.

It is likely that the effect of vehicle on phototoxicity (and penetration) is more complex than generally stated; until all the variables are understood, it is prudent to employ the vehicle intended for human use in the predictive assay. A more realistic evaluation of potential hazard is obtained by also employing an experimental vehicle (such as alcohol) that is likely to release the test compound.

CUTANEOUS METABOLISM

Bergamot dermatitis as a model of phototoxicity can be produced in most humans and in several animal species (see above). It is not known whether special cutaneous metabolic activities are needed to convert bergapten to a toxic material, although it is unlikely. It is possible or even likely that some ordinarily nonphototoxic materials can be converted to toxic materials by individuals having appropriate metabolic machinery. This is a reasonable explanation for the extremely rare person who develops phototoxicity from oral tetracycline. Investigators will have to look for this with topical agents also.

SYSTEMIC EXPOSURE

The classical model of phototoxicity from systemic exposure is demethychlortetracycline (Maibach et al., 1967).

When the drug was first released for human use, certain patients developed an exaggerated sunburn. The mechanism of this and the method of producing it experimentally were not clear. Attempts to show that there was a decreased minimal erythema dose were difficult to reproduce.

Eventually it was found that phototoxicity with this drug could be readily demonstrated by a straightforward procedure. This required exposing subjects to strong UV light (most easily done with natural sunlight) that had been screened of its major erythema rays by an appropriate filter; that is, one that removed wavelengths below 310 nm, such as Mylar type D plastic film or window glass (Sams, 1966).

At a full therapeutic dose most subjects reacted with 4 hr of natural sunlight so administered. The same test method can be used in experimental animals. The guinea pig proved useful for this purpose but it is likely that other animals would be similarly suitable. Caution is required in exposing guinea pigs to natural sunlight (especially when restrained) in the summer, as they are heat-sensitive and may die. This problem is obviated when other appropriate light sources are used (Sams and Epstein, 1967).

Other attempts to investigate similar phenomena by applying test chemicals that will be taken orally or parenterally in humans by a different route have been examined (Kligman and Breit, 1968). They showed that this potential could be demonstrated by injecting certain materials intradermally or applying them at very high concentrations to the skin. These methods identify hazards; care must be used in extrapolating the findings to what will happen with the actual route of exposure.

PHOTOAUGMENTATION

Longwave UV light (UV-A, >320 nm) in modest amounts does not produce erythema, but when UV-A is added to less than a minimal erythema dose of sunburning irradiation (UV-B, 280–320 nm) visible erythema occurs at 24 hr. This is the photoaugmentation phenomenon. The results are the same whether UV-A is given before or after UV-B. Photoaugmentation can be demonstrated after an interval of 6 hr between doses, but not after 24 hr. Photoaugmentation has been demonstrated with coal tar and 8-methoxypsoralen (Kaidbey and Kligman, 1975). It is not unreasonable to suspect that this may be of clinical relevance in chemical phototoxicity.

COMMENT

Research with phototoxic agents relevant to humans has been mainly related to their clinical toxicity potential (bergamot dermatitis) or to attempts to harness their toxic properties for the therapy of vitiligo and psoriasis. This review is concerned mainly with the former. Our insights are related mainly to information gained from bergamot—an obvious form of clinical toxicity that long awaited simple animal or human models for experimental study.

Are there other forms of phototoxicity that are less obvious? One might ask whether there are any melanodermas or cholasmas due to phototoxicity from as yet undelineated chemicals. Will other forms of clothing dermatitis (such as bikini dermatitis) due to phototoxic agents be demonstrated? Those questions should be answered by the alert investigator. The experimental tools are available and await an inquisitive mind.

SUMMARY

Phototoxicity (photoirritation) should be an easy form of toxicity to detect and prevent because of the ease of performing predictive assays in animals and humans. With widespread application of predictive assays, phototoxicity in humans could become a matter of clinical history rather than current concern.

REFERENCES

Akin, F., Rose, A., Chamness, T., and Marlowe, E. 1979. Sunscreen protection against drug-induced phototoxicity in animal models. *Toxicol. Appl. Pharmacol.* 49:219–224.

Bartle, K. D. 1972. The structure and composition of coal tar and pitch. *Rev. Pure Appl. Chem.* 22:79.

Bay, W., Gleiser, C. A., Dukes, T. W., and Brown, R. S. 1970. Experimental production and evaluation of drug-induced phototoxicity in swine. *Toxicol. Appl. Pharmacol.* 17:538–547.

Birkett, D. A., Garretts, M., and Stevenson, C. J. 1969. Phototoxic bullous eruptions due to nalidixic acid. *Br. J. Dermatol.* 81:342.

Bjoernber, A. 1963. Reactions to light in yellow tattoos from cadmium sulfide. *Arch. Dermatol.* 88:267.

Breza, T., Halperin, K., and Taylor, J. 1975. Photosensitivity reaction to vinblastine. *Arch. Dermatol.* 111:1168–1170.

Burdick, K. 1966. Phototoxicity of Shalimar perfume. *Arch. Dermatol.* 93:424–425.

Crow, K. D., Alexander E., Buck, W. H. L., et al. 1961. Photosensitivity due to pitch. *Br. J. Dermatol.* 73:220–231.

Cullen, S. I., Catalano, P. M., and Helman, R. J. 1966. Tetracycline sun activity. *Arch. Dermatol.* 93:77.

El Mofty, A. M. 1948. A preliminary clinical report on the treatment of leukoderma with *Ammi majus*, Linn. *J. R. Egyptian Med. Assoc.* 31:651.

Emmett, E. 1974. Diphenhydramine photoallergy. *Arch. Dermatol.* 110:249–252.

Emmett, E. A., Taphorn, B. R., and Kominsky, J. R. 1977. Phototoxicity occurring during the manufacture of ultraviolet-cured ink. *Arch. Dermatol.* 113:770–775.

Epstein, S. 1939. Photoallergy and primary photosensitivity to sulfanilamide. *J. Invest. Dermatol.* 2:43–51.

Epstein, J. 1972. Photoallergy. *Arch. Dermatol.* 106:741–748.

Feldmann, R. and Maibach, H. 1967. Regional variation in percutaneous penetration of hydrocortisone in man. *J. Invest. Dermatol.* 48:181–183.

Feldmann, R. and Maibach, H. 1970. Absorption of some organic compounds through the skin in man. *J. Invest. Dermatol.* 54:399–404.

Forbes, P. D., Urbach, F., and Davies, R. E. 1977. Phototoxicity testing of fragrance raw materials. *Food Cosmet. Toxicol.* 15:55–60.

Frost, P., Weinstein, C. D., and Gomez, E. C. 1972. Phototoxic potential of minocycline and doxycycline. *Arch. Dermatol.* 105:681.

Gardiner, J. S., Dickson, A., MacLeod, T. M., and Frain-Bell, W. 1974. The investigation of photocontact dermatitis in a dye manufacturing process. *Br. J. Dermatol.* 86:264–271.

Hakim, R., Freeman, R., Griffin, A. C., and Knox, J. 1961. Experimental toxicologic studies on 8-methoxypsoralen in animals exposed to the long ultraviolet. *J. Pharmacol. Exp. Ther.* 131:394–399.

Harber, L. C. 1981. Current status of mammalian and human models for predicting drug photosensitivity. *J. Invest. Dermatol.* 77:65–70.

Harber, L. and Baer, R. 1972. Pathogenic mechanisms of drug-induced photosensitivity. *J. Invest. Dermatol.* 58:327–342.

Harber, L. C., Tromovich, T. A., and Baer, R. L. 1961. Studies on photosensitivity to demethylchlortetracycline. *J. Invest. Dermatol.* 37:189–193.

Harber, L., Bickers, D., Epstein, J., Pathak, M., and Urbach, F. 1974. *Sunlight and man*, ed. T. Fitzpatrick, pp. 559–568. Tokyo: Univ. of Tokyo Press.

Hjorth, N. and Moller, H. 1976. Phototoxic textile dermatitis (bikini dermatitis). *Arch. Dermatol.* 112:1445–1447.

Ison, A. and Davis, C. 1966. Photoxicity of quinoline methanols and other drugs in mice and yeast. *J. Invest. Dermatol.* 52:193–198.

Jarratt, M. 1976. Drug sensitization. *Int. J. Dermatol.* 15:317–325.

J. Invest. Dermatol. 1969. 53:192.

Kaidbey, K. and Kligman, A. 1974. Topical photosensitizers, influence of vehicles on penetration. *Arch. Dermatol.* 110:868–870.

Kaidbey, K. and Kligman, A. 1975. Further studies of photoaugmentation in humans: Phototoxic reactions. *J. Invest. Dermatol.* 65:412–475.

Kaidbey, K. and Kligman, A. 1978. Phototoxicity to a sunscreen ingredient: Padimate A. *Arch. Dermatol.* 114:547–549.

Kligman, A. and Breit, R. 1968. Identity of phototoxic drugs by human assay. *J. Invest. Dermatol.* 51:90–99.

Kobayashi, F., Wada, Y., and Mizuno, N. 1974. Comparative studies on phototoxicity of chemicals. *J. Dermatol.* 1:93–98.

Lerner, A. B., Denton, C. H., and Fitzpatrick, T. B. 1953. Clinical and experimental studies with 8-methoxypsoralen in vitiligo. *J. Invest. Dermatol.* 20:299–314.

Ljunggren, B. and Moller, H. 1976. Phototoxic reaction to chlorpromazine as studied with the quantitative mouse tail technique. *Acta Derm. Venereol.* 56:373–376.

Ljunggren, B. and Moller, H. 1978. Drug phototoxicity in mice. *Acta Derm. Venereol.* 58:125–130.

Maibach, H., Sams, W., and Epstein, J. 1967. Screening for drug toxicity by wave lengths greater than 3100 Å. *Arch. Dermatol.* 95:12–15.

Marzulli, F. N. and Maibach, H. I. 1970. Perfume phototoxicity. *J. Soc. Cosmet. Chem.* 21:685–715.

Morison, W. L., Parrish, J. A., Anderson, R. R., and Harrist, T. J. 1981. Variations in the erythemal response of guinea pig skin. *Photochem. Photobiol.* 33:283–285.

Parrish, J. A., Fitzpatrick, T. B., Tannenbaum, L., and Pathak, M. A. 1974. Photochemotherapy of psoriasis with oral methoxsalen and longwave ultraviolet light. *N. Engl. J. Med.* 291:1207–1211.

Pathak, M. A. and Fitzpatrick, T. B. 1972. Photosensitivity caused by drugs. *Radiat. Drug Ther.* 6:1–6.

Sams, W. 1966. The experimental production of drug phototoxicity in guinea pigs. *Arch. Dermatol.* 94:773–777.

Sams, W. and Epstein, J. 1967. Experimental production of drug phototoxicity in guinea pigs, using sunlight. *J. Invest. Dermatol.* 48:84–94.

Schothorst, A. A., Suurmond, D., and deLijster, A. 1979. A biochemical screening test for the photosensitizing potential of drugs and disinfectants. *Photochem. Photobiol.* 29:531–537.

Stott, C. W., Strasse, J., Bonomo, R., and Campbell, A. 1970. Evaluation of the phototoxic potential of topically applied agents using long-wave ultraviolet light. *J. Invest. Dermatol.* 55:335–338.

Suhonen, R. 1976. Photoepicutaneous testing. *Contact Dermatitis* 2:218–226.

Tannenbaum, L. 1975. Tar phototoxicity and phototherapy for psoriasis. *Arch. Dermatol.* 111:476–480.

Tromovich, T. A. and Jacobs, P. H. 1953. Photosensitivity to oxytetracycline. *Ann. Intern. Med.* 58:529–530.

Yung, C. W., Winston, E. M., and Lorincz, A. L. 1981. Dacarbazine-induced photosensitivity reaction. *J. Am. Acad. Dermatol.* 4:541–543.

Zajdela, F. and Bisagni, E. 1981. 5-Methoxypsoralen, the melanogenic additive in sun-tan preparations, is tumorgenic in mice exposed to 356 nm u.v. *Carcinogenesis* 2:121–127.

Zaynoun, S., Konrad, K., Gschnait, F., and Wolff, K. 1977. The pigmentary response to photochemotherapy. *Acta Derm. Venereol.* 57:431–440.

Zaynoun, S., Aftimos, B., Tenekjian, K., and Kurban, A. 1981. Berloque dermatitis, a continuing cosmetic problem. *Contact Dermatitis* 7:111–116.

ADDITIONAL PERTINENT REFERENCES IN PHOTOTOXICITY

Daniels, F. 1965. A simple microbiological method for demonstrating phototoxic compounds. *J. Invest. Dermatol.* 44:259–263.

Gloxhuber, C. 1970. Phototoxicity testing of cosmetics. *J. Soc. Cosmet. Chem.* 21:825.

Ison, A. and Blank, H. 1967. Testing drug phototoxicity in mice. *J. Invest. Dermatol.* 49:508–511.

Kligman, A. M. and Goldstein, F. P. 1973. Oral dosage in methoxsalen phototoxicity. *Arch. Dermatol.* 107:548-550.

Ljunggren, B. 1978. Drug phototoxicity. Dept. of Dermatology, Univ. of Lund, General Hospital, Malmo, Sweden.

Mitchell, J. C. 1971. Psoralen-type phototoxicity of tetramethylthiurammonosulphide for Candida albicans; not for man or mouse. *J. Invest. Dermatol.* 56:340.

Saunders, D. R., Miya, T., and Mennear, J. H. 1972. Chlorpromazine-ultraviolet interaction on mouse ear. *Toxicol. Appl. Pharmacol.* 21:260–264.

Song, P. S. and Tapley, K. J. 1979. Photochemistry and photobiology of psoralens. *Photochem. Photobiol.* 29:1177–1197.

Special Issue on Photobiology and Photomedicine, 30th Annual Symposium on the Biology of Skin. 1981. *J. Invest. Dermatol.* 77: No. 1.

Verbov, J. 1973. Iatrogenic skin disease. *Br. J. Clin. Pract.* 27:310–314.

Zaynoun, S., Johnson, B., and Frain-Bell, W. 1977. A study of oil of bergamot and its importance as a phototoxic agent. *Br. J. Dermatol.* 96:475–482.

18

photocontact allergy in humans

■ John H. Epstein ■

INTRODUCTION

Adverse photocutaneous reactions to exogenous chemicals have become increasingly prevalent in the last few decades due to enhanced opportunities for sun exposure and the rapidly increasing numbers of photosensitizing chemicals available. The present discussion is concerned primarily with photoallergic reactions induced by topically applied materials in humans. However, a few definitions would appear to be in order before entering into this specific aspect of photoreactivity.

DEFINITIONS

Action Spectrum and Absorption Spectrum

The wavelengths that are responsible for a photobiological response are termed the *action spectrum* for that particular response. Since nonionizing radiation must be absorbed to act, as described by the Grotthuss-Draper law, a chromophore must be present that will absorb this energy to initiate the photoreaction. The wavelengths that any individual molecule or material will absorb is termed its *absorption spectrum*. Thus the action spectrum for a photoreaction induced by a particular molecule or chemical would be expected to parallel its absorption spectrum. Although this is generally true, it is not essential. It is only necessary that the action spectrum be included in at least some part of the absorption spectrum. An example of this discrepancy occurs with a number of psoralen compounds that have peak absorption

This study was supported in part by USPHS grant CA 15605-01.

391

characteristics of wavelengths shorter than 300 nm but produce their phototoxic effects by absorbing rays in the longer UV range (Pathak et al., 1974).

Sun's Spectrum and Photobiological Reactions

The sun's rays that reach the earth's surface range from 290 nm (or 286 nm) in the UV spectrum, through the visible (400–700 nm), into the infrared, and beyond ($>$ 700 nm). Almost all of the photobiological reactions that occur in the skin on absorption of sunlight are produced by rays between 290 and 320 nm (UV-B), which make up about 0.1–0.2% of the total sun's energy that reaches the earth. These are the rays that inhibit DNA, RNA, and protein synthesis, interrupt mitoses, make vitamin D, cause skin cancer, and produce the delayed erythema response that we call "sunburn" (J. H. Epstein et al., 1970; Daniels, 1974). The longer UV rays between 320 and 400 nm (UV-A) produce a few minor photobiological reactions such as immediate pigment darkening and immediate transient erythema responses (Bacheim, 1956). However, these wavelengths are of great importance because they markedly augment the photoinjury induced by the UV-B spectrum (Willis et al., 1972; Parrish et al., 1974), and they are responsible for the vast majority of exogenously photosensitized reactions (both phototoxic and photoallergic) that occur in human skin. UV rays shorter than 290 nm ($<$ 280 nm = UV-C) emitted by artificial light sources do produce a delayed erythema, alter DNA, RNA, and proteins, cause cancer under experimental conditions, and may enter into photosensitivity problems on occasion.

Photosensitivity

Photosensitivity (J. H. Epstein, 1972) is the broad term that is used to describe abnormal or adverse reactions to the sun or artificial light sources. These responses may be phototoxic or photoallergic in nature.

Phototoxicity. The vast majority of adverse cutaneous reactions induced by the sun and/or artificial light sources are phototoxic in nature and are independent of immune or allergic mechanisms. They can occur in everybody if enough light energy and, in the case of photosensitized responses, enough of the photosensitizer is present in the skin. The clinical picture usually consists of a delayed erythema followed by hyperpigmentation and desquamation. Thus they tend to resemble the usual "sunburn" reaction, which is in itself the most common of all the known phototoxic responses. The mechanisms of these reactions are quite complex and vary greatly with the etiology. In certain instances the presence of oxygen is essential, as in the so-called photodynamic reactions (Blum, 1941). In others, photoproducts with nucleic acids are formed or membrane damage is produced. These responses will be dealt with in a subsequent chapter.

Photoallergy. Unlike phototoxicity, photoallergy is uncommon. It repre- sents an acquired altered reactivity to irradiation that is dependent on an antigen-antibody or a cell-mediated hypersensitivity response. Clinically it is characterized by unusual lesions ranging from immediate urticarial (Fig. 1) to delayed papular and eczematous reactions (Fig. 2). Involvement extending beyond the exposed site frequently occurs. A biopsy of the urticarial response usually reveals very little specific change, whereas the delayed reactions show dense perivascular round cell infiltrates in the dermis (Fig. 3). In general, less energy is required to produce photoallergic than phototoxic reactions.

In addition to the clinical and histological features the following criteria are used to help define the presence of a photoallergic reaction: (1) flares of previously exposed sites following irradiation of a distant site, (2) passive and reverse passive transfer of the reactions with serum for antigen-antibody responses, (3) passive transfer with white blood cells for cell-mediated immunity, and (4) the demonstration of an incubation period and spontaneous flare response when the process is produced under controlled conditions.

Photoallergic reactions may be produced by irradiation alone without the presence of known photosensitizers or may be due to exogenous chemicals. "Solar urticaria" responses are immediate, transient wheal and flare reactions to irradiation alone, which clinically suggest the presence of an antigen-antibody reaction. In certain of these responses, induced primarily by UV-B rays, passive transfer and reverse passive transfer studies have confirmed

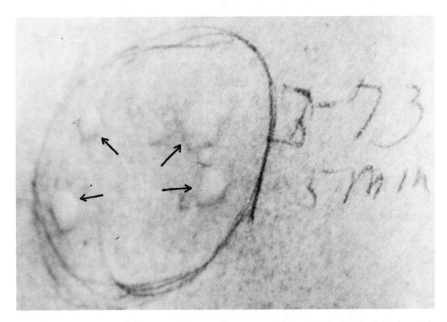

FIGURE 1 Clinical picture of solar urticaria with multiple wheals (J. H. Epstein et al., 1963; reprinted with permission of the American Medical Association).

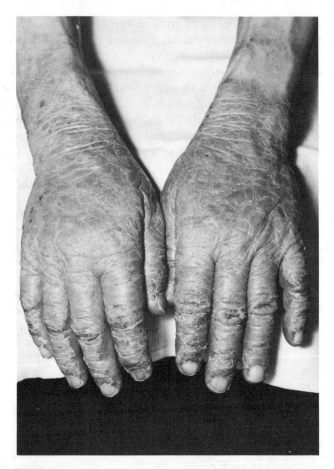

FIGURE 2 Clinical picture of an eczematoid photocontact dermatitis induced by a halogenated salicylanilide (3,5-dibromosali-
cylanilide) (J. H. Epstein, 1972; reprinted with permission of the
American Medical Association).

this relationship (Harber et al., 1963; Sams, 1970). In addition, the clinical
and histologic patterns of the polymorphous light eruptions (PMLEs) strongly
suggest possible CMI responses to UV-B alone (J. H. Epstein, 1966).

Photoallergic reactions induced by exogenous photosensitizers, when
they occur, usually are characterized by delayed reactions, which appear to
depend on cell-mediated immune (CMI) mechanisms. However, Horio (1975)
reported a patient with immediate and delayed photoallergic reactions induced
by chlorpromazine and UV-A. Thus immediate antibody-mediated reactions
may occur. They are very uncommon.

PHOTOALLERGIC CONTACT DERMATITIS

Clinical Picture

Photoallergic contact reactions are clinically identical to any other type of allergic contact dermatitis. Thus the spectrum of the possible responses may range from a simple erythema to a severe vesiculobullous eruption. The most common picture is eczematous in nature (Figs. 2 and 3). When the process is chronic, lichenification results from repeated mechanical trauma (rubbing and scratching). The sun-exposed areas of the skin are involved primarily, as would be expected. However, the eruption may extend to unexposed parts of the body and even become generalized due to conditioned irritability and autoeczematization reactions. Even when this occurs the dermatitis is most notable in the exposed sites.

Adults are much more commonly affected than children. Obviously the reactions will occur in populations that are exposed to sunlight and the photocontactants. Thus reactions to the optical brighteners would more likely be seen in persons who use them, those to chlorpromazine would more likely occur in people who work in mental institutions, and so on. Perhaps the most

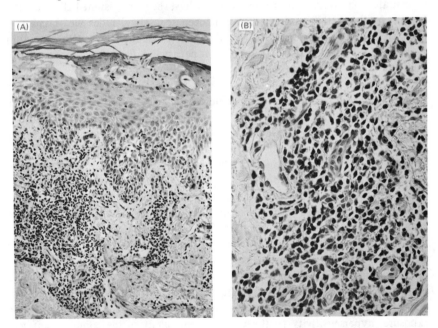

FIGURE 3 (A) Histological appearance of an allergic photocontact reaction showing epidermal edema and vesicle formation and a dense perivascular round cell infiltrate. (B) Higher magnification of the dense perivascular infiltrate. (J. H. Epstein, 1972; reprinted with the permission of the American Medical Association).

extensive statistical data have been compiled on the eruptions induced by the halogenated salicylanilides and related antibacterial compounds because of the large number of people photosensitized by these agents between 1960 and 1970 (Herman and Sams, 1972). The reactions occurred predominantly in men past the age of 40 yr. The reason for this age and sex distribution is unknown. Skin color and race apparently have little influence on the problem, which occurs readily in blacks and Orientals as well as Caucasians.

In general, removal of the offending photosensitizer and related compounds will eliminate the problem once the eruption has subsided. A small percentage of patients who have developed this process will eventuate as persistent light reactors (Jillson and Baughman, 1963). These are people who continue to develop the dermatitis on sun-exposed areas without apparent further contact with the offending agent or related structures. These patients tend to be exquisitely sensitive to the sun and usually have very low UV-B minimal erythema doses. The incidence of this most disturbing problem is unknown, but it probably represents only a small percentage of those who become contact photosensitive. However, up to 25% of patients with photocontact reactions to the halogenated salicylanilides severe enough to necessitate consultation at medical centers have been persistent light reactors. In our studies with the antibacterial halogenated salicylanides we found two types of persistent light reactors: a mild variety that loses its reactivity within $1\frac{1}{2}$ years and a severe type that appears to persist indefinitely (J. H. Epstein et al., 1968).

Chemicals other than the antibacterial halogenated salicylanilides have induced persistent light reactions, including the related antifungal compounds buclosamide (Jadit) (Burry, 1970; Burry and Hunter, 1970), chlorpromazine (Wiskemann and Wulf, 1959; Burdick, 1969), and promethazine (Sidi et al., 1955). Persistent light reactions induced in guinea pigs with sulfonamides have been noted (Schwarz and Speck, 1957), and I have observed a phototoxic persistent light reaction induced by systemic dimethylchlortetracycline that has persisted 3 yr. The mechanism or mechanisms of this persistent light reactivity are not clear. Cross-reactions to unknown photocontactants have been considered. Willis and Kligman (1968a) presented evidence suggesting that the reactions could result from the retention of small amounts of the photosensitizer in the dermis. These authors also reported that the lowered MED in persistent light reactors was a photoallergic reaction, which resembled a sunburn. Other possibilities include the persistence of a sensitized mononuclear infiltrate in the dermis, which will react on minimal antigenic exposure; hypersensitivity to the protein component of the complete antigen, which then becomes an independent photoallergen; or the development of clones of cells that are persistently sensitive to a number of photoallergens (Herman and Sams, 1972). Also, a possible relationship to the chronic eczematous type of polymorphous light eruption (PMLE) has been reported (J. H. Epstein et al., 1968).

Histology

The microscopic anatomy of photocontact reactions is characteristic but not diagnostic. In general, there is some intercellular edema in the epidermis with or without vesicle formation, depending on the clinical pattern. However, the characteristic finding is present in the dermis and consists of a dense perivascular round cell infiltrate, which is identical to that found in any allergic contact dermatitis response (Fig. 3).

Differential Diagnosis

The differential diagnosis includes essentially any eruption that may involve the sun-exposed skin. However, for practical purposes, allergic contact dermatitis, the eczematous type of PMLE, and phototoxic reactions are by far the most important.

Airborne allergens will contact exposed skin primarily. Unlike photo-contact reactions, the airborne contact eruption will be accentuated in fold areas such as the upper eyelids, antecubital fossae, flexural areas of the wrists, and the like because of concentration of the airborne material in these areas. Differentiation from allergic contact reactions to sunscreens, "suntanning" lotions and creams, and medications used to relieve the discomfort of a sunburn is more difficult since they are confined to the sun-exposed areas and are indistinguishable clinically and histologically. The same is true for the eczematous type of PMLE.

Phototoxic reactions induced by topical or systemic exogenous photo-sensitizers will have the same distribution as the photoallergic reactions. The clinical picture and lack of the dermal round cell infiltrate histologically will usually serve to make this differentiation. However, the most useful diagnostic tools available are the patch, photopatch, and phototesting procedures.

Diagnosis

The diagnosis of photocontact dermatitis is suspected by the clinical picture, including the character and distribution of the eruption and the histology. Confirmation and identification of the offending chemical depend on photopatch testing. This is accomplished by the application in duplicate of nonirritating concentrations of the potential photosensitizers in appropriate vehicles (i.e., a 1% concentration of the halogenated salicylanilides in petrolatum). The use of an extra layer of black paper over the patches will help prevent a "masked" positive reaction to the photopatch test (S. Epstein, 1963). This is unnecessary with the use of aluminum patches. Twenty-four hours later one set of patches is irradiated with the UV-A rays. Any light source that emits sufficient amounts of these rays can be utilized, including the sun, hot quartz lamps. fluorescent tubes, xenon arcs, carbon arcs, and monochromatic sources (Harber et al., 1974). Window glass filtration is necessary if there is a significant amount of UV-B emitted by the lamp, as in the case of the hot quartz source. Twenty-four hours after the irradiation, the closed and exposed sites are compared. The reading techniques are identical to those used in evaluation of ordinary patch tests. A positive reaction to the photopatch tests reproduces the clinical lesions morphologically and histologically (Fig. 4). Certain difficulties with patch testing may occur. If the patient is contact allergic to a chemical it may be difficult to determine if he or she is photocontact allergic as well. However, in general, the photopatch test site will be much more reactive than the patch test area in a patient with dual sensitivity.

Another significant problem concerns identifying the potential photoallergen. The history may be helpful in this determination. Unfortunately the patients often do not know what they contacted (except for suntan oils or the like). This is especially true of preservatives and ingredients in soaps. We

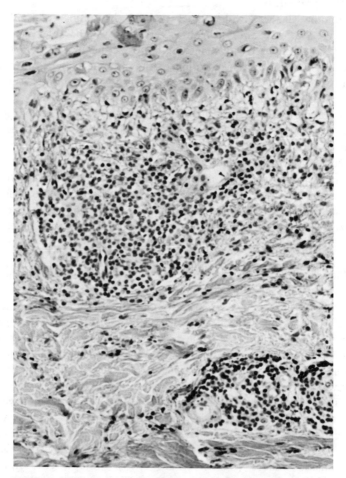

FIGURE 4 Histological appearance of a positive phototest demonstrating the dense perivascular round cell infiltrate.

use the following series of compounds routinely (generally 1% concentrations in white petrolatum) and add whatever can be determined from the history.

1. Dichlorophene
2. Bithionol
3. Hexachlorophene
4. 4,4'-Dichloro-3-(trifluoromethyl) carbanilide
5. 3,4,4'-Trichlorocarbanilide
6. 3,5-Dibromosalicylanilide
7. 4',5-Dibromosalicylanilide
8. 3,4',5-Tribromosalicylanilide
9. 2'3,4',5-Tetrabromosalicylanilide
10. 3,3',4',5-Tetrachlorosalicylanilide
11. Polybromosalicylanilide
12. 6-Methylcoumarin (5% in petrolatum)
13. Musk ambrette (5% in water)

We also routinely patch test with the screening materials suggested by the North American Contact Dermatitis Group (NACDG, 1974) to evaluate other potential contactants and phototest to examine for PMLE (J. H. Epstein, 1966).

Photocontactants

Photoallergic reactions to a number of topically contacted chemicals have been reported. These include sulfonamides (S. Epstein, 1962; Storck, 1965; Schwarz and Speck, 1957), phenothiazines (Sidi et al., 1955; S. Epstein and Rowe, 1957; S. Epstein, 1960a, 1968; Polano, 1964; Storck, 1965; Burdick, 1969), sulfonylcarbamides (Burckhardt and Schwarz-Speck, 1957), men's colognes and after-shave lotions (Starke, 1967), blankophores (optical brighteners) (Burckhardt, 1957), Persian lime rind (S. Epstein, 1956), ragweed (S. Epstein, 1960b), sunscreens (Satulsky, 1950; Sams, 1956; Fitzpatrick et al., 1963; Goldman and Epstein, 1969), diphenhydramine (Emmett, 1974), and psoralens (Sidi and Bourgeois-Cavardin, 1953; Fulton and Willis, 1968).

However, the halogenated salicylanilides and related antibacterial and antifungal compounds represented the most important group of allergic contact photosensitizers. In the 1960s these chemicals were responsible for almost an epidemic of photoallergic reactions. Perhaps tetrachlorosalicylanilide (TCSA) was the most potent photosensitizer of this type. Between 1960 and 1961 it was responsible for an estimated 10,000 cases in England (Wilkinson, 1961) before it was removed from general use. Subsequently, a number of related phenolic compounds were incorporated into soaps and other vehicles to combat infection, reduce body odor, act as preservatives, and destroy fungi. Photocontact reactions were induced by many of these agents, including bithionol, the brominated salicylanilides, hexachlorophene, dichlorophene, the carbanilides, Fentichlor [bis(2-hydroxy-5-chlorophenyl)sulfide], Multifungin (bromochlorosalicylanilide), Jadit (a mixture of buclosamide and salicylic acid) (Herman and Sams, 1972; J. H. Epstein, 1972), and chloro-2-phenylphenol (Adams, 1972).

There has been a rapid decline in the induction of photocontact dermatitis by the halogenated salicylanilides and related compounds since 1968 (Smith and Epstein, 1977). This is most likely due to the removal of the more potent of these photosensitizers from general use. However, within the past 5 yr two new contactants appear to produce primarily, if not exclusively, photoallergic responses. These are the two widely used fragrance compounds 6-methyl-coumarin (Kaidbey and Kligman, 1978; Jackson et al., 1980) and musk ambrette (Raugi et al., 1979; Giovinazzo et al., 1980). In addition, musk ambrette has been reported to be responsible for the induction of a persistent light reactor state similar to that noted with the halogenated salicylanilides (Giovinazzo et al., 1980). The action spectrum for the photoallergic reactions to these fragrances appears to fall in the UV-A range (Giovinazzo et al., 1981; Kaidbey and Kligman, 1978; Jackson et al., 1980).

Mechanism

The clinical appearance, histology, and photopatch test responses strongly suggest that the photoreactions described in this discussion are dependent on a cell-mediated immunity (CMI) process. A number of experimental studies utilizing animal and human models have supported this concept. The animal investigations will be explored by Harber and Shalita (Chap. 14). The present discussion will be limited to human investigations.

Immediate or antibody-mediated hypersensitivity. Herman and Sams (1972), using micro-ouchterlony immune diffusion techniques, could not demonstrate antibodies to 3,5-dibromosalicylanilide (3,5-DBS) protein complexes in the serum of patients photocontact sensitive to this chemical. No binding of fluorescein-tagged goat antihuman IgG, IgA, IgM, complement, or fibrin was noted in positive photopatch test sites with the direct immuno-fluorescence methods. In addition, immunoglobulins in serum from patients photosensitive to TCSA and 3,5-DBS did not bind to cutaneous tissues bathed in these chemicals. Thus no evidence of antibody-mediated hypersensitivity was discovered in patients with photocontact reactions to the halogenated salicylanilides.

Cell-mediated immunity. Photoallergic reactions in human skin characteristic of CMI responses have been induced to a number of agents, including sulfonamides (S. Epstein, 1939), phenothiazines (Burdick, 1969), and the haolgenated salicylanilides (Willis and Kligman, 1968b). Perhaps the most extensive studies have been accomplished with the last of these chemical agents; that is, the halogenated salicylanilides. Willis and Kligman utilized UV-B as well as UV-A exposures plus the chemicals to induce the photosensitivity, but only UV-A and the halogenated salicylanilides were used to elicit the contact allergy.

As noted, animal and human studies have confirmed the CMI mechanism for the photocontact allergy reactions, which appears to be identical to the mechanism of contact allergy itself. However, the nature of the antigen has not been settled. The studies of Schwarz and Speck (1957), Burckhardt and Schwarz-Speck (1957), and Jung and Schwarz (1965) with sulfonilimide and related compounds; Willis and Kligman (1968b, 1969), S. Epstein and Enta (1965), and Jung and Schültz (1968) with the halogenated salicylanilides; and Fulton and Willis (1968) with methoxypsoralen suggested that the haptens were stable photoproducts of these chemicals. Also, *in vitro* binding studies have supported this concept.

An alternative concept was proposed by Jenkins et al. (1964). They concluded that the photoproducts might well be short-lived free radicals, which would attach to the protein carrier within microseconds to form the complete antigen. Support for this theory has developed from clinical observations (Osmundsen, 1969; J. H. Epstein, 1972; Herman and Sams, 1972).

In addition, Jung's studies of postirradiation free radical formation and subsequent binding to albumin and beta-globulin of chlorpromazine (Jung, 1970) and triplet state induction by radiation of triacetyldiphenolisatin (TDI) with deactivation by binding to albumin, γ-globulin, and skin protein (Jung, 1967) present further evidence in favor of the latter concept. The studies of Jung et al. (1968a, 1968b) with Jadit were even more supportive of this second theory immunologically. They were able to demonstrate protein binding *in vitro* after irradiation. This *in vitro* protein complex then acted as a full antigen on plain patch testing of Jadit-photosensitive patients.

As one can see, there is a significant amount of discrepancy in the theories concerning the origin of the antigen in photocontact reactions. Most probably both theories are correct under different circumstances; that is, it is likely that at least some of the subjects experimentally photosensitized by Willis and Kligman (1968b) were actually contact sensitized by stable photoproducts of the chemicals. In contrast, the available evidence suggests that the haptens in the clinically acquired disease are unstable photoproducts, perhaps free radicals, which must be in close proximity to the protein carrier at the time of irradiation.

SUMMARY

Photoallergic contact allergic reactions have become increasingly prevalent over the past several years because of increased opportunities for sun exposure and increasing numbers of photosensitizing chemicals available. The clinical process presents as delayed papular to eczematous eruptions, and histologically it is characterized by a dense perivascular round cell infiltrate in the dermis. The diagnosis is confirmed with photopatch testing techniques, and the action spectrum is usually found in the UV-A range. The clinical picture, histology, and test responses suggest that these reactions are dependent on cell-mediated immunity mechanisms. *In vivo* and *in vitro* experimental studies have confirmed this concept. However, there is a great

402 *Photocontact Allergy in Humans*

deal of discrepancy concerning the nature of the antigen at present. It seems likely that both stable and unstable photoproducts may play a role under different circumstances.

REFERENCES

Adams, R. M. 1972. Photoallergic contact dermatitis to chloro-2-phenyl-phenol. *Arch. Dermatol.* 106:711–714.

Bacheim, A. 1956. Ultraviolet action spectrum. *Am. J. Phys. Med.* 35:177–190.

Blum, H. F. 1941. *Photodynamic Action and Diseases Caused by Light.* New York: Rhinehold.

Burckhardt, W. 1957. Photoallergy eczema due to blankophores (optic brightening agents). *Hautarzt* 8:486–488.

Burckhardt, W. and Schwarz-Speck, M. 1957. Photoallergische Ekzeme durch Nadisan. *Schwiez. Med. Wochenschr.* 87:954–956.

Burdick, K. H. 1969. Prolonged sensitivity to intradermal chlorpromazine. *Cutis* 5:1113–1114.

Burry, J. N. 1970. Persistent light reactions from buclosamide. *Arch. Dermatol.* 101:95–97.

Burry, J. N. and Hunter, G. A. 1970. Photocontact dermatitis from Jadit. *Br. J. Dermatol.* 82:244–249.

Daniels, F., Jr. 1974. Physiological and pathological extracutaneous effects of light on man and mammals not mediated by pineal or other neuroendocrine mechanisms. In *Sunlight and Man*, eds. T. B. Fitzpatrick et al., pp. 247–258. Tokyo: Univ. of Tokyo Press.

Emmett, E. A. 1974. Diphenhydramine photoallergy. *Arch. Dermatol.* 110:249–251.

Epstein, J. H. 1966. Polymorphous light eruption. *Ann. Allergy* 24:397–405.

Epstein, J. H. 1972. Photoallergy: A review. *Arch. Dermatol.* 106:741–748.

Epstein, J. H., Vandenberg, J. J. and Wright, W. L. 1963. Solar urticaria. *Arch. Dermatol.* 133–145.

Epstein, J. H., Wuepper, K. D., and Maibach, H. I. 1968. Photocontact dermatitis to halogenated compounds and related compounds. *Arch. Dermatol.* 97:236–244.

Epstein, J. H., Fukuyama, K., and Fye, K. 1970. Effects of ultraviolet radiation on the mitotic cycle, DNA, RNA and protein synthesis in mammalian epidermis in vivo. *Photochem. Photobiol.* 12:57–65.

Epstein, S. 1939. Photoallergy and primary phototoxicity to sulfanilamide. *J. Invest. Dermatol.* 243–251.

Epstein, S. 1956. Discussion of Sams, W. M. (1956).

Epstein, S. 1960a. Allergic photocontact dermatitis from promethazine (Phenergan). *Arch. Dermatol.* 81:175–180.

Epstein, S. 1960b. Role of dermal sensitivity in ragweed contact dermatitis. *Arch. Dermatol.* 82:48–55.

Epstein, S. 1962. Photoallergy versus phototoxicity. In *Dermatoses Due to Environmental and Physical Factors*, ed. R. B. Rees, pp. 119–135. Springfield, Ill.: Thomas.

Epstein, S. 1963. "Masked" photopatch tests. *J. Invest. Dermatol.* 41:369–370.

Epstein, S. 1968. Chlorpromazine photosensitivity: Phototoxic and photoallergic reactions. *Arch. Dermatol.* 98:354–363.

Epstein, S. and Enta, T. 1965. Photoallergic contact dermatitis. *J. Am. Med. Assoc.* 194:1016–1017.

Epstein, S. and Rowe, R. J. 1957. Photoallergy and photocross-sensitivity to Phenergan. *J. Invest. Dermatol.* 29:319–326.

Epstein, S., Enta, T., and Mehregan, A. H. 1968. Photoallergic contact dermatitis from antiseptic soaps. *Dermatologica* 136:457–476.

Fitzpatrick, T. B., Pathak, M. A., Magnus, I. A., et al. 1963. Abnormal reactions of man to light. *Annu. Rev. Med.* 14:195–214.

Fulton, J. E., Jr., and Willis, I. 1968. Photoallergy to methoxsalen. *Arch. Dermatol.* 98:445–450.

Giovinazzo, V. J., Harber, L. C., Bickers, D. R., Armstrong, R. B., and Silvers, D. N. 1980. Photoallergic contact dermatitis to musk ambrette. *J. Amer. Acad. Dermatol.* 3:384–393.

Giovinazzo, V. J., Ichikawa, H., Kochevar, I. E., Armstrong, R. B., and Harber, L. C. 1981. Photoallergic contact dermatitis to musk ambrette: Action spectrum in guinea pigs and man. *Photochem. Photobiol.* 33:773–777.

Goldman, G. C. and Epstein, E., Jr. 1969. Contact photosensitivity dermatitis from sun-protective agent. *Arch. Dermatol.* 100:447–449.

Harber, L. C., Holloway, R. M., Wheatley, V. R., and Baer, R. L. 1963. Immunologic and biophysical studies in solar urticaria. *J. Invest. Dermatol.* 41:439–443.

Harber, L. C., Harris, H., and Baer, R. L. 1966. Structural features of photoallergy to salicylanilides and related compounds. *J. Invest. Dermatol.* 46:303–305.

Harber, L. C., Bickers, D. R., Epstein, J. H., Pathak, M. A., and Urbach, F. 1974. Report on ultraviolet light sources. *Arch. Dermatol.* 109:833–839.

Herman, P. S. and Sams, W. M., Jr. 1972. *Soap Photodermatitis.* Springfield, Ill.: Thomas.

Horio, T. 1975. Chlorpromazine photoallergy. *Arch. Dermatol.* 111:1469–1471.

Jackson, R. T., Nesbitt, L. T., and DeLeo, V. A. 1980. 6-Methyl coumarin photocontact dermatitis. *J. Amer. Acad. Dermatol.* 2:124–127.

Jenkins, F. P., Welti, D., and Baines, D. 1964. Photochemical reactions of tetrachlorosalicylanilide. *Nature (Lond.)* 201:827–828.

Jillson, V. F. and Baughman, R. D. 1963. Contact photodermatitis from bithionol. *Arch. Dermatol.* 88:409–418.

Jung, E. G. 1967. Photoallergie durch Triacetyldiphenolisatin (TDI) II. Photochemische Untersuchungen zur Pathogenese. *Arch. Klin. Exp. Dermatol.* 231:39–49.

Jung, E. G. 1970. In Vitro-Untersuchungen zur Chlorpromazine (CPZ) Photoallergie. *Arch. Klin. Exp. Dermatol.* 237:501–506.

Jung, E. G. and Schültz, R. 1968. Kontakt- und Photoallergien durch Desinfizienzien. *Dermatologica* 137:216–226.

Jung, E. G. and Schwarz, K. 1965. Photoallergy to "Jadit" with photo cross-reactions to derivatives of sulfanilamide. *Int. Arch. Allergy Appl. Immunol.* 27:313–317.

Jung, E. G., Dümmler, U., and Immich, H. 1968a. Photoallergie durch 4-Chlor-2-hydroxy-benzoesäure-n-butylamid. I. Lichtbiologische Untersuchungen zur Antigenbildung. *Arch. Klin. Exp. Dermatol.* 232:403–412.

Jung, E. G., Hornke, J., and Hajdu, P. 1968b. Photoallergie durch 4-Chlor-2-hydroxy-benzoesäure-n-butylamid. II. Photochemische Untersuchungen. *Arch. Klin. Exp. Dermatol.* 233:287–295.

Kaidbey, K. H. and Kligman, A. M. 1978. Contact photoallergy to 6-methyl coumarin in proprietary sunscreens. *Arch. Dermatol.* 114:1709–1710.

NACDG (North American Contact Dermatitis Group) of the National Program for Dermatology. 1974. *The Role of Patch Testing in Allergic Contact Dermatitis*. New Brunswick, N.J.: Johnson & Johnson.

Osmundsen, P. E. 1969. Contact photoallergy to tribromsalicylanilide. *Br. J. Dermatol.* 81:429–434.

Parrish, J. A., Ying, C. Y., Pathak, M. A., and Fitzpatrick, E. 1974. Erythemogenic properties of long-wave ultraviolet light. In *Sunlight and Man*, eds. M. A. Pathak, L. C. Harber, M. Seiji, and A. Kukita, pp. 131–141. Tokyo: Univ. of Tokyo Press.

Pathak, M. A., Kramer, D. M., and Fitzpatrick, T. B. 1974. Photobiology and photochemistry of furocoumarins (psoralens). In *Sunlight and Man*, eds. M. A. Pathak, L. C. Harber, M. Seiji, and A. Kukita, pp. 335–368. Tokyo: Univ. of Tokyo Press.

Polano, J. K. 1964. Photosensitivity due to drugs. *Excerpta Med. Int. Congr. Ser.* 85:102–107.

Raugi, G. J., Storrs, F. J., and Larsen, W. G. 1979. Photoallergic contact dermatitis to men's perfume. *Contact Dermatitis* 5:251–260.

Sams, W. M. 1956. Contact photodermatitis. *Arch. Dermatol.* 73:142–148.

Sams, W. M., Jr. 1970. Solar urticaria: Studies of the active serum factor. *J. Allergy Clin. Immunol.* 45:295–301.

Satulsky, E M. 1950. Photosensitization induced by monoglycerol paraminobenzoate. *Arch. Dermatol.* 62:711–713.

Schwarz, K. and Speck, M. 1957. Experimentelle Untersuchungen zur Frage der Photoallergie der Sulfonamide. *Dermatologica* 114:232–243.

Sidi, E. and Bourgeois-Cavardin, J. 1953. Mise au point due traitment du vitiligo par l'Ammi Majus. *Presse Med.* 61:436–440.

Sidi, E., Hincky, M., and Gervais, A. 1955. Allergic sensitization and photosensitization to Phenergan cream. *J. Invest. Dermatol.* 24:345–352.

Smith, S. Z. and Epstein, J. H. 1977. Photocontact dermatitis to halogenated salicylanilides and related compounds. *Arch. Dermatol.* 113:1372–1374.

Starke, J. C. 1967. Photoallergy to sandlewood oil. *Arch. Dermatol.* 96:62–63.

Storck, H. 1965. Photoallergy and photosensitivity: Due to systemically administered drugs. *Arch. Dermatol.* 91:469–482.

Wilkinson, D. S. 1961. Photodermatitis due to tetrachlorosalicylanilide. *Br. J. Dermatol.* 73:213–219.

Willis, I. and Kligman, A. M. 1968a. The mechanism of the persistent light reactor. *J. Invest. Dermatol.* 51:385–394.

Willis, I. and Kligman, A. M. 1968b. The mechanism of photoallergic contact dermatitis. *J. Invest. Dermatol.* 51:378–384.

Willis, I. and Kligman, A. M. 1969. Photocontact allergic reactions: Elicitation by low doses of long ultraviolet rays. *Arch. Dermatol.* 110:535–539.

Willis, I., Kligman, A. M., and Epstein, J. H. 1972. Effects of long ultraviolet rays on human skin: Photoprotective or photoaugmentative? *J. Invest. Dermatol.* 59:416–420.

Wiskemann, A. and Wulf, K. 1959. Untersuchungen über den auslösenden Spektralbereich und die direkte Lichtpigmentierung bei chronischen und akuten Lichtauschlägen. *Arch. Klin. Exp. Dermatol.* 209:443–453.

19

the evaluation
of photoallergic contact
sensitizers
in humans

■ Kays Kaidbey ■

INTRODUCTION

Test procedures designed to identify potentially photosensitizing chemicals evolved in the wake of the photosensitivity outbreak caused by the antimicrobial halogenated salicylanilides in the early 1960s (Wilkinson, 1961; Calnan et al., 1961). Photocontact allergy, although relatively uncommon, proved to be particularly troublesome. A minority of affected patients developed a persistent photodermatitis for many years despite avoidance of further contact with the offending chemical (Wilkinson, 1962; Jillson and Baughman, 1963). While removal of the photosensitizing phenolic compounds from the marketplace reduced the incidence of photosensitivity (Smith and Epstein, 1977), it quickly became apparent that other, chemically unrelated substances were also capable of inducing this adverse reaction. There was a clear need for a laboratory test to detect potentially photosensitizing agents.

Most of our knowledge concerning photocontact allergy was, until recently, based on the halogenated salicylanilide class of chemicals. Information was gathered primarily from studies of patients (photopatch testing) and from attempts to induce photosensitization experimentally in guinea pigs (Herman and Sams, 1972). Much remains to be learned about the basic mechanism(s) underlying photocontact sensitivity. It is generally accepted that the process is of the delayed cell-mediated type (Harber et al., 1966; Sams, 1975), although the evidence for this has been criticized (Amos, 1973). The role of ultraviolet (UV) radiation is less clear. Absorption of UV energy by the sensitizer in the skin is required for both induction and elicitation. The most plausible explanation for the role of UV radiation is that absorption of photons of specific energy by the sensitizer leads to the formation of an excited molecule, which, under appropriate conditions, can interact with other molecules normally found in the skin to form an antigen or hapten. Other explanations have been postulated (Amos, 1973).

Test procedures for identifying photocontact allergens have received less attention than methods designed to detect ordinary contact sensitizers. Efforts to induce photocontact sensitivity have involved primarily animals, usually guinea pigs, and have thus far not been standardized. Experience with human testing is even more limited. In theory, the variables that influence ordinary contact sensitization—such as the vehicle, concentration, and frequency of application (Marzulli and Maibach, 1974)—can similarly affect the induction of photosensitization. Furthermore, there is the added and important factor of UV radiation. The wavelength dependence (action spectrum), energy requirements (dose) for both induction and elicitation, and absorption characteristics of the chemical must be determined. For screening of novel agents with unknown action spectra, however, it is necessary to use a UV source with a broad emission spectrum. The sources commonly used in the past were fluorescent tubes such as the FS-20 sunlamp bulbs, with emission primarily in the UV-B region, or black light fluorescent bulbs, which emit primarily in the UV-A range, or a combination of both.

PHOTOMAXIMIZATION TEST

This test is conducted in humans and is essentially a repeated insult technique that entails an exaggerated exposure to both chemical and UV (Kaidbey and Kligman, 1980) and follows a design similar to that of the maximization test (Kligman, 1966). The UV source is a 150-W xenon arc solar simulator. The emission spectrum is continuous, extending from about 290 to 410 nm with a peak at about 350 nm, and closely resembles the UV-B spectrum of midday summer sunlight at 41°N and 70° sun elevation (Berger, 1969).

A 5% concentration of the test agent in an appropriate base (such as Hydrophilic Ointment USP) is delivered to the skin by plastic tuberculin syringes at a concentration of 10 $\mu l/cm^2$. The material is spread uniformly with thin glass rods and the sites covered with nonwoven cotton cloth (Webril, Curity) and sealed to the skin with clear occlusive tape (Blenderm, 3M Co.). Twenty-four hours later, the patches are removed and the sites exposed to three minimal erythema doses (MEDs) from the solar simulator. The MED is individually determined beforehand by exposing the skin sites to 25% increments of radiation. The dose required to produce minimal but uniform erythema with a clear border 24 h after exposure is the MED. After a rest period of 48 h, a similar occlusive application is made to the same site for another 24 h, followed again by exposure to three MEDs. This sequence is repeated for a total of six exposures over a period of 3 wk. The subjects are then challenged after a rest period of 14 d by a single exposure to a fresh skin site. An occlusive application is made with the test agent (1.0% concentration) for 24 h, followed by exposure to 4.0 J/cm^2 UV-A. The UV-A is obtained from the same source by filtering the radiation through a 2-mm Schott WG345 filter (50% transmission at about 345 nm). The sites are examined 48 and 72 h after irradiation. Unirradiated control sites are sealed and then covered with three or four layers of opaque adhesive tape. Development of erythema and edema or a vesicular dermatitis in the irradiated but not the unirradiated sites signifies the induction of photocontact sensitivity. Each substance is usually examined in 25 volunteers.

EVALUATION OF SOME PHOTOCONTACT SENSITIZERS

Halogenated Phenolic Compounds

Several members of this class of compounds, notably those that gave rise to outbreaks of photosensitivity in the past, were identified as photosensitizers by the photomaximization test (Table 1). 3,5-Dibromosalicylanilide (3,5-DBS) and tetrachlorosalicylanilide (TCSA) produced the highest sensitization rates (40 and 32%, respectively). One sample of tribromosalicylanilide (TBS) that contained up to 47% dibrominated derivatives as impurities (sample A) produced photosensitization, while a purer sample (B) containing only 1.2% dibrominated derivative (3,5-DBS) produced no instances of sensitization. TBS may have little or negligible photosensitization potential compared to the dibrominated derivatives. The latter substances have also produced higher sensitization rates than TBS in animals (Morikawa et al., 1974). Jadit and bithionol, which are also known photosensitizers, produced photosensitization, although the rates were lower than with TCSA. Trichlorocarbanilide and

TABLE 1   Induction of Photoallergic Contact Dermatitis by the Photomaximization Test ($n = 25$): Halogenated Phenolic Compounds

Compound	No. of photosensitized subjects
3,3′,4′,5-Tetrachlorosalicylanilide	8
3,4,5-Tribromosalicylanilide (sample A)	2
3,4,5-Tribromosalicylanilide (sample B)	0
4,5-Dibromosalicylanilide	3
3,5-Dibromosalicylanilide	10
5-Monobromosalicylanilide	0
4-Chloro-2-hydroxybenzoic acid *n*-butylamide (Jadit)	3
Bithionol	3
Trichlorocarbanilide	0
Hexachlorophene	0

hexachlorophene (Hex) were inactive. Rare reports of photocontact allergy to Hex and TCC based on positive photopatch tests could have represented cross-photoreactions to some other primary photosensitizers such as TCSA or bithionol. In one such study, for example, all patients who were positive in photopatch tests to Hex also had strong reactions to other halogenated phenolics (Epstein et al., 1968).

Coumarins

The coumarins, which constitute a large class of synthetic and naturally occurring substances, are potentially strong photosensitizing agents. Certain synthetic derivatives were used as optical bleachers (Calnan, 1973), while others were incorporated in toiletries as fragrances (Opdyke, 1974). The photosensitizing properties of coumarins became apparent after outbreaks of photosensitivity among users of sunscreens containing 6-methylcoumarin as a fragrance (Kaidbey and Kligman, 1978). This potential was readily demonstrated in the photomaximization test (Table 2). Other derivatives such as 5,7-dimethoxycoumarin, which is naturally found in bergamot oil, were less photosensitizing, while coumarin itself had no detectable activity. Individuals photosensitized to any one of these substances can develop cross-reactions to other derivatives, even when the latter are not primary inducers (Kaidbey and Kligman, 1981). This underscores the importance of identifying and eliminating the photosensitizing or offending derivatives. Examination of the chemical structures shows that substitution of a methyl group at position 6 or an alkoxy group at position 7 of the benzopyrone ring confers strong photoallergenic activity (Kaidbey and Kligman, 1981; Opdyke, 1981). The coumarins in general are strong UV absorbers.

Of special interest was the observation that certain healthy individuals with no history of photodermatitis or other adverse reactions to sunlight had

TABLE 2   Photosensitization Potential of Coumarin Derivatives and Other Fragrances ($n = 25$)

Compound	No. of photosensitized subjects
6-Methylcoumarin	15
4-Methyl-7-ethoxycoumarin	13
7-Methoxycoumarin	11
7-Methylcoumarin	6
5,7-Dimethoxycoumarin	5
Coumarin	0
Hexahydrocoumarin	0
Octahydrocoumarin	0
Isoeugenol	0
Phthalide	0
Musk ambrette	0

a positive photopatch test to coumarins (Kaidbey and Kligman, 1978b). The significance of this finding is not clear, although it is possible that repeated exposure to coumarins in toiletries or elsewhere in the environment could have led to photosensitization. These may be the individuals who are at risk of developing a photodermatitis on their "first" exposure to a coumarin-containing preparation.

Maurer et al. (1980) were unable to induce photosensitization to 6-methylcoumarin in guinea pigs despite concomitant stimulation with Freund's adjuvant. This could have been due to the low concentration (0.1%) used for induction, since Ichikawa et al. (1981) achieved induction with larger concentrations.

Musk Ambrette

This synthetic fragrance, which is used in aftershave lotions, perfumes, and soaps, was recently identified as a photosensitizer (Raugi et al., 1979). Most commonly affected were middle-aged or elderly men using aftershave lotions containing musk. Sporadic cases, some with persistent photosensitivity, have since been reported (Giovinazzo et al., 1980). We have seen three similarly affected males, one of whom had a persistent photodermatitis; all these patients had positive photopatch tests to pure musk ambrette. Efforts to induce photosensitization to this substance in humans have been unsuccessful, even in a trial in which a 10% concentration was employed and the induction phase extended to 6 instead of 3 wk. Musk ambrette is probably a very weak photosensitizer that cannot be detected by the photomaximization test. Furthermore, shaving may be a factor contributing to induction (Kochever et al., 1979). Other musk derivatives have not yet been examined for their photosensitizing potential, and it is possible that positive photopatch tests in patients may represent cross-reactions to other nitro-musks that are more potent inducers.

Recently, photosensitization to musk ambrette has been induced in guinea pigs by use of special procedures such as stripping (Kochevar et al., 1979) and id injection of Freund's complete adjuvant before induction (Ichikawa et al., 1981). Without such modifications, induction was unsuccessful even at a concentration of 10%, which supports the contention that this substance has a very low potential for photosensitization compared to the agents previously discussed.

Other Photosensitizers

Several other topically applied agents have occasionally been incriminated as photosensitizers on the basis of positive photopatch tests in patients (Table 3). These include certain essential oils (e.g., sandalwood oil), *p*-aminobenzoic acid (PABA), and drugs such as benzocaine and diphenhydramine. PABA did not induce photosensitization in the photomaximization test, and the other agents have not been examined in humans. It is unlikely

TABLE 3   Topically Applied Substances Reported
to Produce Photoallergic Contact Dermatitis in Humans

Halogenated phenolic compounds:
  Fentichlor
  Dichlorophene
  Bromochlorosalicylanilide (Multifungin)
  Chloro-2-phenylphenol
Sunscreens:
  p-Aminobenzoic acid (PABA)
  Glyceryl PABA
  Digalloyl trioleate
  2-Hydroxy-4-methoxybenzophenone (Mexenone)
Phenothiazines:
  Promethazine hydrochloride
  Diphenhydramine
Others:
  Sandalwood oil
  Benzocaine
  8-Methoxypsoralen
  Quindoxin
  Optical brighteners

---

that weak photocontact allergens will be identified as such in routine laboratory screens. There have been few reports of photocontact allergy to such agents as PABA and benzocaine despite their extensive use for many years.

Another substance that was found to induce photocontact allergy by the photomaximization test is sodium omadine. The zinc, magnesium, and sodium compounds of omadine are potentially useful since they have broad-spectrum antibacterial and antifungal properties. Sodium omadine, unlike the zinc derivative, has a significant photoallergenic potential (Table 4). The sodium salt has absorption peaks at about 280 and 330 nm, and little or no significant absorption beyond 360 nm.

Some photocontact sensitizers are also capable of inducing ordinary contact allergy. The halogenated salicylanilides are examples. Contact sensitization developed in 6 of 25 subjects exposed to TCSA in the photomaximization test, while in another 6 a combined contact and photocontact sensitivity was suspected on the basis of a marked accentuation of the patch test reactions by UV-A (Kaidbey and Kligman, 1980). Similar observations were made with DBS and bithionol, although they were far less active. It should be pointed out, however, that the photomaximization test is not designed to assess contact sensitization. Repeated exposures to the chemical and UV during induction may lead to the formation of photoproducts, which can themselves be sensitizing. UV may also alter local reactivity and cellular responses by its well-known effects on lymphoid cells. Nonetheless, the halogenated salicylanilides appear to be strong sensitizers in humans (Marzulli and Maibach, 1973). There is, however, no apparent relation between photo-contact potential and ordinary contact sensitization. Thus the substituted coumarins, which are potent photosensitizers, are weak or poor contact allergens in the maximization test in humans (Opdyke, 1976, 1981). No instances of contact sensitization have been reported with musk ambrette, either clinically or in the maximization test.

PHOTOPATCH TESTING

The interpretation of photopatch test results is usually straightforward. Difficulties arise when there is marked enhancement of a positive or weakly positive reaction to a chemical in the unirradiated site by UV. This has been observed in patients and in experimentally photosensitized humans. In these cases, photopatch testing should be carefully repeated by quantitative methods. Measured amounts of the chemical in a suitable vehicle should be delivered to the skin and the unirradiated sites quickly and rigorously sealed with several layers of opaque material to prevent stray radiation. Small amounts of UV-A can reach the skin surface through ordinary tape and trigger a reaction in the unirradiated patch test sites in highly sensitive individuals. This was observed years ago by Epstein (1963), who termed the reaction a "masked" photopatch test and noted that it can lead to an erroneous diagnosis of contact sensitivity. That exceedingly small doses of UV-A are sufficient to provoke a response in photosensitized individuals has been amply demonstrated, especially when relatively large concentrations of the sensitizers (1.0 or 0.1%) are employed (Epstein et al., 1968; Osmundsen, 1968; Willis and Kligman, 1969). If a definite and clear enhancement is still observed after the above procedures, other explanations must be invoked. These include nonspecific enhancement of contact allergy by UV, as through effects on the

TABLE 4   Induction of Photoallergic Contact Dermatitis: Miscellaneous Compounds ($n = 25$)

Compound	No. of photosensitized subjects
Chlorpromazine[a]	6
Benzoyl peroxide	0
5-Fluorouracil	0
p-Aminobenzoic acid	0
Sulfanilamide	0
Chlorothiazide	0
Sodium omadine[b]	6
Zinc omadine	0

[a]Chlorpromazine was tested in 12 volunteers.

[b]Sodium omadine was tested at 2.5% because of irritancy at higher concentrations.

vasculature, release of inflammatory mediators, modification of local cellular immunologic responses, formation of cross-reacting photoproducts, and so on. Such possibilities have not been adequately investigated. Another explanation is the existence of dual sensitivity: i.e. contact and photocontact allergy. Photopatch testing with serial dilutions of the sensitizer should then be performed. A positive photopatch test at a drug concentration that fails to elicit a response in the unirradiated test site is suggestive of dual sensitization.

ACTION SPECTRUM

Few detailed studies have been made of the action spectrum for elicitation of photocontact allergic dermatitis in sensitized humans. Freeman and Knox (1968) and Cripps and Enta (1970), using narrow wave bands, showed that responses to the halogenated salicylanilides in pretreated skin could be elicited over a relatively wide portion of the UV-A spectrum. Furthermore, a reduction of the threshold erythema dose was found with UV-B wavelengths. Essentially similar findings were obtained with two subjects who were photosensitive to 6-methylcoumarin (Kaidbey and Kligman, 1981), although no responses could be provoked with wavelengths longer than 360 nm. In rare cases, there is narrower spectral reactivity—for example, to UV-B wavelengths in a case of photocontact allergy to diphenhydramine (Emmett, 1974).

Studies involving the wavelength dependence for induction of photo-contact allergy are also very few, and only studies in animals have been reported. Cripps and Enta (1970) found that UV-B was necessary for induction with TCSA, while Horio (1976) was able to induce photosensitivity to TCSA and TBS with UV-A only after pretreating the skin with 20% sodium lauryl sulfate (SLS). We found that simulated solar radiation was more effective than UV-A in inducing photocontact allergy to 6-methylcoumarin. When simulated solar radiation was used during induction, 15 of 25 subjects were sensitized. When UV-B was filtered out from the irradiation system and an equivalent dose of UV-A was used, only 4 of 25 were sensitized (Table 5). For the coumarins, at least, it appears that shorter wavelengths are more efficient for induction. Spectral effectiveness for induction will probably be found to depend on the absorption characteristics of the chemical in the skin.

TABLE 5   Influence of UV Wave Band on Induction
on Photocontact Allergy to 6-Methylcoumarin

Wave band	Incidence of photosensitization (%)
Simulated solar radiation	60
UV-A	16

CONCLUSIONS

The photomaximization test is a useful laboratory procedure for identifying substances that are potentially capable of producing photoallergic contact sensitivity in humans. The test combines exaggerated exposure to the drug and simulated solar radiation. Agents suspected of being photosensitizers on clinical grounds or from photopatch testing can be evaluated for this potential in the laboratory. This is necessary to determine whether the chemical can act as an inducer or merely as a cross-reactant. Although substances can be ranked for their photosensitizing capacity under a defined set of laboratory conditions, the possible incidence of photoallergic reactions with normal usage cannot be predicted. Furthermore, this test has the same limitations as other predictive laboratory methods, such as those designed to evaluate ordinary contact sensitization potential. Very weak or marginally active chemicals may not be detected. Systemically administered photosensitizers cannot be evaluated in this test.

Experience with human testing has been limited. Factors that influence induction, such as concentration, vehicle, and UV dose, need to be further investigated.

REFERENCES

Amos, H. E. 1973. Photoallergy. A critical survey. *Trans. St. John's Hosp. Dermatol. Soc.* 59:147–151.

Berger, D. S. 1969. Specification and design of solar ultraviolet simulators. *J. Invest. Dermatol.* 53:192–199.

Calnan, C. D., Harman, R. R. M., and Wells, G. C. 1961. Photodermatitis from soaps. *Br. Med. J.* 2:1266.

Calnan, C. D. 1973. Hazards of optical bleachers. *Trans. St. John's Hosp. Dermatol. Soc.* 59:275–282.

Cripps, D. J. and Enta, T. 1970. Absorption and action spectra studies on bithionol and halogenated salicylanilide photosensitivity. *Br. J. Dermatol.* 82:730–742.

Emmett, E. A. 1974. Diphenhydramine photoallergy. *Arch. Dermatol.* 110:249–252.

Epstein, S. 1963. "Masked" photopatch test. *J. Invest. Dermatol.* 41:369–370.

Epstein, J. H., Wuepper, K. D., and Maibach, H. I. 1968. Photocontact dermatitis to halogenated salicylanilides and related compounds. *Arch. Dermatol.* 97:236–244.

Freeman, R. G. and Knox, J. M. 1968. The action spectrum of photocontact dermatitis. *Arch. Dermatol.* 97:130–136.

Giovinazzo, V. J., Harber, L. C., Armstrong, R. B., and Kochevar, I. E. 1980. Photoallergic contact dermatitis to musk ambrette. *J. Am. Acad. Dermatol.* 3:384–393.

Harber, L. C., Harris, H., and Baer, R. L. 1966. Photoallergic contact dermatitis. *Arch. Dermatol.* 94:255–262.

Herman, P. S. and Sams, W. M., Jr. 1972. *Soap Photodermatitis: Photosensitivity to Halogenated Salicylanilides.* Springfield, Ill.: Thomas.

Horio, T. 1976. The induction of photocontact sensitivity in guinea pigs without UV-B radiation. *J. Invest. Dermatol.* 67:591–593.

Ichikawa, H., Armstrong, R. B., and Harber, L. C. 1981. Photoallergic contact dermatitis in guinea pigs: Improved induction technique using Freund's complete adjuvant. *J. Invest. Dermatol.* 76:498–501.

Jillson, O. F. and Baughman, R. D. 1963. Contact photodermatitis from bithionol. *Arch. Dermatol.* 88:409–416.

Kaidbey, K. H. and Kligman, A. M. 1978a. Contact photoallergy to 6-methylcoumarin in proprietary sunscreens. *Arch. Dermatol.* 114:1709–1710.

Kaidbey, K. H. and Kligman, A. M. 1978b. Photocontact allergy to 6-methylcoumarin. *Contact Dermatitis* 4:277–282.

Kaidbey, K. H. and Kligman, A. M. 1980. Photomaximization test for identifying photoallergic contact sensitizers. *Contact Dermatitis* 6:161–169.

Kaidbey, K. H. and Kligman, A. M. 1981. Photosensitization by coumarin derivatives: Structure-activity relationships. *Arch. Dermatol.* 117:258–263.

Kligman, A. M. 1966. The identification of contact allergens by human assay. III. The maximization test. A procedure for screening and rating contact sensitizers. *J. Invest. Dermatol.* 47:393–409.

Kochevar, I. E., Zaler, G. L., Einbinder, J., and Harber, L. C. 1979. Assay of contact photosensitivity to musk ambrette in guinea pigs. *J. Invest. Dermatol.* 73:144–146.

Marzulli, F. and Maibach, H. 1973. Antimicrobials. Experimental contact sensitization in man. *J. Soc. Cosmet. Chem.* 24:399–421.

Marzulli, F. and Maibach, H. 1974. Use of graded concentrations in studying skin sensitization in man. *Food Cosmet. Toxicol.* 12:219–277.

Maurer, T. H., Weirich, E. G., and Hess, R. 1980. Evaluation of the photocontact allergenic potential of 6-methylcoumarin in the guinea pig. *Contact Dermatitis* 6:275–278.

Morikawa, F., Nakayama, Y., Fukuda, M., Hamano, M., Yokoyama, Y., Nagura, T., Ishihara, M., and Toda, K. 1974. Techniques for evaluation of phototoxicity and photoallergy in laboratory animals. In *Sunlight and Man*, eds. T. B. Fitzpatrick, M. A. Pathak, L. C. Harber, M. Seiji, and A. Kukita, pp. 529–557. Tokyo: Univ. of Tokyo Press.

Opdyke, D. L. 1974. Monographs on fragrance raw materials: Coumarin. *Food Cosmet. Toxicol.* 12:385–405.

Opdyke, D. L. 1976. Monographs on fragrance raw materials: 6-Methylcoumarin. *Food Cosmet. Toxicol.* 14:605.

Opdyke, D. L. 1981. The structure activity relationships of some substituted coumarins with respect to skin reactions. *Dragoco Rep. (Engl. Ed.)* 2:43–48.

Osmundsen, P. E. 1968. Contact photodermatitis due to tribromosalicylanilide. *Br. J. Dermatol.* 80:228–234.

Raugi, G. J., Storrs, F. J., and Larsen, W. G. 1979. Photoallergic contact dermatitis to men's perfume. *Contact Dermatitis* 5:251–260.

Sams, W. M., Jr. 1975. The immunology of photocontact dermatitis. *Int. J. Dermatol.* 14:251–253.

Smith, S. Z. and Epstein, J. H. 1977. Photocontact dermatitis to halogenated salicylanilides and related compounds. *Arch. Dermatol.* 113:1372–1374.

Wilkinson, D. S. 1961. Photodermatitis due to tetrachlorosalicylanilide. *Br. J. Dermatol.* 73:213–219.

Wilkinson, D. S. 1962. Patch test reactions to certain halogenated salicylanilides. *Br. J. Dermatol.* 74:302–306.

Willis, I. and Kligman, A. M. 1969. Photocontact allergic reactions. Elicitation by low doses of long ultraviolet rays. *Arch. Dermatol.* 100:535–539.

20

photocarcinogenesis

■ Frederick Urbach ■

INTRODUCTION

The high-energy, short-wavelength portion of the solar electromagnetic spectrum (wavelengths shorter than 320 nm) is potentially very detrimental to living cells and tissues. A low concentration of ozone formed in the stratosphere absorbs most of the photons of ultraviolet (UV) radiation and thus prevents most of them from reaching the earth. However, even in the presence of this ozone layer, which varies in thickness at different latitudes and different seasons, a biologically significant amount of UV radiation reaches the surface of the earth.

The major effects on humans of ultraviolet radiation in the UV-B range (320–280 nm) are on the skin and eyes. Acute effects consist of "sunburn," an inflammatory response of the tissues that may be no more than mild redness or slight stinging of the eyes, or may develop into the equivalent of second-degree (blistering) burns. The acute effects of single overdoses of UV-B are transient, heal without scarring, and in the skin lead to adaptive changes of skin thickening and pigmentation, which afford some degree of protection. The only established positive (beneficial) effect of UV-B in humans is the production of vitamin D precursors in the skin, which are absorbed into the bloodstream and prevent rickets, a serious vitamin deficiency disease. Most work has been done on the harmful effects of UV-B and relatively little attention has been given to possible beneficial effects, however.

Repeated UV-B exposure, prolonged over years, can result in chronic degenerative changes in skin, characterized by skin "aging" and the development of premalignant and malignant skin lesions.

EXPERIMENTAL SKIN CARCINOGENESIS

Effects of Long-Term Exposure of Skin to Ultraviolet Radiation

Ultraviolet irradiation induces an inflammatory response and ulceration in the epidermis and the dermis, the latter being infiltrated with leukocytes in the region of the lesions, and to a much lesser extent between them. These lesions ulcerate and the epidermis may disappear for a time in the center. However, peripherally there is particularly active hyperplasia. The basal membrane (between the epidermis and the dermis) may disappear for a time in the regions of these "open" lesions. Between the lesions, the infiltration of leukocytes is relatively slight.

Injury to the epidermis and dermis, brought about by long-term exposure to UV, leads to dermal alteration, fibrosis and elastosis, and to epidermal atrophy. Experimental production of cutaneous elastotic changes in animals by artificial UV irradiation has been reported only rarely. Using histochemical methods, Sams et al. (1964) demonstrated focal dermal elastosis in mice after prolonged exposure to artificial UV radiation. UV-induced changes in connective tissue were seen in rat skin by Nakamura and Johnson (1968).

Tumor Types

Epidermal tumors. The first visible step in UV-induced epidermal tumor formation in animal skin consists of cell proliferation, that is, an increase in the number of squamous cells and cell layers, which gradually become papillomatous in character (Stenbäck, 1978). This is accompanied by an increase in cellular atypia, nuclear enlargement, hyperchromatism, indentation, and prominence of nucleoli. This basically proliferative response is frequently replaced by a dysplastic pleomorphism, occasionally with pseudoepithelio-matous hyperplasia-like features, which ultimately invade the dermis. The tumors first seen are acanthomatous papillomas, with a predominantly epithelial component.

Among malignant tumors that ultimately develop are squamous cell carcinomas of different types, including solid keratin-containing tumors; moderately differentiated, individually keratinizing tumors with distinct inter-cellular bridges; and less differentiated, nonkeratinizing spindle cell tumors, in which ultrastructural analysis reveals squamous cell patterns.

Another type of neoplastic progression seen in mice, particularly after intensive treatment with large doses of UV over a short time, consists of ulceration, scarring, and the subsequent formation of dermal tumors. These tumors begin as aggregates of regularly built, elongated cells with small monomorphic nuclei. Epithelial proliferation is occasionally observed as a secondary phenomenon. The tumors rarely extend grossly through the surface. In the early stages, they appear to be papillomas, although they consist entirely of fibroblastic cells (Stenbäck, 1975a). Sarcoma induction is partly species-specific, as such tumors are not seen in UV-irradiated Syrian golden hamsters (Stenbäck, 1975b) or in hairless mice (Epstein and Epstein, 1963) or guinea pigs, all of which are susceptible to chemical sarcoma induction (Stenbäck, 1969, 1975b).

Adnexal tumor formation is not as common in UV-treated animals (Stenbäck, 1975b) as in, for example, carcinogen-treated rats (Zackheim, 1963; Stenbäck, 1969). Hyperplasia and cystic disorganization of hair follicle walls are common, but rarely progress to grossly visible neoplasia. Even more uncommon are hamartomatous tumors, hair follicle-derived trichofolliculomas, and sebaceous gland tumors.

Action Spectrum for Photocarcinogenesis

Determination of the effective wavelengths or "action spectrum" is one of the primary objectives in the study of photobiological responses. However, data are not available for the action spectrum of UV-induced cancer formation. The paucity of this information for one of the most extensively studied photobiological reactions is due to a number of factors, including the large number of potential wavelengths, the considerable number of animals necessary, the length of time (months or years) required for exposure to each wavelength, the difficulties in immobilizing experimental animals, and the need for an especially good monochromator with practically no stray light contamination. Although the complete curve of the carcinogenic spectrum is not known, certain aspects have been determined by less sophisticated methods. Roffo (1933) reported that window glass filtration eliminated the carcinogenic effects of sunlight on white rats. Thus the offending rays of the sun would be found approximately between 290 and 320 nm. Investigators using mercury arc and fluorescent sunlamps with filters confirmed that, under their experimental conditions, 320 nm represented the longer wavelength limit for cancer formation (Griffin et al., 1955; Blum, 1969). Furthermore, carcinogenic responses have been produced by radiation as short as 230.2 nm (Roffo, 1933), and skin cancer has been induced by UV-C and UV-B. Thus the action spectrum appears to include wavelengths between 230 and 320 nm, but wavelengths between 290 and 320 nm have significantly greater carcinogenic effects than those shorter than 260 nm (Rusch et al., 1941; Blum, 1943; Blum and Lippincott, 1943; Kelner and Taft, 1956).

Freeman (1978) performed experiments to provide more specific comparative data by testing the hypothesis that the action spectrum for carcinogenesis paralleled that for erythema. Squamous cell carcinomas developed at approximately the same rate and frequency, when UV exposure was proportional to that for erythema, with decreasing potency from 300 to 320 nm. No tumors occurred in mice exposed to 290 nm. These cancer-producing wavelengths are responsible for the normal phototoxic sunburn reaction. Longer UV and visible light are neither erythema-producing nor carcinogenic under ordinary conditions.

It cannot be assumed that the action spectra for human skin erythema and mouse skin photocarcinogenesis are similar, unless a common chromophore or action mechanism is involved. Setlow (1974) proposed that the common denominator was the action spectrum for affecting DNA. Making some allowance for the skin transmission of UV radiation, he showed that the shapes of action spectra for DNA, erythema, and possibly skin cancer production were similar and could be made to coincide.

Physical Factors Influencing Photocarcinogenesis

Although the tumor-promoting properties of such physical factors as freezing, scalding, and wounding have been described for chemical carcinogenesis systems, little information is available about the effects of these factors on UV-induced cancer formation. Bain and Rush (1943) reported that increasing the temperature to 35–38°C accelerated the tumor growth rate. The stimulating effects of heat on UV carcinogenesis were confirmed by Freeman and Knox (1964). Heat also enhanced the acute injury response to UV.

Temperature does not affect the photochemical reactions that follow UV irradiation, but it does affect many of the biochemical reactions that follow the initial photochemical change (Blum, 1943, 1969). Although it is known that heat adversely affects photosensitivity (Lipson and Baldes, 1960) and other phenomena of light injury (Bovie and Klein, 1919; Hill and Eidenow, 1923) and that heat alters the effects of X-rays (Carlson and Jackson, 1959), the influence of heat on burns produced by sunlight or UV has rarely been considered (Freeman and Knox, 1964).

High winds and high humidity significantly increase tumor incidence (Zilov, 1971; Owens et al., 1977).

Chemically Enhanced Photocarcinogenesis

A significant problem concerns photoinduced carcinogenesis following the application to the skin of agents that are phototoxic, but not in themselves carcinogenic.

A portion of the sunlight spectrum is carcinogenic, even in the absence of an exogenous photosensitizer. At the current rate of introduction of new compounds into the environment, it has become increasingly important to determine whether a readily demonstrable property such as phototoxicity can be used to predict compounds or treatment regimes that could enhance photocarcinogenesis.

Concepts of chemical interaction with UV-photocarcinogenesis are of recent origin. Blum (1969) and Emmett (1974) reviewed reports dealing with the influence of phototoxic substances on photocarcinogenesis. The results frequently appeared to be in disagreement, a situation possibly reflecting differences in technique—including solvent, route of administration, light source, and criteria for tumor recognition—and in statistical evaluation (Blum, 1969). In addition, characteristics of some compounds (toxicity, carcinogenicity, instability) rendered their interactions with light complex and their analysis difficult.

The relative enhancing effects on photocarcinogenesis of two widely recognized photoactive compounds, 8-methoxypsoralen (8-MOP) and anthracene, were studied by Forbes et al. (1970). Both compounds were phototoxic, but only the 8-MOP solutions markedly enhanced photocarcinogenesis. Thus, the ability of a chemical to induce phototoxicity is not always sufficient to augment photocarcinogenesis.

Interactions between Light and Chemical Carcinogenesis

The fact that UV can alter several phenanthrene carcinogens photochemically has been known for some time. Davies et al. (1972a, 1972b) showed that the carcinogenicity of 7,12-dimethylbenz[a]anthracene (DMBA) was reduced by light according to the demonstrable photochemical lability of the compound. There was evidence that an additional time-dependent factor could influence this effect. At least in the case of DMBA-treated animals, light may contribute in two opposing ways: (1) by degrading the carcinogen to noncarcinogenic products, and (2) by stimulating a phototoxic response that appears to coincide with a relatively increased tumor yield.

Depending on the UV wavelengths used, carcinogens can be photodegraded to a less carcinogenic compound or can induce phototoxicity, which may augment carcinogenesis or cause such a severe local phototoxic reaction that the epithelial skin cells are nearly all destroyed. Thus, either enhancement or inhibition of skin carcinogenesis may occur, depending on ,the carcinogen and the wavelength of the light source used.

Photochemical conversion of sterols to carcinogenic substances has been proposed as an explanation for the cancer-causing effects of light on skin (Black and Douglas, 1973). *In vitro*, one such compound, cholesterol-5α-oxide, which possesses carcinogenic properties (Bischoff, 1969), is formed in human skin exposed to UV (Black and Lo, 1971).

HUMAN SKIN CARCINOGENESIS

Nonmelanoma Skin Cancer

Examination of the sun's role in the production of human skin cancer does not lend itself to direct experimentation. However, extensive astute observations have strongly suggested the etiologic significance of light energy in the induction of these tumors. Skin cancers in Caucasians in general are most prevalent in the geographic areas of greatest insolation and among people who receive the most exposure, that is, men who work outdoors. They are rare in Negroes and other deeply pigmented individuals, who have the greatest protection against UV light injury. Further, the lightest complexioned individuals, such as those of Scottish and Irish descent, appear to be most susceptible to skin cancer formation when they live in geographic areas of high UV exposure. When skin cancers do occur in the darkly pigmented races, they are not distributed primarily in the sun-exposed areas as they are in light-skinned people. The tumors in these pigmented individuals are more commonly stimulated by other forms of trauma, such as chronic leg ulcers, irritation due to lack of wearing shoes, use of a kangri (an earthenware pot filled with burning charcoal and strapped to the abdomen for warmth), wearing of a dhoti (loincloth), and so on. In contrast, the distribution of skin cancer in the Bantu albino and in patients with xeroderma pigmentosum follows sun exposure patterns.

Blum (1959), Urbach et al. (1972), and Emmett (1974) reviewed the evidence supporting the role of sunlight in human skin cancer development. Briefly, the main arguments are:

1. Superficial skin cancers occur most frequently on the head, neck, and hands, parts of the body habitually exposed to sunlight.
2. Pigmented races, who sunburn much less readily than people with light skin, have very much less skin cancer, and when skin cancer does occur it affects areas not exposed to sunlight most frequently.
3. Among Caucasians there appears to be a much greater incidence of skin cancer in those who spend more time outdoors than those who work predominantly indoors.
4. Skin cancer is more common in light-skinned people living in areas where insolation is greater.
5. Genetic diseases resulting in greater sensitivity of skin to the effect of solar UV radiation are associated with marked increases in and premature skin cancer development (albinism, xeroderma pigmentosum).
6. Superficial skin cancers, particularly squamous cell carcinoma of the skin, occur predominantly on the areas that receive the maximum amounts of solar UV radiation and where histological changes of chronic UV damage are most severe.
7. Skin cancer can be produced readily on the skin of mice and rats with repeated doses of UV radiation, and the upper wavelength limit of the most effective cancer-producing radiation is about 320 nm—that is, the same spectral range that produces erythema solare in human skin.

Although these arguments do not constitute absolute proof, there is excellent epidemiologic evidence supporting the role of sunlight in non-melanoma skin cancers.

Malignant Melanoma

Malignant melanoma (MM) is a relatively uncommon tumor, primarily occurring in humans. The sex ratio varies from 1:1 to 1:1.2 (males:females). In contrast to nonmelanoma skin cancer (NMSC), the anatomic distribution of MM does not follow the most UV-exposed sites. About 10% of MM are on the head and neck. This type of lesion most often represents lentigo maligna melanoma (LMM) and has basically the same characteristics as squamous cell carcinoma: location on the most exposed sites of the head and neck, low incidence before age 50, rapid and progressive rise in frequency with advancing age, almost uniform presence of solar elastosis in the adjacent skin, and low aggressiveness (Magnus, 1977).

While NMSC is extremely uncommon in pigmented races, MM occurs about one-fifth as frequently in such people as in light-skinned patients and is mostly found (75–85%) on the foot and lower leg (Oettle, 1963).

Another 6–11% of MM appear to be of genetic origin, as evidenced by familial and multiple lesions and peculiar precursors found early in life (B-K mole) (Clark et al., 1978).

The remaining approximately 75–80% of MM in whites have interesting attributes. The incidence rises sharply from adolescence to early adult life (particularly on the legs of women), levels off through middle age, and rises again in old age (because of the appearance of LMM). The incidence in males and females shows a preponderance of young females (less than 40 yr old), and the sites of greatest incidence differ, being the trunk in males and the lower leg in females (Magnus, 1977). Of interest is the observation that, although the various populations studied live in such disparate areas as Finland (north of 60°N) (Teppo et al., 1978) and Queensland, Australia (25–15°S) (Beardmore, 1972) and thus are exposed to very different amounts of solar UV, the relative proportions of MM affecting various body sites remained quite stable until recently. In at least two areas (Norway and Hawaii) the differences in incidence of MM between males and females on the most affected sites (back in men and legs in women) seem to have been disappearing in the past decade (Hinds and Kolonel, 1980).

Latitude gradients for incidence (and mortality) of MM exist in some countries but not in others. Thus there are real latitude gradients for MM in Norway, Sweden, Great Britain, and the United States (Lee, 1977); less striking or even reversed gradients in Western Australia and central Europe (Crombie, 1979); and a partial latitude gradient in Eastern Australia, where in Queensland the incidence of MM is less in the tropics than in the subtropical areas (Holman et al., 1980).

In contrast to NMSC, the populations most affected are not the outdoor workers, but the white-collar, more educated, more affluent people (Lee and Strickland, 1980), and the concentration of MM in large cities cancels out a latitude gradient in such places as Finland and Western Australia, where this has been investigated (Holman et al., 1980).

The worldwide rapid increase in the incidence of MM (and much slower increase in mortality rates, as if MM were becoming less aggressive) has been attributed to changes in life-style, as greater exposure to solar UV occurs during leisure activities and vacations (Magnus, 1977). The more affluent are considered more likely to participate in such activities, and it is reasoned that men removing their shirts outdoors and women wearing shorter skirts account for the peculiar anatomic distribution of MM (Fears et al., 1976).

The lack of evidence for chronic solar damage of skin in which MM appear, young age of the majority of patients, variation in latitude gradients, anatomic distribution not matching the most exposed skin areas, and preponderance of city dwellers suggest strongly that there is a significant difference in pathogenesis between NMSC and MM, at least as far as the significance of solar UV is concerned.

Except for LMM, MM are certainly not related to chronic, repeated solar UV damage resulting from accumulated dose. Whether acute, intermittent exposure to solar UV, intensity of irradiation, or some interaction of UV with chemicals or precursor lesions is the basis of MM etiology remains to be determined. The absence of a good animal model for MM, at least for the relation of UV to MM, makes such studies difficult.

SUMMARY

Human skin cancers, particularly basal cell and squamous cell carcinomas, are closely associated with chronic, repeated exposure of the skin to solar UV radiation. Individuals who sunburn easily and have considerable exposure to solar UV have a much higher incidence of nonmelanoma skin cancer than those who sunburn rarely, tan easily, and have little exposure to the sun. Pigmented people rarely develop such skin cancers in light-exposed areas unless pigment is missing (albinos).

In addition to natural UV exposure, the interaction of UV and certain photosensitizing chemicals (psoralens, coal tar, etc.) can augment photocarcinogenesis.

Skin tumors similar to squamous cell carcinoma in humans can be regularly induced in rodents by using UV similar to that present in sunlight.

Malignant melanoma, which is considerably rarer than nonmelanoma skin cancer, is more serious because of its ability to metastasize and cause death. There has been a consistent, worldwide increase in the incidence of MM of about 3-7% per year, leading to a doubling of incidence rates in 10-15 yr.

There are striking differences in anatomic distribution between MM and NMSC by sex and site. MM is a disease of younger adults; NMSC occurs primarily in the older population. A relation to chronic insolation, which is so striking in NMSC, is at most doubtful in MM.

REFERENCES

Bain, J. and Rush, H. P. 1943. Carcinogenesis with UV radiation of wavelengths 2800–3400 A. *Cancer Res.* 3:425–430.

Beardmore, G. L. 1972. The epidemiology of malignant melanoma in Australia. In *Melanoma and Skin Cancer*, pp. 39–64. Sydney: New South Wales Government Printer.

Bischoff, F. 1969. Carcinogenic effect of steroids. *Adv. Lipid Res.* 7:165–244.

Black, H. S. and Douglas, D. R. 1973. Formation of a carcinogen of natural origin in the etiology of UV carcinogenesis. *Cancer Res.* 33:2094–2096.

Black, H. S. and Lo, W. B. 1971. Formation of a carcinogen in human skin irradiated in ultraviolet light. *Nature (Lond.)* 234:306–308.

Blum, H. F. 1943. Wavelength dependence of tumor induction by ultraviolet radiation. *J. Natl. Cancer Inst.* 3:533–537.

Blum, H. F. 1959. *Carcinogenesis by Ultraviolet Light.* Princeton, N.J.: Princeton Univ. Press.

Blum, H. F. 1969. Quantitative aspects of cancer induction by UV light. In *The Biological Effects of Ultraviolet Radiation*, ed. F. Urbach, pp. 543–549. Oxford, Pergamon.

Blum, H. F. and Lippincott, S. W. 1943. Carcinogenic effectiveness of UV radiation of wavelength 2537 Å. *J. Natl. Cancer Inst.* 3:211–216.

Bovie, W. T. and Klein, A. 1919. Sensitization to heat due to exposure to light of short wavelengths. *J. Gen. Physiol.* 1:331–336.

Carlson, L. D. and Jackson, B. H. 1959. Combined effects of ionizing radiation and high temperature on longevity of Sprague-Dawley rats. *Radiat. Res.* 11:509–519.

Clark, W. H., Jr., Reiner, R. R., Greene, M., et al. 1978. Origin of familial malignant melanoma from heritable melanocytic lesions. *Arch. Dermatol.* 114:732–738.

Crombie, I. K. 1979. Variation of melanoma with latitude in North America and Europe. *Br. J. Cancer* 40:774–781.

Davies, R. E., Dodge, H. A., and Austin, W. A. 1972a. Carcinogenicity of DMBA under various light sources. *Proc. 9th Int. Congr. Photobiol.*, p. 247 (abstract).

Davies, R. E., Dodge, H. A., and DeShields, L. H. 1972b. Alteration of the carcinogenicity of DMBA by light. *Proc. Am. Assoc. Cancer Res.* 13:14 (abstract).

Emmett, E. A. 1974. Ultraviolet radiation as a cause of skin tumors. *Crit. Rev. Toxicol.* 2:211.

Epstein, J. H. and Epstein, W. L. 1963. A study of tumor types produced by UV light in hairless and hairy mice. *J. Invest. Dermatol.* 41:463–473.

Fears, T. R., Scotto, J., and Schneiderman, M. A. 1976. Skin cancer, melanoma and sunlight. *Am. J. Public Health* 66:461–464.

Forbes, P. D., Davies, R. E., and Urbach, F. 1970. Phototoxicity and photocarcinogenesis: Comparative effects of anthracene and 8-methoxypsoralen in the skin of mice. *Food Cosmet. Toxicol.* 14:243.

Freeman, R. G. 1978. Data on the action spectrum for ultraviolet carcinogenesis. *Natl. Cancer Inst. Monogr.* 50:27–30.

Freeman, R. G. and Knox, J. M. 1964. Ultraviolet-induced corneal tumors in different species and strains of animals. *J. Invest. Dermatol.* 43:431–436.

Griffin, A. C., Dolman, V. S., et al. 1955. The effect of visible light on the carcinogenicity of ultraviolet light. *Cancer Res.* 15:523.

Hill, L. and Eidenow, A. 1923. Biological action of light. I. Influence of temperature. *Proc. R. Soc. London Ser. B.* 95:163–180.

Hinds, M. W. and Kolonel, L. N. 1980. Malignant melanoma of the skin in Hawaii, 1960-1977. *Cancer* 45:811-817.

Holman, C. D. J., Mulroney, C. D., and Armstrong, P. K. 1980. Epidemiology of pre-invasive and invasive malignant melanoma in Australia. *Int. J. Cancer* 25:317-323.

Kelner, A. and Taft, E. B. 1956. The influence of photoreactivating light on the type and frequency of tumors induced by UV radiation. *Cancer Res.* 16:860-866.

Lee, J. A. H. 1977. Current evidence about the causes of malignant melanoma. *Prog. Clin. Cancer* 7:151.

Lee, J. A. H. and Strickland, D. 1980. Malignant melanoma: Social status and outdoor work. *Br. J. Cancer* 41:757-763.

Lipson, R. L. and Baldes, E. J. 1960. Photosensitivity and heat. *Arch. Dermatol.* 82:517-520.

Magnus, K. 1977. Incidence of malignant melanoma of the skin in the five Nordic countries. *Int. J. Cancer* 20:477-485.

Nakamura, K. and Johnson, W. C. 1968. Ultraviolet light induced connective tissue changes in rat skin. *J. Invest. Dermatol.* 51:253-258.

Oëttle, C. H. 1963. Skin cancer in Africa. In *Natl. Cancer Inst. Monogr.* 10:197-214.

Owens, D. W., Knox, J. H., et al. 1977. The influence of wind on chronic ultraviolet light-induced carcinogenesis. *Br. J. Dermatol.* 97:285.

Roffo, A. H. 1933. Cancer y sol. *Boll. Inst. Med. Exp. Estud. Trata Cancer* 10:417-439.

Rusch, H. P., Kline, B. Z., and Bauman, C. A. 1941. Carcinogenesis by UV rays with reference to wavelength and energy. *Arch. Pathol.* 371:135-146.

Sams, W. M., Jr., Smith, J. G., and Burk, P. G. 1964. The experimental production of elastosis with ultraviolet light. *J. Invest. Dermatol.* 43:467.

Setlow, R. B. 1974. The wavelengths in sunlight effective in producing skin cancer: A theoretical analysis. *Proc. Natl. Acad. Sci. U.S.A.* 71:3363-3366.

Stenbäck, F. 1969. Promotion in the morphogenesis of chemically inducible skin tumors. *Acta Pathol. Microbiol. Scand. Suppl.* 208:1-116.

Stenbäck, F. 1975a. Cellular injury and cell proliferation in skin carcinogenesis by UV light. *Oncology* 31:61-65.

Stenbäck, F. 1975b. Species-specific neoplastic progression by ultraviolet light on the skin of rats, guinea pigs, hamsters and mice. *Oncology* 31:209-225.

Stenbäck, F. 1978. Life history and histopathology of ultraviolet light induced skin tumors. *Natl. Cancer Inst. Monogr.* 50:37-70.

Teppo, L., Pakkanen, M., and Hakulinen, T. 1978. Sunlight as a risk factor of malignant melanoma of the skin. *Cancer* 41:2018-2027.

Urbach, F., Rose, D. B., and Bonnem, M. 1972. Genetic and environmental interactions in skin carcinogenesis. In *Environment and Cancer*, pp. 355-371. Baltimore, Md.: Williams & Wilkins.

Zackheim, H. S. 1963. Origin of the human basal cell epithelioma. *J. Invest. Dermatol.* 40:283-297.

Zilov, J. N. D. 1971. In *Ultraviolet Radiation*, pp. 237-241. Moscow: Medicina.

21

cutaneous carcinogenesis

■ Fred G. Bock ■

INTRODUCTION

The production of skin cancer by chemicals was described more than two centuries ago (Potter, 1963). Since that time, we have accumulated a great deal of empirical data by observing this process in experimental animals. Inasmuch as experimental results are being used to develop social decisions aimed at a reduction of human malignant disease, the relationships between carcinogenesis in animals and humans are very important. It is the purpose of this review to explore some of the factors affecting the response of various species exposed to carcinogens. In this way, the significance of animal studies may be easier to determine.

More than one and one-half centuries were required for experimental skin carcinogenesis to be demonstrated at all. However, following the landmark experiment of Yamagiwa and Ichikawa (1918), animal models appeared to be particularly appropriate for the study of human carcinogenesis. It became routine to produce skin cancers in animals by applying the environmental agents that were believed to produce skin cancer in humans (U.S. Public Health Service, 1973). But somewhat later, numerous anomalies were encountered. Carcinogenesis was often organ-specific. Various species exhibited a range of responses. Substances such as glucose or sodium chloride that did not produce cancer in usual circumstances produced this disease when high concentrations were injected into animals. Size and shape of implanted materials were sometimes more important than chemical composition (Autian, 1974). There followed a period of questioning what a carcinogen was and the significance to humans of agents that produced cancer in animal experiments. These questions were of theoretical importance, of course. But they were also cited to impede remedial action directed against very important environmental carcinogenic stimuli. Arriving at the answers is one of the most promising albeit the most challenging problems that faces experimental oncologists, public health officials, and medical practitioners today.

WHAT IS A CARCINOGEN?

A recent definition has been used for development of safety standards (Office of Research Safety, National Cancer Institute, 1975). A "chemical carcinogen is a chemical which has been demonstrated to cause tumors in mammalian species by induction of a tumor type not usually observed, by induction of an increased incidence of the tumor type normally seen, or by the appearance of such tumors at an earlier time than would be otherwise expected." The term can be further refined (Hecker, 1976) to take into account different mechanisms through which a change in tumor incidence is induced. The definitions are explicit and meet the requirements for clarity. Nevertheless, they fail to be completely useful in guiding control of environmental carcinogens. For example, carbon-14 is undoubtedly a carcinogen because it is radioactive. However, one would not mandate avoidance of that carcinogen, which of course is present in all foodstuffs and in the exhaled air of every human being.

To achieve a real understanding of practical carcinogenesis, we must distinguish between a carcinogen and a carcinogenic stimulus. For chemical agents, a carcinogenic stimulus is a material that contains sufficient carcinogen to produce an increase in cancer incidence in a *particular* population. The population may be unique with respect to genetic background or antecedent history. For example, croton oil does not meet the NCI definition of a carcinogen in the strictest sense, and yet a dilute solution of croton oil is a potent carcinogenic stimulus for special populations of mice. It will produce very large numbers of tumors if the animals are previously exposed to very low doses of certain other chemicals (Berenblum and Shubik, 1947; Boutwell, 1964). This distinction between carcinogens and carcinogenic stimuli is very important in limiting human carcinogenesis. We cannot hope to avoid contact with every carcinogen. We can, however, control those that are present under conditions that make them effective carcinogenic stimuli for humans (Gori, 1976).

The concept of carcinogenic stimulus implies acceptance of tumor incidences below some minimally detectable level. This is not to say that there is a threshold of concentration of carcinogen activity. Evidence for such thresholds is not convincing. Indeed, the problems of threshold have led Mantel and Schneiderman (1975) to develop a method to identify acceptable levels of carcinogens for humans. Their proposal provides a valuable point of departure, but was not designed to consider the diversity of genetic backgrounds that exists in human populations.

ULTIMATE CARCINOGEN MOLECULES AND THE
ESSENTIAL CARCINOGENIC STEP

It is now widely accepted that in order to produce cancer, a chemical molecule (positively charged) must react (covalently) with nucleophilic centers (usually DNA) in target molecules within the cell (Miller, 1970). Unfortunately, the classes of carcinogens are more extensive than would be apparent from this evaluation. Many of the first carcinogens discovered showed no apparent chemical activity that could account for their biological properties. These included the prominent cutaneous carcinogens of humans—the polycyclic hydrocarbons of coal tar. The discovery that these substances were metabolized by the host animal into highly reactive intermediates has contributed enormously to our understanding in this field. Consideration of these events now provides a basis for extrapolating animal observations to humans, for comparison of organ sensitivity, and perhaps for identifying the genetic sensitivity of individuals.

The ultimate target of carcinogenesis lies in the genetic mechanism of the affected cell. Most believe that DNA molecules react directly with the ultimate carcinogens. However, the active carcinogens are capable of combining with proteins as well (Heidelberger, 1970) and other plausible mechanisms have been proposed (Pitot and Heidelberger, 1963).

Exposure to a carcinogen results in cancer only after a protracted period. The effects on the target, therefore, appear to be irreversible. The permanence of these changes were measured by conducting two-stage tumor induction experiments in mouse skin. In these studies a single very low dose of 7,12-dimethylbenz[a]anthracene (DMBA) or urethan was followed later by repetitive treatment with a tumor promoter such as croton oil or its active component, 12-O-tetradecanoyl phorbol-13-acetate (TPA). It was found that the tumor-initiating effect of DMBA persisted for the entire period of observation, which was as long as 43 wk (Berenblum and Shubik, 1949) or 56 wk (Van Duuren et al., 1975) in some experiments. These periods are about half of the life-span of mice.

Before we assume that the very first step of carcinogenesis is irreversible, we must consider some possible exceptions. It has been demonstrated that repair of DNA occurs after exposure of cells to certain types of carcinogenic stimuli (Cleaver, 1968; Stich and San, 1971). Cells from xeroderma pigmentosum patients lack the ability to repair DNA after such carcinogen treatment, accounting for the high skin tumor incidence in individuals with this condition. With some carcinogens, therefore, the first carcinogenic event is reversible. With other carcinogens an irreversible second step must follow immediately after the first reversible alteration.

COCARCINOGENESIS

Rous and his colleagues showed that cutaneous carcinogenesis could be divided into at least two separate processes, which they described as "initiation" and "promotion" (Friedenwald and Rous, 1944). This work was refined in a study by Berenblum and Shubik (1947), who further characterized the initiation and promotion phases of tumor development. Except for relatively minor effects, a promoting stimulus must be applied after the initiating stimulus in order to be active. In these two-stage carcinogenesis experiments, the tumor promoters appear to have definite threshold levels of concentration or frequencies of application below which they are ineffective. Cocarcinogenesis and anti-carcinogenesis can be expected to occur through other mechanisms as well as a consequence of the pathways of tumor induction (Berenblum, 1969). We found that the typical tumor-promoter TPA is a strong synergist of benzo[a]pyrene (BP) if it is applied concurrently with the hydrocarbon rather than sequentially (Bock et al., 1974). In this situation TPA is active at concentrations much lower than those required for tumor-promoting activity. Similar synergistic effects probably account for the carcinogenic activity of cigarette smoke condensate in mice (Hoffmann and Wynder, 1971).

Examples of synergistic carcinogenic stimuli in humans are seen in asbestos workers (Selikoff and Hammond, 1972) and uranium miners (Archer et al., 1973) who smoke. It would seem likely that synergisms of carcinogenic stimuli may account for a large proportion of the tumors observed in the general human population.

Many years ago, it was known that caloric restriction would reduce the incidence of tumors. In the skin, at least, this effect involved the promotion stage of carcinogenesis. More recently, a number of food constituents have been shown capable of inhibiting carcinogenesis (Wattenberg, 1980).

DELIVERY OF CARCINOGENS TO THE SKIN

One of the striking features of experimental carcinogenesis is the large variety of active compounds that have been identified. In the compilations of experiments in carcinogenesis by Shubik and Hartwell (1957), about a fifth of all of the chemicals reported gave at least one positive result. The compilers caution that the list is weighted in favor of positive compounds. Nevertheless, the prevalance of carcinogens is startling. Van Duuren et al. (1974b) recently tabulated the variety of chemical carcinogens according to chemical classification. These compounds have been identified in most part by their effects on a variety of organs. In order to understand their potential for cutaneous carcinogenesis, it seems wise to examine them according to the broadest mechanisms by which they could react with appropriate targets within the skin. Ultimate carcinogens could reach such targets by three pathways (Fig. 1; Table 1).

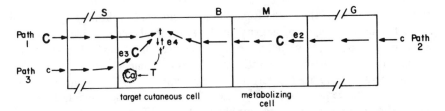

FIGURE 1 Schematic illustration of possible pathways by which ultimate carcinogens reach targets. (Path 1) An already active carcinogen (C) passes through skin surface cells (S) and through target cell cytoplasm to the target molecule (t). (Path 2) A procarcinogen (c), passes through intervening cells (G) to a metabolizing cell (M). There it is activated by an enzyme system (e2) to an ultimate carcinogen. The ultimate carcinogen passes out of M and is transported through the blood (B) to the target cell. (Path 3) A procarcinogen passes through S to the target cell. There it is activated by an enzyme system (e3) to an ultimate carcinogen, which reacts with a target molecule within the same cell. In all three pathways, the target molecule is altered to t' by a reversible step or further to T by an irreversible step. Over a period of time, T will give rise to a malignant cell through a variety of mechanisms, including action of cocarcinogens.

Path 1 will be followed by chemicals that are themselves active carcinogens; that is, those which possess strong electrophilic centers in their molecular structure. The active compounds must traverse a surface layer of cells (S) on route to the target cell. Within the target cell, the active molecules pass through a variable portion of cytoplasm to reach the target molecule (T).

Several characteristics of the carcinogen will affect its activity in either animals or humans (Table 1). First, the carcinogen molecule must be relatively stable in order to survive the period required for it to move through the surface cells and through the cytoplasm of the target cell. Second, the carcinogenic molecule must be relatively active in order to effectively transform the target molecule. This second requirement is the opposite of the

TABLE 1 Sources of Differences in Carcinogenic Response[a]

A. Before initial target reaction

Path 1	Path 2	Path 3
Stability of C	Stability of C	
Transit of S	Transit of G, M, B	Transit of S
Activity of C	Activity of C	Activity of C
	Presence of e2	Presence of e3
Damage to S or other cells	Damage to other organs	

B. After initial target reaction

Availability to T of promoters, other cocarcinogens, or anticarcinogens
Presence of e4

[a]See Fig. 1.

first. Accordingly, the effectiveness of carcinogens following path 1 is restricted by the degree of activity of the electrophilic center. If they are too strongly or too weakly active, compounds will have limited carcinogenic importance. The carcinogenic activity will also depend on the rate at which the molecules move to the target cell. For skin, solubility in lipids should enhance carcinogenic activity. The use of volatile lipid solvents also adds to their effectiveness (Bock and Burnham, 1961). The time required for a carcinogen to pass through the surface layer of cells depends as well on the species and on genetic factors within a species. In mice, the skin is thin and the target cells lie very close to the surface; penetration of lipid materials is enhanced (Bock, 1963). Penetration is much less efficient in humans. Humans should therefore be much less sensitive than mice to percutaneous exposure of path 1 carcinogens.

One would expect that, even in mice, subcutaneous injection of path 1 carcinogens would be more effective than skin painting. Indeed, this is the case (Van Duuren et al., 1974a). In humans, we should expect that these agents would be much more likely to induce cancer in organs where the target cells lie closer to the surface than they do in the skin. This also seems to be the case. After bis(chloromethyl) ether was identified as a carcinogen for mouse skin (Van Duuren et al., 1969), workers exposed to this material were found to have a higher incidence of lung carcinoma (Figueroa et al., 1973; Sakabe, 1973).

A final factor limits the manifestation of path 1 carcinogenic activity. If the carcinogenic molecule causes acute damage to cells other than the target cells, these effects may preclude observation of carcinogenesis. In experimental animals such damage will limit the dose or the length of time the animals can be observed. In either case, a sufficient carcinogenic stimulus might not be achieved. Demonstration of carcinogenic activity in human skin by such materials is particularly unlikely because acute manifestations of toxicity will lead to control of exposure.

Path 2 requires that a carcinogen is metabolized to an ultimate carcinogenic form in a distant organ and is then transported to the skin (Fig. 1). This pathway is as yet hypothetical for cutaneous carcinogenesis, although it is well known with respect to targets in other organs (Miller and Miller, 1974). We can expect that the skin is not immune to the action of such ultimate carcinogenic forms. However, the complex nature of path 2 limits carcinogenesis by this route and will impose great diversity in species and individual sensitivities to such carcinogens.

Many of the same factors that affect path 1 also affect the expression of carcinogenic activity by compounds following path 2. If the ultimate carcinogen molecule is very strongly active, it will survive and be effective only in the vicinity of its production. Many ultimate carcinogens are produced in the liver and exert their greatest activity there (Miller and Miller, 1974). To be effective as cutaneous carcinogens, the active molecules must successfully pass out of the metabolizing cells (M) through the blood stream (B) to the skin. The longer path places stricter upper limits on the activity of the ultimate carcinogen target cells than does path 1. Again, however, reaction with target molecules depends on the activity of the ultimate carcinogenic forms. It is not surprising that clear examples of skin carcinogenesis by this mechanism are not yet available. Oral administration of hydrocarbon carcinogens is also an effective stimulus of skin carcinogenesis and tumor initiation (Poel, 1963; Boutwell, 1964). It was not shown whether the agent was transported to the skin in the unchanged or metabolically activated form. After gastric intubation, unchanged hydrocarbons can be transported to distant lipid depots (Bock and Dao, 1961). It seems likely that the experimental results are a consequence of path 3 rather than path 2.

Path 2 will entail variability among species and individuals according to the presence of enzyme systems (e2) required to generate the ultimate carcinogenic forms from the precursor carcinogen molecules. Differences in species sensitivity to aromatic amine carcinogens are well known (Miller et al., 1964). Species-related factors such as diet and anatomic structure may also affect response to path 2 carcinogens. Finally, as in the case of path 1, we can expect that an effective carcinogenic stimulus will be impossible if the active agent causes such severe acute toxicity that adequate dosage is precluded.

In some cases, a procarcinogen may be metabolized to a proximal form, which can then be transported without substantial degradation to a distant site where the more active ultimate carcinogen is produced. The presence or absence of enzyme systems to carry out such steps has been proposed as an explanation for species differences in response to oral administration of carcinogenic aromatic amines (Lower and Bryan, 1979). Such a mechanism that combines elements of paths 2 and 3 has not been proposed for skin carcinogenesis.

Path 3 for carcinogen delivery to the skin is the one with which we are most familiar. In this situation, the compound in contact with the skin surface is not carcinogenic in itself. The compound must pass through the surface cells (S) to the target cell. There it is metabolized to an ultimate carcinogenic form within the skin. These compounds include the polycyclic hydrocarbons, which are formed by incomplete combustion of organic matter. They are metabolized by a complex system of enzymes that are found in the endoplasmic reticulum of most, if not all, organs and in most, if not all, species. It appears likely that the ultimate carcinogenic forms of aromatic hydrocarbons are bay region dihydrodiol epoxides (Conney et al., 1979). These compounds possess the necessary electrophilic activity and epoxide-forming enzymes are present in the skin in many strains of mice and in other species (Kinoshita and Gelboin, 1972; Pyerin and Hecker, 1975).

Because the chemically active ultimate carcinogens do not have to pass through a large volume of nontarget material before they reach the target cell, skin carcinogenesis by path 3 is the type most commonly observed in humans.

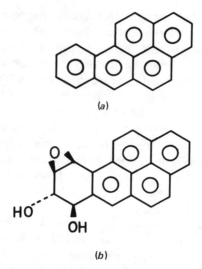

(a)

(b)

FIGURE 2 *(a)* Structure of benzo-[*a*]pyrene **(BP)**. *(b)* Structure of benzo[*a*]pyrene-7,8-dihydrodiol-9,10-epoxide, which may be the ultimate carcinogenic form of BP.

The compounds to which the skin surface is exposed are not themselves active, and effective carcinogenic stimuli will not cause damage to the surface cells or to other organs in the body. Exposure is not restricted within practical limits by acute toxicity. There is no strict upper limit on the activity of the ultimate carcinogenic molecule because the transit time from its site of production to its target within the same cell is very short. These factors, together with the widespread distribution of hydrocarbon-activating enzymes among species and in most organs, have caused these carcinogens to produce tumors in a very broad range of experiments.

Several factors contribute to species and individual differences in response to these agents. Transit of the hydrocarbon through the surface cells depends on the chemical properties of the hydrocarbon itself. Penetration of the skin by aromatic hydrocarbons is enhanced by solubility in less polar solvents (Bock, 1964). Penetration of hydrocarbons into mouse skin depends on the genetic constitution through mechanisms that have not been determined. Active participation by the mouse is not important; penetration is equally effective in dead mice. By far the most important factor affecting penetration into the cutaneous targets is skin thickness (Bock, 1963). This factor, no doubt, accounts in a large part for the high susceptibility of mouse skin to topically applied carcinogens.

Another important cause of variation in species and individual sensitivity to aromatic hydrocarbons is the level of metabolizing enzyme in the skin. The ultimate carcinogens appear to be dihydrodiol epoxides. The enzyme systems leading to their formation are complex (Wiebel et al., 1973). Furthermore, the same enzyme systems may ultimately lead to inactivation of the epoxides once they are formed (Wood, quoted in Wislocki et al., 1976). The level of enzymes within the tissues is a function of a basal level already present and the amount of enzyme induced by exposure to any of several substrates. Both the basal level and the extent of induction appear to be under genetic control (Kodama and Bock, 1970; Benedict et al., 1973). In some reports, the level of enzyme is correlated with the sensitivity of mice to carcinogenic treatment (Kouri et al., 1973; Thomas et al., 1973), but in other studies this is not the case (Benedict et al., 1973; Nebert et al., 1972). The level of enzyme in humans is also under genetic control (Kellermann et al., 1973a; Paigen et al., 1977). It has been reported (Kellermann et al., 1973b) that the incidence of human lung cancer is related to the inducibility of the enzyme. However, later work failed to confirm those observations (Paigen et al., 1977b).

At least two important factors will affect carcinogenesis as soon as the primary reaction between the target and ultimate carcinogen has occurred. Repair of affected DNA is under enzymic control (e4), which, in turn, is genetically determined (Cleaver, 1968; Stich and San, 1971). Agents that affect this system or the genetic variation of its effectiveness will affect the response of exposed individuals to carcinogens. A greater source of variation is the availability of cocarcinogens or anticarcinogens to the transformed target (T). The existence of such effects has been documented extensively in animal experiments (Berenblum, 1969). Cocarcinogenesis appears to play a role in human cancer as well (Selikoff and Hammond, 1972; Archer et al., 1973). Cocarcinogenesis could be expected to play a very important role in human skin cancer because everyone has been exposed to subthreshold levels of a number of carcinogens. Under such conditions, a cocarcinogen would deliver an effective carcinogenic stimulus and would not be distinguishable from a true carcinogen.

TUMOR PROMOTION

The production of tumors from initiated cells requires a substantial period of time and appears to be reversible (Boutwell, 1964). The most active tumor promoters are phorbol esters. Repeated applications of 0.5 nmol 12-tetradecanoylphorbol-13-acetate (TPA) are sufficient to promote tumors in mice previously "initiated" with carcinogenic hydrocarbons. Anthralin, an unrelated polyphenol, is active when doses of 100 nmol or greater are employed (Bock and Burns, 1963). Tumor-promoting activity is exhibited in many other types of compounds, albeit only with much greater concentrations. These include simple phenols (Boutwell and Bosch, 1959), iodoacetic acid (Rusch et al., 1955), peracetic acid (Bock et al., 1975), some detergents (Setälä, 1960), saturated aliphatic hydrocarbons (Bock and Chortyk, 1970), and fatty alcohols (Bock and Tso, 1976). These various compounds are, in general, either potent skin irritants or else agents that might be expected to affect the lipid-rich areas of cell membrane. Among the skin irritants, the phorbol esters bind to membrane receptors of a variety of cells including mouse epidermis (Driedger and Blumberg, 1980; Shoyab and Todaro, 1980; Ashendel and Boutwell, 1981). On the other hand, other skin irritants with promoting activity do not bind to those receptors (Driedger and Blumberg, 1980).

A number of changes in tissue treated with phorbol esters appear to be related to the promoting activity of these compounds. These include numerous changes that may be a consequence of alteration of epidermal cell membranes (Weinstein, 1980). Morphological changes induced by TPA in cultured 3T3 cells do not depend on the presence of the nucleus (Nagle and Blumberg, 1980), further suggesting that reactions with the cell membrane are the first critical step in tumor promotion by the phorbol esters. It has also been suggested that tumor promotion involves changes in nucleic acid metabolism (Paul and Hecker, 1969), DNA repair (Gaudin et al., 1972), or the release of reactive oxygen species from phagocytic cells activated by exposure to promoters (Goldstein et al., 1981). As yet, no consensus concerning the essential components of the promotion process has been achieved.

Understanding the nature of tumor promotion is made even more difficult by the demonstration that promotion itself can be divided into stages (Boutwell, 1964; Slaga et al., 1980). Either turpentine or mezerein can carry out the later stages of promotion but not the early stages.

Because of the complexity of promotion and other cocarcinogenic mechanisms as well, agents that do not cause cancer in controlled experimental environments may prove to be very significant carcinogenic stimuli for humans. The best example is arsenic. There is abundant evidence that inorganic arsenic compounds cause cancer in human skin as well as other organs (Konetzke, 1974). On the other hand, arsenical solutions were not effective carcinogenic stimuli in very sophisticated laboratory tests (Baroni et al., 1963). The latter studies employed hydrocarbons or urethan as primary carcinogens. This inconsistency may be resolved by examining other systems of carcinogenesis. Jung et al. (1969) reported that arsenate treatment caused a temporary fall in the DNA repair activity of human skin. Such an effect would enhance the carcinogenic activity of UV light because the first effect of UV light on DNA is largely reversible. In contrast, the first observed carcinogenic effects of DMBA and urethan are irreversible and less likely to be affected by DNA repair mechanisms. By and large, laboratory mice are protected from UV exposure. If arsenic owes its carcinogenic properties to inhibition of DNA repair, it would be the first clear example of a human carcinogenic stimulus provoked by an external agent that was not by itself carcinogenic.

Another material that plays a role in the manifestation of carcinogenesis is vitamin A or its analogs. The record here is also rather inconsistent. In the hamster respiratory tract elevated dietary vitamin A is reported to inhibit (Saffiotti et al., 1967) or enhance (Smith et al., 1975) the carcinogenic effects of benzpyrene. Vitamin A inhibits keratinization of rabbit keratoacanthomas and enhances the skin tumorigenic effect of DMBA in that species (Prutkin, 1968). Retinoids also inhibit the malignant transformation of cultured cells by 3-methylcholanthrene (Merriman and Bertram, 1979). It seems possible that these effects of vitamin A analogs are due to inhibition of tumor promotion (Bollag, 1972; Bollag, 1975; Verma et al., 1979). Retinoids inhibit TPA-stimulated ornithine decarboxylase activity in both intact mouse skin (Verma and Boutwell, 1977) and mouse skin organ cultures (Verma and Boutwell, 1980). They also inhibit formation of the superoxide anion radical in TPA-treated polymorphonuclear leukocytes (Witz et al., 1980).

In humans, the incidence of lung cancer is inversely related to the reported dietary levels of vitamin A (Mettlin et al., 1979). It is significant that cigarette smoke appears to act like a tumor promoter in humans (Doll and Peto, 1978).

The results with arsenic show the limitations of using negative animal experiments as an indication of safety for humans. We must also consider that many identified carcinogens at subthreshold levels can act as cocarcinogens or synergists with each other. Thus, any carcinogen exposure that is not an effective carcinogenic stimulus by itself may have this effect when imposed on a subject with past, present, or future exposure to low levels of other carcinogens. There is a real need for very careful monitoring of the human population—especially populations at high risk because of coexisting exposure to low levels of known carcinogens.

CONCLUSIONS

Several factors have been considered to determine whether animal carcinogenesis studies can be extrapolated to human skin. These include the path by which the ultimate carcinogen reaches the target and the future environment of the target after the initial carcinogenic event. A number of specific conclusions can be reached.

1. Agents that must be metabolized elsewhere to an active form, which is then transported to the skin, are most unlikely to be recognized as carcinogenic stimuli for human skin. Limitations on chemical activity and the likelihood of acute toxicity militate against sufficient exposure for significant skin carcinogenesis in the general population.

2. Agents that are already in the ultimate carcinogenic form are likely to be very effective when administered by the subcutaneous route. They are less likely to be active in mouse skin because losses incurred

in movement to the target site impose limitations on chemical activity. They are still less likely to cause skin cancer in humans or thick-skinned animals because of the longer path to the target. Acute toxicity of these materials will also limit exposure of humans, so that effective carcinogenic stimuli may not be encountered.

3. Agents that are themselves inactive but are transformed in the skin to active forms are most likely to be effective carcinogenic stimuli for human or mouse. Once again, human skin will be more resistant because the longer path will reduce the amount of carcinogen that reaches the target. Acute toxicity, however, will not be an important protective device.

4. Agents that do not cause cancer in controlled laboratory experiments may be serious carcinogenic stimuli for humans. Likewise, apparently subthreshold levels of carcinogens may serve as cocarcinogens. Careful monitoring of human populations is necessary to prevent avoidable cancers. Laboratory study, alone, is not sufficient.

We do not know, with certainty, the target molecule affected by carcinogenesis. Nor do we fully understand how cocarcinogens play a role in tumor development. Ultimately this knowledge will permit more precise assessment of human risk. Until then, we can achieve a measure of success by relating experimental results with chemical structure and the route by which the carcinogen arrived at the target organ.

REFERENCES

Archer, V. E., Wagoner, J. K., Hyg, S. D. and Lundin, F. E., Jr. 1973. Uranium mining and cigarette smoking effects on man. *J. Occup. Med.* 17:204–211.

Ashendel, C. L. and Boutwell, R. K. 1981. Direct measurement of specific binding of highly lipophilic phorbol diester to mouse epidermal membranes using cold acetone. *Biochem. Biophys. Res. Commun.* 99:543–549.

Autian, J. 1974. Film carcinogenesis. *Proc. 11th Int. Cancer Congr.* 2:94–101.

Baroni, C., Van Esch, G. J. and Saffiotti, U. 1963. Carcinogenesis tests of two inorganic arsenicals. *Arch. Environ. Health* 7:668–674.

Benedict, W. F., Considine, N. and Nebert, D. W. 1973. Genetic differences in aryl hydrocarbon hydroxylase induction and benzo[a]pyrene-produced tumorigenesis in the mouse. *Mol. Pharmacol.* 9:266–277.

Berenblum, I. 1969. A re-evaluation of the concept of cocarcinogenesis. *Progr. Exp. Tumor Res.* 11:21–30.

Berenblum, I. and Shubik, P. 1947. A new quantitative approach to the study of the stages of chemical carcinogenesis in the mouse's skin. *Br. J. Cancer* 1:383–391.

Berenblum, I. and Shubik, P. 1949. The persistence of latent tumour cells induced in the mouse's skin by a single application of 9:10-dimethyl-1:2-benzanthracene. *Br. J. Cancer* 3:384–386.

Bock, F. G. 1963. Species differences in penetration and absorption of chemical carcinogens. *Natl. Cancer Inst. Monogr.* 10:361–375.

Bock, F. G. 1964. Early effects of hydrocarbons on mammalian skin. *Progr. Exp. Tumor Res.* 4:126–168.

Bock, F. G. and Burnham, M. 1961. The effect of experimental conditions upon the concentration of hydrocarbons in mouse skin after cutaneous application. *Cancer Res.* 21:510–515.

Bock, F. G. and Burns, R. 1963. Tumor-promoting properties of anthralin (1,8,9-anthratriol). *J. Natl. Cancer Inst.* 30:393–397.

Bock, F. G. and Chortyk, O. T. 1970. Tumor promoting activity of aliphatic hydrocarbons. *Proc. Am. Assoc. Cancer Res.* 11:9.

Bock, F. G. and Dao, T. L. 1961. Factors affecting the polynuclear hydrocarbon level in rat mammary glands. *Cancer Res.* 21:1024–1029.

Bock, F. G. and Tso, T. C. 1976. Tumor promoting activity of agriculture chemicals. In *Smoking and health. I. Modifying the risk for the smoker,* Publ. No. (NIH) 76-1221, eds. E. L. Wynder, D. Hoffmann, and G. B. Gori, pp. 175–189. Washington, D.C.: Department of Health, Education and Welfare.

Bock, F. G., Bross, I. D. J. and Priore, R. L. 1974. Synergistic action of benzo[a]pyrene and tetradecanoyl phorbol acetate when applied concurrently. *Abstr. 11th Int. Cancer Congr.* 2:43.

Bock, F. G., Myers, H. K. and Fox, H. W. 1975. Cocarcinogenic activity of peroxy compounds. *J. Natl. Cancer Inst.* 55:1359–1361.

Bollag, W. 1972. Prophylaxis of chemically induced benign and malignant epithelial tumors by vitamin A acid (retinoic acid). *Eur. J. Cancer* 8:689–693.

Bollag, W. 1975. Prophylaxis of chemically induced epithelial tumors with an aromatic retinoic acid analog (Ro 10-9359). *Eur. J. Cancer* 11:721–724.

Boutwell, R. K. 1964. Some biological aspects of skin carcinogenesis. *Progr. Exp. Tumor Res.* 4:207–250.

Boutwell, R. K. and Bosch, D. K. 1959. The tumor-promoting action of phenol and related compounds for mouse skin. *Cancer Res.* 19:413–424.

Cleaver, J. E. 1968. Defective repair replication of DNA in xeroderma pigmentosum. *Nature (Lond.)* 218:652–656.

Conney, A. H., Levin, W., Wood, A. W., Yagi, H., Lehr, R. E. and Jerina, D. M. 1979. Biological activity of polycyclic hydrocarbon metabolites and the bay-region theory. *Adv. Pharmacol. Toxicol.* 9:41–52.

DeYoung, L. M., Helmes, C. T., Chao, W.-R., Young, J. M. and Miller, V. 1981. Paradoxical effect of anthralin on 12-O-tetradecanoylphorbol-13-acetate-induced mouse epidermal ornithine decarboxylase activity, proliferation, and tumor promotion. *Cancer Res.* 41:204–208.

Driedger, P. E. and Blumberg, P. M. 1980. Specific binding of phorbol ester tumor promoters. *Proc. Natl. Acad. Sci. U.S.A.* 77:567–571.

Figueroa, W. G., Raszkowski, R. and Weiss, W. 1973. Lung cancer in chloromethyl methyl ether workers. *N. Engl. J. Med.* 288:1096–1097.

Friedenwald, W. F. and Rous, P. 1944. The initiating and promoting elements in tumor production. *J. Exp. Med.* 80:101–125.

Gelboin, H. V. 1980. Benzo[a]pyrene metabolism, activation and carcinogenesis: Role and regulation of mixed-function oxidases and related enzymes. *Physiol. Rev.* 60:1107–1166.

Goldstein, B. D., Witz, G., Amoruso, M., Stone, D. S. and Troll, W. 1981. Stimulation of human polymorphonuclear leukocyte superoxide anion radical production by tumor promoters. *Cancer Lett.* 11:257–262.

Gori, G. B. 1976. Low-risk cigarettes: A prescription. *Science* 194:1243–1246.

Hecker, E. 1976. Definitions and terminology in cancer (tumor) etiology—An analysis aiming at proposals for a current internationally standardized terminology. *Int. J. Cancer* 18:122–129.

Heidelberger, C. 1970. Cellular and molecular mechanisms of hydrocarbon carcinogenesis. *Eur. J. Cancer* 6:161–172.

Hoffmann, D. and Wynder, E. L. 1971. A study of tobacco carcinogenesis. XI Tumor initiators, tumor accelerators, and tumor promoting activity of condensate fractions. *Cancer* 27:848–864.

Jung, E. G., Trachsel, B. and Immich, H. 1969. Arsenic as an inhibitor of the enzymes concerned in cellular recovery (dark repair). *Ger. Med. Mon.* 14:614–616.

Kellermann, G., Luyten-Kellermann, M. and Shaw, C. R. 1973a. Genetic variation of aryl hydrocarbon hydroxylase in human lymphocytes. *Am. J. Hum. Genet.* 25:327–331.

Kellermann, G., Shaw, C. R. and Luyten-Kellermann, M. 1973b. Aryl hydrocarbon hydroxylase inducibility and bronchogenic carcinoma. *N. Engl. J. Med.* 289:934–937.

Kinoshita, H. and Gelboin, H. V. 1972. The role of aryl hydrocarbon hydroxylase in 7,12-dimethylbenz(α)anthracene skin tumorigenesis: On the mechanism of 7,8-benzoflavone inhibition of tumorigenesis. *Cancer Res.* 32:1329–1339.

Kodama, Y. and Bock, F. G. 1970. Benzo[*a*]pyrene-metabolizing enzyme activity of livers of various strains of mice. *Cancer Res.* 30:1846–1849.

Konetzke, G. W. 1974. Die kanzerogene Wirkung von Arsen und Nickel. *Arch. Geschwulstforsch.* 44:16–22.

Kouri, R. E., Ratrie, H. and Whitmire, C. E. 1973. Evidence of a genetic relationship between susceptibility to 3-methylcholanthrene-induced subcutaneous tumors and inducibility of aryl hydrocarbon hydroxylase. *J. Natl. Cancer Inst.* 51:197–200.

Lower, G. M. and Bryan, G. T. 1979. Etiology and carcinogenesis: Natural systems approaches to causality and control. In *Management of urologic cancers*, ed. N. Javadpour, pp. 29–53. Baltimore, Md.: Williams & Wilkins.

Mantel, N. and Schneiderman, M. A. 1975. Estimating "safe" levels, a hazardous undertaking. *Cancer Res.* 35:1379–1386.

Merriman, R. L. and Bertram, J. S. 1979. Reversible inhibition by retinoids of 3-methylcholanthrene-induced neoplastic transformation in C3H/10T$\frac{1}{2}$ clone 8 cells. *Cancer Res.* 39:1661–1666.

Mettlin, C., Graham, S. and Swanson, M. 1979. Vitamin A and lung cancer. *J. Natl. Cancer Inst.* 62:1435–1438.

Miller, E. C. and Miller, J. A. 1974. The metabolic activation and reactivity of carcinogenic aromatic amines and amides. *Proc. 11th Int. Cancer Congr.* 2:3–8.

Miller, E. C., Miller, J. A. and Enomoto, M. 1964. The comparative carcinogenicities of 2-acetylaminofluorene on its N-hydroxy metabolite in mice, hamsters, and guinea pigs. *Cancer Res.* 24:2018–2032.

Miller, J. A. 1970. Carcinogenesis by chemicals: An overview—G. H. A. Clowes memorial lecture. *Cancer Res.* 30:559–576.

Nagle, D. S. and Blumberg, P. M. 1980. Activity of phorbol ester tumor promoters on enucleated Swiss 3T3 cells. *Cancer Res.* 40:1066–1072.

Nebert, D. W., Benedict, W. F., Gielen, J. E., Oesch, F. and Daly, J. W. 1972.

Aryl hydrocarbon hydroxylase, epoxide hydrase, and 7,12-dimethyl-benz[a]anthracene-produced skin tumorigenesis in the mouse. *Mol. Pharmacol.* 8:374–379.

Office of Research Safety, National Cancer Institute. 1975. National Cancer Institute safety standards for research involving chemical carcinogens. *DHEW Publ. No. (NIH) 76-900.*

Paigen, B., Gurtoo, H. I., Minowada, J., Houten, L., Vincent, R., Paigen, K., Parker, N. B., Ward, E. and Hayner, N. T. 1977a. Questionable relation of aryl hydrocarbon hydroxylase to lung-cancer risk. *N. Engl. J. Med.* 297:346–350.

Paigen, B., Gurtoo, H. L., Minowada, J. and Paigen, K. 1977b. Heritability of aryl-hydrocarbon hydroxylase in the human population. In *Proceedings of the 3rd international symposium on microsomes and drug oxidations*, eds. V. Ullrich, I. Roots, A. Hildebrandt, R. Estabrook and A. Conney. Oxford: Pergamon Press, in press.

Paul, D. and Hecker, E. 1969. On the biochemical mechanism of tumorigenesis in mouse skin. II. Early effects on the biosynthesis of nucleic acids induced by initiating doses of DMBA and by promoting doses of phorbol-12,13-diester TPA. *Z. Krebsforsch.* 73:149–163.

Pitot, H. D. and Heidelberger, C. 1963. Metabolic regulatory circuits and carcinogenesis. *Cancer Res.* 23:1694–1700.

Poel, W. E. 1963. Skin as a test site for the bioassay of carcinogens and carcinogen precursors. *Natl. Cancer Inst. Monogr.* 10:611–625.

Potter, M. 1963. Percivall Pott's contribution to cancer research. *Natl. Cancer Inst. Monogr.* 10:1–13.

Prutkin, L. 1968. The effect of vitamin A acid on tumorigenesis and protein production. *Cancer Res.* 28:1021–1030.

Pyerin, W. G. and Hecker, E. 1975. Epoxide hydrase activity in mouse skin epidermis. *Z. Krebsforsch.* 83:81–83.

Rusch, H. P., Bosch, D. and Boutwell, R. K. 1955. The influence of irritants on mitotic activity and tumor formation in mouse epidermis. *Acta Unio. Int. Contra Cancrum* 699–703.

Saffiotti, U., Montesano, R., Sellakumar, A. R. and Borg, S. A. 1967. Experimental cancer of the lung. Inhibition by vitamin A of the induction of tracheobronchial squamous metaplasia and squamous cell tumors. *Cancer* 20:857–864.

Sakabe, H. 1973. Lung cancer due to exposure to bis(chloromethyl) ether. *Ind. Health* 11:145–148.

Selikoff, I. and Hammond, E. C. 1972. Environmental cancer in the year 2000. *Proc. 7th Natl. Cancer Conf.* 687–696.

Shoyab, M. and Todaro, G. J. 1980. Specific high affinity cell membrane receptors for biologically active phorbol and ingenol esters. *Nature (Lond.)* 288:451–455.

Shubik, P. and Hartwell, J. L. 1957. Survey of compounds which have been tested for carcinogenic activity. *Public Health Serv. Publ. No. 149, Suppl. 1.*

Slaga, T. J., Fischer, S. M., Nelson, K. and Gleason, G. L. 1980. Studies on the mechanism of skin tumor promotion: Evidence for several stages in promotion. *Proc. Natl. Acad. Sci. U.S.A.* 77:3659–3663.

Smith, D. M., Rogers, A. E., Herndon, B. J. and Newberne, P. M. 1975. Vitamin A (retinyl acetate) and benzo(a)pyrene-induced respiratory tract carcinogenesis in hamsters fed a commercial diet. *Cancer Res.* 35:11–16.

Stich, H. F. and San, R. H. C. 1971. Reduced DNA repair synthesis in xeroderma pigmentosum cells exposed to the oncogenic 4-nitroquinoline-1-oxide and 4-hydroxy-amino-quinoline-1-oxide. *Mutat. Res.* 13:279–282.

Thomas, P. E., Hutton, J. J. and Taylor, B. A. 1973. Genetic relationship between aryl hydrocarbon hydroxylase inducibility and chemical carcinogen induced skin ulceration in mice. *Genetics* 74:655–659.

U.S. Public Health Service. 1973. *Survey of compounds which have been tested for carcinogenic activity, 1970–1971 volume.* Washington, D.C.: Government Printing Office.

Van Duuren, B. L., Goldschmidt, B. M., Katz, C., Langseth, L., Mercado, G. and Sivak, A. 1969. Alpha-haloethers: A new type of alkylating carcinogen. *Arch. Environ. Health* 16:472–476.

Van Duuren, B. L., Goldschmidt, B. M., Katz, C., Seidman, I. and Paul, J. S. 1974a. Carcinogenic activity of alkylating agents. *J. Natl. Cancer Inst.* 53:675–700.

Van Duuren, B. L., Witz, G. and Sivak, A. 1974b. Chemical carcinogenesis. In *Physiopathology of cancer*, 3rd ed., eds. F. Homburger and P. Shubik, vol. 1, pp. 1–63. Basel: Karger.

Van Duuren, B. L., Sivak, A., Katz, C., Seidman, I. and Melchionne, S. 1975. The effect of aging and interval between primary and secondary treatment in two-stage carcinogenesis on mouse skin. *Cancer Res.* 35:502–505.

Verma, A. K. and Boutwell, R. K. 1977. Vitamin A acid (retinoic acid), a potent inhibitor of 12-O-tetradecanoyl-phorbol-13-acetate-induced ornithine decarboxylase activity in mouse epidermis. *Cancer Res.* 37:2196–2201.

Verma, A. K. and Boutwell, R. K. 1980. An organ culture of adult mouse skin: An *in vitro* model for studying the molecular mechanism of skin tumor promotion. *Biochem. Biophys. Res. Commun.* 96:854–862.

Verma, A. K., Shapas, B. G., Rice, H. M. and Boutwell, R. K. 1979. Correlation of the inhibition by retinoids of tumor promoter-induced mouse epidermal ornithine decarboxylase activity and of skin tumor promotion. *Cancer Res.* 39:419–425.

Wattenberg, L. W. 1980. Inhibitors of chemical carcinogens. *J. Environ. Pathol. Toxicol.* 3:35–52.

Weinstein, I. B. 1980. Studies on the mechanism of action of tumor promoters and their relevance to mammary carcinogenesis. In *Cell biology of breast cancer*, pp. 425–450. New York: Academic Press.

Wiebel, F. J., Leutz, J. C. and Gelboin, H. V. 1973. Aryl hydrocarbon (benzo[a]pyrene) hydroxylase: Inducible in extrahepatic tissue of mouse strains, not inducible in liver. *Arch. Biochem. Biophys.* 154:292–294.

Wislocki, P. G., Wood, A. W., Chang, R. L., Levin, W., Yagi, H., Hernandez, O., Dansette, P. M., Jerina, D. M. and Conney, A. H. 1976. Mutagenicity and cytotoxicity of benzo(a)pyrene arene oxides, phenols, quinones, and dihydrodiols in bacterial and mammalian cells. *Cancer Res.* 36:3350–3357.

Witz, G., Goldstein, B. D. Amoruso, M., Stone, D. S. and Troll, W. 1980. Retinoid inhibition of superoxide anion radical production by human polymorphonuclear leukocytes stimulated with tumor promoters. *Biochem. Biophys. Res. Commun.* 97:883–888.

Wood, A. W., Wislocki, P. G., Chang, R. L., Levin, W., Lu, A. Y. H., Yagi, H., Hernandez, O., Jerina, D. M. and Conney, A. H. 1976. Mutagenicity and cytotoxicity of benzo(a)pyrene benzo-ring epoxides. *Cancer Res.* 36:3358–3366.

Yamagiwa, K. and Ichikawa, K. 1918. Experimental study of the pathogenesis of carcinoma. *J. Cancer Res.* 3:1–29.

22

detection
of environmental
depigmenting chemicals

Gerald A. Gellin ▪ Howard I. Maibach

INTRODUCTION

The "white skin syndrome" may have several causes (Lerner, 1971). A most perplexing aspect of human medicine is delineating the cases due to vitiligo (an idiopathic entity) and those due to a chemical (acquired leukoderma). Until more specific and simple diagnostic techniques become available, the latter is identified by chemical history (handling of known chemical depigmenters) and epidemiology (clustering of cases). New chemical causes of leukoderma can also be identified by prospective appropriate screening in animals and humans.

HISTORY

Occupational leukoderma due to skin contact with a chemical substance was reported for the first time more than 40 years ago (Oliver et al., 1939). The depigmentation, which resembled vitiligo, was produced by monobenzyl ether of hydroquinone (MBEH). Several congeners of MBEH were subsequently demonstrated to produce leukoderma—intentionally, accidentally, and experimentally. MBEH was used to depigment hyperpigmented skin in humans (Lerner and Fitzpatrick, 1953; Becker and Spencer, 1962). Its parent compound, hydroquinone (HQ), has been used commercially for two decades for this purpose (Spencer, 1961; Arndt and Fitzpatrick, 1965).

Reports from Japan, Russia, Holland, and the United States between 1960 and 1971 indicated that unexpected leukoderma was appearing among

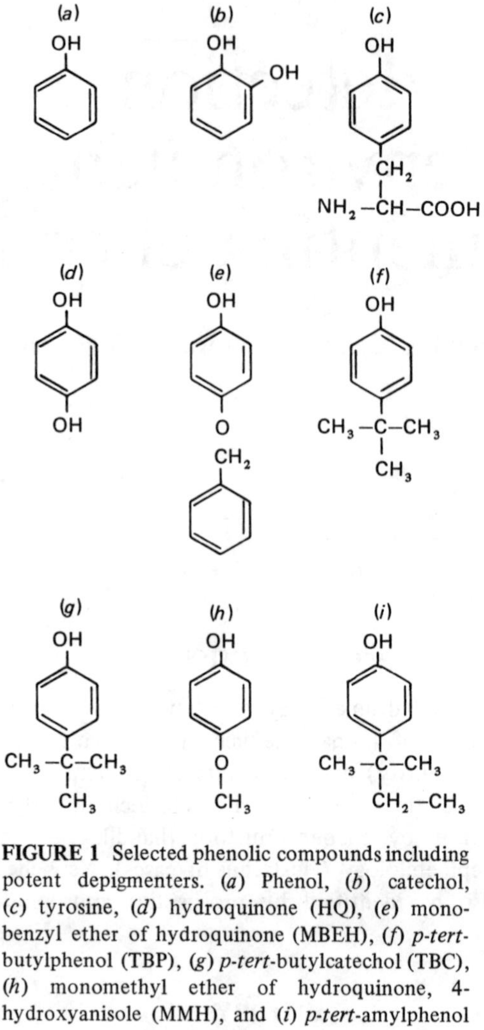

FIGURE 1 Selected phenolic compounds including potent depigmenters. (*a*) Phenol, (*b*) catechol, (*c*) tyrosine, (*d*) hydroquinone (HQ), (*e*) monobenzyl ether of hydroquinone (MBEH), (*f*) *p-tert*-butylphenol (TBP), (*g*) *p-tert*-butylcatechol (TBC), (*h*) monomethyl ether of hydroquinone, 4-hydroxyanisole (MMH), and (*i*) *p-tert*-amylphenol (TAP).

industrial workers. The unifying feature was exposure to phenolic and catecholic compounds. HQ and MBEH are in this family of compounds (Fig. 1). They are used in the manufacture of plastics, resins, synthetic rubber, paint, gasoline, and petroleum products. Functionally, they are antioxidants or rust inhibitors. They are chemical intermediates or end products in the broad field of phenolic chemistry.

Experimental work to study chemically induced depigmentation in animal models has been conducted by Brun (1960, 1967, 1974), Riley (1969a, 1969b), Fitzpatrick and co-workers (Arndt and Fitzpatrick, 1965; Frenk et al., 1968; Bleehen et al., 1968; Jimbow et al., 1974), Lerner (1971), and Shelly and Raque (1972), and in our laboratories. These studies were supplemented by clinical reports, cited above, which involved confirmatory work on animals. The major review article was by Malten et al. (1971). Kahn (1970) and Gellin et al. (1970a, 1970b) reported on clinical and laboratory studies in the United States.

Animals chosen for the screening of depigmenting action by chemicals have included black goldfish (Chavin, 1963); brown, wild-colored, and black guinea pigs; brown and black cats (Oettell, 1936); black rabbits; and black mice.

Gellin et al. (1970a, 1970b) studied four cases of leukoderma following exposure to *p-tert*-butylcatechol (TBC). This antioxidant and rust inhibitor was the sole additive in an assembly lubricating fluid handled by 75 workers in a factory making automobile tappets (valve lifters). The use concentration of TBC was 0.005%. Leukoderma began on the hands in the three Caucasian men and one woman. In three distant body sites depigmentation occurred. In these three cases positive patch tests were elicited, demonstrating allergic sensitization. In one of these, the positive patch test depigmented and remained leukodermatous over 20 mo. The irritant nature of TBC was noted by a 60% incidence of contact dermatitis among co-workers who eschewed protective clothing. When TBC was removed from the assembly oil the incidence of dermatitis fell.

ANIMAL MODELS

The animal models utilized are in Table 1. We extensively examined the guinea pig and mouse system (Gellin et al., 1979).

Guinea Pigs

Randomly bred adult male and female black guinea pigs were studied. Most observations were based on groups of five guinea pigs. Chemicals studied

TABLE 1   Animal Models Utilized to Study Experimental
Induction of Depigmentation

Animal	Reference
Guinea pig	Bleehen et al., 1968; Brun, 1960, 1972, 1974; Gellin et al., 1970b, 1979; Jimbow et al., 1974; Kahn, 1970; Malten et al., 1971; Mansur et al., 1978; Riley, 1970; Riley et al., 1975; Snell, 1964
Mouse	Dewey et al., 1977; Frenk et al., 1968; Hara and Nakajima, 1969; Hara and Uda, 1966; Hoshino et al., 1981; Ikeda et al., 1970; Ito et al., 1968; Rodermund et al., 1975
Cat	Malten et al., 1971; Oettell, 1936
Goldfish	Chavin, 1963
Rabbit	Chumakov et al., 1962

included industrially or commercially used phenols and catechols, their congeners, and antioxidants used as food preservatives.

Chemicals tested were butylated hydroxyanisole (BHA), butylated hydroxytoluene (BHT), catechol, MBEH, phenol, o-phenylphenol, p-phenylphenol, n-propyl gallate, p-tert-amylphenol (TAP), p-tert-butylphenol (TBP), TBC, isopropyl catechol (IPC), HQ, monomethyl ether of hydroquinone or p-hydroxyanisole (MMH), nordihydroguaiaretic acid (NGDA), dilauryl thiodiproprionate, nonyl phenol, octyl phenol, tocopherol (D-α-tocopherol acid succinate), ethoxyquin, gum guaiac, diethylamine hydrochloride, and octyl gallate.

The following solvents were used: acetone, petrolatum, hydrophilic ointment, Eucerin, dimethyl sulfoxide (DMSO) in concentrations of 30–100%, propylene glycol, chloroform, and ethyl alcohol in concentrations of 70, 90, and 100%.

The dorsal surface of the guinea pig was epilated weekly with an electric shaver. Eight dorsal sites, 3×3 cm, and the unepilated skin of ears and nipples were used. Each test area received 0.1-ml aliquots with either a micropipette or a syringe. Solvent control sites included at least one sector on the back, an ear, and one nipple. The test material was rubbed in with a glass rod or rubber-gloved finger. Applications and observations were made each weekday for 1–6 mo. If significant irritation developed, application was curtailed until irritation subsided.

Chemical concentrations ranged from 0.01 to 1.0 M for liquid solvents. Most observations were made with 0.1, 0.25, and 0.5 M. For solid ointment bases, concentrations ranged from 0.1 to 10%. Most observations were based on concentrations of 1, 5, and 10%.

The criteria for assessing depigmentation and irritation, as visually observed, are listed in Table 2.

Mice

Black adult mice were used for comparison with the depigmenting potency as observed in guinea pigs with known depigmenters. Groups of 10 were used for each test substance and for solvent controls.

The chemicals compared were TBC, TBP, HQ, octyl phenol, MBEH, and o-phenylphenol. The concentrations used were 0.1, 0.25, 0.5, and 1.0 M. Solvents used were acetone and DMSO (in 10% increments) from 30 to 90%.

Limited by size, the entire dorsal surface of the mouse was the application site. Ears and nipples were not tested. The surface was unepilated, for the skin of black mice is white except for a few black spots. (The hair is black.) Each mouse received 0.1-ml aliquots with a micropipette. Applications and observations were made each weekday for 2–4 mo. If significant irritation developed, application was curtailed until irritation subsided.

The criteria for assessing depigmentation and irritation were identical to those for the guinea pig (Table 2).

TABLE 2 Criteria for Assessing Irritancy and Depigmentation[a]

Observation	Assigned degradation	Degree of irritancy or depigmenting potency
Scoring of irritancy		
No reaction	0	Nonirritating
Erythema[b] and scaling	1+	Mildly irritating
Erythema and edema beyond area of application	2+	Moderately irritating
Eschar formation	3+	Severely irritating
Scoring of depigmentation		
No visible depigmentation; skin color similar to that of control areas	0	Absent
Small spots or speckles of depigmentation	±	Definite, but weak
Uniform hypopigmentation	+	Definite, but moderate
Complete depigmentation	++	Very strong

[a]Criteria after Bleehen et al.,(1968).
[b]Erythema was difficult to detect on gray-black skin of the guinea pig.

Complete depigmentation on all test sites was achieved with MMH and TBC in the black guinea pig (Figs. 2–4; Table 3). Less pronounced pigment loss was noted with these chemicals in black mice. TAP and MBEH were able to fully depigment only the back and nipple, respectively, of the black guinea pig. Moderate depigmentation followed the application of IPC, HQ, TBP,

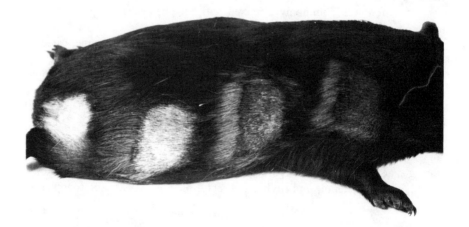

FIGURE 2 Back of black guinea pig after 122 d of application of MMH in acetone in different concentrations (left to right): 1.0, 0.5, 0.25, and 0.1 *M*.

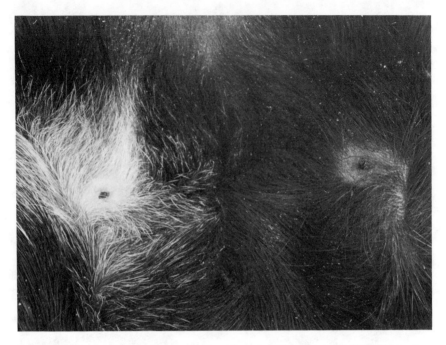

FIGURE 3 Nipple of black guinea pig after 73 d of application of 0.1 *M* MMH in acetone. The acetone control is on the opposite nipple.

phenol, and catechol (Tables 3–5). There was considerable variation in the duration of application to achieve partial or complete depigmentation (Tables 4 and 5). Not only was this true from one chemical to another, but the concentration and solvent were important variables (Tables 4 and 5).

Irritation was commonly observed with all phenols. It played a role in the production of pigment loss. Solvents affected the degree of irritation produced with and without subsequent depigmentation. For example, catechol and phenol produced uniform depigmentation in hydrophilic ointment and DMSO, respectively. However, no pigment loss was induced with these parent compounds, regardless of concentration, in acetone, DMSO, and propylene glycol (for catechol) and acetone, hydrophilic ointment, and propylene glycol (for phenol).

No depigmentation was induced with the following substances in black guinea pigs and black mice: BHA, BHT, octyl and propyl gallate, ethoxyquin, gum guaiac, diethylamine hydrochloride, dilauryl thiodiproprionate, nonyl phenol, *o*-phenylphenol, *p*-phenylphenol, octyl phenol, NDGA, and tocopherol.

Onset of Depigmentation

The minimum time for the appearance of depigmentation at any site from daily applications was 7 d with 0.5 *M* TBC in DMSO, 12 d with 0.25 *M*

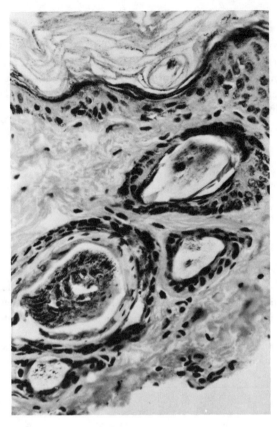

FIGURE 4 Back of black guinea pig, untreated control
site, ×125.

TABLE 3 Regional Variation of Maximal
Depigmenting Activity of Selected Alkyl
Phenols in Black Guinea Pig

Chemical	Body site[a]		
	Back	Ear	Nipple
MMH	++	++	++
TBC	++	++	++
TAP	++	±	0
MBEH	0	±	++
HQ	+	±	+
TBP	+	+	0
Phenol	+	+	0
Catechol	+	+	+

[a]See Table 2 for scoring of depigmentation.
Each data point represents the average for a minimum of five animals.

MMH in acetone, and 23 d with 0.25 M TBP in DMSO—all on the black guinea pig ear. Tables 4 and 5 show the minimal interval for complete or maximum depigmentation to be produced by the chemicals studied. Average figures are given. The longest time required to induce maximal depigmentation in a single guinea pig was 119 d for 0.25 M MMH in acetone on the ear and 112 d for 1 M TBP in acetone on the back (Figs. 2 and 3).

Depigmentation at Distant Sites

Despite the production of complete depigmentation with MMH in four black guinea pigs, repeated application at the three body sites chosen produced no pigment loss at any untreated area. Daily applications were continued for 119–175 d.

Histological Findings

Reduction to complete absence of melanin was noted with hematoxylin & eosin (H&E) and silver stains of skin specimens with clinically observed hypopigmentation and/or depigmentation (Figs. 4 and 5). Acanthosis was a concomitant finding. An increase of mononuclear-histiocytic cells appeared in

TABLE 4 Vehicles and Degree of Irritation in Association with Complete Depigmentation (++ Gradation) at Different Body Sites in Black Guinea Pig Produced by Selected Alkyl Phenols

Chemical	Site	Minimal eliciting concentration and vehicle	Grade of irritation[a]	Minimal interval for complete depigmentation to be observed (d)
MMH	Back	0.25 M acetone	1	33
		0.5 M DMSO	2	18
		10% hydrophilic ointment	2	12
	Ear	1.0 M acetone	2	62
		5% hydrophilic ointment	2	33
	Nipple	0.25 M acetone	1	49
TBC	Back	0.5 M propylene glycol	3	64
		10% hydrophilic ointment	3	29
	Nipple	0.25 M acetone	2	49
		5% hydrophilic ointment	3	29
	Ear	1.0 M acetone	2	20
TAP	Back	0.25 M DMSO	2	18
MBEH	Nipple	0.5 M propylene glycol	2	45

[a]See Table 2 for gradation of irritation. Each data point represents the average for a minimum of five animals.

TABLE 5 Vehicles and Degree of Irritation in Association with Uniform
Hypopigmentation (+ Gradation) at Different Body Sites in Black Guinea Pig
Produced by Selected Alkyl Phenols

Chemical	Site	Minimal eliciting concentration and vehicle	Grade of irritation[a]	Minimal interval for uniform hypopigmentation to be observed (d)
HQ	Back	0.5 *M* DMSO	2	30
	Nipple	5% hydrophilic ointment	3	15
TBP	Back	0.25 *M* DMSO	3	23
		10% hydrophilic ointment	3	74
	Ear	0.25 *M* DMSO	2	23
Phenol	Back	0.5 *M* DMSO	2	43
	Ear	0.25 *M* DMSO	1	43
Catechol	Back	10% hydrophilic ointment	3	46
	Ear	5% hydrophilic ointment	2	14
	Nipple	5% hydrophilic ointment	2	14
IPC	Back	1% petrolatum	3	30

[a]See Table 2 for gradation of irritation. Each data point represents the average for a minimum of five animals.

the upper and middle dermis, some with engulfed pigment (melanophages). These findings were similar regardless of the chemical that produced the leukoderma.

Confirmation of the depigmenting action of selected alkyl phenols was achieved. Unequivocal leukoderma with several solvents was noted with MBEH, MMH, TAP, and TBC.

In view of the ubiquity of organic antioxidants in industry and the home, some of which are chemically similar to these potent depigmenters, a variety were studied. Commercial uses of the phenols and catechols in this study include manufacture of paint, plastics and varnishes, soaps and germicidal detergent disinfectants, de-emulsifiers of oil, motor and lubricating oil additives, synthetic rubber manufacture, insecticides, and deodorants (Fisher, 1976b; Gellin et al., 1970a; Kahn, 1970). The antioxidants BHA and BHT are used in topical medications and foods (Fisher, 1975, 1976a; Roed-Petersen and Hjorth, 1976). Consumer products containing these substances are adhesive tapes, latex glues, rubber products ("falsies," condoms, stockings, girdles, bandages, cosmetic facial sponges), shoes, and wristwatch straps (Fisher, 1976b). BHA and BHT (commonly used in pharmaceuticals and

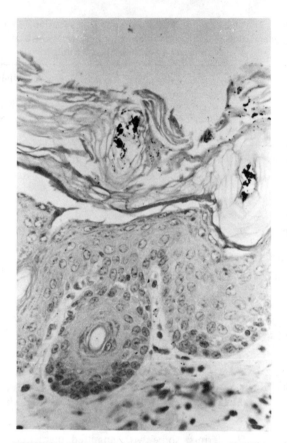

FIGURE 5 Back of black guinea pig after 0.1 *M* TBC in
DMSO, showing hyperkeratosis and absent pigment in
basal layer with increase in dermal mononuclear cells,
×125.

foods) did not induce leukoderma even when the concentration, solvent, and
test site were varied and application continued up to 10 wk (Maibach et al.,
1975). Failure to depigment mammalian skin was noted with another food
antioxidant, *n*-propyl gallate, which Kahn et al. (1974) reported as a
sensitizer.

Since there is widespread use of vitamin E in over-the-counter preparations for oral and topical use, this biological antioxidant was screened. With
acetone as the solvent, no depigmentation was induced on the three test sites
of the black guinea pig, although moderate irritation was seen. Brun (1960)
also failed to induce depigmentation with tocopherol (vitamin E) on the
nipples of brown guinea pigs.

No one solvent could be endorsed as appropriate for all substances. A
certain solvent may be irritating with one chemical but not another; for

instance, BHA in acetone is highly irritating while BHT in acetone is slightly irritating. As Kaidbey and Kligman (1974) noted in their study of suitable vehicles for topical photosensitizers, each substance has to be approached separately for its optimal solvent, should similar experimental studies be conducted. False positive results—that is, decreased depigmentation resulting from marked irritation per se—were seen with catechol, phenol, and DMSO in concentrations over 70%. False negatives or equivocal depigmentation were observed with known depigmenters: MMH in propylene glycol, hydroquinone in acetone and propylene glycol (Arndt and Fitzpatrick, 1965; Jimbow et al., 1974); MBEH in acetone (Becker and Spencer, 1962; Schwartz, 1947; Snell, 1964); TBP in acetone and propylene glycol (Babanov and Chumakov, 1966; Kahn, 1970; Malten et al., 1971); and octyl, nonyl, and phenyl phenols in the same solvents (Ikeda et al., 1970; Ito et al., 1968; Malten et al., 1971). The fault lies with the solvent system, or possibly the animal model, per se.

Solvents

Almost all substances were tested in acetone, propylene glycol, hydrophilic ointment, and 100% DMSO. DMSO was tested in 10% increments from 30 to 90% in mice only.

Acetone is easy to apply, readily absorbed into the skin, and dissolves most lipophilic chemicals. The disadvantages are that it evaporates readily if the container is not tightly closed, which raises the molarity of the solute, and that it has given false negative results with known depigmenters such as MBEH. MBEH was the first alkyl phenol shown to depigment human skin (Oliver et al., 1939).

Propylene glycol dissolves some test substances. It has the disadvantages that it is difficult to apply to animal skin due to its viscosity, not quickly absorbed so that it tends to spread beyond application sites, and more irritating than acetone or hydrophilic ointment.

DMSO is readily absorbed through animal skin. Test materials are easily incorporated into it. Its disadvantages include its offensive smell; slower absorption on animal skin compared to acetone, resulting in some of the solution rolling away from sites of application; and irritant action, at concentrations of 70% or more (Kligman, 1965).

Hydrophilic ointment is mildly irritating. It is difficult to deliver exact amounts in replicate studies. It tends to spread away from sites of application with animal movements such as rubbing against the cage and scratching, and it promotes retention of scales because of its occlusive nature.

Body Sites

No one body site seemed preferable. However, the nipples and ears were more susceptible than the back to depigmentation for most chemicals. For example, MBEH depigmented nipples (in propylene glycol) but did not depigment the back (in acetone or hydrophilic ointment). Depigmentation was induced at all three areas chosen. Brun (1960) studied the nipple almost exclusively in brown guinea pigs. Its histological similarity to human skin is a major advantage. Most prior investigations have been performed on the back of the black guinea pig or mouse.

Back. Major advantages include the relatively large surface area, which is easily accessible for multiple chemical applications and biopsies. Disadvantages include the need for repeated shaving or epilation, the confusion of grading that results from remaining hair, and the tendency for gray scales to accumulate, mimicking mild depigmentation.

Ear. Its advantages are the absence of hair, simplicity of applying test substances, and ease of rating depigmentation and taking biopsies.

Nipple. In addition to its histological resemblance to human skin, it is hairless. The disadvantages are its relative inaccessibility due to its location, which is sometimes hidden by hair, and the limitation of the number of chemicals that may be applied—only one to an animal.

Test Animals

The black guinea pig is a satisfactory choice for the study of chemically induced leukoderma. The hair and skin are black, and multiple anatomic sites can be chosen for grading a series of dilutions or substances simultaneously. Problems encountered include limited supply, since they are not widely bred; limitations of space, since animals were housed individually; the need for shaving weekly; removal of test substance by shaking, rubbing, or chewing off; and too frequent premature deaths of animals in the first 2 wk in the laboratory due to respiratory and/or gastrointestinal infection. Up to 20% died in some lots received from commercial breeders. Salmonellosis affects some strains commonly.

Black mice have the following advantages: they may be housed in groups, are readily obtained from animal supply houses, and require no shaving, and the results are visually reproducible. Disadvantages include rubbing off or spreading of applied chemicals; limitation to only one substance and/or dilution per animal; and the presence of hair, which may mask readings of irritation (although the hair was black, the skin was unpigmented).

MECHANISM OF ACTION

Chemically induced depigmentation results from a selective melano-cytotoxic action on functional melanocytes (Bleehen et al., 1968; Hoshino et al., 1981; Jimbow et al., 1974; McGuire and Hendee, 1971). The potent depigmenters studied have a structural similarity to tyrosine, which is probably relevant (Brun, 1972; Riley, 1969a) (Fig. 1). Competitive inhibition of the enzyme tyrosinase has been suggested (Denton et al., 1952). Inhibition of tyrosinase activity has been demonstrated (Usami et al., 1980). These compounds are incorporated into melanogenic cells in culture (Riley, 1969b). Riley showed that semiquinone free radicals are formed, initiating lipid peroxidation, which is a chain reaction, leading to destruction of lipoprotein membranes of the melanocyte and its consequent death (Riley, 1970, 1971; Riley et al., 1975).

Optimal depigmenting action is seen when the 4 (or *para*) position on the phenolic or catecholic ring has an alkyl side chain (Bleehen et al., 1968).

In addition to the hazard of skin irritation, sensitization, and depigmentation induced by certain phenols and catechols, reports from West Germany suggested that TBP has produced hepatosplenopathy and diffuse thyroid enlargement among workers (Rodermund et al., 1975). The imputed route of exposure was inhalation. The finding of abnormal liver function tests among six men with severe TBP-induced leukoderma has been noted (James et al., 1977).

The role of delayed hypersensitivity in chemically induced leukoderma was explored. Numerous animals that were depigmented were skin-tested. No evidence of delayed hypersensitivity was obtained (data unpublished). That melanocytes can be destroyed *in vitro* suggests that sensitization may not be requisite for depigmentation (Mansur et al., 1978).

PROPOSED MODEL FOR SCREENING
IN GUINEA PIGS

On the basis of these studies, we believe that we know how to avoid certain pitfalls in proposing a model to be used in predictive screening. If many chemicals are to be examined, the back of the black guinea pig allows at least six chemicals to be assayed per animal. Although there is individual variation, five animals per compound would be adequate to identify any of the agents studied here.

Solvent variability was significant. With unknown chemicals we would use two solvents, such as acetone and hydrophilic ointment. Either alone might produce a false negative response. DMSO is useful, but the concentration must be less than 70% to avoid irritation. Solvent controls should be run routinely for a background estimate of irritancy-induced depigmentation.

The duration of the assay should be at least 60 d. This should be sufficient to identify all chemicals studied here.

Any animal model has the inherent risk of not being clinically relevant. False positive results seen in our studies serve to emphasize this. Any new agent found to be a depigmenter in this type of predictive assay should not be discarded for commercial or industrial use, as sufficient data do not exist to permit the assumption that this will occur in humans. A cautiously performed human trial should offer minimal risk, as application can be limited to a small noncosmetic (covered) test area (Maibach et al., 1975).

We suspect that when large-scale screening assays are performed, additional compounds will be found that depigment skin and have not been clinically suspected. We emphasize that chemically induced leukoderma is clinically indistinguishable from vitiligo.

ALTERNATIVE ROUTES AND METHODS
OF ADMINISTRATION OF DEPIGMENTERS

Brun worked exclusively with the nipples of brown guinea pigs. Animal feeding experiments were unsuccessful with wild-colored guinea pigs and cats (Malten et al., 1971). Japanese workers succeeded in their depigmenting studies by feeding black C-57 mice TBP, p-octylphenol, o-phenylphenol, or p-phenylphenol (Hara and Nakajima, 1969; Ito et al., 1968). Riley (1969a, 1969b) was also unsuccessful in feeding black guinea pigs p-hydroxyanisole (monomethyl ether of hydroquinone). Oettell (1936) produced gray hair on black cats fed HQ.

Daily subcutaneous administration to black rabbits produced gray hair in 10–14 d when TBP was used (Chumakov et al., 1962; Babanov and Chumakov, 1966). Parenteral injections (sc) of TBP and p-octylphenol also led to depigmentation in black C-57 mice 12 wk after beginning injections with the former chemical and 9 wk after with the latter (Hara and Uda, 1966; Hara and Nakajima, 1969).

IN VITRO STUDIES

In vitro cell systems have been studied. One extensive investigation included rat liver cells and their mitochondria, human erythrocytes, and black guinea pig epidermis; the effects of three structural isomers of hydroxyanisole were studied (Riley, 1969b; Riley et al., 1975). TBC has also been evaluated with harvested melanocytes from the ears of black guinea pigs (Mansur et al., 1978). The effects of HQ, MBEH, and p-hydroxypropiophenone and other substituted phenols on Harding-Passey mouse melanoma cells and on melanin formation have been studied (Bleehen, 1976; Dewey et al., 1977; Denton et al., 1952).

PATHOGENESIS OF CHEMICAL LEUKODERMA

The probable mechanism of action of alkyl phenols is a toxic effect on functional melanocytes (Bleehen et al., 1968; Jimbow et al., 1974). Jimbow et al. (1974) observed three changes in melanocytes by electron microscopy: (1) inhibition of melanogenesis by affecting tyrosinase activity, (2) abnormal melanization, and (3) increased degradation of melanosomes.

Other investigators showed that semiquinone free radicals are formed, initiating lipid peroxidation, a chain reaction that leads to destruction of lipoprotein membranes of the melanocyte and its consequent death (Riley, 1971; Riley et al., 1975).

Among the phenols and catechols studied thus far it has been repeatedly demonstrated that optimal depigmenting action occurs when the 4 position is the site of the alkyl group (Bleehen et al., 1968; Gellin et al., 1979).

In recent *in vitro* studies with harvested melanocytes obtained from the ears of black guinea pigs and incubated with TBC, abnormal cytologic changes were induced in as brief a period as 1 h. The changes seen included irregular cell contour, beaded dendrites, rounding of cell bodies, formation of electron-lucent areas in melanosomes, and wavy intracellular microfilaments. The ultimate effect was the death of melanocytes (Mansur et al., 1978).

CONCLUSION

Only a systematic investigation of chemicals that touch human skin will clarify how many patients with vitiligo have, in fact, chemical leukoderma. We believe that the model systems described here present an admirable solution to the problem.

REFERENCES

Arndt, K. A. and Fitzpatrick, T. B. 1965. Topical use of hydroquinone as a depigmenting agent. *J. Am. Med. Assoc.* 194:965–967.

Babanov, G. P. and Chumakov, N. N. 1966. Etiology and pathogenesis of occupational "vitiligo." *Vest. Dermatol. Venerol.* 40:44–48.

Becker, S. W., Jr. and Spencer, M. C. 1962. Evaluation of monobenzone. *J. Am. Med. Assoc.* 180:279–284.

Bleehen, S. S. 1976. Selective lethal effect of substituted phenols on cell cultures of malignant melanocytes. In *Pigment Cell*, ed. V. Riley, vol. 2, pp. 108–115. Basel: Karger.

Bleehen, S. S., Pathak, M. A., Hori, Y. and Fitzpatrick, T. B. 1968. Depigmentation of skin with 4-isopropyl catechol, mercaptoamines, and other compounds. *J. Invest. Dermatol.* 50:103–117.

Brun, R. 1960. Zur experimentellen depigmentierung. *J. Soc. Cosmet. Chem.* 11:571–580.

Brun, R. 1967. Effect of ethyl ethers of hydroquinone on pigmentation and on the cells of Langerhans. *Dermatologica* 134:125–128.

Brun, R. 1972. Apropos de l'étiologie du vitiligo. *Dermatologica* 145:169–174.

Brun, R. 1974. The presumptive role of amino acid derivatives and catechol-amines in the etiology of vitiligo. *J. Soc. Cosmet. Chem.* 25:61–66.

Chavin, W. 1963. Effects of hydroquinone and of hypophysectomy upon the pigment cells of black goldfish. *J. Pharmacol. Exp. Ther.* 142:275–290.

Chumakov, N. N., Babanov, G. P., and Smirnov, A. G. 1962. Vitiliginoid dermatoses in workers of phenol-formaldehyde resin works. *Vest. Dermatol. Venerol.* 36:3–8.

Denton, C. R., Lerner, A. B. and Fitzpatrick, T. B. 1952. Inhibition of melanin formation by chemical agents. *J. Invest. Dermatol.* 18:119–135.

Dewey, D. L., Butcher, F. W. and Galpine, A. R. 1977. Hydroxyanisole induced regression of the Harding-Passey melanoma in mice. *J. Pathol.* 122:117–127.

Fisher, A. A. 1975. Contact dermatitis due to food additives. *Cutis* 16:961–966.

Fisher, A. A. 1976a. Reactions to antioxidants in cosmetics and foods. *Cutis* 17:21–28.

Fisher, A. A. 1976b. Vitiligo due to contactants. *Cutis* 17:431–448.

Frenk, E., Pathak, M. A., Szabo, G. and Fitzpatrick, T. B. 1968. Selective action of mercaptoethylamines on melanocytes in mammalian skin—experimental depigmentation. *Arch. Dermatol.* 97:465–477.

Gellin, G. A., Possick, P. A. and Davis, I. H. 1970a. Occupational depigmentation due to 4-tertiary butyl catechol (TBC). *J. Occup. Med.* 12:386–389.

Gellin, G. A., Possick, P. A. and Perone, V. B. 1970b. Depigmentation from 4-tertiary butyl catechol—an experimental study. *J. Invest. Dermatol.* 55:190–197.

Gellin, G. A., Maibach, H. I., Misiaszek, M. H. and Ring, M. 1979. Detection of environmental depigmenting substances. *Contact Dermatitis* 5:201–213.

Hara, I. and Nakajima, T. 1969. Studies on the leucoderma caused by alkylphenols. *Proc. 16th Int. Congr. Occup. Health, Tokyo,* pp. 635–637.

Hara, I. and Uda, K. 1966. Pathological studies of leucoderma caused by alkyl phenols. I. Subcutaneous injection experiment. *Jpn. J. Ind. Health* 8:211.

Hoshino, S., Nishimura, M., Fukuyama, K., Gellin, G. A. and Epstein, J. H. 1981. Effects of 4-tertiary butyl catechol on melanocytes of hairless mice. *J. Invest. Dermatol.* 76:231–238.

Ikeda, M., Ohtsuji, H. and Miyahara, S. 1970. Two cases of leucoderma, presumably due to nonyl—or octyl—phenol in synthetic detergents. *Ind. Health* 8:192–196.

Ito, K., Nishitani, K. and Hara, I. 1968. A study of cases of leucomelano-dermatosis due to phenyl-phenol compounds. *Bull. Pharm. Res. Inst.* 76:6–13.

James, O., Mayes, R. W. and Stevenson, C. J. 1977. Occupational vitiligo induced by *p*-tertiary butyl phenol, a systemic disease? *Lancet* ii:1217–1219.

Jimbow, K., Obata, H., Pathak, M. A. and Fitzpatrick, T. B. 1974. Mechanism of depigmentation by hydroquinone. *J. Invest. Dermatol.* 62:436–449.

Kahn, G. 1970. Depigmentation caused by phenolic detergent germicides. *Arch. Dermatol.* 102:177–187.

Kahn, G., Phanuphak, P., and Claman, H. N. 1974. Propyl gallate: Contact sensitization and orally-induced tolerance. *Arch. Dermatol.* 109:506–509.

Kaidbey, K. H. and Kligman, A. M. 1974. Topical photosensitizers: Influence of vehicles on penetration. *Arch. Dermatol.* 110:868–870.

Kligman, A. M. 1965. Topical pharmacology and toxicology of dimethyl sulfoxide. *J. Am. Med. Assoc.* (Part 1) 193:796–804; (Part 2) 193:923–928.

Lerner, A. B. 1971. On the etiology of vitiligo and gray hair. *Am. J. Med.* 51:141–147.

Lerner, A. B. and Fitzpatrick, T. B. 1953. Treatment of melanin hyperpigmentation. *J. Am. Med. Assoc.* 152:577–582.

Maibach, H. I., Gellin, G. and Ring, M. 1975. Is the antioxidant butylated hydroxytoluene a depigmenting agent in man? *Contact Dermatitis* 1:295–296.

Malten, K. E., Seutter, E., Hara, I. and Nakajima, T. 1971. Occupational vitiligo due to paratertiary butyl phenol and homologues. *Trans. St. John's Hosp. Dermatol. Soc.* 57:115–134.

Mansur, J. D., Fukuyama, K., Gellin, G. A. and Epstein, W. L. 1978. Effects of 4-tertiary butyl catechol on tissue cultured melanocytes. *J. Invest. Dermatol.* 70:275-279.

McGuire, J. and Hendee, J. 1971. Biochemical basis for depigmentation of skin by phenolic germicides. *J. Invest. Dermatol.* 57:256-261.

Oettell, H. 1936. Die hydrochinonvergiftung. *Arch. Exp. Pathol. Pharmacol.* 183:319-362.

Oliver, E. A., Schwartz, L. and Warren, L. H. 1939. Occupational leukoderma: Preliminary report. *J. Am. Med. Assoc.* 113:927-928.

Riley, P. A. 1969a. Hydroxyanisole depigmentation: *In vivo* studies. *J. Pathol.* 97:185-191.

Riley, P. A. 1969b. Hydroxyanisole depigmentation: *In vitro* studies. *J. Pathol.* 97:193-206.

Riley, P. A. 1970. Mechanism of pigment cell toxicity produced by hydroxyanisole. *J. Pathol.* 101:163-169.

Riley, P. A. 1971. Acquired hypomelanosis. *Br. J. Dermatol.* 84:290-293.

Riley, P. A., Sawyer, B. and Wolff, M. A. 1975. The melanocytotoxic action of 4-hydroxyanisole. *J. Invest. Dermatol.* 64:86-89.

Rodermund, O.-E., Jörgens, H., Müller, R. and Marstellar, H.-J. 1975. Systemische veränderungen bei berufsbedingter vitiligo. *Hautarzt* 26:312-316.

Roed-Petersen, J. and Hjorth, N. 1976. Contact dermatitis from antioxidants: Hidden sensitizers in topical medications and foods. *Br. J. Dermatol.* 94:233-241.

Schwartz, L. 1947. Occupational pigmentary changes in the skin. *Arch. Dermatol. Syphilol.* 56:592-600.

Shelley, W. B. and Raque, C. J. 1972. Delayed patterned hair depigmentation in CBA mice following application of laundry ink. *J. Invest. Dermatol.* 59:202-205.

Snell, R. S. 1964. Monobenzyl-ether of hydroquinone—its effect on the activity of epidermal melanocytes. *Arch. Dermatol.* 90:63-70.

Spencer, M. C. 1961. Hydroquinone bleaching. *Arch. Dermatol.* 84:131-134.

Usami, Y., Landau, A. B., Fukuyama, K. and Gellin, G. A. 1980. Inhibition of tyrosinase activity by 4-tert-butylcatechol and other depigmenting agents. *J. Toxicol. Environ. Health* 6:559-567.

23

chloracne (halogen acne)

■ K. D. Crow ■

INTRODUCTION

Chloracne is always a symptom of systemic poisoning and not just a cutaneous infection (Goldmann, 1973). Such systemic absorption, however small, must always occur—for all chloracnegens are absorbed through the skin (May, 1973). Since chloracne appears a most sensitive indicator of poisoning in the human subject (Moore, 1978), in most cases the systemic levels of chloracnegen are insufficient to cause target organ damage, either clinically or as assessed by laboratory investigation. There are two factors that probably make up this equation: the relation between dose and route of absorption on the one hand, and chloracne and systemic effects on the other. Much work remains to be done in this field, but one thing is certain: animal experiments demonstrate conclusively that the effects of an arbitrary amount of any chloracnegenic toxin are less severe as a single dose than if given in divided doses over a longer period. The effects of route of absorption will be discussed.

Definition

Chloracne is defined as an acneiform eruption due to poisoning by halogenated aromatic compounds having a specific molecular shape (Poland and Glover, 1977). Since bromination renders such a compound more acnegenic than chlorination (Echobichon et al., 1977), halogen acne may be a more specific term, but the word chloracne is too well established to be abandoned.

Chloracnegens

Only the following substances have been unequivocally proved to have caused chloracne in humans; some have also caused it in experimental animals.

Chloronaphthalenes (CNs)
Polychlorinated biphenyls (PCBs)
Polybrominated biphenyls (PBBs)
Polychlorinated dibenzofurans (PCDFs)
Polychlorinated dibenzodioxins (PCDDs)
Tetrachloroazobenzene (TCAB)
Tetrachloroazoxybenzene (TCAOB)

Bromination of certain naphthalenes, biphenyls, and dibenzofurans has been achieved and their acnegenicity confirmed in experimental animals (Kimbrough et al., 1977a). So far, only brominated biphenyls, mainly 2,4,5,2',4',5'-hexabromobiphenyl, have caused chloracne in human subjects (I. J. Selikoff, personal communication); this occurred in Michigan in 1973, when cattle feed was accidentally contaminated with hexabromobiphenyl manufactured as a flame retardant (Landrigan et al., 1979).

No fewer than four of the chloracnegens on the list above are found mainly as contaminants formed accidentally during the manufacture of other materials. Thus the dioxins occur in chlorinated phenols; the chlorodibenzofurans occur in chlorobiphenyls and chlorophenols (Taylor, 1979); and 3,3',4,4'-tetrachlorazo- and azoxybenzenes are formed during the manufacture of 3,4-dichloroaniline and occur in various end products and chemical processes involving its use or formation (Taylor et al., 1977).

The degree of halogenation does not necessarily determine toxicity; the position of the halogen atoms on the outside of the molecule (isomerism) is vital (McConnell et al., 1978a). A full knowledge of the nature and quantity of the isomers of any single chloracnegen is essential before its possible toxicity can be predicted. Great advances in analytical chemistry by conventional methods and, more recently, radioimmunoassays have made this possible (Albro et al., 1979).

CUTANEOUS MANIFESTATIONS

Distribution

The distribution of chloracne lesions is of considerable diagnostic importance. The most sensitive areas of the human skin are below and to the outer side of the eye (the so-called malar crescent) and behind the ear. They frequently may be affected when the rest of the skin is normal. Furthermore, they are the areas most likely to show residual lesions years after more extensive chloracne has faded. Next in frequency are the cheeks, forehead, and neck, but the nose is almost invariably spared. This should cause us to reflect when we consider the sebaceous gland development of this region, for the pathological basis of chloracne is squamous metaplasia of sebaceous glands into keratin-forming cysts. The genitalia—both penis and scrotum, but particularly the latter—are sensitive regions. With increasing toxicity the spread of the lesions is to the shoulders, chest, and back and eventually the buttocks and abdomen. The hands, forearms, feet, legs, and thighs are involved usually only in the worst cases. One curious quirk of distribution is axillary lesions (Jirasek et al., 1974), which have been commonly seen only in patients for whom ingestion or inhalation was the only route or a major route of absorption, as in Japan in 1968 (Yusho poisoning) or at Seveso, Italy, in 1976, where axillary lesions were seen only in the few children who were actually enveloped in the toxic cloud.

Morphology

The basic lesion of chloracne is the comedone, and in the mildest cases these may be the only lesions present (Fig. 1). If so, they are likely to involve only the sensitive areas—that is, the malar crescents and behind the ears—and as few as a dozen lesions on each side may be diagnostic. One must be careful with older patients to distinguish the so-called senile comedones, which are often seen in the malar areas, or with younger patients acne vulgaris, which may exactly mimic chloracne. The distinction may be clinically impossible, but consideration of other factors should decide the issue. Thus, apart from the distribution, factors such as unusual age of onset, clustering of similar cases in a factory, involvement of a specific occupation or even a township, presence of known chloracnegens or chemicals with a similar molecular shape, and absence of other external causes of acne such as pitch, tar, and mineral oils, considered together, make the diagnosis fairly straightforward. When doubt still remains, histology is conclusive.

In all but the mildest cases, pale yellow cysts, from the size of a pinhead to a lentil, mingling with the comedones, make up the characteristic picture of typical chloracne (Fig. 2) (Crow, 1970). As the severity of the disease increases, the lesions become more numerous and, in the worst cases, comedones, some no larger than pinpoints, may involve every follicle, giving the appearance of grayish sheets. These lesions are to be distinguished from the equally profuse, but pale, follicular hyperkeratoses, yet to be described.

In the most severe cases inflammatory lesions begin to appear, and with them larger cysts and even cold abscesses (Fig. 3). As ever wider areas become involved the picture may come to resemble that of severe cystic acne, but with much less inflammation than in the latter disease. Such gross lesions are most often seen on the back of the neck, trunk, and buttocks (Fig. 4). Widespread changes resembling solar elastosis have been described in chloracne associated with 2,4,5-trichlorophenol manufacture (Jirasek et al., 1973), and such changes were present in some of more than 116 patients examined in

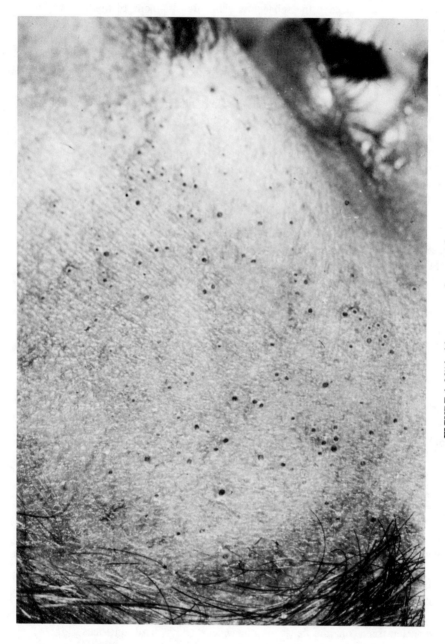

FIGURE 1 Mild chloracne: malar comedones.

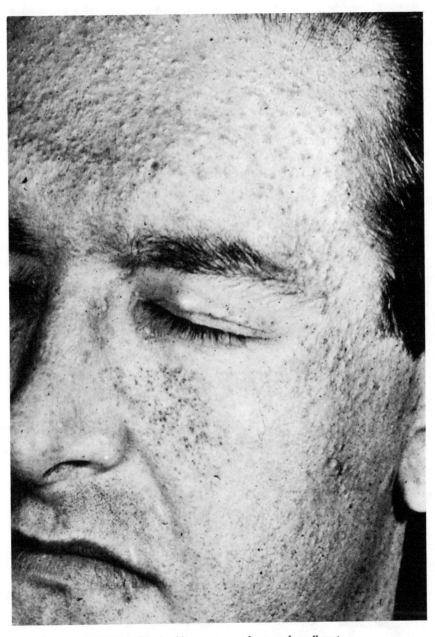

FIGURE 2 Classic chloracne: comedones and small cysts.

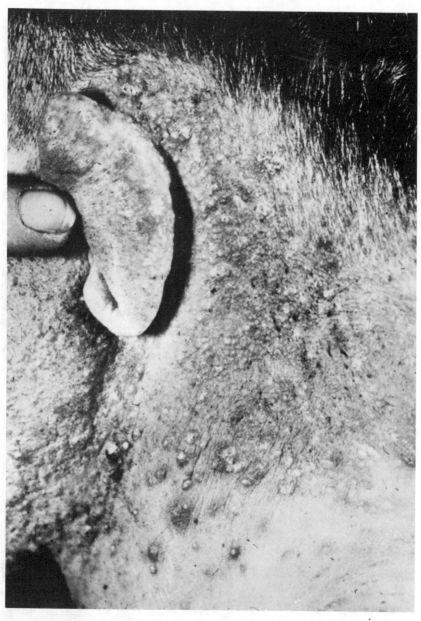

FIGURE 3 Severe chloracne: comedones, cysts, and inflammatory lesions.

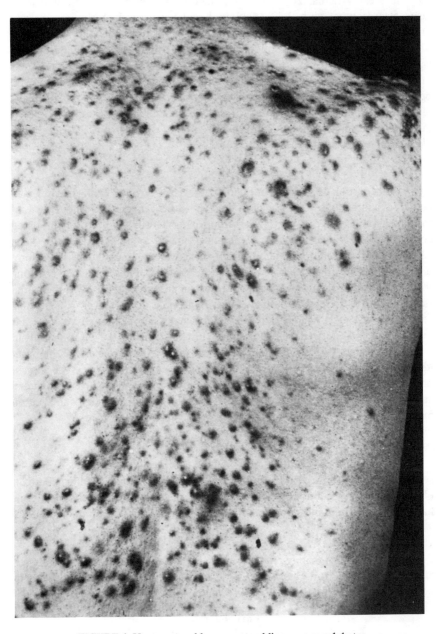

FIGURE 4 Very severe chloracne resembling acne conglobata.

1979 in West Virginia, 20–30 yr after their initial severe chloracne and some years after contact with 2,4,5-trichlorophenol had ceased. A similar case was presumably due to hexachlorodioxins from pentachlorophenol manufacture. The histology was that of chloracne. Scarring, absent in the mildest cases, varies from fine pitting, as in atrophoderma vermiculare, to extensive lesions of the sort that follow severe cystic acne. In the worst cases lesions may still be present after 30 yr, usually only in the malar region and behind the ears. Mild cases may clear up a few months after contact ceases (as at Seveso) (V. Puccinelli, personal communication), and after 2–3 yr all but 20% or so are likely to have resolved.

Pigmentation

Pigmentation is largely confined to the face, but in the worst cases may be more widespread, and has been known to be generalized. About 70% of the Japanese victims of Yusho, a mass poisoning due to the use of a rice-based cooking oil (Kuratsune et al., 1972) accidentally contaminated with large amounts of tetrachlorobiphenyl, itself heavily contaminated with chlorodibenzofurans (Rappe et al., 1977), exhibited a curious pigmentation affecting the nails, lips, gingival and buccal mucosae, and conjunctivae. Such pigmentation was also described in a similar mass poisoning in Taiwan in 1979 (Wong and Hwang, 1981). Pigmentation affecting nails and conjunctivae only has been found in industrial PCB poisoning (Fischbein et al., 1979), but only in 2–3% of the cases. This difference may be a dose or racial effect, or both. Yusho and the Taiwan disaster are the only recorded instances of human poisoning where external contact and inhalation can be positively excluded and a direct comparison made with toxicological animal feeding or intubation experiments.

Hypertrichosis

Hypertrichosis, a rare finding, mainly confined to the temples, may be secondary to the hepatic prophyria caused by tetrachlorodibenzodioxin (TCDD), but it has undoubtedly been present in patients whose uroporphyrins have been measured and remained constantly normal (Jirasek et al., 1974).

Sweating

Hyperhidrosis, mainly of the palms and soles, has been reported (Jirasek et al., 1974; Goto and Higuchi, 1969; Lee et al., 1980), but it is difficult to be sure that it was not overlooked elsewhere.

Phrynoderma

Follicular hyperkeratosis, to be distinguished from comedones, may be widespread and even generalized in rare cases, with usually severe accompanying chloracne (Crow, 1978). Despite its usual rarity, no fewer than 70% of the Japanese Yusho and 20% of the Taiwan victims developed a similar fine follicular hyperkeratosis on the upper trunk, neck, and, most unusual of all, the flexural areas (Goto and Higuchi, 1969; Cheng and Liu, 1981). It is interesting to speculate on whether this is due wholly or in part to the exclusively gastrointestinal route of poisoning in these cases. Cutaneous findings in stillborn infants and neonates born to Yusho and Taiwanese mothers poisoned with PCBs and PCDFs have been of great interest. Instead of chloracne, the entire skin was hyperpigmented and covered with grayish scales (Higuchi, 1976, pp. 116-117; Wong and Hwang, 1981). Several months after birth the skin became normal. The histology showed an atrophic epidermis with hyperkeratosis and dilatation of follicles, which were filled with keratin. These findings are clinically and histologically similar to those in cattle poisoned with penta- and hexachloronaphthalenes in 1947 (Olafson, 1947) and with hexabromobiphenyl in Michigan in 1973. Similar changes were observed in horses poisoned with TCDD in Missouri in 1971 (Kimbrough et al., 1977b).

Ophthalmic Changes

Conjunctivitis has sometimes been noted in severe poisoning with various chloracnegens, but has been seen in extreme form only in Yusho and Taiwan victims, whose meibomian glands were converted into squamous cysts filled with a cheesy keratinous material (Higuchi, 1976, pp. 115-116; Lee et al., 1980). In ingestion experiments, similar lesions were induced in rhesus monkeys by chlorodibenzodioxins, chlorodibenzofurans, and 3,4,3',4'-tetra-chlorobiphenyl (McConnell et al., 1978b; McNulty et al., 1981). They appear to have been an even more sensitive indicator of poisoning in the rhesus than chloracne in the Yusho patients. Where poisoning has been mainly by external contact, however, chloracne is much more common than meibomian gland changes, almost certainly indicating the importance of route of absorption in determining the clinical spectrum.

Erythema

The erythematous changes that may occasionally be associated with the onset of chloracne (Jirasek et al., 1974; May, 1973) have been a source of confusion. Because such erythema is confined exclusively to exposed areas, it has been wrongly ascribed to photosensitivity. Telegina and Biklulatuva (1970), describing an outbreak of severe chloracne and systemic poisoning during the manufacture of (2,4,5-trichlorophenoxy)acetic acid esters, established that the affected individuals had reduced sensitivity to ultraviolet light. A few cases of erythema preceding the severe chloracne resulting from massive internal exposure to probable chloronaphthalenes are genuine, but the other recorded cases have all occurred during chlorophenol manufacture. Such erythema has never been recorded from PCBs, even in the massive Yusho and Taiwan poisonings, nor from TCAB or TCAOB.

Exposure to chloracnegens in chlorophenol manufacture implies exposure to sodium salts of chlorophenols (Suskind, 1978; Joint NIEHS/IARC Working Group, 1978) as well as to the dioxins and dibenzofurans. The corrosiveness of adequate amounts of the sodium salts on damp skin is unquestioned; there was every reason to believe that erythema was likely to have been caused by sodium chlorophenate burns. The Seveso accident, however, provided abundant evidence to support this theory.

SEVESO

The main purpose of the Icmesa factory at Seveso was to produce 2,4,5-trichlorophenol by alkaline hydrolysis of 1,2,4,5-Tetrachlorobenzene. On July 10, 1976, the full reactor began an exothermic reaction (Reggiani, 1980), terminating in an explosion that discharged its contents in a vertical jet into the air. The cloud of finely dispersed reactor contents, mainly the potentially corrosive sodium 2,4,5-trichlorophenate, drifted slowly downwind on a slight southeast breeze. July 10 was a hot summer day, and those who were caught in the cloud with sweaty skins, or who handled objects covered with the discharge, suffered chemical burns. Some of those who ate contaminated food had nausea, vomiting, and diarrhea due to chlorophenols and not to dioxin. Of 447 adults and children examined within days after the explosion, 76% had erythema on the exposed areas of skin. In many cases it was severe enough to cause blistering. The small children who were contaminated suffered most. By far the most severe burns were suffered by eight children who were caught in the chemical cloud.

An examination of several of the most severely burned children at the end of July revealed typical chemical burns affecting the face, neck, forearms, and arms below the clothing as well as the legs and lower part of the thighs. In the burned areas there were many curious circumscribed raised lesions like small coins, mainly confined to the hands, forearms, and legs. That these were part of the chemical burns and nothing more esoteric was confirmed as they subsided with the rest of the lesions. A follicular hyperkeratosis affecting virtually every follicle in the burned area heralded the first sign of chloracne. As the burns faded, leaving hyperpigmentation, the chloracne developed. With the occasional exception of the axillae, it affected few covered areas. There were in all 8 severely and 11 moderately burned children with a curious type of chloracne, which in the more severe cases formed diffuse thick hyperkeratotic sheets as every follicle had formed a small keratinous cyst. Four months later this diffuse crusting was already separating, leaving small atrophoderma vermiculare-like scarring scattered with comedones.

There were 168 other cases of chloracne, all mild to minimal in extent. Unlike the children, fewer than 5% of the adults who had received caustic burns developed chloracne, and this was of a very minor degree. It seems likely that the major contact at Seveso was external, since there were cases where the chloracne was limited to odd-shaped areas of pigmented skin where burns had previously been present, the intervening skin being unaffected. Some ingestion and/or inhalation could not, of course, be excluded. Despite extensive and continuing investigation, there has at no time been any clear evidence of systemic poisoning in any of the Seveso cases, again consistent with a largely external contact. Nevertheless, V. Puccinelli (personal communication) theorizes that chloracne at Seveso resulted from ingestion and/or inhalation of TCDD, although others disagree. However, Seveso is the finest example of chloracne being the most sensitive marker of human TCDD poisoning, for no cases of systemic toxicity have yet been discovered, whereas chloracne, mostly mild, was widespread.

ROUTES OF ABSORPTION

Experimental data do not indicate whether variation of the route of absorption of a chloracnegen alters the distinctive features of poisoning, but circumstantial evidence suggests that this may be so to a minor degree. A comparison of the Yusho and Taiwan poisonings, where the chloracnegens were ingested without dermal contact or inhalation, shows certain differences from industrial poisonings where contact is known to be by contact and inhalation. Capacitor workers with gross skin contact and inhalation have blood PCB levels as high as the Yusho cases, but no signs of toxicity except chloracne and respiratory changes. In industry, generally, contact appears to make chloracne the most sensitive marker (Kimmig and Schulz, 1957; Crow, 1970; May, 1973; Taylor et al., 1977); pigmentation, ophthalmic signs, and many of the subjective symptoms (often presenting complaints in Japanese and Chinese cases) occur only in severe cases with severe chloracne. It seems possible that these differences and many others may be due not only to different chloracnegens but also to the route of absorption. Nevertheless, it is well to bear in mind that even in the Yusho and Taiwan cases chloracne and/or meibomian gland metaplasia (chloracne equivalent) affected nearly 90%, so that alleged poisoning by chloracnegens in the absence of chloracne or meibomian changes should be viewed with some suspicion.

SOME PROPERTIES OF ALL CHLORACNEGENS

Acnegenic potential of all chloracnegens can be equated with overall toxicity. This is supported both by animal experiments in which the LD50 was determined and by an ingenious experimental method based on a characteristic of all chloracnegenic toxins—their ability to induce various microsomal drug-metabolizing enzymes, of which liver cells are a particularly rich source. The most useful of these has been aryl hydrocarbon hydroxylase (AHH) (Poland and Kende, 1976), which is responsible for the initial rupture of the aromatic nucleus to an arene oxide and therefore the first step in the metabolism of these compounds. The most powerful inducer of AHH is

2,3,7,8-tetrachlorodibenzo-*p*-dioxin, which animal experiments have shown to be not only the most toxic small molecule known but also the most powerful of all chloracnegens. Thus we have a simple method of determining the relative toxicity and therefore acnegenicity of any chemical and its isomers. This technique has enabled the structure-activity relations of many possible chloracnegenic isomers to be determined (Poland and Glover, 1977). All such isomers, while varying greatly in overall toxicity, share the characteristic of attacking the same target organs of various animal species (Moore et al., 1979). The biological basis of chloracne, in particular its predilection for certain areas of skin, is unknown. Investigation is hampered by the lack of an analytical method sufficiently sensitive to study the material in comedones and cysts.

ANIMAL MODELS

Chloracne, or something very like it clinically and histologically, has been produced in only three experimental animals: the rhesus monkey (affecting the face with loss of hair and disruption of meibomian glands, as in humans), the hairless mouse, and, most important, the rabbit (inner surface of the ear) (Adams et al., 1941). It is not possible to produce chloracne on any other part of the rabbit's skin. Even systemic absorption of chloracnegens by the rabbit produces chloracne only on the inner surface of the ear (V. K. Rowe, personal communication). Thus there is a clear parallel to the curious sensitivity of the malar crescents and ears in human subjects. The rabbit ear appears to be the most sensitive biological surface known, reacting to as little as 1 μg of the most potent known chloracnegen.

HISTOLOGY

Where exposure has been severe, histological changes may begin within 5 d. Initially, there is stimulation of the epithelium of the outer root sheath and sebaceous gland ducts (Hambrick, 1957). It seems likely that the subsequent disappearance of the sebaceous glands is due to squamous metaplasia of sebaceous forming cells. The sebaceous gland is inevitably replaced by a keratinous cyst, which always has an attachment to the epidermis. The exit is tiny in some lesions, while others are little more than a shallow trough. Inflammatory changes are minimal in most lesions. The squamous metaplasia of meibomian glands (which are modified sebaceous glands) is identical to that in the skin and is clearly a modified chloracne. This rapid and total transformation of sebaceous glands into squamous cysts appears to be pathognomonic to poisoning with chloracnegens and is therefore of the greatest diagnostic value.

CLINICAL SIGNS AND SYMPTOMS
IN NONCUTANEOUS SYSTEMS

Because of cutaneous absorption (which has been estimated as half the applied epidermal dose for TCDD) (Schwetz et al., 1973), possible ingestion, and/or inhalation, all cases of chloracne must be submitted to careful clinical and laboratory investigations designed to detect the following abnormalities.

Weight

Weight loss is one of the most sensitive indicators of poisoning in experimental animals, especially the rhesus monkey, but in most human poisonings wasting has not been carefully monitored or, where it has, it has been found only in more severe cases (Jirasek et al., 1974).

Hepatic Effects

Liver damage has been considered one of the classic signs of systemic poisoning from chloracnegens, but the facts do not support this. Liver damage does occur (Goldmann, 1973; Jirasek et al., 1974) in some severely poisoned cases, but apparently not in others (Joint NIEHS/IARC Working Group, 1978). This is presumably a function of dose and route of absorption. It is important not to assume that liver enlargement necessarily means detectable liver damage. The increase in size and weight may be due, as in the rat, to a large increase in smooth endoplasmic reticulum (Higuchi, 1976, p. 94), which is thought to be an indication of increased enzyme induction.

Lipoproteins

Lipoprotein abnormalities are most important because there is a possible (although as yet unconfirmed) association with cardiovascular disease. The only consistent abnormality in animals and human subjects is an increased triglyceride level. Cholesterol is variable but usually normal, as are high-density lipoprotein (HDL)/cholesterol levels, where these have been measured. Work with TCDD in guinea pigs revealed raised triglycerides and unchanged cholesterol and HDL (Gasiewicz et al., 1979). The cause of the triglyceride increase is much debated, but two mechanisms may be involved, separately or together. Evidence for increased hepatic enzyme activity might support increased triglyceride synthesis. Alternatively, there may be a decrease in removal of plasma triglycerides due to a decrease in plasma lipoprotein lipase activity, as revealed in Yusho patients (Higuchi, 1976, p. 98).

Neurological (Central) Effects

The reported symptoms of central nervous system (CNS) involvement, being subjective, are most difficult to evaluate, but a combination of headache, fatigue, irritability, insomnia, impotence, and loss of libido has occurred so often that they are unquestionably genuine symptoms. It cannot be stressed too strongly that they were reported only in cases of severe poisoning (Suskind, 1978; Jirasek et al., 1974; Goldmann, 1973) before the terms chloracne, TCDD, and so on became household words after the Seveso accident. Furthermore, these symptoms arose during the worst of the poisoning and not after a symptomless interval of several years.

Neurological (Peripheral) Effects

Peripheral sensory nerves, particularly in the legs, may be affected; again, this occurs in severe cases, almost always associated with halogenated dioxin poisoning. The neuritis may cause lower limb pains of disabling severity, together with patchy numbness. This neuropathy may be confirmed by biopsy, which shows demyelination, or more easily by measurement of conduction velocity, which is found to be lowered. Motor nerves are rarely affected, and then only after sensory involvement.

Pulmonary Effects

Pulmonary changes are frequent and persistent bronchitis with effort dyspnea is well documented, but the recent discovery that there is a lowering of vital capacity is particularly interesting, for in PCB poisoning it may be the only sign of toxicity (Warshaw et al., 1979).

Porphyrins

Porphyria of the hepatic type has been described only twice in human poisoning, each time for TCDD in 2,4,5-T manufacture (Bleiberg et al., 1964; Jirasek et al., 1974). Patients exhibited in exposed areas hyperpigmentation, hypertrichosis, traumatic and actinic bullae, milia, and scars. TCDD also produces porphyria in experimental animals (Rose et al., 1976), whereas the closely related 2,3,7,8-tetrachlorodibenzofuran appears not to do so (Oishi et al., 1978). PCBs have produced porphyria in animals and also an excess of porphyrins in the liver tissue of Yusho victims. Urinary uroporphyrin levels are only moderately raised in most cases. The enormous induction by powerful chloracnegens of δ-aminolevulinic acid synthetase in liver microsomes made it seem likely that this was the cause of the porphyria. TCDD inhibits the enzyme uroporphyrinogen decarboxylase, which is almost certainly the cause of the hepatic porphyria (Jones and Sweeney, 1977). Rapid poisoning seems to be ineffective, long-term moderate doses being apparently necessary to produce overt porphyric changes.

Gastrointestinal Effects

Nausea, vomiting, and diarrhea seem to be confined to acute poisoning and may therefore be due to associated chlorophenols. On the other hand, these symptoms occurred in 20% of Yusho victims.

Musculoskeletal Effects

Rarer still is bursitis, usually of the olecranon or prepatellar bursae, and edema of all four limbs (Kuratsune et al., 1972; Baader and Bauer, 1951).

Immunological Effects

Immunological deficiencies have been indicated in animals of various species, but the results are confusing and of doubtful significance. In human subjects a decrease in circulating T cells has been demonstrated in poisoning from hexabromobiphenyl (Bekesi et al., 1978).

Teratogenicity and Fetotoxicity

Teratogenicity has been demonstrated in rats and mice, but the far greater fetotoxic effect of chloracnegens is clearly a limiting factor. Neither of these effects has yet been demonstrated in the only two episodes of poisoning with chloracnegens in which women were involved equally with men—Seveso and Yusho (Japan and Taiwan).

Miscellaneous

The actual cause of death from chloracnegens is unknown (McConnell et al., 1978b), but even when the minimal lethal dose is greatly increased, the time to death, 14-21 d, remains unchanged. Attribution of rapid deaths to chloracnegens must therefore be seriously questioned and other causes sought. Both in animal toxicology and with the human subject it is even more difficult when severe poisoning is present to distinguish lesions that are purely secondary to severe illness from those that are specifically due to the toxin. The symptoms and signs described so far have occurred in a sufficient number of poisonings from different chloracnegens to be certainly specific. Other findings that have been recorded, such as cardiac, renal, pancreatic, and other changes, await confirmation.

CARCINOGENICITY

Numerous mutagenicity studies have yielded somewhat equivocal results, but careful lifetime feeding studies on rats (Kociba et al., 1978) and mice (Holmes et al., 1978) with TCDD and the two most toxic hexachlorodioxin isomers have revealed that malignant tumors can be induced, but only by doses large enough to produce a state of chronic toxicity, low doses having no effect. Skin painting (Holmes et al., 1978) suggested that dioxins are complete carcinogens—that is, initiators and promoters—but other experimental evidence suggests that they are cocarcinogens. PCBs fed to rodents throughout their lives produced liver tumors, whose true malignancy was not fully established. Against this background, what are the human data?

Seventy men who suffered chloracne and severe poisoning with TCDD during 2,4,5-T manufacture were followed up for 25 yr and showed an increase in stomach cancer in one age group only (Goldmann, 1973). Seventy-nine cases of chloracne from TCDD following the explosion of a 2,4,5-T reactor in 1968 had, 10 yr later, no excessive evidence of malignant neoplasms (May, 1978). Yusho victims have shown in an increased mortality from malignant neoplasms (4 of 11 autopsied), but this is not considered statistically significant and the survey is being continued (Urabe et al., 1979). A follow-up of 121 men who had severe chloracne and severe poisoning from TCDD, again after the explosion of a 2,4,5-T reactor, showed 9 cancer deaths compared to an expected figure of 9.04 (29 yr later) (Zack and Suskind, 1980).

Apart from controversial work by Hardell and Sandstrom (1979), there have been reports of five cases of soft-tissue sarcomas in workers exposed to TCDD. While the data so far are only circumstantial, potentially exposed persons must be monitored with care for the occurrence of such tumors (Zack and Suskind, 1980; Honchar and Halperin, 1981; Cook, 1981; Moses and Selikoff, 1981). The evidence suggests that severe and lifelong toxicity in rodents may produce excess malignancies, but so far statistical evidence of similar lesions in human subjects is not forthcoming. There is no reliable evidence so far of any increase in cardiovascular disease. The increase in triglycerides in the apparent absence of lowered HDL suggests that all such data will have to be most carefully evaluated.

SOURCES OF CHLORACNEGENS

Manufacture (Primary)

The formation of halogenated dioxins, dibenzofurans, TCABs, and TCAOBs during chemical manufacture of chlorinated phenols and chlorinated biphenyls has already been mentioned. Although these are closed processes, they have certain well-known points at which exposure can occur. Thus, the repair and servicing of pipework, valves, and reactors with spillage; laboratory checks of reaction masses; and the removal of highly toxic reaction residues may all entail contact, often at points in the reaction where there are high contaminant levels. Laboratory workers have been poisoned while synthesizing highly toxic chloracnegens.

Manufacture (Secondary)

Some materials, such as chlorophenols (containing PCDDs and PCDFs) and 3,4-dichloroaniline (containing TCAB and traces of TCAOB), may be used as chemical intermediates. Thus, 2,4,5-trichlorophenol can be reacted to form numerous herbicidal esters; 3,4-dichloroaniline (3,4-DCA) may be further reacted to form the herbicides diuron, linuron, and propanil and many other substances. Depending on the reaction, the final products may contain the chloracnegenic contaminant, but usually in very small amounts since they are reduced during primary manufacture. Exceptions are linuron and 3,4-DCA, some samples of which (manufactures differ greatly) have high TCAB levels.

USES OF FINAL PRODUCTS

With one major exception (chlorinated naphthalenes), chloracne in users of final products is extremely rare; it mostly occurred years ago, when contaminant levels were not controlled and in some batches may have been very high indeed (Londono, 1966). Some early PCBs appear to have been very acnegenic, but systemic toxicity was apparently rare (Puccinelli, 1954). Moderate but prolonged heating, as when PCBs are used as heat exchanger fluids, may greatly increase the PCDF content, posing a toxic risk if they are handled or ingested (Meigs et al., 1954). Chloronaphthalenes, the only toxic forms of which are the penta- and hexa- ones, were once widely used in hot, molten form (for dipping) as dielectrics. The fumes were highly acnegenic, but systemic toxicity seemed to be rare. They have been largely replaced but may still be encountered.

PYROLYSIS

Fire, either accidental or deliberate (municipal incinerators), may form PCDDs from chlorophenols and PCDFs from chlorobiphenyls. As yet, this has not been proved to be an environmental hazard. We cannot evaluate it until we have complete details concerning the presence and quantity of toxic isomers.

ENVIRONMENTAL EXPOSURE

There are five unquestioned and two doubtful examples of human exposure to chloracnegenic toxins in the environment. Seveso has been discussed. In Missouri in 1971 three horse training arenas and a farm road were accidentally sprayed with the massive quantity of 33 ppm TCDD and larger amounts of chlorophenols. Despite intimate contact of children and adults with the sprayed soil, only domestic animals, birds, and horses were fatally poisoned; human symptoms and signs were confined to chloracne.

The Japanese and Chinese Yusho disasters have been described. Interest in these cases is due to the severity and longevity of the poisoning. Workers handling large quantities of PCBs daily in the capacitor industry have PCB blood levels higher than in the Yusho cases but no signs of toxicity (Ouw et al., 1976). The presence in Yusho oils of PCDFs and polychlorinated quaterphenyls may explain the difference, but this idea is still speculative.

Large numbers of residents of Michigan ingested various amounts of 3,4,5,3',4',5'-hexabromobiphenyl in 1973, and again a (less severe) Yusho-like syndrome resulted.

The remaining two incidents, involving defoliant spraying in Vietnam and the correct use of phenoxyacid and ester herbicides by spraying, cannot be said to have caused adequately proved disease at the time of this writing.

To sum up, without chloracne the possibility of human poisoning of any degree by chloracnegens is exceedingly small, but whenever chloracne is encountered a full personal and environmental investigation must be made and continued.

REFERENCES

Adams, Irish, D. D., Spencer, H. C., and Rowe, U. K. 1941. The response of rabbit skin to compounds reported to have caused acneiform dermatitis. *Ind. Med. Surg.* 2:1–4.

Albro, P. W., Luster, M. I., Chae, K., Chaudhary, S. K., Clark, G., Lawson, L. D., Corbett, S. T., and McKinney, S. D. 1979. A radio-immunoassay for chlorinated dibenzo-*p*-dioxins. *Toxicol. Appl. Pharmacol.* 50:137–146.

Baader, H. C. E. and Bauer, H. J. 1951. Industrial intoxication due to pentachlorophenol. *Ind. Med. Surg.* 20:286–292.

Bekesi, J. G., Holland, J. F., Anderson, H. A., Fischbein, A. S., Rom, W., Wolff, M. S., and Selikoff, I. J. 1978. Lymphocyte function of Michigan dairy farmers exposed to polybrominated biphenyls. *Science* 199:1207–1209.

Bleiberg, J., Wallen, M., Brodkin, R., Applebaum, I. L. 1964. Industrially acquired porphyria. *Arch. Dermatol.* 89:793–799.

Cheng, P. C. and Liu, K. Y. 1981. PCB poisoning. Special issue. *Clin. Med. (Taipei)* 7:41–45 (Chinese).

Cook, R. R. 1981. Dioxin, chloracne, and soft tissue sarcoma (letter). *Lancet* i:618–619.

Crow, K. D. 1970. Chloracne: A critical review including a comparison of two series of cases of acne from chloronaphthalene and pitch fumes. *Trans. St. John's Hosp. Dermatol. Soc.* 56:79–99.

Crow, K. D. 1978. Chloracne: The chemical disease. *New Sci.* April 13, pp. 78–80.

Echobichon, D. J., Hansell, M. M., and Safe, S. 1977. Halogen substituents at the 4 and 4′ positions of biphenyl; influence on hepatic function in the rat. *Toxicol. Appl. Pharmacol.* 42:359–366.

Fischbein, A., Wolff, M. A., Lilis, R., Thornton, J., and Selikoff, I. J. Clinical findings among PCB-exposed capacitor manufacturing workers. *Ann. N.Y. Acad. Sci.* 320:703–715.

Gasiewicz, T. A., Swift, L. L., Dunn, G. D., Soulé, R. D., and Neal, R. A. 1979. TCDD in lipid metabolism in guinea pigs. *Pharmacologist* 21:143.

Goldmann, P. J. 1973. Severe acute chloracne, a mass intoxication by 2,3,6,7-tetrachlorodibenzodioxin. *Hautarzt* 24:149–152.

Goto, M. and Higuchi, K. 1969. The symptomatology of Yusho (chloro-biphenyl poisoning) in dermatology. *Fukuoka Acta Med.* 60:409–431.

Hambrick, G. S. 1957. The effect of substituted naphthalenes on the pilosebaceous apparatus of rabbit and man. *J. Invest. Dermatol.* 28:89–103.

Hardell, L. and Sandstrom, A. 1979. Case-control study; Soft tissue sarcoma and exposure to phenoxy acetic acids or chlorophenols. *Br. J. Cancer* 39:711–717.

Higuchi, K. 1976. *PCB Poisoning and Pollution.* London: Academic.

Holmes, P. A., et al. 1978. Long term effects of TCDD and HCDD in mice and rats. *N.Y. Acad. Sci. Sci. Week,* June 21–30, abstract 26.

Honchar, P. A. and Halperin, W. E. 1981. 2,4,5-T, trichlorophenol and soft tissue sarcoma. *Lancet* i:268.

Jirasek, L., Kalensky, J., Kubec, K., Pazderova, J., and Lukas, E. 1973. Acne chlorina, porphyria cutanea tarda and other manifestations of general intoxication during the manufacture of herbicides. Part I. *Cesk. Dermatol.* 48:306–317.

Jirasek, L., Kalinsky, J., Kubec, K., Pazderova, J., and Lukas, E. 1974. Acne chlorina, porphyria cutanea tarda and other manifestations of general intoxication during the manufacture of herbicides. Part II. *Cesk. Dermatol.* 49:145–157.

Joint NIEHS/IARC Working Group. 1978. *Long-term hazards of polychlorinated dibenzodioxins and polychlorinated dibenzofurans, p. 39. Lyon: International Agency for Research in Cancer.*

Jones, K. C. and Sweeney, G. D. 1977. Association between induction of aryl hydrocarbon hydroxylase and depression of uroporphyrinogen decarboxylase activity. *U.S. Environ. Prot. Agency Pestic. Abstr.* 10:707.

Kimbrough, R. D., Burse, U. W., and Liddle, J. A. 1977a. Toxicity of polybrominated biphenyl. *Lancet* ii:602.

Kimbrough, R. D., Carter, C. D., and Liddle, J. A. 1977b. Epidemiology and pathology of a tetrachlorodibenzo-*p*-dioxin poisoning episode. *Arch. Environ. Health* 3:77–85.

Kimmig, J. and Schulz, K. H. 1957. Berufliche akne (sog Chlorackne) durch Chlorierte aromatische zyklische Ather. *Dermatologica* 115:540–553.

Kociba, R. J., Keyes, D. G., Beyer, J. E., Carreon, R. M., Wade, C. E., Dittenber, D. A., Kalnins, R. P., Frauson, L. E., Park, C. N., Barnard, S. D., Hummel, R. A., and Hummiston, C. G. 1978. Results of a two year chronic toxicity and oncogenicity study of 2,3,7,8-tetrachlorodibenzo-*p*-dioxin in rats. *Toxicol. Appl. Pharmacol.* 46:279–303.

Kuratsune, M., Yoshimura, T., Matsuzaka, J., and Yamaguchi, A. 1972. Epidemiologic study of Yusho, a poisoning caused by ingestion of a rice oil contaminated with a commercial brand of polychlorinated biphenyls. *Environ. Health Perspect.* 1:119–128.

Landrigan, P. J., Wilcox, K. R., Silva, J., Jr., Humphrey, H. E., Kauffman, C., and Heath, C. W., Jr. 1979. Cohort study of Michigan residents exposed to polybrominated biphenyls: Epidemiologic and immunologic findings. *Ann. N.Y. Acad. Sci.* 320:295–307.

Lee, Y. Y., Wong, P. N., Lu, Y. C., Sun, C. C., Wu, Y. C., Yin, B. L., Jee, S. H., Ng, K. Y., and Yeh, H. P. 1980. An outbreak of PCB poisoning. *J. Dermatol.* 7:435–441.

Londono, F. 1966. Chloracne from weedkillers. *Med. Cutanea* 1:225.

May, G. 1973. Chloracne from the accidental production of tetrachlorodibenzodioxin. *Br. J. Ind. Med.* 30:276–283.

McConnell, E. E., Moore, J. A., and Dalgard, D. W. 1978a. Toxicity of 2,3,7,8-tetrachlorodibenzo-*p*-dioxin in rhesus monkeys (*Macaca mulatta*) following a single oral dose. *Toxicol. Appl. Pharmacol.* 43:175–187.

McConnell, E. E., Moore, J. A., Haseman, J. K., and Harris, M. W. 1978b. The comparative toxicity of chlorinated dibenzo-*p*-dioxin isomers in mice and guinea pigs. *Toxicol. Appl. Pharmacol.* 44:335–336.

McNulty, W. P., Pomerantz, I., and Farrell, T. 1981. Chronic toxicity of

2,3,7,8-tetrachlorodibenzofuran for rhesus macaques. *Food Cosmet. Toxicol.* 19:57–65.

Meigs, J. W., Albom, J. J., and Kartin, B. L. 1954. Chloracne from an unusual exposure to Arachlor. *J. Am. Med. Assoc.* 154:1417.

Moore, J. A. 1978. Toxicity of 2,3,7,8-tetrachlorodibenzo-*p*-dioxin. Ramel C (ed) chlorinated phenoxy acids and their dioxins. *Ecol. Bull.* (Stockholm) 27:134–144.

Moore, J. A., McConnell, E. E., Dalgard, D. W., and Harris, M. W. 1979. Comparative toxicity of three halogenated dibenzofurans in guinea pigs, mice and rhesus monkeys. *Ann. N.Y. Acad. Sci.* 320:151–163.

Moses, M. and Selikoff, I. J. 1981. *Lancet* in press.

Oishi, S., Morita, M., and Fukuda, H. 1978. Comparative toxicity of poly-chlorinated biphenyls and dibenzofurans in rats. *Toxicol. Appl. Pharmacol.* 43:13–22.

Olafson, P. 1947. Hyperkeratosis (x-disease) of cattle. *Cornell Vet.* 48:135–138.

Ouw, K. H., Simpson, G. R., and Siyali, D. S. 1976. Use and health effects of Aroclor 1242, a polychorinated biphenyl in an electrical industry. *Arch. Environ. Health* 2:189–194.

Poland, A. and Glover, E. 1977. Chlorinated biphenyl induction of aryl hydrocarbon hydroxylase activity; a study of the structure activity relationships. *Mol. Pharmacol.* 13:924–938.

Poland, A. and Kende, A. 1976. 2,3,7,8-Tetrachlorodibenzo-*p*-dioxin; environ-mental contaminant and molecular probe. *Fed. Proc.* 35:2404–2418.

Puccinelli, V. 1954. Chloracne from pentachlorodiphenyl. *Med. Lav.* 45:131–145.

Puccinelli, V., et al. 1977. Skin disorders in the Seveso area during the first year after the accident at the Icmesa plant. Report to meeting of the Chloracne Panel, Commission of the European Communities, Health and Safety Directorate, Luxembourg, July 11–12, Milan, Document 4383, p. 39.

Rappe, C., Gara, A., Buser, H. A., and Bosshardt, H. P. Analysis of polychlorinated dibenzofurans in Yusho oil using high resolution gas chromatography–mass spectrometry. *Chemosphere* 5:231–236.

Reggiani, G. 1980. Human exposure. In *Topics in Environmental Health. Halogenated Biphenyls, Terphenyls, Naphthalenes, Dibenzodioxins and Related Compounds,* chap. 2. Amsterdam: Elsevier Biomedical. In press.

Rose, J. Q., Ramsey, J. C., Wentzler, T. H., Hummel, R. A., and Gehring, P. J. 1976. The fate of 2,3,7,8-tetrachlorodibenzo-*p*-dioxin following single and repeated oral doses to the rat. *Toxicol. Appl. Pharmacol.* 36:209–220.

Schwetz, B. A., et al. 1973. Toxicology of chlorinated dibenzo-*p*-dioxins. *Environ. Health Perspect.* 5:87–100.

Suskind, R. R. 1978. Chloracne and associated health problems in the manufacture of 2,4,5-T. Report of the Joint Conferences, National Institute of Environmental Health Sciences and International Agency for Research on Cancer, Lyon, France, Jan. 11.

Taylor, J. S. 1979. Environmental chloracne: Update and overview. *Ann. N.Y. Acad. Sci.* 320:295–307.

Taylor, J. S., Wuthrick, R. C., Lloyd, K. M., and Poland, A. 1977. Chloracne from manufacture of a new herbicide. *Arch. Dermatol.* 113:616–619.

Telegina, K. A. and Biklulatuva, M. 1970. Affection of the follicular apparatus of the skin in workers occupied in production of butyl ester of 2,4,5-trichlorophenoxy acetic acid. *Vestn. Dermatol. Venerol.* 44:35–39.

Urabe, H., Koda, H., and Asaki, M. 1979. Present state of Yusho patients. *Ann. N.Y. Acad. Sci.* 320:273–276.

Warshaw, R., Fischbein, A., Thornton, J., Miller, A., and Selikoff, I. J. 1979. Decrease in vital capacity in PCB exposed workers in a capacitor manufacturing facility. *Ann. N.Y. Acad. Sci.* 320:277–283.

Wong, K. C. and Hwang, M. Y. 1981. PCB poisoning. Special issue. *Clin. Med. (Taipei)* 7:83–88 (Chinese).

Zack, J. and Suskind, R. R. 1980. The mortality experience of workers exposed to tetrachlorodibenzo-*p*-dioxin in a trichlorophenol process accident. *J. Occup. Med.* 22:11–20.

24

reactions to systemic exposure to contact allergens

■ Torkil Menné ■

INTRODUCTION

Systemic reactions to ingested allergens occur in patients previously sensitized by percutaneous absorption of an allergen. Until recently, such reactions have mainly been of theoretical interest when they were occasionally observed in patients sensitized to a topically applied medicament who later developed widespread dermatitis when treated with the same medicament systemically.

Contact sensitivity to nickel, chromium, and cobalt is frequent and is often associated with chronic hand eczema (Fregert et al., 1969). As these metals occur in small amounts in our food, it is possible that systemic contact dermatitis is a common phenomenon.

CLINICAL PICTURE

Pompholyx Hand Eczema

This consists of recurring itching eruptions with deep-seated vesicles and some or no erythema localized on the palms, volar aspects, and sides of the fingers. Exacerbations occur at intervals of weeks to months without any obvious external reason.

Flare-ups of Earlier Patch Test and Contact Dermatitis Reactions

This phenomenon has been observed experimentally in provocation studies with nickel and chromium in patients sensitized to these metals and in patients sensitized to medicaments. Periodic flare-up reactions in earlier positive patch tests have not been observed in clinical practice.

Generalized Maculopapular-vesicular Rash

This consists of a symmetric eruption localized to the elbow flexure, axillae, eyelids, side of the neck, and genital area. The pattern seems characteristic of the systemic contact dermatitis reaction.

Vasculitis

Circular excoriations on the back, buttocks, and thighs were observed in nickel-sensitive women (Hjorth, 1976). Similar excoriations were noticed in two nickel-sensitive patients treated with a nickel chelating drug (Kaaber et al., 1979). Histopathology shows superficial allergic vasculitis.

Systemic Symptoms

In relation to positive oral provocation with nickel and medicament, general symptoms such as headache and malaise occur. In neomycin- and chromate-sensitive patients oral provocation with the hapten produces nausea, vomiting, and diarrhea (Ekelund and Möller, 1969; Pirilä, 1970; Kaaber and Veien, 1977).

NICKEL

Environmental exposure to nickel and nickel metabolism have been described in detail (National Academy of Sciences, 1975; Nriagu, 1980; Underwood, 1977; Brown and Sunderman, 1980). Daily nickel intake varies from 100 to 800 μg. The highest nickel content is found in vegetables, whole wheat or rye bread, and shellfish. Nickel release from stainless steel cooking utensils during the preparation of food with a low pH value causes additional exposure (Christensen and Möller, 1978; Brun, 1979). Nickel exposure from drinking water and air pollution is usually negligible, although important exceptions occur (Fregert, 1971).

Most ingested nickel remains unabsorbed in the gastrointestinal tract. Only 1-10% is absorbed. The nickel concentration in urine ranges from 1 to 10 μg per day. The concentration in sweat is high, ranging from 7 to 270 μg per day. Thus sweating may be an important route of excretion of nickel from the body.

Oral provocation with 5.6 mg nickel as the sulfate to 12 nickel-sensitive female patients with pompholyx hand eczema resulted in a flare of the dermatitis with fresh vesicles in 9 of the patients. The reaction appeared within 2 to 16 h (Christensen and Möller, 1975). This observation has been confirmed (Kaaber et al., 1978; Veien et al., 1979b; Christensen, 1981). Cronin et al. (1980) observed exacerbation of pompholyx hand eczema in 5 of 5, 3 of 5, and 2 of 5 patients after oral doses of 2.5, 1.25, and 0.6 mg nickel, respectively.

Jordan and King (1979) gave 10 nickel-sensitive women with chronic vesicular hand dermatitis 0.5 mg nickel twice as a supplement to the regular diet. Only one of the women experienced worsening of her hand eczema. Burrows (1980) gave 22 nickel-sensitive patients with hand eczema 2 mg and then 4 mg nickel on two successive days, twice over 2 wk, with lactose as a placebo in a double-blind study. No difference was found between the two periods.

The clinical significance of these findings is a matter of discussion. The nickel dosages used in the provocation studies often exceed the figures given for the normal daily intake of nickel. In experimental studies we have often observed flare reactions at the site of an earlier nickel patch test. This phenomenon does not appear in clinical practice. After oral provocation with 0.6-5.6 mg nickel, a nonphysiological high urinary nickel value was observed on the following days (20-200 $\mu g/l$) (Christensen and Lagesson, 1981; Cronin et al., 1980; Menné et al., 1978; Veien et al., 1979b). In two studies including four patients (Menné and Thorboe, 1976; de Yongh et al., 1978) there was a tendency for higher nickel excretion in the urine to be related to active hand dermatitis, but the urinary nickel level was far from the high concentrations measured on the days after oral nickel provocation.

These observations do not exclude the possibility that systemic exposure to nickel is important for the chronic occurrence of hand eczema related to nickel sensitivity. Undoubtedly, the daily nickel intake will sometimes exceed 0.6 mg, and 2 of 5 patients reacted to this dose in the study of Cronin et al. (1980). A diet with a low nickel content diminished the activity of hand eczema in 9 of 17 patients (Kaaber et al., 1978), and after the diet was abandoned 7 of the 9 experienced a flare of their hand eczema.

A systemic contact dermatitis reaction in nickel-sensitive people can also be provoked by treatment with nickel chelating drugs. The drug of choice in the treatment of nickel carbonyl poisoning is diethyldithiocarbamate (DDC) (Sunderman, 1979). Antabuse (tetraethylthiuram disulfide) is metabolized to DDC after absorption in the gastrointestinal tract. Treatment with these drugs at a daily dosage of 50-400 mg has been effective in the treatment of nickel hand eczema (O. B. Christensen and M. Kristensen, personal communication; Kaaber et al., 1979; Menné et al., 1980; Spruit et al., 1978).

Antabuse treatment of nickel hand eczema was evaluated in a double-blind study (K. Kaaber et al., unpublished observation). During the treatment, 5 of 11 in the Antabuse group healed completely, compared with 2 of 13 in the placebo-treated group. There was a statistically significant decrease in the number of flare and scaling reactions in the Antabuse-treated group. Regarding the other parameters—area of dermatitis, redness, and number of vesicles—the difference between the Antabuse and placebo groups was not statistically significant. In the placebo group the weekly amount of steroid ointment was 5.3 g, compared with 1.6 g in the Antabuse group. Even with a dose of 50 mg Antabuse a day, some patients had a severe flare of their dermatitis during the first weeks of treatment. This effect was not due to increased nickel absorption, since Antabuse has nickel chelating properties after it has been absorbed and metabolized.

If nickel is given iv to nickel-sensitive patients, 1-3 μg may elicit a severe systemic contact dermatitis reaction. This has been observed in patients treated with iv infusions through a cannula releasing traces of nickel (Stoddart, 1960; Smeenk and Teunissen, 1977).

Indomethacin (Spruit, 1979) increases absorption of nickel, whereas adverse reactions are possible in nickel-sensitive patients. Nickel associates with a variety of natural occurring proteins and amino acids (Nriagu, 1980). Thus flare of dermatitis in a nickel-sensitive patient may not always be caused by increased oral exposure to nickel, but could be caused by metabolic and pharmacological reactions.

CHROMIUM

Chromium metabolism and toxicology have been described in detail (National Academy of Sciences, 1974; Underwood, 1977). The chromium intake in the United States varies from 5 to 400 μg per day. Exact figures for absorption are difficult to give because they depend on the source of chromium. Inorganic chromium compounds are poorly absorbed; among them, hexavalent chromium is more easily absorbed than trivalent chromium, the absorption ranging from 1 to 25% of an oral dose. Most meats are good sources of chromium; fish and most vegetables are poor ones.

Sidi and Melki (1954) suggested that oral intake of dichromate by chromate-sensitive patients might be of importance for the chronicity of the dermatitis. Fregert (1965) challenged five patients sensitive to chromium with 0.05 mg potassium dichromate. Within 2 h they developed severe vesiculation of the palms. One of the patients experienced acute exacerbation of a generalized dermatitis. Schleiff (1968) observed a flare in chromate dermatitis in 20 patients challenged with 1-10 mg potassium dichromate contained in a homeopathic drug. Some of the patients also experienced a flare in a previously positive dichromate patch test.

Kaaber and Veien (1977) studied the significance of oral intake of dichromate by chromate-sensitive patients in a double-blind study. Thirty-one patients were challenged orally with either 2.5 mg potassium dichromate or a placebo tablet. Nine of 11 patients with pompholyx hand eczema reacted with a flare of the dermatitis within 1 or 2 d, but did not react to placebo. The patients with another morphology reacted to a lesser degree. A few reacted to placebo. Three patients developed vomiting or abdominal pains and transient diarrhea after the chromate provocation, but not after the challenge with placebo.

A systemic contact dermatitis reaction to chromium may also occur after inhalation of chromium contained in welding fumes (Shelley, 1964).

COBALT

Cobalt metabolism is described in Underwood (1977). Daily intake of cobalt ranges from 0.14 to 1.77 mg in the United States. Among individual types of foods, green-leafed vegetables and shellfish have the highest cobalt contents. Unlike nickel and chromium, cobalt salts are easily absorbed in the gastrointestinal tract. The absorption in humans ranges from 20 to 95% of an oral dose. Most of it is excreted in the urine. Cobalt is an essential trace element, but its function other than as part of the vitamin B_{12} molecule is unknown.

In nature, cobalt is usually found together with nickel. Cobalt sensitivity has often been found in association with nickel sensitivity in females and chromate sensitivity in males (Fregert and Rorsman, 1966). Isolated cobalt sensitivity is rare (Rystedt, 1979). Cronin (1980) found an isolated cobalt reaction relevant in only 20% of males and 45% of females. Most cases among the females were due to jewelry dermatitis. The possibility of a systemic contact dermatitis reaction in cobalt-sensitive patients has not been systematically examined. Veien and Kaaber (1979) challenged patients who had negative standard patch tests and pompholyx hand eczema with 1 mg cobalt as the chloride. Two of 16 reacted to the oral dose with a flare in the original dermatitis.

Clendenning (1971) observed a 49-yr-old housewife with persistent eczema of the palms and an isolated cobalt allergy. After the removal of metal dentures made of a cobalt-chromium alloy (Vitallium) the dermatitis cleared. The patient had not had any local symptoms in the mouth. After the removal of the prostheses she noticed a return of her appetite, the loss of which had been a definite symptom during the entire period of the dermatitis.

Because cobalt is so well absorbed, it may play a greater role in systemic contact dermatitis than nickel or chromium. If this is the case, it could explain why hand eczema related to combined sensitivity to nickel-cobalt or chromium-cobalt has a more unfavorable prognosis than that related to isolated nickel or chromate sensitivity (Christensen, 1981; Förström et al., 1969; Menné, 1980).

REACTIONS TO IMPLANTED METAL PROSTHESES

Implantation of metal alloys is used with increasing frequency in orthopedic reconstructive surgery. The most commonly used alloys are stainless steel (15–20% chromium, 0% cobalt, 10–14% nickel) and Vitallium (27–30% chromium, 60.65% cobalt, 0–4% nickel). Both alloys include molybdenum in small concentrations, and vanadium and copper may be present. As an alternative to these two alloys, titanium 318 can be used.

Often the implant is a joint replacement with two surfaces articulating against each other. This is either a metal-to-metal or, more commonly now, a metal-to-plastic contact. In patients with metal-to-metal prostheses elevated concentrations of chromium and cobalt have been found in blood and urine (Coleman et al., 1973) and in the tissues adjacent to the joint prostheses (Evans et al., 1974). In patients with metal-to-plastics prostheses the metal concentrations are normal in blood and urine and only slightly elevated in the tissues (Coleman et al., 1973; Evans et al., 1974).

The sensitization potential of implanted metal alloys has been evaluated in retrospective and prospective clinical studies. The significance of these studies is difficult to interpret because metal allergy is a common phenomenon in the general population. The prevalence of nickel allergy in females approaches 10% (Menné, 1978; Peltonen, 1979; Prystowsky et al., 1979), with the highest value in those 15–30 yr old. The high prevalence is due to the common use of nickel-plated alloys in direct skin contact, for instance, through ear piercing and costume jewelry. The prevalence of nickel allergy is 0.8–0.9% in man (Peltonen, 1979; Prystowsky et al., 1979). It is commonly thought that cobalt allergy is often related to nickel allergy. In clinical studies of hospital patients, 53% of the nickel-sensitive women, not including those who were also chromium-sensitive, were also sensitive to cobalt (Fregert and Rorsman, 1966). This high figure is probably due to a sampling bias, because most patients referred to hospital departments have had eczema and not just a dermatitis related to skin contact with metal. In an investigation of unselected female twins, only 6 of 63 nickel-sensitive twins were also cobalt-sensitive. Four of the six had hand eczema (Menné, 1980). Thus cobalt allergy in the general population is rare compared to nickel allergy and the prevalence probably does not exceed 1%. Chromium is mainly an industrial sensitizer and is seen in bricklayers, masons, and workers in the metal industries.

In retrospective studies of patients with metal-to-metal prostheses (cobalt, chromium), a high incidence of metal sensitivity was found. In 14 patients with loose prostheses 9 were sensitive to either cobalt or chromium. In 24 patients with a normally functioning prosthesis, none were sensitive to metal (Evans et al., 1974). Elves et al. (1975) studied 50 patients with metal-to-metal prostheses (cobalt, chromium). Of the 50 patients, 23 had a nontraumatic failure of the prostheses. Fifteen of these were sensitive to metals: seven to cobalt, three to cobalt and nickel, two to nickel, two to chromium, and one to both nickel and vanadium. Of the other 27 patients with stable prostheses or with a traumatic failure, only four were metal-sensitive. Benson et al. (1975) found an incidence of 28% metal sensitivity in patients with metal-to-metal prostheses. Among 34 patients with pain and loosening of the prostheses, Munro-Ashman and Miller (1976) found 16 with metal sensitivity. Thirteen were sensitive to cobalt, four to nickel, and two to chromium. The results of these studies are similar, and even though the studies are retrospective they suggest that at least cobalt sensitization occurs as a consequence of systemic exposure to the metal from an implanted metal alloy.

In patients with an internal metal-to-plastic prosthesis the number who are metal-sensitive does not exceed that in nonoperated patients (controls) (Benson et al., 1975). In prospective studies involving similar patients whose preoperative status was evaluated by patch testing, no evidence was found of sensitization to the implanted metal alloys (Carlsson et al., 1980; Deutman et al., 1977; Nater et al., 1976; Rooker and Wilkinson, 1980) when the patients were retested months to years after the operation. In the retrospective part of the study by Carlsson et al. (1980) a statistically significant increased number of metal-sensitive patients was found among those with loose prostheses. Among the patients studied prospectively only few had complications with pain and loosening of the prostheses. Rooker and Wilkinson (1980) studied 69 patients prospectively. Before the operation six patients were metal-sensitive, but only one remained so afterwards. Rooker and Wilkinson suggest that the minimal systemic exposure to the hapten led to immunological tolerance. The safety of the metal-to-plastic prostheses with respect to sensitization is in agreement with the small amounts of metal released from this type of prosthesis (Coleman et al., 1973; Evans et al., 1974).

Sensitization from metal prostheses has been reported mostly in patients with loosening of the prostheses. This does not prove that the allergy is the cause of the loosening; alternatively, the loosening may cause the allergy. The available evidence supports the latter exploration (Lead article, *Br. Med. J.,* 1980; Lead article, *Lancet,* 1980).

Skin symptoms in patients who have undergone implantation of metal prostheses are rare. They occur in two forms: as a dermatitis localized to the skin that covers the area of the metal prosthesis (Cramers and Locht, 1977; Munro-Ashman and Miller, 1976), or as a generalized dermatitis (Barranco and Solomon, 1973; Deutman et al., 1977; Elves et al., 1975; Foussereau and Laugier, 1966; Oleffe and Wilmet, 1980). One patient first had a localized dermatitis and then developed a generalized dermatitis (Grimalt and Romaguera, 1980).

It is noteworthy that in none of the patients with a dermatitis caused by a metal hip or knee prosthesis was it necessary to remove the prosthesis, as the symptoms were transient (Deutman et al., 1977; Elves et al., 1975; Munro-Ashman and Miller, 1976). Those who develop rashes from osteosynthesis screws have a more persistent disease and removal of the screws has been followed by rapid clearing of the dermatitis (Barranco and Solomon, 1973; Cramers and Locht, 1977; Grimalt and Romaguera, 1980; Oleffe and Wilmet, 1980).

The limited number of patients with allergic reactions due to implanted metal prostheses does not indicate that all patients should be patch-tested preoperatively. Carlsson et al. (1980) recommend that patients with a history of metal allergy should be examined by a dermatologist and patch-tested. If metal allergy is found, stainless steel can be used in patients with an isolated cobalt allergy, and vitallium in those with isolated nickel allergy. Otherwise, titanium alloys should be used. Only long-term prospective studies can determine whether it is necessary to take any precautions at all.

Localized lesions or generalized dermatitis caused by allergic reactions due to metals used in dentistry have not been discussed here. The subject has been reviewed by Fisher (1974).

MEDICAMENTS

Systemic contact dermatitis due to medicaments has been reviewed by Cronin (1972) and Fisher (1973). Usually, sensitization occurs through topical application of the drug and the patient later has a systemic reaction when the drug is taken orally or parenterally. The opposite situation can occur, with a patient first having an exanthema due to an antibiotic and later developing a localized dermatitis when the drug is applied topically (Girard, 1978). Pirilä (1970) termed this phenomenon primary endogenic contact eczema.

The most commonly used topical antibiotics are neomycin, bacitracin, and chloramphenicol. Ekelund and Møller (1969) challenged 12 patients with leg ulcers sensitized to neomycin with an oral dose of the hapten. Ten of the 12 had a reaction. Five developed a flare-up of the original dermatitis. Six had a flare-up at the site of the earlier positive patch test. Three developed pompholyx hand eczema. Four had nausea, and one vomited. Pililä (1970) made a similar study and also observed diarrhea. It is noteworthy that the pompholyx eczema of the hands occurred as a primary event after the systemic administration of the hapten and did not represent a flare-up of the original dermatitis. The gastrointestinal symptoms are signs of a systemic contact dermatitis reaction.

Systemic contact dermatitis to penicillin has occurred in patients who were sensitized by topical treatment with penicillin and later exposed to very small amounts of penicillin in milk (Vickers et al., 1958). Similarly, nurses contact-sensitized to streptomycin have had systemic reactions during parenteral desensitization with streptomycin (Wilson, 1958).

The pharmacological effectiveness of topically applied antihistamines is questionable. The ethanolamine and ethylenediamine antihistamines are the most common contact-sensitizing antihistamines in the United States (Fisher, 1976). Ethylenediamine-derived antihistamine may elicit reactions in patients sensitized to ethylenediamine from the use of Mycolog cream. In the San Francisco area 0.43% of the general population are sensitized to ethylenediamine (Prystowsky et al., 1979). Aminophylline, containing theophyllamine and ethylenediamine, elicits systemic reactions in ethylenediamine-sensitized patients (Provost and Jillson, 1967).

During the World War II sulfonamides were the most important antibacterial drugs. Many soldiers were sensitized by topical applications and later developed a local flare-up reaction and a generalized maculopapular rash when the drugs were given orally. Park (1943, 1944) found that the severity of the eruption varied with the sensitivity of the subject and the size of the dose. Sulzberger et al. (1947) frequently found cross-reactions between the different antibacterial sulfonamides.

Sidi and Dobkevitch-Morrill (1951) studied cross-reactions between the para-amine compounds. Systemic reactions were seen after oral provocation with procaine in primary sulfonamide-sensitized patients, to p-aminophenylsulfamide in primary procaine-sensitized patients, and to p-aminophenylsulfamide and procaine in primary p-phenylenediamine-sensitized patients. Baer and Leider (1949) challenged 20 p-phenylenediamine-sensitive patients with an oral dose of 15 to 210 mg azodyes. Seven of the 20 had a flare of their dermatitis. A similar response occurred in two of 20 controls. The possible clinical significance of this observation has not been evaluated.

Antabuse is used as a rubber chemical, fungicide, and in the treatment of chronic alcoholism. Cross-reactions to other carbamates may occur. In sensitized patients treatment with Antabuse can lead to a systemic contact dermatitis (Pirilä, 1957). Subcutaneous implantation of Antabuse led to sensitization in two patients (Lachapelle, 1975). Subsequent oral Antabuse led to a systemic contact dermatitis in one of the patients, while the other tolerated the drug.

Acetylsalicyclic acid (aspirin) is a rare contact sensitizer. One patient sensitized to methyl salicylate developed a systemic contact dermatitis when treated with aspirin. Patch tests were negative with aspirin but positive with sodium salicylate. Hindson (1977) suggested that the common intermediate metabolite was the cause of the systemic reaction.

In a pharmaceutical factory 14 cases of allergic contact dermatitis to the β-adrenergic blocking agent alprenolol (Aptine) occurred. One man had pruritus and widespread dermatitis after oral provocation with 100 mg of the drug (Ekenvall and Forsbeck, 1978).

Merthiolate is a preservative used in sera and vaccines. In the Scandinavian countries the prevalence of merthiolate sensitivity approaches 7–16% in the young age groups (Förström et al., 1980; Hansson and Möller, 1970). Forty-five merthiolate-sensitive patients were tested sc with 0.5 ml 0.01% merthiolate solution, equal to the dose contained in a tetanus toxoid shot. One developed generalized dermatitis and fever (Förström et al., 1980).

Propylene glycol is a vehicle in topical medicaments and cosmetics and a food additive. The Food and Agriculture Organization/World Health Organization (FAO/WHO) have accepted a daily intake of up to 20 mg per kilogram of body weight. Propylene glycol is both a sensitizer and a primary irritant. Hannuksela and Förström (1978) challenged 10 patients with a positive patch test to 2% propylene glycol with 2–15 ml. Eight reacted with an exanthema

3–16 h after the ingestion, in seven of these the rash disappeared within 24–48 h without treatment. This observation differs from the picture of a systemic contact dermatitis reaction in some respects. Local flare-up of earlier dermatitis and earlier positive patch tests was not seen, and the rapid disappearance of the rash indicates a pharmacological effect rather than an immunologically mediated process.

A positive patch test to a drug usually contraindicates further use of the drug. Accidental oral exposure will often lead to a severe systemic contact dermatitis reaction.

OTHERS

In hyposensitizing persons against rhus dermatitis, Kligman (1958a) observed systemic contact dermatitis reactions. Half of the moderately to severely sensitive patients experienced either pruritus or a rash. Flares at healed contact dermatitis sites occurred with a frequency of 10%. Dyshidrosis of the palms and erythema multiforme were rare. Pruritus ani occurred in 10% of the highly sensitive.

Sensitization to balsam of Peru often leads to sensitivity to flavors and orange peel (Hjorth, 1961). Hjorth (1961) observed two children who were sensitive to balsam of Peru whose dermatitis flared after they ate fruits and ices. Hjorth (1965) also described a doctor with severe hand eczema for 10 yr who, because he reacted to balsam of Peru on patch testing, was told to avoid orange peel. To test the validity of the advice he ate a jar of orange marmalade. After 12 h he experienced the most severe attack of hand eczema he had ever had. By avoiding perfumes, cola drinks, vermouth, throat lozenges, cinnamon, and similar items, he has since been free of dermatitis.

Pentadecyl catechols, the sensitizers in poison ivy, cross-react with oil of cashew nuts (Kligman, 1958b). Five patients who had been sensitized to poison ivy had a widespread dermatitis after eating 150–450 g raw cashew nuts purchased in a health food store. The dermatitis involved the palms, medial aspects of the arms, axillae, bathing trunk area, and posterior parts of the legs (Ratner et al., 1974). Test with commercially available dry roasted cashew nuts did not produce any symptoms.

The antioxidant butylated hydroxyanisole (BHA), which is permitted in both foods and topical preparations, caused systemic contact dermatitis in two patients (Roed-Petersen and Hjorth, 1976). Both patients had a flare of hand eczema after oral intake of 5–10 mg BHA for 4 d. Other rare sensitizers, vitamin B_1 (Hjorth, 1958) and vitamin C (Metz et al., 1980), have given rise to systemic contact dermatitis.

MECHANISM

The clinical observation of rapid onset (within hours) of the effect of oral exposure to haptens in sensitized individuals suggests that mechanisms other than the allergic type 4 reaction are involved. It is not unusual for a nickel-sensitive patient who is exposed to nickel to develop a systemic rash within hours and a flare of hand dermatitis after 12–48 h.

Veien et al. (1979a) investigated 14 patients with a positive nickel patch test. All were challenged orally with 2.5 mg nickel. After 6–12 h five of them developed widespread erythema. Three of the five demonstrated precipitating antibodies in serum against a nickel-albumin complex in a passive immuno-diffusion assay. In the area with erythema no clinical dermatitis developed. The same phenomenon was observed in chromium-sensitized guinea pigs (Polak and Turk, 1968b). The response began 6–8 h after an injection of chromate. Histologically, at 24 h there was marked dilatation of the super-ficial capillaries in the upper dermis, but without any obvious perivascular infiltration. Like Veien et al. (1979), Polak and Turk suggested that circulat-ing immune complexes were the triggering mechanism.

Christensen et al. (1981) studied flare-up reactions in 4- to 7-wk-old positive nickel patch tests in five patients after oral provocation with 5.6 mg nickel. The histological picture was that of acute dermatitis. Direct immuno-fluorescence examination for deposits of immunoglobulin G (IgG), IgA, IgM, complement 3, and fibrinogen were negative. The histological picture of flare-up reactions in chromate-sensitive guinea pigs after an iv injection of chromate shows a perivascular infiltration with polymorphonuclear leukocytes (Polak and Turk, 1968b).

Veien et al. (1979b) studied lymphocyte stimulation after oral provoca-tion with 4 mg nickel in eight nickel-sensitive patients. They found a statistically significant increase over controls in the lymphocytic transforma-tion test. The response was independent of the severity of the skin symptoms. There is clinical and experimental evidence that systemic reactions to ingested haptens can be mediated by both a type 3 and a type 4 immunologic reaction. Both types of reactions can be seen in the same patient. The immunologic reactivity, judged from an increase in the lymphocytic trans-formation test, can be maintained by oral ingestion of a hapten.

DIAGNOSIS

Usually, patients with a systemic reaction to ingested haptens have a positive patch test. This is not surprising, because it is a positive patch test that confirms the diagnosis. But patch testing is not always a reliable diagnostic procedure in systemic contact dermatitis.

Veien and Kaaber (1979) investigated 16 patients with pompholyx hand eczema and negative routine patch tests. Two of them had an aggravation of their hand eczema after oral provocation with 2.5 mg chromium and two with 1.0 mg cobalt. None reacted to placebo.

Veien et al. (1981), in an open study, challenged 109 patients who had pompholyx hand eczema with a tablet containing 2.5 mg nickel, 1 mg cobalt, and 2.5 mg chromium as salts of the respective metals. Of the 109 patients, 39 reacted to the mixture of metals and 29 of those to the individual metal salts. Three were considered placebo reactions. Seven patients were not challenged with the individual salts. Males reacted primarily to chromate and cobalt, and females to nickel and cobalt.

Menné (1981) investigated monozygotic twins who both had a history of nickel allergy and a pompholyx hand eczema. One of the twins had a negative patch test to 5% nickel sulfate in petrolatum, repeated twice. In spite of this, oral provocation with 2.5 mg nickel caused a rash in the axillae and the genital area and a recurrence of the hand eczema.

The occurrence of a systemic contact dermatitis reaction and a negative patch test was demonstrated experimentally in guinea pigs. Polak et al. (1970) studied dichromate contact-sensitive animals which had been made permanently tolerant with respect to contact sensitivity by iv injections of dichromate followed by epicutaneous application of dichromate. When the animals were later given a systemic injection of dichromate, a flare-up at old positive skin test sites followed.

Therefore oral provocation with haptens may be considered diagnostic in patients with a negative patch test and a clinical picture of systemic contact dermatitis. In nickel-sensitive patients we start with a dose of 0.6 mg, after 2 d 1.25 mg, and after another 2 d 2.5 mg nickel as the sulfate. If the patient reacts we do not go on with a higher dose. Using this schedule, we have not had any severe reactions. With chromium and cobalt, 2.5 and 1.0 mg as the dichromate and the chloride, respectively, have been used. Studies with lower doses (e.g., Fregert, 1965) are desirable. Guidelines for challenge with medicaments are difficult to give, but to exclude a systemic contact dermatitis reaction it is necessary to challenge with a therapeutic dose. In patients with a history of urticaria or any other anaphylactic reaction, systemic exposure to a hapten may cause a life-threatening reaction, and small amounts must be used for the initial dose.

TOXICOLOGICAL ASSAYS

The many examples of contact-sensitizing chemicals that can also give rise to systemic contact dermatitis reactions make it necessary to include this possibility when the safety of new chemicals and topical drugs is evaluated.

If a chemical is a topical sensitizer in humans or experimental animals, future systemic reactions are a possibility. In evaluating safety it is necessary to include data on the occurrence of the chemicals in foodstuffs or in drugs for systemic use. Data on absorption and metabolism should be considered. A high degree of absorption would suggest the possibility of future systemic reactions.

Polak and Turk (1968a, 1968b) and Polak et al. (1970) observed systemic reactions and local flare-ups after parenteral administration of dichromate to dichromate-sensitized guinea pigs. This model may be valuable for comparing the ability of different chemicals to elicit systemic contact dermatitis reactions.

Everyone agrees that systemic contact dermatitis reactions occur, but the relevance of the phenomenon in daily clinical practice is still a matter of discussion. Many patients suffer from long-standing dermatitis, especially chronic hand eczema. In the United States (O'Quinn et al., 1972) and Denmark (Menné and Bachmann, 1979), among all skin diseases, allergic contact dermatitis is the most common cause of vocational disability. Analyses of the Danish figures show that hand eczema due to nickel was predominant in women, and hand eczema due to chromate in men. These alarming figures may be an indication of systemic contact dermatitis reactions.

REFERENCES

Baer, R. L. and Leider, M. 1949. The effects of feeding certified food azo dyes in paraphenylenediamine-hypersensitive subjects. *J. Invest. Dermatol.* 13:223–232.

Barranco, V. P. and Solomon, H. 1973. Eczematous dermatitis caused by internal exposure to nickel. *South. Med. J.* 66:447–448.

Benson, M. K., Goodwin, P. G., and Brostoff, J. 1975. Metal sensitivity in patients with joint replacement arthroplasties. *Br. Med. J.* 4:374–375.

Brown, S. S. and Sunderman, F. W., Jr., eds. 1980. *Nickel Toxicology.* New York: Academic.

Brun, R. 1979. Nickel in food: The role of stainless-steel utensils. *Contact Dermatitis* 5:43–45.

Burrows, D. 1980. A double-blind trial on the effect of oral nickel in patients with nickel dermatitis. Presented at the 5th International Symposium on Contact Dermatitis, Barcelona.

Carlsson, Å. S., Magnusson, B., and Möller, H. 1980. Metal sensitivity in patients with metal-to-plastic total hip arthroplasties. *Acta Orthop. Scand.* 51:57–62.

Christensen, O. B. 1981. Nickel allergy and hand eczema in females. Thesis, Department of Dermatology, University of Lund, Malmö, Sweden.

Christensen, O. B. and Lagesson, V. 1981. Nickel concentration of blood and urine after oral administration. *Ann. Clin. Lab. Sci.* 8:184–189.

Christensen, O. B. and Möller, H. 1975. External and internal exposure to the antigen in the hand eczema of nickel allergy. *Contact Dermatitis* 1:136–141.

Christensen, O. B. and Möller, H. 1978. Release of nickel from cooking utensils. *Contact Dermatitis* 4:343–346.

Christensen, O. B., Lindström, G. C., Löfberg, H., and Möller, H. 1981. Micromorphology and specificity of orally induced flare-up reactions in nickel-sensitive patients. *Acta Derm.-Venereol.*, in press.

Clendenning, E. W. 1971. Allergy to cobalt in metal denture as cause of hand dermatitis. *Contact Dermatitis Newslett.* 10:225–226.

Coleman, R. F., Harrington, J., and Scales, J. T. 1973. Concentrations of wear products in hair, blood, and urine after total hip replacement. *Br. Med. J.* i:527–529.

Cramers, M. and Locht, U. 1977. Metal sensitivity in patients treated for tibial fractures with plates of stainless steel. *Acta Orthop. Scand.* 48:245–249.

Cronin, E. 1972. Reactions to contact allergens given orally or systematically. *Br. J. Dermatol.* 86:104–107.

Cronin, E. 1980. *Contact Dermatitis.* Edinburgh: Churchill Livingstone.

Cronin, E., DiMichiel, A. D., and Brown, S. S. 1980. Oral challenge in nickel-sensitive women with hand eczema. In *Nickel Toxicology*, eds. S. S. Brown and F. W. Sunderman, Jr., pp. 149–155. New York: Academic.

Deutman, R., Mulder, T. J., Brian, R., and Nater, J. P. 1977. Metal sensitivity before and after total hip arthroplasty. *J. Bone Jt. Surg.* 59A:862–865.

Ekelund, A.-G. and Möller, H. 1969. Oral provocation in eczematous contact allergy to neomycin and hydroxy-quinolines. *Acta Derm.-Venereol.* 49:422–426.

Ekenvall, L. and Forsbeck, M. 1978. Contact eczema produced by a β-adrenergic blocking agent (alprenolol). *Contact Dermatitis* 4:190–194.

Elves, M. W., Wilson, J. N., Scales, J. E., and Kemp, H. B. S. 1975. Incidence of metal sensitivity in patients with total joint replacements. *Br. Med. J.* 4:376–378.

Evans, E. M., Freeman, M. A. R., Miller, A. J., and Vernon-Roberts, B. 1974. Metal sensitivity as a cause of bone necrosis and loosening of the prosthesis in total joint replacement. *J. Bone Jt. Surg.* 56B:626–642.

Fisher, A. A. 1973. *Contact Dermatitis*, 2d ed. Philadelphia: Lea & Febiger.

Fisher, A. A. 1974. Allergic reactions due to metals used in dentistry. *Cutis* 14:797–800.

Fisher, A. A. 1976. Antihistamine dermatitis. *Cutis* 18:329–336.

Foussereau, J. and Laugier, P. 1966. Allergic eczema from metallic foreign bodies. *Trans. St. John's Hosp. Dermatol. Soc.* 52:220–225.

Fregert, S. 1965. Sensitization to hexa- and trivalent chromium. In *Pemphigus, Occupational Dermatosis due to Chemical Sensitization*, pp. 50–55. Budapest.

Fregert, S. 1971. Nickel in tap water. *Contact Dermatitis Newslett.* 9:202.

Fregert, S. and Rorsman, H. 1966. Allergy to chromium, nickel and cobalt. *Acta Derm.-Venereol.* 46:144–148.

Fregert, S., Hjorth, N., Magnusson, B., Bandmann, H.-J., Calnan, C. D., Cronin, E., Malten, K., Meneghini, C. L., Pirilä, V., and Wilkinson, D. S. 1969. Epidemiology of contact dermatitis. *Trans. St. John Hosp. Derm.* 55:17–35.

Förström, L, Pirilä, V., and Huju, P. 1969. Rehabilitation of workers with cement eczema due to hypersensitivity to bichromate. *Scand. J. Rehabil. Med.* 1:95–100.

Förström, L., Hannuksela, M., Kausa, M., and Lehmuskallio, E. 1980. Merthiolate hypersensitivity and vaccination. *Contact Dermatitis* 6:241–245.

Girard, J. P. 1978. Recurrent angioneurotic oedema and contact dermatitis due to penicillin. *Contact Dermatitis* 4:309.

Grimalt, F. and Romaguera, C. 1980. Acute nickel dermatitis from a metal implant. *Contact Dermatitis* 6:441–447.

Hannuksela, M. and Förström, L. 1978. Reactions to peroral propylene glycol. *Contact Dermatitis* 4:41–45.

Hansson, H. and Möller, H. 1970. Patch test reactions to merthiolate in healthy young subjects. *Br. J. Dermatol.* 83:349–356.

Hindson, C. 1977. Contact eczema from methyl salicylate reproduced by oral aspirin (acetylsalicylic acid). *Contact Dermatitis* 3:348.

Hjorth, N. 1958. Contact dermatitis for vitamin B_1 (thiamine). *J. Invest. Dermatol.* 30:261–264.

Hjorth, N. 1961. *Eczematous Allergy to Balsams*, thesis. Copenhagen: Munksgaard.

Hjorth, N. 1965. Allergy to balsams. *Spectrum Int.* 7:97–101.

Hjorth, N. 1976. Nickel vasculitis. *Contact Dermatitis* 2:356–357.

Jordan, W. P. and King, S. E. 1979. Nickel feeding in nickel-sensitive patients with hand eczema. *J. Am. Acad. Dermatol.* 1:506–508.

Kaaber, K. and Veien, N. K. 1977. The significance of chromate ingestion in patients allergic to chromate. *Acta Derm.-Venereol.* 57:321–323.

Kaaber, K., Veien, N. K., and Tjell, J. C. 1978. Low nickel diet in the treatment of patients with chronic nickel dermatitis. *Br. J. Dermatol.* 98:197–201.

Kaaber, K., Menné, T., Tjell, J. C., and Veien, N. 1979. Antabuse treatment of nickel dermatitis. Chelation—a new principle in the treatment of nickel dermatitis. *Contact Dermatitis* 5:221–228.

Kligman, A. M. 1958a. Hyposensitization against rhus dermatitis. *Arch. Dermatol.* 78:47–72.

Kligman, A. M. 1958b. Cashew nut shell oil for hyposensitization against rhus dermatitis. *Arch. Dermatol.* 78:359–363.

Lachapelle, J. M. 1975. Allergic "contact" dermatitis from disulfiram implants. *Contact Dermatitis* 1:218–220.

Lead article. 1980. Can metal sensitivity loosen joint replacements? *Lancet* ii:1284–1285.

Lead article. 1980. Metal allergy: A false alarm? *Br. Med. J.* 281:1303–1304.

Menné, T. 1978. The prevalence of nickel allergy among women. *Dermatosen Beruf Umwelt* 26:123–124.

Menné, T. 1980. Relationship between cobalt and nickel sensitization in females. *Contact Dermatitis* 6:337–340.

Menné, T. 1981. Nickel allergy—reliability of patch test. *Dermatosen Beruf Umwelt*, in press.

Menné, T. and Bachmann, E. 1979. Permanent disability from hand dermatitis in females sensitive to nickel, chromium and cobalt. *Dermatosen Beruf Umwelt* 27:129–135.

Menné, T. and Thorboe, A. 1976. Nickel dermatitis—nickel excretion. *Contact Dermatitis* 2:353–354.

Menné, T., Mikkelsen, H. I., and Solgaard, P. 1978. Nickel excretion in urine after oral administration. *Contact Dermatitis* 4:106–108.

Menné, T., Kaaber, K., and Tjell, J. C. 1980. Treatment of nickel dermatitis. *Ann. Clin. Lab. Sci.* 10:160–164.

Metz, J., Hundertmark, U., and Pevny, I. 1980. Vitamin C allergy of the delayed type. *Contact Dermatitis* 6:172–174.

Munro-Ashman, D. and Miller, A. J. 1976. Rejection of metal prosthesis and skin sensitivity to cobalt. *Contact Dermatitis* 2:65–67.

Nater, J. P., Brian, R. G., Deutman, R., and Mulder, T. J. 1976. The development of metal hypersensitivity in patients with metal-to-plastic hip arthroplasties. *Contact Dermatitis* 2:259–261.

National Academy of Sciences. 1974. *Chromium. Medical and Biological Effects of Environmental Pollutants.* Washington, D.C.: National Academy of Sciences.

National Academy of Sciences. 1975. *Nickel. Medical and Biologic Effects of Environmental Pollutants.* Washington, D.C.: National Academy of Sciences.

Nriagu, J. O. 1980. *Nickel in the Environment.* New York: Wiley.

Oleffe, J. and Wilmet, J. 1980. Generalized dermatitis from an osteosynthesis screw. *Contact Dermatitis* 6:365.

O'Quinn, S. E., Cole, J., and Many, H. 1972. Problems of disability and rehabilitation in patients with chronic skin diseases. *Arch. Dermatol.* 105:35–41.

Park, R. G. 1943. Cutaneous hypersensitivity to sulphonamides. *Br. Med. J.* 2:69–72.

Park, R. G. 1944. Sulphonamide allergy. *Br. Med. J.* 1:781–782.

Peltonen, L. 1979. Nickel sensitivity in the general population. *Contact Dermatitis* 5:27–33.

Pirilä, V. 1957. Dermatitis due to rubber. *Acta Derm.-Venereol. Proc. 11th. Int. Congr. Dermatol.* 2:252–255.

Pirilä, V. 1970. Endogenic contact eczema. *Allerg. Asthma* 16:15–19.

Polak, L. and Turk, J. L. 1968a. Studies on the effect of systemic administration of sensitizers in guinea-pigs with contact sensitivity to inorganic metal compounds. *Clin. Exp. Immunol.* 3:245–251.

Polak, L. and Turk, J. L. 1968b. Studies on the effect of systemic administration of sensitizers in guinea-pigs with contact sensitivity to inorganic metal compounds. *Clin. Exp. Immunol.* 3:253–262.

Polak, L., Frey, J. R., and Turk, J. L. 1970. Studies on the effect of systemic administration of sensitizers to guinea-pigs with contact sensitivity to inorganic metal compounds. *Clin. Exp. Immunol.* 7:739–744.

Provost, T. T. and Jillson, O. F. 1967. Ethylenediamine contact dermatitis. *Arch. Dermatol.* 96:231–234.

Prystowsky, S. D., Allen, A. M., Smith, R. W., Nonomura, J. H., Odon, R. B., and Akers, W. A. 1979. Allergic contact hypersensitivity to nickel, neomycin, ethylenediamine and benzocaine. *Arch. Dermatol.* 115:959–962.

Ratner, J. H., Spencer, S. K., and Grainge, J. M. 1974. Cashew nut dermatitis. *Arch. Dermatol.* 110:921–923.

Roed-Petersen, J. and Hjorth, N. 1976. Contact dermatitis from antioxidants. *Br. J. Dermatol.* 94:233–241.

Rooker, G. D. and Wilkinson, J. C. 1980. Metal sensitivity in patients undergoing hip replacement. *J. Bone Jt. Surg.* 62B:502–505.

Rystedt, I. 1979. Evaluation and relevance of isolated test reactions to cobalt. *Contact Dermatitis* 5:233–239.

Samitz, M. H. and Katz, S. A. 1975. Nickel dermatitis hazards from prostheses. *Br. J. Dermatol.* 92:287–290.

Schleiff, P. 1968. Provokation des Chromatekzems zu Testzwechen durch interne Chromzufuhr. *Hautarzt* 19:209–210.

Shelley, W. B. 1964. Chromium in welding fumes as a cause of eczematous hand eruption. *J. Am. Med. Assoc.* 189:772–773.

Sidi, E. and Dobkevitch-Morrill, S. 1951. The injection and ingestion test in cross-sensitization to the para group. *J. Invest. Dermatol.* 16:299–310.

Sidi, E. and Melki, G. R. 1954. Rapport entre dermatitis de cause externe et sensibilisation par voi interne. *Sem. Hop. Paris* 30:1560–1565.

Smeenk, G. and Teunissen, P. C. 1977. Allergische reacties op nikkel uit infusie-toedieningssystemen. *Ned. Tijdschr. Geneeskd.* 121:4–9.

Spruit, D. 1979. Increased nickel absorption following indomethacin therapy. *Contact Dermatitis* 5:62.

Spruit, D., Bongaarts, P. J. M., and de Yongh, G. F. 1978. Dithiocarbamate therapy for nickel dermatitis. *Contact Dermatitis* 4:350–358.

Stoddart, J. C. 1960. Nickel sensitivity as a cause of infusion reactions. *Lancet* ii:741–742.

Sulzberger, M. B., Kanof, A., Baer, R. L., and Lowenberg, C. 1947. Sensitization by topical application of sulphonamides. *J. Allergy* 18:92–103.

Sunderman, F. W. 1979. Efficacy of sodium diethyldithiocarbamate (dithiocarb) in acute nickel carbonyl poisoning. *Ann. Clin. Lab. Sci.* 9:1–10.

Underwood, E. J. 1977. *Trace Elements in Human and Animal Nutrition.* New York: Academic.

Veien, N. K. and Kaaber, K. 1979. Nickel, cobalt and chromium sensitivity in patients with pompholyx (dyshidrotic eczema). *Contact Dermatitis* 5:371–374.

Veien, N. K., Christiansen, A. H., Svejgaard, E., and Kaaber, K. 1979a. Antibodies against nickel-albumin in rabbits and man. *Contact Dermatitis* 5:378–382.

Veien, N. K., Svejgaard, E., and Menné, T. 1979b. *In vitro* lymphocyte transformation to nickel: A study of nickel-sensitive patients before and after epicutaneous and oral challenge with nickel. *Acta Derma.-Venereol.* 59:447–451.

Veien, N., Hattel, T., Justesen, O., and Nørholm, A. 1981. Oral challenge with nickel, cobalt, and chromate of patients with eczema. Presented at the joint meeting of the Dowling Club and the Danish Dermatological Society.

Vickers, H. R., Bagratuni, L., and Alexander, S. 1958. Dermatitis caused by penicillin in milk. *Lancet* i:351–352.

Wilson, H. T. H. 1958. Streptomycin dermatitis in nurses. *Br. Med. J.* i:1378–1382.

de Yongh, G. F., Spruit, D., Bongaarts, P. J. M., and Duller, P. 1978. Factors influencing nickel dermatitis. I. *Contact Dermatitis* 4:142–148.

25

drug- and chemical-induced hair loss

John R. T. Reeves ▪ Howard I. Maibach

INTRODUCTION

Increased shedding of hair (effluvium) and noticeable hair thinning or baldness (alopecia) are increasingly cited as side effects of drug therapy. In this report we review the drugs implicated, discuss the mechanisms that may be responsible, describe criteria for defining the mechanism, and propose animal and human assay models.

MECHANISM OF HAIR PRODUCTION

As cells of living skin approach the exterior surface they undergo a complicated maturation and degenerative process (keratinization) resulting in the formation of a tough, fibrous, impermeable substance, keratin. Similarly, living cells of the hair root, or follicle, sacrifice themselves to become part of the keratinous hair shaft. As more cells are added to the deep end of the shaft it is lengthened and forced farther above the skin surface by the cell proliferation forces behind it. In concert, the hair follicles of one individual produce each day approximately 100 ft of hair, composed largely of protein (Pillsbury et al., 1956). The intense metabolic activity of the hair matrix cells responsible for this feat is unmatched in the body, except perhaps by the bone marrow or gastrointestinal tract (Rook et al., 1968; Van Scott, 1964).

This process of rapid cell proliferation and hair production does not occur continuously during the life of the follicle, but rather is subject to fairly orderly cycles of growth and regression. Biologically active materials may exert toxic effects in various ways during these cycles to result in an increase of hair loss. It is necessary to examine the cycles of hair production more closely to understand these effects.

HAIR CYCLE

Every hair follicle on the human body, whether present on the scalp, brow, or trunk, moves through three phases (Kligman, 1959).

Anagen

Anagen is the phase during which a mature hair is being produced. On the scalp and beard areas this phase lasts 2-6 yr, but it may last much longer in certain individuals. With hair growth occurring at a rate of approximately 0.35 mm/day (or $\frac{1}{2}$ in./month) this means that human scalp hair attains a length of 12-36 in. before being shed. Those persons—mainly women—enjoying a 6 yr anagen will have untrimmed hair reaching the buttock—in the manner portrayed in the rendition of Lady Godiva. On the brow, trunk, or elsewhere the growth period does not exceed 6 months, resulting in a uniform untrimmed hair length of a few inches or less.

Catagen

Anagen is followed by a brief involutional phase called catagen. Here the follicular cells cease division and the hair root shrivels to a small group of cells ascending toward the surface, pushing the inert hair shaft ahead of it.

Telogen

The resting telogen phase now occurs with the hair shaft and attached bulb of cells lying loosely in the dormant follicle. Mild trauma, such as brushing or shampooing, dislodges these "club hairs" with their terminal white bulb. The duration of catagen and telogen is unknown but is not longer than a few months. It is followed by the redevelopment of an anagen follicle below the telogen one, which dislodges the club hair if it still remains.

In humans these cycles occur in a relatively random fashion in the follicles at various sites of the body. In certain animals (e.g., the mouse or rabbit) the hair cycle is largely synchronized, with regional waves of growth and loss leading to readily discernible areas of hair loss. Other animals are more mosaic (like humans) in their cycles. It is likely that patterns of cycling occur in humans; the anterior hair line is one probable candidate. Identifying these minor areas of synchrony in humans has been difficult.

In the scalp about 85-95% of the follicles are in anagen at any given time, while 5-15% are in the telogen phase of shedding. On the average, 40-100 hairs are lost from the scalp each day. In the eyebrow, in contrast, anagen lasts only 10 wk, while telogen persists for 9 months, so that a greater percentage of eyebrow hairs are in telogen rather than anagen. Areas with a higher percentage of anagen follicles, such as scalp or beard, will be more susceptible to agents affecting rapidly dividing cells, and the higher telogen areas will be relatively resistant. This accounts for the scalp-beard pattern of hair loss seen, for example, with cytotoxic agents.

NON–CHEMICAL–RELATED HAIR LOSS

Few endogenous events affecting hair growth are delineated. Extreme starvation or protein deprivation may result in the formation of sparse and brittle hair, through diminished mitotic activity of the hair bulb (Goette and Odom, 1975). An unusually large percentage of hair follicles may be thrown into an untimely telogen phase by a major systemic insult such as high fever, major surgery, illness, or trauma. Telogen may also be precipitated by sudden hormonal fluctuations, such as those following childbirth. The shedding resulting from this telogen synchronization (or "telogen effluvium") occurs about 3 months after the insult, reflecting the time required for the full telogen state to be reached. This statement represents a generalization only. All hairs in telogen effluvium rarely synchronize. They gradually increase in loss frequency, reaching a crescendo, and then gradually decrease to a normal level. The patient notices the loss at varying times up to its peak.

ANAGEN VERSUS TELOGEN HAIR LOSS

Chemicals or medications may cause excessive hair shedding by precipitating telogen development, may directly poison the anagen root, or may work in other, undetermined ways.

IDENTIFICATION OF ANAGEN AND TELOGEN

The phase of hair loss may be determined by examining the shed or easily plucked (abnormally loose) hairs. The anagen hair will have at its proximal end an elongated translucent sheath (representing layers of the living follicle), with a pigmented tip, unless the hair is very light in color (Fig. 1). Generally, when in anagen hair loss, the majority of hairs have so severe a mitotic inhibition that the hair shaft breaks, leaving the bulb in the scalp. These broken hairs are almost always tapered, revealing a diagnostic artifact of anagen effluvium (Maibach and Maguire, 1964). The only condition mimicking this is the acutely spreading phase of generalized alopecia areata (alopecia totalis).

The club hair of a telogen follicle possesses on its proximal end the familiar nonpigmented spherical bulb (Fig. 2). Biopsy of the hair-bearing skin may be helpful in verifying the relative frequency of telogen versus anagen follicles, or with severe toxicity may show actual necrosis of the follicle.

PLUCKING: GENTLE PULL TEST VERSUS PLUCK TEST

The above description refers to the appearance of shed hair or that about to be shed. The sample is obtained from the comb, pillow, clothing, or shampoo, or by gently pulling at several areas of the scalp (without a forceps)

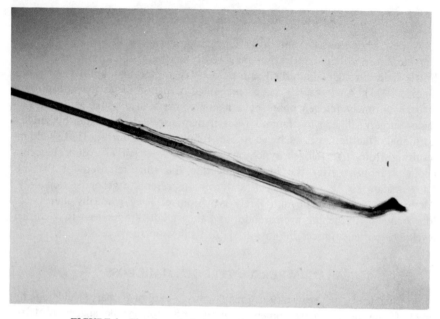

FIGURE 1 The elongated pigmented anagen root sheath (×13).

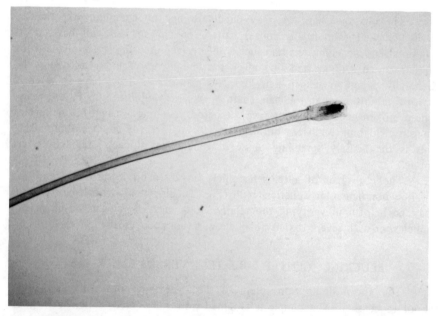

FIGURE 2 The familiar nonpigmented spherical telogen root sheath (×13).

(Fig. 3). With minimal clinical experience and knowledge of when the hair was last shampooed, the frequency and extent of combing and brushing, and in general the number of hairs in the scalp, it is possible to make a shrewd assessment of whether an abnormal amount of hair is shed. This examination, lasting but a minute or two and requiring only a good light source and several powers of magnification, is all that is required in most instances.

An alternate method of demonstrating the anagen-telogen ratio is more direct but unfortunately more cumbersome, time- and equipment-consuming, and hence less frequently performed (Van Scott, 1964). Here one takes a rubber-tipped forceps, grasping 30–100 hairs (near the scalp) in its grip (Fig. 4). A rapid, forceful pluck yields all hairs—anagen and telogen. Placing these in a petri dish with a thin layer of water for viewing with a binocular dissecting microscope at low magnification permits accurate enumeration of the number of anagen, catagen (uncommon), and telogen hairs. Cutting of the extraneous hair on the other side of the grasping forceps simplifies manipulation of the bulbs in the dish. Any hair whose shaft is broken is considered as anagen—with its bulb being too securely fixed in the scalp to remove it. If the hair is not jerked quickly, but extended gradually instead, discomfort is increased and bulb artifacts produced (Maguire and Kligman, 1964).

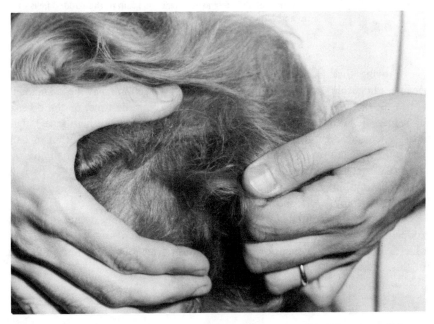

FIGURE 3 The pull test: the investigator gently pulls on locks of hair from several sites on the scalp.

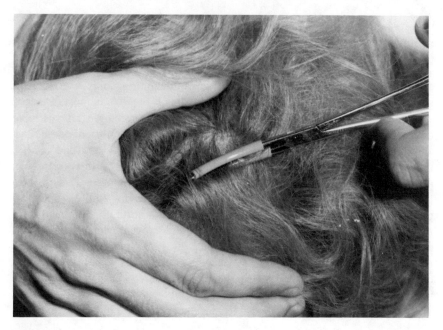

FIGURE 4 The pluck test: a lock of hair is grasped near the scalp in the padded jaws of a clamp and removed by a rapid foreceful pluck.

DIAGNOSTIC CRITERIA

Proving that alopecia in an individual is caused by a drug is difficult because idiopathic hair shedding, which is very common, may be coincident with drug therapy, other drugs may be in use at the same time, or the disease for which the drug is being given may produce hair loss (e.g., high fever). The most conclusive demonstration of drug-related hair loss is reproduction of hair loss with repeated administration of the drug. Some drugs cause hair loss so uniformly that even a small series with few patients will convince the observer of the relationship. Less convincing are isolated cases "proved" by regrowth of hair when therapy is discontinued.

Medications reputed to cause hair shedding will be discussed below, grouped, as well as possible, by probable mechanism of action on the hair follicle. The last group mentioned will be those drugs only tenuously culpable for this side effect.

ANAGEN-TYPE HAIR LOSS

This refers to hair loss within days to weeks of drug administration, which is due to inhibition of follicular mitoses and subsequent keratinization. Examination of a shed or pulled hair reveals a tapered broken shaft, or an anagen sheath (which is much less common).

Antimitotic Agents

Hair loss occurs following the use of cancer chemotherapeutic agents of all types: alkylating agents, alkaloids, and antimetabolites. Colchicine, an antimitotic used in the treatment of gout, has similar effects. Shedding of hair begins after only 1-2 wk of therapy, but as it occurs gradually it may be several weeks longer before thinning of the hair is noticed by the patient (Falkson and Shulz, 1964). Hair growth resumes 2 months after therapy has stopped. The loss affects the anagen but not telogen hairs; thus eyebrow and body hair is relatively spared.

The effect of these drugs on the rapidly dividing hair matrix cells is directly toxic, leading to hair loss in two ways (Crounse and Van Scott, 1960). If the matrix itself suffers a severe and/or prolonged insult, then much of the hair follicle is affected, so that hairs may be easily removed with the necrotic anagen sheath adhering to them. This is a true anagen effluvium.

If the insult is less severe, or of brief duration, then mitotic activity will only temporarily decrease, which will result in continued growth of the hair, but with a weak constricted area in the shaft. When this weak point grows above the surface of the skin it will break with minor trauma and appear to the observer as a type of hair shedding. This tapered hair is the hallmark of anagen effluvium (Maibach and Maguire, 1964).

Phenyl Glycidyl Ether (? Topical)

Lee et al. (1977) report alopecia in rats exposed to a vapor of phenyl glycidyl ether, a material used in industry to stabilize halogenated compounds. Oral administration of this agent causes profound systemic symptoms and death from central nervous system depression. Controlled exposure to various levels of vapor caused no systemic effects in rats and dogs, but there was hair loss in the rats, predominantly in females. The hair loss was due to damage to anagen follicles, which caused abnormal keratinization of the hair shaft, and to increased conversion to telogen follicles. Lee et al. postulate that the effect was from percutaneous and follicular absorption, not from inhalation.

Dixyrazine

Dixyrazine is a phenothiazine major tranquilizer produced in Belgium (Esucos UCB) and used primarily in Europe. Poulsen (1981) reports that four patients who took this drug developed a syndrome of blepharoconjunctivitis, ichthyosis, depigmentation of hair, and hair loss. The hair loss was of both the anagen and telogen types. In addition to its psychotropic qualities, dixyrazine interferes with cholesterol synthesis. It is of interest that the syndrome it induces is similar to that produced by the anticholesterol agent triparanol (see below), but that drug caused alopecia only of the telogen type.

MEDICATIONS PRECIPITATING TELOGEN

This refers to hair shedding that occurs 2–4 months after drug administration. The shed hairs bear telogen bulbs and are easily teased from the scalp. There is an increased conversion of anagen to telogen follicles.

Oral Contraceptives

Pregnancy increases the percentage of anagen hairs found in the scalp. When pregnancy is concluded there is an excess conversion of hair follicles to the telogen phase, resulting in hair loss 2–3 months later, indeed a common finding in the postpartum state. Hair loss occasionally follows cessation of oral contraceptive therapy by 2–3 months, and the loss is of the telogen type. Griffiths (1973) confirms this finding, but points out that previous studies have shown that hair cycle changes similar to those found in pregnancy are not found during oral contraceptive use, so the mechanism of telogen induction is unknown.

Griffiths also considers the reports that hair loss may be increased during the time oral contraceptives are used. He studied women presenting to his clinic with hair loss and could find no statistical relationship to the usage of oral contraceptives.

Anticoagulants

Increased hair shedding has been induced by all forms of anticoagulants (Tudhope et al., 1958): heparin, heparinoids, dextran, and coumarins. The scalp is most commonly involved, although the brows, axillae, and suprapubic regions may be affected. Regardless of the drug involved, hair loss is of the telogen type, usually occurring more than 1 month after onset of therapy. Very small doses have induced hair loss, but severe alopecia (noticeable balding) is associated with higher doses (Tudhope et al., 1958).

Tudhope et al. (1958) point out that the toxic effects of dextran (alopecia, diarrhea, thrombocytopenia) mimic those of X-irradiation or antimetabolites, and that heparin is antimitotic. These actions might suggest a cytotoxic effect on the follicle, but anagen hair shedding has not yet been recorded.

Propranolol

Martin et al. (1973) convincingly related a telogen effluvium—involving hair of the scalp, trunk, and extremities—to the ingestion of propranolol, a beta-adrenergic blocker, in one patient. The telogen hair bulbs and portions of the shafts were found to be dysplastic when examined by polarized microscopy. The authors stated that three cases of alopecia were reported to the manufacturer during clinical trials of the drug. The latter cases were not documented in detail.

Martin et al. considered whether the telogen effluvium was secondary to the basic cardiac disease or was caused by the drug. They proceeded to settle the issue. Stopping the drug led to noticeable hair regrowth and cessation of increased hair loss. This still did not rule out the possibility that the previous loss was related to the patient's cardiac disease. The final step was cautious drug challenge (with the patient's informed consent)—leading to another wave of telogen loss.

Two more recent reports (Scribner, 1977; Hilder, 1979) also describe telogen effluvium 3 or 4 wk after starting propranolol, but rechallenge was not performed.

Triparanol

Winkelmann et al. (1963) noted hair loss in 5 of 19 patients receiving triparanol (MER-29), with shedding beginning 5 wk to 14 months after onset of therapy. It did not appear to be a dose-related phenomenon, and regrowth occurred with cessation of therapy. The hairs shed were of the telogen type. Triparanol, long ago withdrawn from the market because of cataract induction, interferes with cholesterol synthesis, but the mechanism by which it acts on the hair follicle is unknown.

Winkelmann et al. stated that another lipid-lowering drug, nicotinic acid, can induce a telogen effluvium, but the statement was not documented.

Thallium

This element (usually as the sulfate salt) was used for its depilatory effect for the treatment of ringworm of the scalp. It is currently not found in any medications, but is still available in the United States in rodent poisons, and accidental poisoning may occur from contaminated grains (Reed et al., 1963) and other foods (Steinberg, 1961).

Thallium interferes with the incorporation of cystine into the keratin molecule, and its toxic effect can be blocked by the administration of cystine (Schwartzman and Kirshbaum, 1962). In humans, hair loss begins 10 days after ingestion of thallium, and is complete in 1 month. Scalp hair is primarily affected, with sparing of the trunk, axillary, and brow hair. The hairs show an accumulation of air bubbles in the shaft, through which areas breakage occurs. The follicles themselves show on biopsy dyskeratosis, necrosis, parakeratosis, spongioform abscess formation, and increased number of telogen follicles.

The follicular changes are those of an incomplete telogen (A. M. Kligman, personal communication). The hairs are thrown into an imperfect catagen and become incomplete club hairs, and the follicular column retracts only slightly. Anagen begins in 3–4 wk. About 5–10% of the hairs show a temporary inhibition of growth, a constriction of the shaft.

Phenyl Glycidyl Ether

See above under Anagen. Hair loss is of the anagen and telogen types.

Dixyrazine

See above under Anagen. Hair loss is of the anagen and telogen types.

Selenium Disulfide (Topical)

Selenium disulfide is the active ingredient in several popular antidandruff shampoos. In the United States the 2.5% strength requires a prescription, and the 1% preparation is available over the counter. Wirth et al. (1980) induced significant telogen hair loss in guinea pigs by applying a 2.5% solution of selenium disulfide 6 times a day at 3-d intervals. The material was not washed off and exposure was very intense, so it is difficult to compare this exposure to use of the material by humans as a shampoo, but Wirth et al. mention "isolated observations of diffuse hair loss" after such use.

MEDICATIONS CAUSING HAIR LOSS OF UNKNOWN TYPE

In this category, hair loss has reliably been noted to occur, but the mechanisms either are unknown or have not been studied.

Antithyroid Drugs

When hypothyroidism occurs, either spontaneously or from overuse of antithyroid medications, the hair may become thin, dry, and brittle. It has also been reported, however, that hair thinning may occur during antithyroid therapy even though the patient remains euthyroid. This effect has been noted during therapy with iodine, thiouracil, and carbimazole (Papadopoulos and Harden, 1966). The mechanism of this effect is unknown, but the timing of the hair loss during carbimazole therapy suggests a telogen effluvium.

Clofibrate

This antihyperlipemic agent, now used extensively throughout the world, has been occasionally reported to cause hair loss (De Gennes et al., 1965). This medication interferes with cholesterol synthesis in the liver, but has other effects, as reflected by its ability to lower serum triglycerides. Hair loss occurs after several months of therapy and is reversible. The brochure that accompanies the drug states that dry, brittle hair has been noted in female patients taking the drug.

Boric Acid

A recent case report by Stein et al. (1973) documents increased hair shedding due to the ingestion of enormous quantities of boric acid-containing mouthwash. The mechanism of the hair loss is unknown but is presumed to be toxic, with hair growth resuming after cessation of borate ingestion. Stein et al. did not record whether this was an anagen or telogen effluvium. Toxic amounts of boric acid can be absorbed through the skin from topical applications of boric acid compresses or powder, and the American Academy of Pediatrics has recommended that all such applications in children be curtailed (Press, 1960). Hair loss has not been reported from such exposure. Stein et al. provide on request a list of more than 400 over-the-counter and prescription products containing boric acid (in 1972).

There is one report of hair loss due to occupational exposure to borax, or sodium borate (Tan, 1970). The mechanism of the hair loss was unknown, but was presumed toxic. Boron is in the same family as thallium in the periodic table.

Vitamin A

Diffuse alopecia is a commonly noted side effect in hypervitaminosis A, and is presumably due to interference with keratinization (Flesch, 1963), although again the exact mechanism is unknown. In contrast to the effect of more toxic agents, the hair loss occurs only after several months of continuous ingestion of excessive amounts of vitamin A. The commonest causes of hypervitaminosis A are excessive ingestion of foods high in the substance (cod liver oil, polar bear liver) or vitamin A therapy for various diseases (acne, Darier's disease, pityriasis rubra pilaris).

Thiamphenicol

This antibiotic, related to chloramphenicol, exerts its effects on bacteria by inhibiting protein synthesis. Moeschlin et al. (1974) observed ten cases of alopecia (two to complete baldness) in 155 patients receiving this drug, which they assumed was due to inhibition of protein synthesis by follicular cells. In the *Year book of dermatology* (Malikinson and Pearson, 1975), however, the editors point out that mitosis is also inhibited when protein synthesis is blocked, which might contribute to the overall suppression of hair growth. Thus, the mechanism of hair shedding is not clear-cut. Simple observation of the shed hair (telogen versus broken tapered hairs) will settle this issue.

This medication is unavailable in the United States.

Valproic Acid

Valproic acid is a new anticonvulsant drug that is not chemically related to earlier ones. Partial and transient hair loss has been reported (Browne, 1980) during therapy with valproic acid, but its incidence and mechanism have not been studied and many of the patients were taking other drugs as well.

Bromocriptine

Bromocriptine is an ergot derivative used in the treatment of hyperpro-lactinemia, acromegaly, and Parkinson's disease. Blum and Leiba (1980) administered the drug to 14 women and 10 men. All the women complained of hair loss, the severity of which varied with the dose of bromocriptine used. The effect was not quantitated nor was the mechanism examined, but the authors suggested a relation to the drug's vasoconstrictive properties. There has been a report of alopecia due to the vasoconstrictor methysergide (see below).

MEDICATIONS POSSIBLY ASSOCIATED WITH HAIR LOSS

Trimethadione

There is one report (Holowach and Sanden, 1960) of two patients who noticed diffuse hair loss while taking trimethadione, with subsequent regrowth after cessation of therapy. No mechanism is suggested.

Amphetamines

Amphetamines in the form of weight-reducing pills have been reported to cause hair loss (Eckert et al., 1967), but other causes were not excluded, and no mechanism was postulated.

L-Dopa

Two female patients with Parkinson's disease developed diffuse alopecia 6 and 12 wk after starting levodopa therapy (Marshall and Williams, 1971). No mention was made of concomitant seborrheic dermatitis, which may be very severe in Parkinsonians, nor were the shed hairs studied. Alopecia persisted for several months while therapy was continued.

Allopurinol

Severe rashes or erythroderma are major side effects of this drug, and hair shedding may occur with such marked cutaneous inflammation. The one report in the literature imputing hair shedding in noninflamed skin to allopurinol is far from convincing (Auerbach and Orentreich, 1968).

Methysergide

This antimigraine medication has been implicated in one case of hair shedding (Sadjadpour, 1974), but other causes were not excluded. The package insert for Sansert mentions alopecia as a rare side effect.

Gentamycin

The one patient presented in the literature in whom Gentamycin-induced hair shedding is suggested had many other probable causes of that finding (Yoshioka and Matsuda, 1970). The shed hairs and scalp were not examined.

Salicylates

While studying patients with idiopathic hair loss, Rawnsley and Shelly (1968) found urinary evidence of salicylate ingestion. Further investigations found salicylate products in 9 of 12 patients with hair loss, compared to 3 of 21 controls. The hair loss, they postulated, could be a result of the disease for which the salicylate was being taken, or of the anemia frequently seen with salicylate ingestion (from intestinal blood loss), or could be a possible toxic effect of salicylate itself on the hair follicle. These findings have not been studied further.

Lithium Carbonate

In two studies (Zall et al., 1968; Vacaflor et al., 1970) in which a total of 120 patients were given lithium for mental disorders, thinning of hair was mentioned as a side effect in two patients. No studies were performed on the hair or scalp.

Ibuprofen

Meyer (1979) reported increased shedding of hair in 15 of 21 arthritis patients who were being treated with the nonsteroidal anti-inflammatory drug ibuprofen. Hair growth returned to normal when the patients were switched to other anti-inflammatory drugs. Hair counts and other quantitative tests were not mentioned.

Cimetidine

Shmad (1979) reported one patient who had profuse effluvium when she was given cimetidine on two separate occasions. Since both episodes occurred after worsening of duodenal ulcer symptoms, for which the H_2 antihistamine was being given, the effluvia could have been secondary to systemic illness.

Pyridostigmine Bromide

Pyridostigmine bromide is an oral cholinesterase inhibitor used to treat myasthenia gravis. Field (1980) reported one patient who had profuse effluvium on the two occasions when she was given the drug.

Gold

Rosenbaum and Rosenbaum (1979) state that "partial or complete hair loss" occurs rarely in patients being treated with gold. The cases were not described, and it is known that alopecia may occur in rheumatoid diseases, for which gold is used.

ANIMAL MODELS

The past history of toxicology adequately warns us that once we know the existence of a potential hazard from an animal model, we are more likely to identify that phenomenon in human trials. We know of no pharmaceutical or toxicological laboratory presently including a systematic examination of hair growth and loss in its profile in drug preclinical evaluation. We believe that it is time that such an evaluation be considered. It is not unreasonable to suspect that once this is initiated, we will identify other drugs and chemicals producing hair loss. Anagen effluvium is dramatic and not as likely to be missed by the patient or physician; telogen effluvium is far from obvious. The several boron toxicity patients (Stein et al., 1973; J. Herndon, personal communication) with severe hair loss resulting in a marked alopecia did not have a sign on their scalp identifying the chemical or its source for the patient. It took the investigators' shrewd detective work to make the association. When we have a list of chemicals and drugs (and approximate potencies) productive of hair loss (and mechanism), we will know where and when to look in humans. Will each study show that a significant portion of "typical" male pattern hair loss or diffuse alopecia of women is, in fact, secondary to drug or other chemical dosing?

Animal Choice

This is moot at present. An inexpensive, conveniently handled animal would be valuable for screening, with less convenient animals such as the monkey reserved for special studies. An animal that is a mosaic, similar to humans, may be more realistic for humans than an animal (like the mouse) having synchronous waves. At present the guinea pig would appear suitable in terms of cost, handling, and similarity to humans. The experimental design should include control (vehicle)-treated animals since many factors, including season, nutrition, intercurrent disease, etc., may influence hair growth dynamics in animals. If the animals become otherwise toxic, the usual maneuvers used in toxicology must be employed to ascertain whether this is a drug effect or secondary to the animals' general status. Dose response studies, temporal relationships, and toxicity controls will be helpful in this regard.

Observations

Gross hair observations include the presence or absence of spotty or diffuse alopecia, and excessive shedding noted in the cage. Only potent agents might be expected to produce a loss significant for observation in this gross observation.

Pull tests and pluck tests should reveal more subtle changes. This will require careful record-keeping and sampling. If no one in the laboratory is experienced in observations of the anagen, catagen, and telogen, they can be rapidly trained to perform the pull test and pluck test—placing the samples in envelopes for forwarding to a laboratory experienced in hair bulb morphology. It is preferable that the hair be forwarded in coded fashion; control animals must be included.

HUMAN MODELS

The mensuration of hair growth and loss has been studied. The reader is referred to a review for details (Maibach, 1974). The same principles used in the animal model are appropriate to humans. Any chemical or drug producing hair loss in the animal must not be excluded from consideration for human use without careful examination of the data. It is possible that drugs producing hair loss in animals will not do so in humans—at the dose levels used by the latter.

REFERENCES

Auerbach, R. and Orentreich, N. 1968. Alopecia and ichthyosis secondary to allopurinol. *Arch. Dermatol.* 98:104.

Blum, I. and Leiba, S. 1980. Increased hair loss as a side effect of bromocriptine treatment. *N. Engl. J. Med.* 303:1418.

Browne, T. R. 1980. Valproic acid. *N. Engl. J. Med.* 302:661.

Crounse, R. G. and Van Scott, E. J. 1960. Changes in scalp hair roots as a measure of toxicity from cancer chemotherapeutic drugs. *J. Invest. Dermatol.* 35:83.

De Gennes, J. L., Maunand, B., Salmon, L. P. and Truffert, J. 1965. Résultats du traitement par l'atromide on CPIB avec on sans androstérone dans les hyperlipidemies (110 essais thérapeutiques sur deux ans). *Bull. Mem. Soc. Med. Hop. Paris* II:759.

Eckert, J., Church, R. E., Ebling, F. J. and Munro, D. S. 1967. Hair loss in women. *Br. J. Dermatol.* 79:543.

Falkson, G. and Schulz, E. J. 1964. Skin changes caused by cancer chemotherapy. *Br. J. Dermatol.* 76:309.

Field, L. M. 1980. Toxic alopecia caused by pyridostigmine bromine. *Arch. Dermatol.* 116:1103.

Flesch, P. 1963. Inhibition of keratinizing structures by systemic drugs. *Pharmacol. Rev.* 15:653.

Goette, D. K. and Odom, R. B. 1975. Profuse hair loss. *Arch. Dermatol.* 111:930.

Griffiths, W. A. D. 1973. Diffuse hair loss and oral contraceptives. *Br. J. Dermatol.* 88:31.

Hilder, R. J. 1979. Propranolol and alopecia. *Cutis* 24:63.

Holowach, J. and Sanden, H. V. 1960. Alopecia as a side effect of treatment of epilepsy with trimethadione. *N. Engl. J. Med.* 263:1187.

Kligman, A. M. 1959. The human hair cycle. *J. Invest. Dermatol.* 33:307.

Lee, K. P., Terrill, J. B. and Henry, N. W. 1977. Alopecia induced by inhalation exposure to phenyl glycidyl ether. *J. Toxicol. Environ. Health* 3:859.

Maguire, H. C. and Kligman, A. M. 1964. Hair plucking as a diagnostic tool. *J. Invest. Dermatol.* 43:77.

Maibach, H. I. 1974. In *The first human hair symposium*, ed. A. C. Brown, p. 399. New York: Med Com Press.

Maibach, H. I. and Maguire, H. C. 1964. Acute hair loss from drug-induced abortion. *N. Engl. J. Med.* 270:1112.

Malikinson, F. D. and Pearson, R. W. eds. 1975. *The year book of dermatology, 1975*, p. 116. Chicago: Year Book Medical Publishers.

Marshall, A. and Williams, M. J. 1971. Alopecia and levodopa. *Br. Med. J.* 2:47.

Martin, C. M., Southwick, E. G. and Maibach, H. I. 1973. Propranolol induced alopecia. *Am. Heart J.* 86:236.

Meyer, H. C. 1979. Alopecia associated with ibuprofen. *J. Am. Med. Assoc.* 242:142.

Moeschlin, S., Novotny, Z., Koller, E. and Reufli, P. 1974. Cystostatic side effects of thiamphenicol: Alopecia and reversible cytopenia. *Schweiz. Med. Wochenschr.* 104:384.

Papadopoulos, S. and Harden, R. Mc. G. 1966. Hair loss in patients treated with carbimazole. *Br. Med. J.* 2:1502.

Pillsbury, D. M., Shelly, W. S. and Kligman, A. M., eds. 1956. Hair. In *Dermatology*, p. 45. Philadelphia: Saunders.

Poulsen, J. 1981. Hair loss, depigmentation of hair, ichthyosis, and blepharoconjunctivitis produced by dixyrazine. *Acta Derm.-Venereol. (Stockh.)* 61:85.

Press, E., chairman. 1960. Report of Subcommittee on Accidental Poisoning— Statement on hazards of boric acid. *Pediatrics* 26:884.

Rawnsley, H. M. and Shelly, W. B. 1968. Salicylate ingestion and idiopathic hair loss. *Lancet* I:567.

Reed, D., Crawley, J., Faro, S. N., Pieper, S. J. and Kurland, L. T. 1963. Thallotoxicosis, acute manifestations and sequelae. *J. Am. Med. Assoc.* 183:516.

Rook, A., Wilkinson, D. S. and Ebling, F. J. G., eds. 1968. Hair. In *Textbook of dermatology*, p. 1355. Philadelphia: Davis.

Rosenbaum, E. E. and Rosenbaum, R. B. 1979. Chrysotherapy. *Arch. Intern. Med.* 139:1316.

Sadjadpour, K. 1974. Methysergide alopecia. *J. Am. Med. Assoc.* 229:639.

Schwartzman, R. M. and Kirshbaum, J. O. 1962. The cutaneous histopathology of thallium poisoning. *J. Invest. Dermatol.* 39:169.

Scribner, M. D. 1977. Propranolol therapy. *Arch. Dermatol.* 113:1303.

Shmad, S. 1979. Cimetidine and alopecia. *Ann. Intern. Med.* 91:930.

Stein, K. M., Odom, R. B., Justice, G. R. and Martin, G. C. 1973. Toxic alopecia from ingestion of boric acid. *Arch. Dermatol.* 108:95.

Steinberg, H. J. 1961. Accidental thallium poisoning in adults. *South. Med. J.* 54:6.

Tan, T. G. 1970. Occupational toxic alopecia due to borax. *Acta Derm. Venereol. (Stockh.)* 50:55.

Tudhope, G. R., Cohen, H. and Meikle, R. W. 1958. Alopecia following treatment with dextran sulfate and other anticoagulant drugs. *Br. Med. J.* 1:1034.

Vacaflor, L., Lehmann, H. E. and Ban, T. A. 1970. Side effects and teratogenicity of lithium carbonate treatment. *J. Clin. Pharmacol.* 10:387.

Van Scott, E. J. 1964. Physiology of hair growth. *Clin. Obstet. Gynecol.* 7:1062.

Winkelmann, R. K., Perry, H. O., Achor, R. W. P. and Kirby, T. J. 1963. Cutaneous syndromes produced as side effects of triparanol therapy. *Arch. Dermatol.* 87:372.

Wirth, H., Dunsing, W. and Gloor, M. 1980. Telogenes effluvium nach anwendung von selendisulfid beim meerschweinshen. *Hautarzt* 31:502.

Yoshioka, H. and Matsuda, I. 1970. Loss of hair related to Gentamycin treatment. *J. Am. Med. Assoc.* 211:123.

Zall, H., Therman, P. G. and Myers, J. M. 1968. Lithium carbonate: A clinical study. *Am. J. Psychiatry* 125(4):141.

26

drug- and heavy metal-induced hyperpigmentation

Richard D. Granstein ▪ Arthur J. Sober

INTRODUCTION

Many therapeutic agents are associated with the induction of various types of hyperpigmentation. The dermatologist must be familiar with these situations in order to differentiate them from disorders of hyperpigmentation resulting from other etiologies. This review is organized by category of therapeutic agent. The mechanism of hyperpigmentation, nature of the pigment, and anatomic location are discussed, when known. Most agents producing primarily epidermal hyperpigmentation also produce some dermal deposition of pigment.

Dermal hyperpigmentation may result from several different mechanisms. A variety of drugs and pharmacologic agents can lead to deposition of pigment within the dermis. Some of these agents stimulate the formation of melanin. Others produce nonmelanin pigments, which may be either the agent itself or a metabolic product of the agent. Some drugs produce dermal pigmentation by both drug deposition and increased melanin deposition. Because of the Tyndall effect, blue-gray or blue-black pigmentation is observed clinically. In some instances, abnormal epidermal and dermal pigment may coexist. Fixed drug reactions that have dermal pigment (melanin) deposition are covered first.

Supported in part by the Marion Gardner Jackson Trust.

Presented in part at the International Conference on Dermatology and Cosmetic Science, October 8–9, 1980, Tokyo, Japan.

FIXED DRUG ERUPTION

Fixed drug eruptions produce clinically circumscribed lesions that recur at the same site with each challenge of the offending agent. Erythematous, eczematous, or occasionally even bullous eruptions are produced that resolve, leaving pigmented areas. Fixed drug eruptions are most commonly associated with phenolphthalein, barbiturates, and tetracycline, although numerous other drugs have been reported to be associated with these eruptions (Table 1). Histopathologic analysis reveals vacuolar alteration of the basal cell layer with subsequent pigmentary incontinence, resulting in the presence of large amounts of melanin within macrophages in the upper dermis (N. P. Sanchez and M. C. Mihm, personal communication).

Patch testing at the site of a fixed drug eruption with the responsible agent gives positive results in some cases, but negative results in others, notably with phenolphthalein (Stritzler and Kopf, 1960). This can be interpreted as indicating that phenolphthalein requires modification by passage through the gastrointestinal tract or liver before it becomes antigenic. Other agents may require no modification or may become complete antigens by passage through the skin epicutaneously. Transplantation experiments have been done to try to identify the anatomic site within the skin that is involved in the fixed drug eruption. Some of these studies have indicated that the site of sensitivity can be moved by transplantation of full-thickness skin. Other studies show that the skin of involved areas, when transplanted to normal areas, reacts initially but subsequently fails to react when challenged with the agent, while normal skin transplanted to the original site of the eruption becomes reactive. The first group of experiments suggests that the superficial tissues and vessels are the relevant site of reaction in a fixed drug eruption,

TABLE 1   Pharmacologic Agents Associated with Production
of Fixed Drug Eruptions[a]

Acetaminophen	Cinchophen	Phenacetin
Acetanilide	Dapsone	Phenolphthalein
Aminopyrine	Emetine	Phenylbutazone
Anovulatory agents	Gold salts	Quinacrine
Antimony salts	Iodides	Quinidine
Antipyrine	Isoaminile citrate	Quinine
Arsenicals	Meprobamate	Salicylates
Barbiturates	Mercury	Sulfonamides
Bismuth	Nystatin	Tetracycline
Bromides	Oxyphenbutazone	
Chlordiazepoxide	Oxytetracycline	
8-Chlorotheophylline	p-Aminosalicylic acid	
Chlortetracycline	Penicillin	

[a]Wintroub et al., 1979; Beerman and Kirshbaum, 1975; Baker, 1979; Pareek, 1980.

while the second group of experiments indicates that the site of reaction resides in deeper vessels and tissues.

Sanchez and Mihm (personal communication) present one hypothesis to account for the prominent postinflammatory pigmentation found at the site of a fixed drug eruption. They suggest that the drug may act as a hapten, using a melanocyte carrier protein. The melanocyte becomes the target of sensitized lymphocytes. Lymphokines released along the course of dendrites affecting adjacent keratinocytes may explain the clustering of damaged keratinocytes seen in fixed drug eruptions. Gimenez-Camarasa et al. (1975) showed that blast transformation of lymphocytes from patients with fixed drug eruptions occurred with the addition of autologous serum taken at the time of clinical reaction. Addition of the responsible drug increased the degree of blast transformation severalfold. Addition of the drug alone did not cause blast transformation. This serum blast transforming factor spontaneously diminishes or disappears a few days after clinical exacerbation.

HEAVY METALS

Heavy metals were commonly reported as a cause of drug-induced hyperpigmentation in the older literature. Recent reports on these agents are infrequent. Several of the agents used therapeutically can cause increases in dermal pigmentation (Table 2).

Mercury

Facial creams containing inorganic mercury compounds such as mercurous chloride, ammoniated mercury, and mercurous oxide were widely used as skin bleaches early in this century. Prolonged use of these topical preparations was found to cause a "slate-gray" pigmentation. This pigmentation is increased in skin folds. Generally the pigmentation is most pronounced on the eyelids, in the nasolabial folds, and in the folds of the neck (Lamar and Bliss, 1966). Percutaneous absorption of mercury is thought to occur exclusively via the skin appendages (Calvery et al., 1946).

Histopathology of these lesions reveals numerous coarse brown-black granules in the dermis. The Prussian blue reaction for iron is negative and melanin is excluded by decoloration of the pigment with 10% sodium sulfide (Lamar and Bliss, 1966). The granules are concentrated in the upper dermis, some appearing in macrophages, some located about capillaries, and some lying free in the dermis (Burge and Winkelmann, 1970). Increased melanin in the basal layer of the epidermis has also been reported. Dark-field microscopy shows the granules to be brilliantly refractile. Neutron activation analysis and histochemical techniques confirmed the presence of mercury in tissue from one patient (Burge and Winkelmann, 1970). Electron microscopy on that patient's tissue showed the granules to be small, electron-dense particles appearing to aggregate into larger coarse granules with diameters up to 340

TABLE 2 Heavy Metal Pigmentation

Agent	Color	Regions involved	Nature of pigment	Histopathologic site of deposition
Mercury	Slate-gray	Increased in skin folds (topical administration); gingival hyperpigmentation (systemic administration)	1. Mercury granules (brown-black) up to 340 nm; irregular granules; EM-14 nm particles in aggregates up to 340 nm	1. Upper dermis about capillaries; associated with elastic fibers or among collagen fibers; some within macrophages
			2. May have increased melanin	2. Basal layer of epidermis; dermal melanophages
Silver	Slate-gray	Increased in sun-exposed areas; sclera, nails, and mucous membranes may be involved; decreased in skin folds	1. Silver granules (brown-black) less than 1 μm in diameter; fairly uniform size; EM-13 to 1000 nm aggregates	1. Silver granules in membrana propria of sweat glands and in connective tissue sheaths about hair follicles and sebaceous glands; may be found in collagen just below basement membrane; predilection for elastic fibers
Bismuth	Blue-gray	Generalized skin; conjunctiva and oral mucosa; blue-black gingival line	Bismuth granules	Small granules in papillary and reticular dermis
Arsenic	Bronze	Most prominent on trunk	Arsenic; melanin	—
Gold	Blue-gray	Limited to sun-exposed areas; more pronounced about the eyes; skin folds less involved	Gold granules	Small round or oval black granules, irregular in size located around blood vessels and in dermal macrophages; granules larger than silver
Lead	"Lead hue" pallor and lividity	Generalized, gingival line	Lead	—

nm. The granules were frequently associated with elastic fibers, free among collagen fibers, and also were found within macrophages. The increased pigmentation probably results from a combination of the tattoo effect of the mercury granules and increased amounts of melanin in the epidermis and in dermal macrophages. No mercury granules are found in the epidermis, and the ultrastructure of melanocytes there is normal.

Systemic administration of mercury has been reported to result in gingival hyperpigmentation similar to that produced by lead and bismuth (Everett, 1979).

Silver (Argyria)

Ingestion of silver compounds or their application to mucous membranes as medicaments was once common. It is well recognized that these practices may result in slate-gray pigmentation of the skin. Although silver is not absorbed by the intact skin, it can be readily absorbed by the mucosal tissues as such or in an insoluble form as oxide, sulfide, or metallic silver (Mehta et al., 1941). Argyria in furnace men resulting from industrial exposure to molten silver has also been reported (Bleehen et al., 1981). The resulting hyperpigmentation is most prominent in sun-exposed areas of the skin, with relative sparing of skin folds. Sclerae, nails, and mucous membranes may become hyperpigmented. Pigmentation is usually noted months to years after ingestion.

Histologic findings in involved areas show silver granules on the membrana propia of the sweat glands, on the connective tissue membrane about sebaceous glands, and in relation to the basal lamina of the epidermis, hair follicles, and small blood vessels. These appear brilliantly refractile when examined with the dark-field microscope (Hill and Montgomery, 1941). Silver granules are also found free in the collagen just below the basement membrane. Elastic tissue stains reveal predilection of silver granules for elastic fibers. Scant deposits of silver may also be seen in the connective tissue of the liver and spleen, in the basement membrane surrounding renal glomerular capillaries and the glomerular capsule, and in the basement membrane around the seminiferous tubules (Prose, 1963). No deposits of silver are found in the epidermis. Electron microscopy reveals the silver deposits to be round or oval bodies 13-1000 nm in diameter (Prose, 1963). These are most numerous in relation to the basal lamina of the secretory coil of the eccrine sweat glands. The inner structure of most bodies can be resolved into aggregated granules 3-70 nm in diameter, occasionally dispersed into concentric rings (Prose, 1963). The granules are localized within the cytoplasm of fibroblasts (Mehta et al., 1941; Bleehen et al., 1981) inside lysosome-like bodies. X-ray micro-analysis has been performed on these granules and demonstrates the presence of silver in the cases of industrial exposure (Bleehen et al., 1981). In addition, the same granules contain sulfur and selenium (Bleehen et al., 1981). In occasional granules, variable amounts of mercury, titanium, and/or iron were found. Presumably, the patients were also exposed to the fumes of these metals. Melanocytic activity is stimulated by deposits of silver in the dermis. The increase in pigmentation in sun-exposed areas is difficult to explain. It has been suggested that there is increased deposition of silver granules in areas of solar elastosis, but this mechanism has been rejected as inadequate to explain the increase in pigmentation in sun-exposed areas in most patients (N. P. Sanchez and M. C. Mihm, personal communication).

Localized argyria from topical exposure to silver salts over long periods of time may also occur (Buckley, 1963). Histopathologic findings in one case showed pigment only at the dermoepidermal junction or in the papillary body directly adjacent to the epidermal portion of the sweat duct. Electron microprobe X-ray analysis demonstrated silver ion only at these sites, suggesting that silver enters the skin through the sweat ducts.

Bismuth

Bismuth compounds were once used parenterally in the treatment of venereal diseases. Rarely, generalized blue-gray pigmentation resembling argyria occurs from systemic bismuth use. The conjunctivae and oral mucosa may also become pigmented, and a distinctive blue-black line may occur at the gingival margin. Histology of involved skin shows small metallic granules in the papillary and reticular layers of the dermis (Lueth et al., 1936). One author stated that the prominent oral coloration is secondary to hydrogen sulfide, formed from the action of bacteria on organic matter in the mouth reacting with the bismuth compound to produce deposition of a blue-black granular substance within the subjacent connective tissues and capillary endothelial cells (Dummett, 1964).

Arsenic

Pentavalent organic and trivalent inorganic salts of arsenic were used systemically for many conditions in the past, including psoriasis, and also as a general health "tonic." Water supplies may be contaminated with arsenic, and occupational exposures may occur. Prolonged ingestion of inorganic arsenic may result in a diffuse macular bronze pigmentation, most prominent on the trunk, where it may produce the "raindrop" appearance from small areas of normal or depigmented skin within the larger areas of hyperpigmentation (Levantine and Almeyda, 1973). These findings occur 1–20 yr after exposure. There is nearly always concomitant hyperkeratosis of the palms and soles. The color is partly due to the metal itself and partly to increased melanin synthesis (Levantine and Almeyda, 1973).

Gold

Chrysiasis is a rare, permanent cutaneous hyperpigmentation, similar to argyria, that occurs after exposure of the skin to ultraviolet light in patients who are receiving parenteral gold therapy. Clinically, the pigmentation differs from that of argyria in that gold-induced pigment is more pronounced about the eyes and is limited to exposed areas. Skin folds are less involved. An inflammatory dermatitis may or may not precede pigmentation. The hyperpigmentation occurs months to years after exposure.

Microscopic examination reveals small round or oval black granules, irregular in size, located around blood vessels and in dermal macrophages (Everett, 1979). Distribution may be similar to that of silver (Caseos, 1936). On dark-field examination, the granules of gold are larger and more irregular than those of silver (Birmingham, 1979). The color is mainly due to the metal itself (Levantine and Almeyda, 1973).

Lead

Chronic lead poisoning can produce the so-called lead hue. This is a mixture of pallor and lividity of the skin. In addition, a lead line at the gingival margin may mimic that associated with bismuth. This is due to a subepithelial deposit of lead granules, which is converted to lead sulfide (Birmingham, 1979).

Iron Salts

At one time, the application of solutions of iron salts was used in the treatment of *Rhus* poisoning. A number of cases of permanent dark brown discoloration at the sites of application were subsequently reported. This phenomenon occurred only in areas where skin had been eroded. Histologic examination revealed pigment deposition around blood vessels and between the collagen fibers of the upper corium (Traub and Tennen, 1936). Perls' stain shows hemosiderin to be present. This pigmentation is most probably a tattoo.

ANTIMALARIAL DRUGS

The antimalarials, a group of acridines and 4-aminoquinolines used in the treatment of a variety of disorders, cause pigmentary changes in up to 25% of patients receiving them for periods of more than 3 or 4 mo (Levantine and Almeyda, 1973). The drugs most commonly cited are quinacrine, chloroquine, and hydroxychloroquine. Amodiaquine also may produce diffuse pigmentation, but less frequently. The color varies from a yellow-brown to gray and is accentuated in light-exposed areas (Campbell, 1960).

Tuffanelli et al. (1963) found that 25 of 300 patients receiving antimalarial drugs for a collagen vascular disease had localized deposition of pigment (Table 3). Eighteen patients had pretibial pigment, which was bilateral, patchy, irregular, and varied in color from gray to blue-black. Early lesions resembled ecchymoses (Levantine and Almeyda, 1973). Nine had palatal involvement with a sharp line demarcating the soft and hard palates. Four had diffuse facial pigmentation and four had subungual hyperpigmentation. Transverse bands of blue-black pigmentation may occur (Levantine and Almeyda, 1973) on the nails. The duration of antimalarial treatment prior to

TABLE 3   Clinical Findings in Patients with
Antimalarial Hyperpigmentation[a]

Observation	Frequency
Pretibial pigment, bilateral, patchy, irregular, gray to blue-black	18/300
Line between soft and hard palate	9/300
Diffuse facial pigmentation	4/300
Subungual pigmentation	4/300

[a]Tuffanelli et al., 1963.

the appearance of pigmentation varied from 4 to 70 mo. Seven patients received chloroquine only, one received quinacrine only, one hydroxychloroquine only, and the rest received two or more drugs. Cessation of therapy led to decreased intensity of pigmentation but no patient cleared completely.

Histologic examination reveals both intracellular and extracellular yellow to dark brown pigment granules in the dermis, primarily in the deeper layers (Table 4). Stains for melanin and hemosiderin demonstrate hemosiderin around capillaries and melanin in the deeper layers. Analysis of chloroquine levels in normal and pigmented skin showed increased lesional content in one of three patients tested. There is evidence that chloroquine binds to melanin (Sams and Epstein, 1965). Increased incidence of retinopathy in patients with the cutaneous hyperpigmentation is noted; 4 of 21 such patients had retinopathy (Tuffanelli et al., 1963). The same authors noted that only 5 of 300 other patients receiving antimalarials developed retinopathy.

Quinacrine also causes a well-known diffuse lemon-yellow coloration of the skin. This occurs in most patients who take the drug and fades in 1–4 mo after the drug is discontinued. The pigmentation is felt to be secondary to direct staining of the tissues by the medication (Lutterloh and Shallenberger, 1946). Staining of the sclerae is slight or absent, distinguishing the coloration of quinacrine from that of jaundice.

PHENOTHIAZINES

Phenothiazine drugs given chronically can, on occasion, produce hyper-pigmentation of the skin, particularly in sun-exposed areas. Chlorpromazine is the most commonly associated drug. Patients affected have taken high doses of the drug for long periods of time. Women are most frequently affected (Greiner and Berry, 1964; Satanove, 1965). Pigmentation occurs only on sun-exposed areas and varies in color from a diffuse violet to a deep purple-gray metallic color. The sun exposure requirement is highlighted by the frequent sparing of facial wrinkles and the cleft below the lower lip. Areas most commonly involved include the forehead, cheeks, nose, dorsal aspect of the hands and upper extremities, and exposed parts of the lower extremities.

Nail beds are involved in several cases (Satanove, 1965). The pigmentation is cumulative, fading only slightly in winter. The color is originally tan, becomes slate-gray with further sun exposure, and eventually becomes purple. Ocular manifestations have been noted only in patients with hyperpigmentation of the skin. Ocular findings include hazy brown discolorations of exposed sclera and cornea, and dark brown central lens opacities. Slit lamp examination in two cases showed the corneal lesion to consist of stromal yellow-white granules located mainly in the posterior half of the cornea. The lens opacity consists of discrete yellow-white dots concentrated centrally in the anterior subcapsular pole.

Light microscopic examination reveals pigment present in macrophages throughout the dermis, particularly around capillaries in the superficial layers.

TABLE 4 Nature of Pigment and Histopathologic Findings

Agent	Pigment	Histopathology
Antimalarials	Yellow to dark brown pigment granules	Granules located intra- and extracellularly throughout dermis but especially in deep dermis; hemosiderin around capillaries; melanin in deep dermis
Phenothiazines	Granules have staining properties of melanin; chlorpromazine metabolite and/or chlorpromazine-melanin polymer	Pigment in dermal macrophages, especially around capillaries in the superficial dermis; EM—many melanosome complexes within lysosomes of dermal macrophage; electron-dense round or irregularly shaped bodies 0.2–3 nm in diameter in macrophages, endothelial cells, pericytes, Schwann cells, and fibroblasts (presumed to be melanin-chlorpromazine complexes)
ACTH	Melanin	Synthesis and transfer of melanin from basilar melanocytes to epidermal keratinocytes
Amiodarone	? Lipofuscin	Histiocytes, often around capillaries, containing aggregates of finely granular yellow-brown pigment
Clofazimine: Early, red Late, black-brown	Drug itself ? Ceroid-like pigment	Present in fat and reticuloendothelial cells Present in macrophages of dermis and subcutaneous tissue, rimming fat globules within cytoplasm of macrophage
Oral contraceptives	Melanin	Epidermal ± dermal
Psoralens	Melanin	Synthesis and transfer of melanin from basilar melanocytes to epidermal keratinocytes

Stains for hemosiderin are negative; the pigment has the staining properties of melanin (Table 4) (Satanove, 1965).

Electron microscopic studies (Hashimoto et al., 1966) show increased numbers of melanin granules in all layers of the epidermis. In the basal cell layer and lower stratum spinosum, membrane-bound melanin granules, either intact or partially disintegrated, are noted. Also, within the membrane-bound granules numerous fine electron-dense particles are noted. The upper and middle dermis contain aggregations of large macrophages, mainly in a perivascular location. These cells contain in their lysosomes intact and/or fragmented melanin granules, electron-dense particles as noted, and round to oval bodies of various electron densities measuring up to 3 μm in diameter. Endothelial cells show numerous pinocytotic vesicles along the vascular lumen and also contain bodies of various sizes and electron densities. No dopa-positive cells were present in the dermis (Hashimoto et al., 1966).

Satanove (1965), using the skin window technique, demonstrated transport of pigment in inflammatory cells from dermis of sun-exposed skin to the bloodstream. Blue-green granules were noted in the cytoplasm of polymorphonuclear leukocytes and mononuclear cells. These granules stain black with Fontana stain and are dopa-positive with dopa stains. Buffy coat studies revealed the presence of a few circulating blood cells containing these granules. Transport via the bloodstream was postulated to account for the generalized melanosis.

Brown pigment can be demonstrated in cells of the reticuloendothelial system and in parenchymal cells of the liver, myocardium, kidney, lung, and brain of patients treated with chlorpromazine (Van Woert, 1968). Van Woert (1968) was able to extract two brown pigments from the liver of a patient treated with chlorpromazine. These pigments were not found in liver tissue from a patient who did not receive phenothiazines. The pigments were thought to be chlorpromazine polymers produced by the action of ultraviolet radiation on chlorpromazine. Electron paramagnetic resonance (EPR) spectroscopy showed that both naturally occurring and synthetic chlorpromazine pigments are stable free radicals. These findings suggest that chlorpromazine polymers may account in part for the pigmentary abnormalities found with phenothiazine use and would account for the prominence in sun-exposed areas. The electron-dense bodies seen in the endothelial cells and dermal macrophages may represent a chlorpromazine metabolite (Hashimoto et al., 1966). Chlorpromazine has also been found to bind *in vivo* to melanin (Blois, 1965). White light without an ultraviolet component is also capable of producing free radicals from chlorpromazine. A major portion of the drug appears to be bound reversibly to melanin, although a small portion may be permanently incorporated. The chlorpromazine-melanin complexes are not metabolized by the body (Lever and Schaumburg-Lever, 1975).

One report attributes to imipramine pigmentation similar to that seen with chlorpromazine. The patient's history of medication is not clear, and he had taken chlorpromazine for a short time 10 yr earlier (Hare, 1970).

TETRACYCLINES

Tetracycline Hydrochloride

Since the introduction of tetracycline therapy for acne, reports of bluish pigmentation of cutaneous osteomas occurring in previously inflamed skin have appeared (Basler et al., 1974) (Table 5). Other reports mention antibiotics without specifying type (Jewell, 1971; Gropen, 1977). Osteoma cutis is an uncommon complication of acne vulgaris which is thought to result from deposition of calcium in areas of acne-damaged skin (Walter and Macknet, 1979). In one patient "blue dots" appeared on the face after 4 yr of intermittent tetracycline use (Walter and Macknet, 1979). Examination of the osteoma from this patient with 365-nm light demonstrated yellow fluorescence consistent with tetracycline deposition. No additional pigmented lesions appeared after the tetracycline was discontinued.

Methacycline (Rondomycin)

Methacycline, another tetracycline derivative, was reported to cause gray-black pigmentation of light-exposed areas of the skin and yellow-brown pigmentation of exposed parts of conjunctivas in seven patients (Dyster-Aas, 1974) (Table 5). These cases were from a group of 250 patients similarly treated, giving a frequency of approximately 3%. Duration of therapy in the affected patients ranged from 2 to 7.5 yr. Cumulative doses ranged from 420 to 1575 g. Four of the patients had taken another form of tetracycline previously. Involved were face, with enhancement at malar eminences, lateral forehead, and dorsa of hands. Six patients had both skin and conjunctival involvement; one had only conjunctival involvement. In one patient, who had worn shorts during

TABLE 5 Pigmentary Changes Associated with the Tetracyclines

Drug	Clinical findings	Histopathology
Tetracycline hydrochloride	Blue cutaneous osteomas	
Methacycline	Gray-black pigmentation of light-exposed areas; yellow-brown pigmentation of exposed parts of conjunctiva	Hyperpigmentation of basal cell layer ($\uparrow$ melanin); elastotic degeneration of upper and middle dermis; dermal macrophages containing pigment
Minocycline:		
Localized	Blue-black pigmentation in areas of acne scarring	Electron-dense material noted in dermal macrophage; fine particles 50–100 nm and coarse granules up to 1.5 μm; stain positive for iron
Diffuse	Blue-gray hyperpigmentation most prominent in sun-exposed areas	Pigment in basal layer of epidermis; brown-black pigment scattered in macrophages of the upper dermis; negative for iron; positive for melanin

the summer, skin involvement was limited to the shins. Pigmentation of the conjunctivas was limited to the area bounded by the palpebral fissures. Slit-lamp examination showed yellow-brown granules in involved conjunctivas. In one patient "dust-fine" pigmentation was noted on the corneal endothelium; in another patient there was a thin subepithelial deposit of dust-fine pigment, and in three patients similar pigment was found on the anterior lens capsule.

Histopathologic examination of involved skin reveals moderate basal hyperpigmentation with staining properties consistent with melanin. The upper and intermediate dermis show elastotic degeneration of the connective tissue. Among the elastotic fibers are (1) moderate number of pigmented macrophages that stained variably positive with Masson-Fontana stain and (2) occasional large, highly refractile bodies. These granules are much smaller than those seen within the macrophages, do not fluoresce at any wavelength, and stain black with von Kossa's stain. By electron microscopy, the epidermal pigment has the characteristics of melanin. The dermal pigmented cells contain structures very similar to epidermal melanin granules in various states of degradation and are at least partly contained within membrane-limited structures. The collagen fibers are normal, though reduced in number. The elastic fibers show few microfibrils and consist of an amorphous substance of moderate electron density. In this substance are streaks of osmiophilic, dark material containing large numbers of irregularly shaped granules of great electron density, often surrounded by a clear halo and without discernible inner structure.

Minocycline (Minocin)

Minocycline, a tetracycline derivative, is a popular and effective therapy for acne vulgaris. Basler and Kohnen (1978) reported a case of blue-black pigmentation in areas of previous acne scarring. At the time of onset of pigmentation, the patient was taking minocycline. The significance of this association was not initially appreciated. Basler (1979) noted that he had received anecdotal reports of similar pigmentation within acne scars, occurring only in patients receiving long-term minocycline therapy, as had the patient he reported (Table 5). Gray-green discoloration of teeth and a generalized "muddy" hue to the skin were also noted.

Potassium ferricyanide stains of histologic sections reveal scattered iron-containing aggregates consistent with hemosiderin in the middle and upper dermis. Electron microscopic studies reveal electron-dense material within dermal macrophages, corresponding to the iron-positive material seen on light microscopy. This material was present in two forms, fine particles 50 to 100 nm in diameter consistent with ferritin, and larger aggregates of coarse, granular material up to 1.5 μm in diameter consistent with hemosiderin. Noteworthy is the black-colored thyroid gland found at autopsy in a patient who took minocycline for 1 yr (Attwood and Dennett, 1976). Histology of this gland showed iron-free, nonfluorescent pigment granules associated with lipofuscin in colloid and within most follicular cells. Thick Paragon-stained sections revealed the presence of a black and a green pigment. The black pigment was present as discrete droplets or, less commonly, within green droplets. The green droplets were numerous and were present singly or in clumps. The same patient had blue-black pigmentation of the ala nasi, dark costal cartilages, and yellow-brown parietal bones. Black pigmentation of monkey and rat thyroid glands following minocycline has also been noted (McGrae and Zelickson, 1980). In dogs, minocycline accumulates in brain, bone, and thyroid. The pigmentation described was attributed to specific concentrations of minocycline within the thyroid and to lipofuscin deposition (Attwood and Dennett, 1976). Minocycline deposition in the skin may account in part for the cutaneous pigmentation. No explanation for localization to sites of scarring has been offered.

Recently, three men were described who had developed brown-gray or blue-black discoloration of the anterior legs while on minocycline (McGrae and Zelickson, 1980). Light microscopic findings were identical in these patients. Histopathology revealed brown-black granules most prominent below the upper papillary dermis, concentrated in perivascular mononuclear cells, which were increased in number. Perls' test for iron was positive, and the Fontana-Masson silver method stained the pigment granules. Electron microscopic findings were similar to those of Basler and Kohnen (1978) with electron-dense particles located within macrophages, mainly limited by unit membranes. The material was finely particulate, but in places formed larger masses. This material did not resemble melanosomes. The authors concluded that the material is related to minocycline.

Generalized cutaneous dark blue-gray hyperpigmentation in a white female being treated with minocycline has also been reported (Simons and Morales, 1980). Pigmentation was most prominent in sun-exposed areas. Partial resolution of the pigmentation occurred after the drug was discontinued. Histology of involved areas revealed increased pigment in the basal layer of the epidermis and a brown-black pigment scattered in the macrophages of the upper dermis. The staining properties of melanin were observed with the Fontana-Masson technique. The Prussian blue reaction for hemosiderin was negative (Table 5).

CHEMOTHERAPEUTIC AGENTS

Hyperpigmentation has been associated with the administration of several chemotherapeutic agents. The site and mechanism of this hyperpigmentation await study, but from clinical appearances the deposition appears primarily epidermal (Table 6).

Cyclophosphamide (Cytoxan)

Alkylating agents are widely used in the treatment of internal malignancies. Cyclophosphamide has been reported to produce skin and nail

TABLE 6 Pigmentary Disturbances Related to Antitumor Agents

Agent	Clinical appearance	Mechanism/histopathology
Busulfan	Diffuse brownish pigmentation of face, forearms, chest, and abdomen	Basilar epidermal melanin; melanin in dermal macrophages
Bleomycin	Streaks of hyperpigmentation on trunk and over pressure points on extremities	Unknown
Doxorubicin	Pigment in palmar and inter-phalangeal creases; diffuse uniform black-brown hyperpigmentation of palms and soles	Increased melanin deposition in epidermis; increased melanocytes in the basal layer
5-Fluorouracil	Uniform increased pigment in sun-exposed areas May overlie veins used for infusion	Unknown
Mechlorethamine (topical)	Epidermal hyperpigmentation	Possible alteration of melanosome aggregation or functional impairment of keratinocytes
BCNU (topical)	Epidermal hyperpigmentation	Enlarged melanocytes; (?) increased numbers of melanocytes and increased pigment production; (?) postinflammatory

hyperpigmentation (Solidoro and Saenz, 1966). Shah et al. (1978) reported five cases of black pigmentation of the nails. The cumulative doses of the drug prior to the onset of the pigmentation ranged from 1.2 to 12.3 g, and the duration of the treatment ranged from 10 d to 26 wk. The pattern of pigmentation varied from diffuse to horizontal or longitudinal streaks. One patient had involvement of palmar and digital creases and the dorsa of the hands. Nail pigmentation starts proximally, extends distally, and, when the drug is stopped, clears proximally first, suggesting that a disturbance of the nail plate is involved in the disorder (Table 7). No histopathology is available.

There is also a brief report in the literature of a brown line on the teeth at the junction of the gingiva in one patient taking cyclophosphamide (Harrison and Wood, 1972).

Busulfan (Myleran)

Busulfan, another alkylating agent, is commonly associated with hyper-pigmentation (Table 6). Three of 19 patients treated with busulfan developed diffuse brownish pigmentation of the face, forearms, chest, and abdomen, which resolved over 3 mo (Galton, 1953). In another study, 39 of 788 patients receiving busulfan for chronic granulocytic leukemia developed hyperpigmentation (Kyle et al., 1961). This pigmentation is brown, generalized, and most prominent on the trunk, face, and hands. With the exception of one report of a linear deposit of pigment on the gingiva, the mucous membranes have been spared. Palmar creases are not hyperpigmented. The incidence of pigmentation is higher in dark-skinned patients and lower in those who are light-skinned (Burns et al., 1971). In one patient, pigmentation regressed after discontinuation of the drug and recurred when the drug was resumed. In some patients, this hyperpigmentation is associated with weakness, fatigue, weight loss, anorexia, and nausea. Endocrine evaluation in patients with this "Addison's disease-like" syndrome is normal (Kyle et al., 1961).

Histopathologic examination reveals increased melanin in the basal layer of the epidermis and in dermal macrophages. No increase in the number of melanocytes is seen. Stains for iron are negative.

Kyle et al. (1961) speculated that busulfan inactivates sulfhydryl groups in the skin by "dethiolation," thus removing an inhibitor of tyrosinase with subsequent hyperpigmentation. Topical busulfan failed to cause hyperpigmentation when applied twice a day for 4 wk.

Melphalan (Alkeran)

The alkylating agent melphalan was reported to cause dark pigmentation of the nail beds in a patient being treated for malignant melanoma (Malacarne and Zaragli, 1977) (Table 7). However, pigmented banding has been reported in patients with metastatic melanoma without chemotherapy (Adrian et al., 1980). The pigmentation regressed after discontinuation of the melphalan, suggesting an etiologic association (Malacarne and Zaragli, 1977). No histopathology was reported, and the mechanism of pigmentation is unknown.

TABLE 7 Nail Disturbance Related to Chemotherapeutic Agents

Agent	Nail findings	Mechanism
Cyclophosphamide	Black pigmentation of nail beds and plate; onset in proximal nail fold and progresses distally	Unknown
Melphalan	Dark pigmentation of nail bed	Numerical increase of melanin granules present in basal layer melanocytes of nail bed
Bleomycin	One case (patient also on vinblastine); pigment in nail bed and not nail plate	Unknown
Doxorubicin	Horizontal pigment banding of nails in black patients; gray, brown, and black longitudinal bands also reported	Unknown
Daunorubicin	Transverse brown-black bands that move distally as nails grow	Unknown

Daunorubicin (Cerubidine)

Daunorubicin is an antibiotic whose greatest utility is in the treatment of acute leukemias. This drug has been associated with production of pigmented transverse bands of the fingernails and toenails (de Marinis et al., 1978) (Table 7). Histopathology has not been done, and the mechanism is unknown.

Bleomycin

Bleomycin is an antibiotic, derived from *Streptomyces verticillus*, used in the treatment of several malignancies. In mice, the highest concentration of the drug after ip instillation is found in skin and lung (Werner and Thornberg, 1976). Cutaneous toxicity is high in human patients. The incidence of hyperpigmentation has varied from 8 to 20% (Blum et al., 1973). Commonly reported findings are linear bands of hyperpigmentation on the chest and back and pigmentation over small joints of the hands and, occasionally, over the elbows and knees (Table 6). This hyperpigmentation is usually reversible when the drug is stopped. Cumulative drug doses at the time of onset of the pigmentation have ranged from 90 to 285 mg (Cohen et al., 1973).

Full-thickness dermoepidermal histology has not been reported. Dopa staining of an epidermal sheet taken from a hyperpigmented area shows larger melanocytes with larger and more complex dendrites and enhanced tyrosinase activity compared to adjacent nonhyperpigmented skin.

One case of pigmented banding of the nails was reported in association with bleomycin (Shetty, 1977) (Table 7). That patient was also on vinblastine.

Doxorubicin (Adriamycin)

Doxorubicin is an anthracycline antibiotic with broad antitumor activity. Reports of both horizontal and longitudinal pigmented banding of nails associated with its use have been published (Morris et al., 1977; Priestman and James, 1975) (Table 7). The horizontal bands occur 6–8 wk after the start of therapy. Pigment appears to be in the nail plate. The mechanism of production of this pigment is unknown. Pratt and Shanks (1974) reported increased pigmentation in nails, nail beds, and phalangeal creases of the dorsa of the fingers in children. These findings appear to be more common in blacks than in whites; 5 of 13 blacks and 6 of 39 whites had such pigmentation. A report of black pigmentation of the tongue in two of eight black and none of two nonblack children taking doxorubicin was observed in another study (Rao et al., 1976); this pigmentation cleared over 2 wk. Rothberg et al. (1974) reported a case of diffuse, uniform black-brown hyperpigmentation of the palms, soles, and proximal nails with similar but less intense changes on the dorsa of the knuckles (Table 6). Several small hyperpigmented spots were also present on the buccal mucosa. These changes occurred after 6 wk of treatment, at which time 148 mg doxorubicin had been given. The pigmentation cleared over 2 mo when the drug was discontinued. The nail pigmentation grew out as a horizontal band. Histopathology of hyperpigmented skin over a knuckle showed increased melanin deposition with an increased number of melanocytes in the basal layer of the epidermis.

5-Fluorouracil

5-Fluorouracil is a pyrimidine analog used in the treatment of several varieties of carcinoma. This drug has been associated with hyperpigmentation in 2-5% of all patients treated (Hrushesky, 1976; Bateman et al., 1971). The hyperpigmentation usually occurs uniformly on sun-exposed areas of the body (Table 6). There is one report of increased pigmentation over veins in which 5-fluorouracil had been infused (Hrushesky, 1976). The veins underlying this pigmentation were not tender, thrombosed, or sclerosed. No histopathology was done.

Mechlorethamine (Mustargen)

Mechlorethamine, the first of the nitrogen mustard alkylating agents to be introduced into clinical medicine, can be dissolved in water and applied to the skin topically for the treatment of mycosis fungoides. In both whites and blacks exposed to mechlorethamine topically the skin may become hyperpigmented (Table 6). The hyperpigmentation may occur in the absence of clinical signs of irritation or inflammation (Flaxman et al., 1973). By electron microscopy of hyperpigmented skin, increased numbers of melanocytes were found (Flaxman et al., 1973). Striking changes were found in the aggregation of melanosomes within the keratinocytes. In normal Caucasian skin, melanosomes are arranged in membrane-bound groups of two or more within keratinocytes. The size of these melanosomes is 0.3-0.5 μm. In normal blacks the melanosomes are larger, varying in size from 0.5 to 0.8 μm, and are mainly nonaggregated. In the hyperpigmented skin of whites treated with nitrogen mustard, melanosomes were increased in number and were no longer arranged in membrane-bound groups but were mainly nonaggregated. The largest size of these melanosomes was 0.5 μm. In blacks, increased numbers of normally nonaggregated melanosomes of normal size were found. Mechanisms proposed to account for these findings include: (1) a continuous toxic effect of mechlorethamine causing keratinocytes to be functionally impaired, and (2) a selective effect of mechlorethamine on the aggregation mechanism (Flaxman et al., 1973).

BCNU

1,3-Bis(chlorethyl)-1-nitrosourea (BCNU) has been shown to cause hyperpigmentation when applied topically to the skin. This was first noted by physicians and nurses who accidentally spilled some on their own skin (Frost and DeVita, 1966). Frost and DeVita felt that postinflammatory hyperpigmentation was a likely explanation for this phenomenon. In a study of hairless mice treated topically with BCNU, spotty pigmentation appeared by the fifth day (Hilger et al., 1974). Histopathologic examination of the induced hyperpigmentation revealed an increase in melanocyte number and in pigment-containing keratinocytes (Hilger et al., 1974). Patients given BCNU parenterally do not appear to develop hyperpigmentation.

MISCELLANEOUS MEDICATIONS

Adrenocorticotropic Hormone (ACTH)

Administration of ACTH can produce diffuse bronze skin coloration from increased epidermal melanin formation (Cass et al., 1964) (Table 4). ACTH is known to have melanocyte stimulating hormone (MSH)-like activity. In 122 patients with multiple sclerosis treated with 120 U intramuscular ACTH per day for 21 d, followed by a tapering dosage, 6 cases of hyperpigmentation occurred. Five developed pigmentation during the tapering phase and one while on a maintenance dosage of 20 U/d. Pigmentation was reversible in all cases by decreasing the ACTH dose and administering dexamethasone.

Amiodarone

Amiodarone, a coronary vasodilator, has been used in Europe since 1964. After 1967, reports appeared of a yellow-brown granular pigmentation of the cornea in patients treated with this agent (Delage et al., 1975) (Table 4). Electron microscopic study of these corneas revealed numerous lysosomal inclusions, probably lipofusin, in the cytoplasm of the basal and intermediary cells. The reported frequency of corneal pigmentation ranges from 7 to 76% (Delage et al., 1975). After 1970, numerous reports of gray-blue pigmentation of the face and other light-exposed areas of the skin in association with amiodarone therapy appeared (Delage et al., 1975). Yellow-brown granules in the cytoplasm of dermal histiocytes are described. Electron microscopic studies of affected skins reveal membrane-bound dense bodies, believed to be lipofuscin, in the cytoplasm of dermal histiocytes. Dosage and duration of treatment are directly related to both corneal and cutaneous pigmentation. Doses of 400 to 800 mg/d seem necessary to produce the condition. Onset of corneal pigmentation has been reported as early as 13 d into therapy. Skin deposits are observed 6-39 mo after onset of therapy. In most cases, a photosensitivity reaction in light-exposed areas occurs before pigmentation. Discontinuance of amiodarone results in the slow disappearance of both corneal and cutaneous pigmentation. Skin pigmentation may persist for up to 1 yr.

Histopathology reveals small numbers of histiocytes, often located around capillaries, containing aggregates of finely granular yellow-brown pigment in their cytoplasm (Delage et al., 1975). Staining is moderately positive for periodic acid–Schiff (PAS); strongly positive for Ziehl-Neelsen, 8-h and 18-h Fontana's stain; and negative for Turnbull blue (Delage et al., 1975). The epidermis is normal. Electron microscopy reveals numerous dense bodies within the cytoplasm of histiocytes, measuring 250 to 2,500 nm in diameter, composed of dense, slightly granular osmiophilic material within a single membrane. Sometimes a clear halo can be seen between the membrane and the electron-dense material. The authors of this study suggest that the osmiophilic material is probably lipofuscin and not amiodarone itself (Delage et al., 1975). They further speculate that amiodarone may accelerate normal cellular autophagocytosis with increased formation of lipofuscins.

Clofazimine (Lamprene)

Clofazimine, a synthetic phenazine dye, is an effective drug in the treatment of leprosy. The most frequent side effect of this drug is abnormal coloration of the skin. This can be divided into two types (Pettit, 1969): (1) initial redness occurring within 1–4 wk of starting the drug; (2) black-brown or violaceous-brown pigmentation that develops during the 2d and 3d mo of treatment, limited mainly to lesional areas (Table 4). The red pigmentation is thought to be secondary to accumulation of the drug itself, mainly in the reticuloendothelial cells and subcutaneous fat, since the drug is highly fat-soluble (Sakurai and Skinsnes, 1977). Studies in mice have shown coloration of fat throughout the animal and red-orange bodies within macrophages in several organs (Conalty and Jackson, 1962). With prolonged exposure, these bodies are replaced by bright red crystals in the macrophages. Similar findings occur in rats and guinea pigs. Autopsy studies in humans have shown internal organs, especially adipose tissue, turning yellow-orange and finally orange-red within minutes of exposure to air (Mansfield, 1974). In three of four autopsies, the highest concentration of drug was found in fat. Organs with large reticuloendothelial components, such as spleen, lymph nodes, and lung, also had high concentrations.

The dark pigmentation seen mainly in lesional areas has been attributed to increased melanin in the basal layer of the epidermis, associated in some cases with pigment incontinence into the upper dermis (Pettit et al., 1967). Skin biopsies performed in a later study (Sakurai and Skinsnes, 1977) showed diffuse brown coloration throughout the dermis and subcutaneous tissue. Histology of unstained sections showed yellow-brown pigment forming a rim around fat globules within the cytoplasm of macrophages throughout the dermis and subcutaneous fat. Histochemical stains showed this material to be acid-fast, positive for lipid stains even after extraction by fat solvents, and positive or weakly positive for the Schmorl reaction and chrome alum hematoxylin stain. Sakurai and Skinsnes (1977) interpreted these findings as evidence that the pigment is a ceroidlike substance rather than lipofuscin. They hypothesized that the ceroid probably originates from unsaturated fatty acids of the leprosy bacilli through oxidation or their binding with the drug. One of three cases studied showed some increased melanin in the basal layer of the epidermis. Melanin incontinence was seen in some instances.

Oral Contraceptives

Melasma is known to occur with the use of oral contraceptives. In one study, 29% of patients taking oral contraceptives were affected (Resnik, 1967). Eighty-seven percent of these patients also had melasma during pregnancy. Both combination and sequential oral contraceptives produced melasma with similar frequencies. Whether estrogens or progestins cause the melasma is not known. Decreased doses of estrogen did not lower the incidence of melasma. After stopping oral contraceptives, melasma may remain or may remit only partially.

Histopathology reveals increased melanin in the basal layer of the epidermis with a normal number of melanocytes (Table 4). The melanocytes, however, are larger than normal. Recent studies suggested that in some cases the pigmentation is both dermal and epidermal (M. A. Pathak, personal communication).

Psoralens

In recent years, psoralens and long-wave ultraviolet radiation (UV-A, 320–400 nm) have been exploited in the treatment of proliferative disorders of the epidermis, especially psoriasis, and diseases marked by benign or malignant collections of lymphocytes in the skin, such as mycosis fungoides. In addition, for many years psoralens have been used in the treatment of vitiligo, and it is well recognized that increased pigmentation of normal skin occurs. Using dopa- and silver-stained, as well as hematoxylin and eosin-stained histologic sections, Jimbow et al. (1974) showed that exposure to UV-A plus 8-methoxypsoralen causes an increase in the number of functional melanocytes, increased synthesis of melanosomes, and increased transfer of melanosomes to keratinocytes (Table 4). Addition of 8-methoxypsoralen enhanced the rate of synthesis, degree of melanization, and transfer of melanosomes without causing changes in the size or distribution pattern of melanosomes in melanocytes and keratinocytes. Enhanced dermal pigmentation may also be seen in some cases.

Carotenoids

β-Carotene (carotenemia). β-Carotene is a yellowish lipochrome that is found naturally in many vegetables and fruits in addition to carrots, in which it was first recognized. This substance is a precursor of vitamin A, but conversion occurs at relatively slow rates. When the serum concentration of carotene exceeds 250 μg/dl, the skin becomes deep yellow. Pigmentation appears first on the top of the nose, palms, soles, nasolabial folds, and forehead. Once ingestion ceases, the skin color returns to normal in 2-6 wk since little carotene is stored. β-Carotene may be of therapeutic value in the treatment of erythropoietic protoporphyria (Mathews-Roth et al., 1970), but this use has not been accepted universally (Pollitt, 1975).

Carotene is generally thought to be present in stratum corneum (Lascari, 1981) (although experimental evidence is meager) (Greenberg et al., 1958) and in subcutaneous fat (Lascari, 1981). Vitamin A-like autofluorescence was found within the sebum and epidermis when the serum carotene level was raised to three to four times normal (500–750 μg/dl) (Greenberg et al., 1958). No fluorescence was found within sweat glands or ducts. In subjects in whom the serum carotene level was raised one- to twofold or less, the vitamin A-like autofluorescence was found only in the sebaceous glands (Greenberg et al., 1958).

The differential diagnosis of carotenemia includes lycopenemia, jaundice, and pigmentation due to ingestion or percutaneous absorption of other chemicals. Lycopene is an isomer of β-carotene present in tomatoes, beets, rose hips, bittersweet berries, and chili beans. If elevated levels occur in the blood, usually from ingestion of large quantities of tomatoes or tomato juice, the skin may become pigmented. However, the color is usually more orange than that seen with β-carotene. Sclerae and mucous membrane sparing in carotenemia aids in differentiation from jaundice. Ingestion or percutaneous absorption of quinacrine, dinitrophenol, saffron, and picric acid can also produce yellow pigmentation of the skin (Lascari, 1981).

Canthaxanthin. Canthaxanthin is a synthetic carotenoid with no pro-vitamin A activity. Alone in oral doses similar to those of carotene, it imparts a deep salmon pink color to the skin (Pollitt, 1975). When added to β-carotene, the resultant color resembles natural tanning (Pollitt, 1975). Outside the United States it has been used as an oral artificial suntanning agent (Alonso, 1980) and as a food coloring (FAO-WHO, 1974). Canthaxanthin has also been tried in the treatment of porphyrias (Pollitt, 1975; Eales, 1978).

In chickens fed canthaxanthin, distribution of the pigment was analyzed with highest levels found in leg skin, followed by viscera, nonleg skin, and muscles in descending order (Alonso et al., 1980).

REFERENCES

Adrian, R. M., Hood, A. F., and Skarin, A. T. 1980. Mucocutaneous reactions to antineoplastic agents. *Cancer* 90:143–157.

Alonso, A., Martin, M., and Gomez, R. 1980. Absorption and fate of canthaxanthin in chicken. *Rev. Exp. Fisiol.* 36:49–52.

Attwood, H. D. and Dennett, X. 1976. A black thyroid and minocycline treatment. *Br. Med. J.* 2:1109–1110.

Baker, H. 1979. Drug reactions. In *Textbook of Dermatology*, eds. A. Rook et al., pp. 1111–1149. Oxford: Blackwell.

Basler, R. S. W. 1979. Minocycline therapy for acne. *Arch. Dermatol.* 115:1391.

Basler, R. S. W. and Kohnen, P. W. 1978. Localized hemosiderosis as a sequela of acne. *Arch. Dermatol.* 114:1695–1697.

Basler, R. S. W., Taylor, W. B., and Peacor, D. R. 1974. Post-acne osteoma cutis: X-ray diffraction analysis. *Arch. Dermatol.* 110:113–114.

Bateman, J. R., Pugh, R. P., Cassidy, D. R., Marshall, G. J., and Irwin, L. E. 1971. 5-Fluorouracil given once weekly: Comparison of intravenous and oral administration. *Cancer* 28:907–913.

Beerman, H. and Kirshbaum, B. A. 1975. Drug eruptions (dermatitis medicamentosa). In *Dermatology*, eds. S. L. Moschella et al., pp. 350–384. Philadelphia: Saunders.

Birmingham, D. J. 1979. Cutaneous reactions to chemicals. In *Dermatology in General Medicine*, ed. 2, eds. T. B. Fitzpatrick et al., pp. 995–1007. New York: McGraw-Hill.

Bleehen, S. S., Gould, D. J., Harrington, C. I. et al. 1981. Occupational argyria; light and electron microscopic studies and x-ray microanalysis. *Br. J. Dermatol.* 104:19–26.

Blois, M. S. 1965. On chlorpromazine binding *in vivo*. *J. Invest. Dermatol.* 45:475–481.

Blum, R. H., Carter, S. K., and Agre, K. 1973. A clinical review of bleomycin—a new antineoplastic agent. *Cancer* 31:903–914.

Buckley, W. R. 1963. Localized argyria. *Arch. Dermatol.* 88:531–539.

Burns, W. A., McFarland, W., and Matthews, M. J. 1971. Toxic manifestations of busulfan therapy. *Med. Ann. D.C.* 40:567–572.

Burge, K. M. and Winkelmann, R. K. 1970. Mercury pigmentation: An electron microscopic study. *Arch. Dermatol.* 102:51–61.

Calvery, H. O., Draize, J. H., and Laug, E. P. 1946. The metabolism and permeability of normal skin. *Physiol. Rev.* 26:495–540.

Campbell, C. H. 1960. Pigmentation of the nail-beds, palate and skin occurring during malarial suppressive therapy with "camoquin." *Med. J. Aust.* 1:956–960.

Cascos, A. 1936. Etude comparative des pigmentations metallique, argyrose et chryose. *Acta Derm.-Venereol.* 7:751–762.

Cass, L. C., Alexander, L., Frederick, W. S., and Ireland, P. 1964. ACTH-induced melanoderma in man. *Curr. Ther. Res. Clin. Exp.* 6:601–607.

Cohen, I. S., Mosher, M. B., O'Keefe, E. J., Klaue, S. N., and DeConti, R. C. 1973. Cutaneous toxicity of bleomycin therapy. *Arch. Dermatol.* 107:553–555.

Conalty, M. L. and Jackson, R. D. 1962. Uptake by reticulo-endothelial cells of the rimino-phenazine B663 (2-*p*-chloroaniline-5-*p*-chlorophenyl-3:5-dihydro-3-isopropylinophenazine). *Br. J. Exp. Pathol.* 43:650–654.

Delage, C., Lagacé, R., and Huard, J. 1975. Pseudocyanotic pigmentation of the skin induced by amiodarone: A light and electron microscopic study. *Can. Med. Assoc. J.* 112:1205–1208.

de Marinis, M., Hendricks, A., and Soltzner, G. 1978. Nail pigmentation with daunorubicin therapy. *Ann. Intern. Med.* 89:516–517.

Dummett, C. O. 1964. Oral mucosal discolorations related to pharmacotherapeutics. *J. Oral Ther.* 1:106–110.

Dyster-Aas, K., Hansson, H., Miorner, G., Moller, H., and Rausing, A. 1974.

Pigment deposits in eyes and light exposed skin during long-term methacycline therapy. *Acta Derm.-Venereol. (Stockh.)* 54:209–222.

Eales, L. 1978. The effects of canthaxanthin on the photocutaneous manifestations of porphyria. *S. Afr. Med. J.* 54:1050–1052.

Everett, M. A. 1979. Metal discolorations. In *Clinical Dermatology*, eds. D. J. Demis et al., unit 11-14, p. 4. Hagerstown: Harper & Row.

FAO-WHO. 1974. *Evaluation of Certain Food Additives*, Tech. Rep. 557, p. 15. Geneva: World Health Organization.

Flaxman, B. A., Sosis, A. C., and Van Scott, E. J. 1973. Changes in malanosome distribution in caucasoid skin following topical application of nitrogen mustard. *J. Invest. Dermatol.* 60:321–326.

Frost, P. and DeVita, V. T. 1966. Pigmentation due to a new antitumor agent. Effects of topical application of BCNU (1,3-bis(chlorethyl)-1-nitrosourea). *Arch. Dermatol.* 94:265–268.

Galton, D. A. G. 1953. Myleran in chronic myeloid leukemia. *Lancet* 264:208–213.

Gimenez-Camarasa, J. M., Garcia-Calderon, P., and de Moragas, J. M. 1975. Lymphocyte transformation test in fixed drug eruption. *N. Engl. J. Med.* 292:819–821.

Greenberg, R., Cornbleet, T., and Jaffay, A. I. 1958. Accumulation and excretion of vitamin A-like fluorescent material by sebaceous glands after the oral feeding of various carotenoids. *J. Invest. Dermatol.* 32:599–604.

Greiner, A. C. and Berry, K. 1964. Skin pigmentation and corneal and lens opacities with prolonged chlorpromazine therapy. *Can. Med. Assoc. J.* 90:663–665.

Gropen, J. 1977. Facial osteoma. *Cutis* 19:254–256.

Hare, P. J. 1970. "Visage mauve" from imipramine. *Br. J. Dermatol.* 83:420.

Harrison, B. M. and Wood, C. B. S. 1972. Cyclophosphamide and pigmentation. *Br. Med. J.* 2:352.

Hashimoto, K., Weiner, W., Albert, J., and Nelson, R. G. 1966. An electron microscopic study of chlorpromazine pigmentation. *J. Invest. Dermatol.* 47:296–306.

Hilger, R., Fukuyama, K., Zackheim, H. S., and Epstein, J. H. 1974. Increased melanocytes in hairless mice following topical treatment with carmustine (BCNU) and nitrogen mustard (NM). *Clin. Res.* 22:159A.

Hill, W. R. and Montgomery, H. 1941. Argyria with special reference to the cutaneous histopathology. *Arch. Dermatol.* 44:588–599.

Hrushesky, W. J. 1976. Serpentine supravenous 5-fluorouracil (NSC-19893) hyperpigmentation. *Cancer Treat. Rep.* 60:639.

Jewell, E. W. 1971. Osteoma cutis. *Arch. Dermatol.* 103:553–555.

Jimbow, K., Kaidbey, K. H., Pathak, M. A., Parrish, J. A., Kligman, A. M., and Fitzpatrick, T. B. 1974. Melanin pigmentation stimulated by UV-B, UV-A, and psoralens. *J. Invest. Dermatol.* 62:548.

Kyle, R. A., Schwartz, R. S., Oliner, H. L., and Damestek, W. 1961. A syndrome resembling adrenal cortical insufficiency associated with long-term busulfan (Myleran) therapy. *Blood* 18:497–510.

Lamar, L. M. and Bliss, B. O. 1966. Localized pigmentation of the skin due to topical mercury. *Arch. Dermatol.* 93:450–453.

Lascari, A. D. 1981. Carotenemia. *Clin. Pediatr.* 20:25–29.

Levantine, A. and Almeyda, J. 1973. Drug induced changes in pigmentation. *Br. J. Dermatol.* 89:105–112.

Lever, W. F. and Schaumburg-Lever, G. 1975. *Histopathology of the Skin*, ed. 5, pp. 240–241. Philadelphia: Lippincott.

Lueth, H. C., Sutton, D. C., McMullen, C. J., and Muehlberger, C. W. 1936. Generalized discoloration of skin resembling argyria following prolonged oral use of bismuth: A case of "bismuthia." *Arch. Intern. Med.* 57:1115–1124.

Lutterloh, C. C. and Shallenberger, P. L. 1946. Unusual pigmentation developing after prolonged suppressive therapy with quinacrine hydrochloride. *Arch. Dermatol. Venereol.* 53:349–354.

Malacarne, P. and Zavagli, G. 1977. Melphalan-induced melanonychia striata. *Arch. Dermatol. Res.* 258:81–83.

Mansfield, R. E. 1974. Tissue concentrations of clofazimine (B663) in man. *Am. J. Trop. Med. Hyg.* 23:1116–1119.

Mathews-Roth, M. M., Pathak, M. A., Fitzpatrick, T. B., et al. 1970. Beta-carotene as a photoprotective agent in erythropoietic protoporphyria. *N. Engl. J. Med.* 282:1231–1234.

McGrae, J. D. and Jelickson, A. S. 1980. Skin pigmentation secondary to minocycline therapy. *Arch. Dermatol.* 116:1262–1265.

Mehta, A. C., Dawson-Butterworth, K., and Woodhouse, M. A. 1941. Argyria, electron microscopic study of a case. *Br. J. Dermatol.* 44:588–599.

Morris, D., Aisner, J., and Wiernik, P. H. 1977. Horizontal pigmented banding of the nails in association with Adriamycin chemotherapy. *Cancer Treat. Rep.* 61:499–501.

Pareek, S. S. 1980. Nystatin-induced fixed eruption. *Br. J. Dermatol.* 103:679–680.

Pettit, J. H. S. 1969. B663 (Lamprene) in mycobacterial infections. *Br. J. Dermatol.* 81:794–795.

Pettit, J. H. S., Rees, R. J. W., and Ridley, D. S. 1967. Chemotherapeutic trials in leprosy. 3. Pilot trial of a riminophenazine derivative, B663, in the treatment of lepromatous leprosy. *Int. J. Lepr.* 35:25–33.

Pollitt, N. 1975. Beta-carotene and the photodermatoses. *Br. J. Dermatol.* 93:721–724.

Pratt, C. B. and Shanks, E. C. 1974. Hyperpigmentation of nails from doxorubicin. *J. Am. Med. Assoc.* 228:460.

Priestman, T. J. and James, K. W. 1975. Adriamycin and longitudinal pigmented banding of fingernails. *Lancet* i:1337–1338.

Prose, P. H. 1963. An electron microscopic study of human generalized argyria. *Am. J. Pathol.* 42:293–299.

Rao, S. P., Potnia, A. V., Sobrinho, T. C., and Brown, A. K. 1976. Pigmentation of the tongue after treatment with Adriamycin. *Cancer Treat. Rep.* 60:1402–1404.

Resnik, S. 1967. Melasma induced by oral contraceptive drugs. *J. Am. Med. Assoc.* 199:601–605.

Rothberg, H., Place, C. H., and Shteir, O. 1974. Adriamycin (NSC-123127) toxicity: Unusual melanotic reaction. *Cancer Treat. Rep.* 58:749–751.

Sakurai, I. and Skinsnes, O. K. 1977. Histochemistry of B663 pigmentation: Ceroid-like pigmentation in macrophages. *Int. J. Lepr.* 45:343–354.

Sams, W. M. and Epstein, J. H. 1965. The affinity of melanin for chloroquine. *J. Invest. Dermatol.* 45:482–488.

Satanove, A. 1965. Pigmentation due to phenothiazines in high and prolonged dosage. *J. Am. Med. Assoc.* 191:263–268.

Shah, P. C., Rao, K. R. P., and Patel, A. R. 1978. Cyclophosphamide induced nail pigmentation. *Br. J. Dermatol.* 98:675–680.

Shetty, M. R., 1977. Case of pigmented banding of the nail caused by bleomycin. *Cancer Treat. Rep.* 61:501–502.

Simons, J. J. and Morales, A. 1980. Minocycline and generalized cutaneous pigmentation. *J. Am. Acad. Dermatol.* 3:244–247.

Solidoro, A. and Saenz, R. 1966. Effects of cyclophosphamide on 127 patients with malignant lymphoma. *Cancer Treat. Rep.* 50:265–270.

Stritzler, C. and Kopf, A. W. 1960. Fixed drug eruption caused by 8-chloro-theophylline in Dramamine with clinical and histologic studies. *J. Invest. Dermatol.* 34:319–330.

Traub, E. F. and Tennen, J. S. 1936. Permanent pigmentation following application of iron salts. *J. Am. Med. Assoc.* 106:1711–1712.

Tuffanelli, D., Abraham, R. K., and Dubois, E. I. 1963. Pigmentation from antimalarial therapy: Its possible relation to the ocular lesions. *Arch. Dermatol.* 88:419–426.

Van Woert, M. H. 1968. Isolation of chlorpromazine pigments in man. *Nature (Lond.)* 219:1054–1056.

Walter, J. F. and Macknet, K. D. 1979. Pigmentation of oesteoma cutis caused by tetracycline. *Arch. Dermatol.* 115:1087–1088.

Werner, Y. and Thornberg, B. 1976. Cutaneous side effects of bleomycin therapy. *Acta Derm.-Venereol. (Stockh.)* 56:115–158.

Wintroub, B. U., Shiffman, N. J., and Arndt, K. A. 1979. Adverse cutaneous reactions to drugs. In *Dermatology in General Medicine,* ed. 2, eds. T. B. Fitzpatrick et al., pp. 555–567. New York: McGraw-Hill.

27

cutaneous granulomas as a toxicologic problem

■ William L. Epstein ■

INTRODUCTION

Chronic inflammation accompanies a wide range of skin diseases. Granuloma formation is one type of chronic inflammatory response, which must be differentiated from the others. Table 1 is an outline of granulomatous inflammation in skin with selected examples (Epstein, 1982). The toxicologist, unlike the dermatologist, will see relatively few cutaneous problems associated with granuloma formation, but granulomas appearing elsewhere, as in the lungs, liver, and other organs, may pose some knotty problems. This brief review presents a concept of the biology of granuloma formation. Although it is based on studies of cutaneous granulomas, the proposal is relevant to granulomas where they occur in the body.

Definition

A granuloma is a tissue response to injury caused by a poorly soluble substance (Epstein, 1967). The material stays at the site of injury and stimulates an influx of cells from the mononuclear phagocyte system (a term coined to replace reticuloendothelial system) (van Furth et al., 1973). The granuloma consists primarily of mononuclear cells, which proliferate and differentiate in the tissue in response to the injury.

This work was supported by the Department of Health, Education, and Welfare, Public Health Service grant AM 07939.

TABLE 1   Classification of Cutaneous Granulomas

Type	Example
Foreign body	Keratin, tattoo
Infectious	Coccidiodomycosis and other deep fungi, gumma, cat scratch disease, lepromatous leprosy, etc.
Immunogenic	Sarcoidosis, tuberculosis, tuberculoid leprosy
Associated with tissue injury	Necrobiosis, granuloma annulare
Not associated with tissue injury	Multicentric reticulohistiocytosis

Clinical Appearance

Clinically, a granuloma is a chronic, tumid, focal lesion; it may or may not ulcerate, and the patient generally does not have subjective complaints such as itching, burning, or pain at the site. Granulomatous inflammation usually heals with scarring, whether or not the lesion ulcerates.

MONONUCLEAR PHAGOCYTE SYSTEM

The mononuclear phagocyte system, as conceptualized by Spector (1974), is shown in Fig. 1. Histologically, granulomas are characterized by the

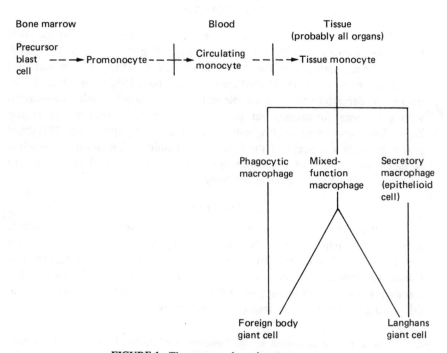

FIGURE 1   The mononuclear phagocyte system.

presence of mononuclear cells, epithelioid cells, and giant cells, which represent the main effector cells of the mononuclear phagocyte system. Sometimes, mononuclear cells in tissue are called histiocytes, but this is redundant and confusing and the term should be dropped from our lexicon. In addition, other cells may appear in the lesion, such as polymorphonuclear leukocytes, eosinophils, and basophils from the bone marrow; lymphocytes and plasma cells from the lymphoid tissues; and fibroblasts from the connective tissue. Also, small blood vessels may at times permeate the inflammatory mass to the point where it resembles granulation tissue, which explains some of the early confusion about nomenclature (Virchow, 1864–1865) and partially accounts for the apathy and delay in unraveling the true nature of granulomatous inflammation.

PATHOPHYSIOLOGY OF GRANULOMA FORMATION

The outline in Table 1 provides a conceptual basis for understanding the dynamics of granuloma formation. In this section foreign body and immunogenic granulomas are compared and contrasted as polar examples of the proliferative and differentiative potential of the mononuclear phagocyte system. Furthermore, the idea of low- and high-turnover granulomas is presented with its ramifications.

Foreign Body Granulomas

In skin, foreign body reactions represent the most common type of granuloma seen (Epstein, 1980) and mechanistically can be likened to the irritant type of contact dermatitis, as compared to the more complex allergic contact dermatitis. They are caused by biologically inert substances infused into the skin in some manner. Pathologically, one sees a macrophage response with simple phagocytosis of the foreign body. If the material is macroscopic in size, foreign body giant cells may appear, and sometimes with continuing tissue breakdown or acute insults polymorphonuclear leukocytes can be observed. During healing, fibroblasts and small blood vessels become prominent. The prototype for foreign body granulomas in skin is the keratin granuloma as it occurs in acne—perhaps the single most common granuloma in the skin.

From the standpoint of the toxicologist, all manner of foreign substances can be inflicted on the skin, in accidents occurring at work or otherwise. Thus, a cactus granuloma in a tender spot conjures up a vision of a horseback riding mishap in the Southwest, whereas gravel and dirt tattoo granulomas occur with a wide variety of activities. Lead pencil tattoos are seen most commonly with schoolchildren and office personnel. More serious are blast injuries from gunpowder and grease guns. Purposeful inoculations, such as tattoos, are readily recognized and generally produce few medical complications (Beerman and Lane, 1954), while others, such as paraffin and silicone granulomas, can cause a diagnostic dilemma. Rarely, injections of drugs or vaccination may lead to granulomatous inflammation, which, if complicated by the onset of an allergic reaction, may be very difficult to recognize. Also, insect bites are responsible for diagnostic problems because they frequently lead to a complex histologic pattern, probably because of the toxins released into the tissue at the time of the bite and, in some instances, the advent of a secondary allergic response.

Silica granulomas in skin produce one of the most puzzling types of foreign body responses. Experimental injection of small particles of silica intracutaneously leads to a straightforward foreign body granuloma (Epstein et al., 1963), which, except for the size of the particles, is comparable to the granulomas seen after sandblasting injuries. More serious granulomas may be produced by embedded glass, quartz, or crude siliceous dust. Only a few of these cases have been reported (Eskeland et al., 1974), but there appears to be a long, asymptomatic latent period between the time of the injury and the advent of a granuloma. Thus the original injury may be overlooked in attempting to explain the fairly sudden appearance of a granuloma that may have tuberculoid features. However, careful examination of the tissue reveals the presence of large amounts of silica, and the cells in the infiltrate are not truly organized into an epithelioid cell granuloma. We studied a patient like this, testing him for granulomatous hypersensitivity to silica, and found that none existed (Epstein, 1971). However, the patient showed extensive phagocytic activity of the injected silica, and on the basis of this observation and similar cases experimentally produced with zirconium we coined the term "immune phagocytosis" to explain the enhanced phagocytic activity of the macrophages under these circumstances (Epstein, 1971).

Inhaled silica also produces an unusual pulmonary response, which should be considered not allergic or immunogenic in nature, but rather uniquely toxic. It was shown several years ago (Kessel et al., 1963) that release of the silica, which stimulates the influx of more mononuclear cells, ultimately results in proliferation of fibroblasts and connective tissue and terminates in the fibrotic changes of advanced silicosis. In recent years, a nonsiliceous factor that can lead to the same changes has been extracted from macrophages (Kilroe-Smith et al., 1973), and the late events of silicosis now can be stimulated in the test tube (Aalto et al., 1976). It is now recognized that macrophages release biologically active proteins very much like lymphocytes (Nelson, 1973), so-called macrokines. Further work will be required to determine whether one of these macrokines is the toxic substance released under the influence of silica ingestion.

It should be emphasized that infectious granulomas are initiated by the same basic macrophage response of the mononuclear phagocyte system, but the main cell usually is a mixed-function macrophage, although purely phagocytic and secretory macrophages may also be seen. In addition, the histologic pattern is altered by other responses, such as acute inflammation, which is the body's first line of defense against most bacteria and fungi, and cell-mediated and/or humoral immune responses elicited by antigens released by the invading organisms. Furthermore, the macrophage response frequently does not contain the invading organism, and the lesion grows progressively and may spread to other sites.

Immunogenic Granulomas

In this type of granuloma, in contrast to the foreign body reaction, the material, while still foreign, "activates" the mononuclear cells of the mononuclear phagocyte system. Conceptually, it is the counterpart of allergic contact dermatitis in contrast to irritant dermatitis, in that it is less frequent but causes more disability. In immunogenic granulomas the full spectrum of the mononuclear macrophage system is displayed—namely monocytes, secretory macrophages (epithelioid cells), and giant cells—and the hallmark in humans is the organized epithelioid cell response. Instead of acting as simple macrophages, the mononuclear cells proliferate in the tissue and differentiate into epithelioid cells, which organize to form tubercles. Clinically, the lesions generally appear more extensive than foreign body granulomas, but may present as localized, tumid lesions. The biopsy, however, shows the characteristic organized epithelioid cell granuloma, with epithelioid cells in the center and mononuclear cells outside forming new foci. The epithelioid cells are readily recognized by their gigantic nuclei with dustlike chromatin, delicate nuclear membrane, and extensive, vesicular cytoplasm taking up massive amounts of space, compared to the mononuclear cells, which are very much smaller and have dense chromatin in their nuclei.

The organized epithelioid cell granuloma is a fairly common type of granuloma in clinical diseases such as tuberculosis, sarcoidosis, and tuberculoid leprosy. Although it was thought long ago that these reactions might be allergic in nature, the proof of this came from the study of patients with axillary granulomas produced by zirconium-containing deodorant sticks (Shelley and Hurley, 1958). Shelley and Hurley (1958) showed that injection of tiny amounts of zirconium salts intradermally, in patients who were allergic to the deodorant sticks, produced a nodule at the injection site; when biopsied, the nodule reproduced the histology of the axillary lesions, namely an organized epithelioid cell granuloma.

Subsequently, it was shown (Epstein et al., 1963) that repeated injections of large amounts of zirconium lactate could induce altered tissue reactivity in humans. Initially, all the subjects showed foreign body responses to the injected zirconium, but once they had become sensitized the biopsy showed organized epithelioid cell granulomas and injections of small amounts of zirconium salts would now elicit pure epithelioid cell granulomas. Furthermore, the reaction was specific for zirconium salts; the sensitized subjects gave merely foreign body responses to injections of other metals, including silica. This finding, then, satisfied the criteria for allergy, namely that the reaction is an acquired, altered tissue reaction different from the response seen in a normal person and specific for the sensitizing metal. Attempts to develop an animal model of granulomatous hypersensitivity to metals have generally failed (Epstein, 1971). A report of success with zirconium in guinea pigs (Turk et al., 1978) is not reproducible and the reaction probably represented an effluorescent foreign body response (Epstein, 1971).

Toxicologists will see very few cutaneous problems involving organized epithelioid cell granulomas, but keep in mind that clinical observation alone cannot reliably distinguish foreign body from immunogenic granulomas; a biopsy must be secured to settle the issue. Metal-induced lesions provide the major source of industrial immunogenic granulomas. Pulmonary berylliosis remains a significant problem in certain industries (Hasan and Kazemi, 1964) and the increasing use of beryllium requires strict safeguards to protect workers. Beryllium oxide is a very potent inducer of granulomatous hypersensitivity; 0.1 ml of a 1% concentration injected id once sensitized four of five volunteers (Epstein, 1971). Cutaneous berylliosis, as developed from broken fluorescent lights (Dutra, 1949), has not been seen for many years, but each new projected use for beryllium and its salts must be carefully scrutinized for potential harm to the public.

The next most important offender is zirconium and its salts. As noted above, zirconium lactate in roll-on stick deodorants was responsible for an outbreak of axillary granulomas in the mid-1950s (Shelley and Hurley, 1958). Removal of the offending chemical led to a sharp decrease in the frequency of axillary granulomas seen by dermatologists. However, in the 1960s zirconium salts were introduced into over-the-counter poison ivy/oak medications and cases of zirconium granulomas began to be seen again (Epstein, 1967, 1971). Fortunately, the number has been small, probably because zirconium is a much weaker sensitizer than beryllium. Repeated injections of 4% zirconium lactate sensitized less than 1% of a large number of volunteers (Epstein, 1971). Nevertheless, zirconium-containing lotions are no more help than calamine in treating poison ivy dermatitis, and on a benefit/risk basis they probably should be dropped from the market. At present, zirconium complexed with aluminum salts with and without glycine is available in several deodorants. Most of these have been tested in zirconium-sensitive subjects and found not to elicit granuloma formation, even when applied under occlusion to damaged skin (W. L. Epstein, unpublished results). Apparently, a complex is formed that makes zirconium unavailable as an antigen. The nature of the complex is not known.

Very rarely, other metals such as cobalt and chromium have been implicated in immunogenic granuloma formation.

Low- and High-Turnover Granulomas

This is an important concept, which is related biologically to how the mononuclear phagocyte system handles an insoluble irritant. If the foreign body is truly inert and relatively easily ingested, the macrophage may simply sequester the material and hold it for years, essentially out of the body's homeostatic economy. Most tattoos behave in this fashion. Experimentally, carrageenin has been shown to produce low-turnover granulomas in animals (Spector, 1974). Rapid turnover of cells in the granuloma occurs when the irritant stirs up more of an inflammatory response, as seen with BCG injections in animals (Ando et al., 1972) and the hepatic granulomas experimentally produced by schistosome eggs (Nishimura et al., 1981). Very few data on humans have been collected, but we believe pulmonary silicosis is a high-turnover lesion because of the cellular injury produced by ingested material. Using tritiated thymidine, we found labeled epitheloid cells regularly 2 wk after injection (Epstein, 1971) but almost never after 4 or 5 wk.

DIAGNOSTIC WORK-UP OF SUSPECTED GRANULOMAS IN SKIN

When confronted with such cases, the first step is to ascertain whether one is dealing with a medical or a toxicological problem. Dermatologic consultation may prove rewarding if there is a unique clinical pattern, but more often a biopsy will be required. Make sure the tissue is evaluated by a histopathologist knowledgeable in the vagaries and complexities of cutaneous granulomas. The toxicologists' contribution is to keep in mind the potential role of foreign substances, because even the most experienced histopathologists frequently overlook this in their interpretations. Since foreign bodies are often coated with mucoglycoproteins before ingestion, it may prove useful to initially ask for special stains, such as toluidine blue, which stains silica metachromatically, or a periodic acid-Schiff (PAS) diastase, which stains many fungi and plant spicules. Also, examining the tissue under polarized light, especially toluidine blue-stained sections, will quickly indicate the presence of foreign objects such as misplaced keratin or silica. Alternatively, phase microscopy can be used. Sometimes microincineration of the tissue sections will help. More drastic manipulations such as those involved in direct chemical analysis and X-ray diffraction have their place, and the toxicologist should know where such facilities are available in the community. Recently, analytic electron microscopy has become more generally available (Mehard and Epstein, 1981; Andres et al., 1980), and if one is careful about interpretation (Mehard and Epstein, 1981) the findings can be especially helpful in the toxicological work-up of granulomatous lesions.

The presence of an immunogenic granuloma should arouse suspicions of a medical problem, and most of the time the undiagnosed immunogenic granuloma will prove to be sarcoidosis. But an awareness of the regional distribution of sarcoid reactions (James, 1972) will prevent embarrassment.

And every now and again the alert toxicologist will uncover a new cause of metal-induced immunogenic granulomas.

REFERENCES

Aalto, M., Potila, M., and Kulonen, E. 1976. The effect of silica-treated macrophages on the synthesis of collagen and other proteins *in vitro. Exp. Cell Res.* 97:193.

Ando, M., Newberg, A. M., and Shima, K. 1972. Macrophage accumulation, division, maturation, and digestive and microcidal capacities in tuberculous lesions. *J. Immunol.* 109:8.

Andres, T. L., Vallyathan, N. V., and Madison, J. F. 1980. Electron-probe microanalysis: Aid in the study of skin granulomas. *Arch. Dermatol.* 116:1272.

Beerman, H. and Lane, R. A. G. 1954. Tattoo. *Am. J. Med. Sci.* 227:444.

Dutra, F. R. 1949. Beryllium granulomas of the skin. *Arch. Dermatol.* 60:1140.

Epstein, W. L. 1967. Granulomatous hypersensitivity. *Prog. Allergy* 11:36.

Epstein, W. L. 1971. Metal-induced granulomatous hypersensitivity in man. *Adv. Biol. Skin* 11:313.

Epstein, W. L. 1980. Foreign body granulomas. In *Basic and Clinical Aspects of Granulomatous Diseases,* eds. D. Boros and H. Yoshida, pp. 181–197. Amsterdam: Elsevier/North Holland.

Epstein, W. L. 1982. Granulomas of the skin. In *Pathology of Granulomas,* ed. H. Ioachim. New York: Raven. In press.

Epstein, W. L., Shahen, J. R., and Krasnobrod, H. 1963. The organized epithelioid cell granuloma: Differentiation of allergic (zirconium) from colloidal (silica) types. *Am. J. Pathol.* 43:391.

Eskeland, G., Langmark, F., and Husby, G. 1974. Silica granuloma of the skin and subcutaneous tissue. *Acta Pathol. Microbiol. Scand. Suppl.* 248:69.

Hasan, F. M. and Kazemi, H. 1974. Chronic beryllium disease: A continuing epidemiologic hazard. *Chest* 65:289.

James, D. G. 1972. All that glitters is not sarcoidosis. *Trans. St. John's Hosp. Dermatol. Soc.* 58:17.

Kessel, R. W. I., Monaco, L., and Marchisio, M. A. 1963. The specificity of the cytotoxic action of silica. *Br. J. Exp. Pathol.* 44:351.

Kilroe-Smith, T. A., Webster, I., van Drimmelman, M., et al. 1973. An insoluble fibrogenic factor in macrophages from guinea pigs exposed to silica. *Environ. Res.* 6:298.

Mehard, C. W. and Epstein, W. L. 1981. The diagnosis of zirconium induced skin granuloma by X-ray microanalysis. In *Analytical Electron Microscopy,* ed. R. H. Geiss, pp. 79–86. San Francisco: San Francisco Press.

Nelson, D. S. 1973. Production by stimulated macrophages of factors depressing lymphocyte transformation. *Nature (Lond.)* 246:306.

Nishimura, M., Fukuyama, K., and Epstein, W. L. 1981. Epithelioid cell granuloma autografts in mouse skin. *Clin. Res.* 29:502A.

Shelley, W. B. and Hurley, H. J. 1958. The allergic origin of zirconium deodorant granulomas. *Br. J. Dermatol.* 70:75.

Spector, W. G. 1974. The macrophage: Its origins and role in pathology. *Pathobiol. Annu.* 4:33.

Turk, J. L., Badenoch-Jones, P., and Parker, D. 1978. Ultrastructural observations on epithelioid cell granulomas induced by zirconium in the guinea-pig. *J. Pathol.* 124:45.

van Furth, R., Cohn, Z. A., Hirsch, J. G., et al. 1973. The mononuclear phagocyte system. *Bull. WHO* 49:845.

Virchow, R. 1864–1865. *Vorlesungen uber Pathologie*, vol. 3, part 2, *Onkologie*, p. 385. Berlin: Hirschwald.

28

eye irritation

T. O. McDonald ▪ Van Seabaugh ▪ John A. Shadduck
▪ Henry F. Edelhauser ▪

INTRODUCTION

Ocular irritation testing represents an important step in the safety evaluation of many substances. Significant advances in reliability, predictability, and reproducibility have been made. Marzulli and Simon (1971) reviewed this subject.

Historical Perspective on Eye Irritancy Evaluation

In 1944, two groups of investigators described methods for grading reactions of eyes to ocular irritants. Friedenwald et al. (1944) studied the effect of various acidic and basic solutions on eyes of rabbits and recorded their observations using a numerical grading system in which reactions of cornea, conjunctiva, and iris were evaluated. Brief descriptions were provided which correlated the nature of the reaction with the number used for scoring. Lesions of increasing severity received higher scores. Carpenter and Smyth (1946) also described an ocular scoring system for grading and comparing ocular lesions in rabbits. The system was devised independently of Friedenwald et al. but was similar to their system in some respects. Since Carpenter

The assistance of A. R. Borgmann, C. A. Robb, H. Hugh Harroff, Beverely Britton, Katherine Kasten, Stan Gregg, and Ron Hervey is gratefully acknowledged. The Pharmaceutical Development Department and Word Processing Center of Alcon Laboratories contributed significantly.

The contents of this chapter represent the individuals' viewpoint and not that of any federal agency.

and Smyth tested many industrial materials, their scores were designed for recording corneal necrosis but conjunctival changes were not scored.

Draize et al. (1944) described an eye irritancy grading system for use in evaluating the potential ocular irritative effect of drugs and other materials intended for use in or around the eye. Numerical scores (somewhat different from those of Friedenwald et al.) were given for reactions of cornea, conjunctiva, and iris. Brief verbal descriptions were provided to guide the observer in converting the changes noted to the numerical score. The authors also specified the number of animals (albino rabbits) to be used and provided techniques for application (frequency and route of administration) of the irritants. This paper had a profound influence on ocular irritation testing and subsequently became the official Food and Drug Administration (FDA) test method.

The Draize scoring system (Draize et al., 1944) provided numerical equivalents for brief subjective statements of ocular reactions seen in cornea, conjunctiva, and iris. For example, corneal reactions were scored according to the density of corneal opacities and the area of the cornea involved on a scale of 0-4. Iridal reactions and conjunctival responses had similar numerical scores. The total ocular irritation score was calculated by a formula that gave very heavy weight (80 of 110 points) to corneal changes. The evaluation of ocular responses by Draize et al. (1944) was done without the aid of magnification devices, although Friedenwald et al. (1944) employed a loupe or slit lamp to grade corneal edema.[1]

Studies of ocular irritation induced by many different substances have subsequently been reported. Hazelton (1952) used the Draize scoring system to evaluate the irritative effect of several surfactants. Hazelton demonstrated wetting agents which, if foamed well, would probably be irritants. Cationic materials appeared to precipitate protein and were accompanied by generalized irritation and a high incidence of corneal opacity. The nonprotein-coagulating surfactants, primarily in the nonionic groups, produced less severe corneal opacities. The data were interpreted as indicating that the order of irritation for detergents was cationic > anionic > nonionic. These results were supported later in an *in vitro* study of bovine corneas in which the order of effectiveness in reducing electrical resistance, increasing the rate of potassium exchange, and increasing hydration was shown to be cationic > anionic > nonionic detergents (Carter et al., 1973).

Kay and Calandra (1962) evaluated the Federal Hazardous Substances Act (FHSA) criteria of pass or fail. They used the ocular scoring scheme of Draize et al. (1944) to devise descriptive eye irritation ratings for nonirritating

---

[1] It should be noted here that Draize et al. (1944) not only described a scoring system but also gave several regimens for applying materials and recommended the number of rabbits to be used. We use the term "Draize scoring system" here to refer to the scoring system without implying that other parts of the original methods were used.

to maximally irritating in a total of eight grades. They noted that many cosmetic products would require labeling as eye irritants by the FHSA criteria, but in their system some separation of various levels of severity was possible. They stressed the difficulty of devising a numerical system for scoring or classifying eye irritants which is totally adequate.

Russell and Hock (1962) submitted shampoos to several laboratories and noted marked variability among the results reported. There was some disagreement for two sets of three rabbits treated with identical test samples at the same laboratory. The scores for the cornea, iris, and conjunctiva covered wide ranges when one laboratory was compared to the next. Verbal descriptions of the effects induced by the same formulation were variable among laboratories with ratings of the same sample ranging from a mild to a moderate ocular irritant. They believed results would be improved if standard methods were available to instill materials into eyes and if a "standard irritant" existed against which to compare other materials.

Gaunt and Harper (1964) concluded that a fairly consistent pattern of ocular responses was obtained regardless of the test method used. They noted that dilution was a critical factor and substantial dilution with water prior to instillation into the eye could prevent expression of the full irritancy of the formulation. They recommended that eyes should be irrigated with water after ocular instillation of the test irritant.

Battista and McSweeney (1965) developed approaches for quantitation of methods for testing of eye irritation. They noted that substances which were quite severely irritating were damaging to the rabbit eye and were readily recognized. It was more difficult to test materials that were nonirritating or mildly irritating or to compare the eye irritancy of related formulations. The methods available were unreliable and yielded erroneous or ambiguous data. In an attempt to partially control this, they developed a corneal applicator for the dispensing of the test formulation onto the cornea in a uniform manner.

Battista and McSweeney (1965) noted that inclusion of discharge and chemosis in conjunctiva scores was a source of variation. Numerical scores for these lesions were of little value unless it was clearly established that the results were not influenced by factors such as ocular infection. The authors concluded that iris, cornea, and conjunctiva should be considered individually and the maximum response alone, rather than the area involved, be used in estimating the severity of ocular injury.

Beckley (1965a) reviewed the literature and sent questionnaires to various laboratories and manufacturers of drugs, cosmetics, and household products asking for methods used to perform and interpret tests for eye irritancy. This paper summarized the results obtained from his questionnaire and contained a list of comments and recommendations for improving the FHSA for eye irritancy evaluation. He recommended the use of a set of reference standards for irritation. Beckley also concluded that at least two animal species, the rabbit and either the dog or the monkey, should be included in eye irritancy testing.

Alexander (1965) reported one incident in 1951 in which a product was marketed that had passed eye irritation tests in rabbits and yet produced minor ocular lesions in some persons.

Bonfield and Scala (1965) evaluated 13 shampoos. Only one shampoo was free of ocular irritative effects 14 days after instillation and even it produced irritation in irrigated eyes 7 days after instillation. They considered the Draize eye test as a useful tool in screening materials for eye irritancy but suggested that other means or methods should be utilized before new material is thoroughly evaluated in humans.

The *Illustrated guide for grading eye irritation by hazardous substances* appeared in 1965 (FDA, 1965). It provided color illustrations and short descriptions of the effects noted in rabbit eyes following instillation of an irritant. The color photographs provided an important reference for standardization of ocular irritation test scores. Scores for individual ocular changes were based on Draize's system (Draize, 1959) but were recorded individually and not summed.

Weltman et al. (1965) combined the Draize (1959) procedures and additional techniques such as photographic collection of data and opthalmoscopic and histologic observations. The objective was to reduce subjective errors and improve evaluation and assessment of eye irritation. They also considered the role of population size, the time of release of the lids after topical ocular instillations, and other factors that might affect the course of the eye irritation. They observed that the individual scoring or subjective errors were a relatively minor influence, but could not rule out the possibility that variations among scores recorded by differently trained individuals from two laboratories may be considerable. The study also demonstrated that one could have considerable differences between total mean scores of various test groups with studies containing 4, 8, or 24 eyes. Statistical analysis demonstrated the greater validity of values based on samples of sufficient population size. Weltman et al. felt that increasing the number of rabbits used in the standard Draize test would be helpful in avoiding the pass-fail errors that can occur by chance when small populations are employed. They concluded that eight eyes was a substantial number. Their data indicated that early release of the lids had an ultimately beneficial effect, which was attributed to eye wash by lacrimation. They noted that the techniques of different laboratories relative to the release of the lids after topical ocular instillation varied and this could contribute to the variability noted among laboratories.

Variability among laboratories has not been resolved. Weltman et al. (1965) stated that the greatest variability was due to the animal itself. Unfortunately there were (and still are) no standard strains of rabbit used for eye tests. In the rabbit, they felt that age, sex, and strain differences could affect the resistance of the laboratory animal to either chemical or physical states of stress. This aspect has yet to be investigated and still warrants attention. In attempting to interpret the usefulness of photographic, ophthalmoscopic, and histologic methods for assessing eye irritation, they noted that the photographic method could permanently record the external appearance and the physical state of the eye within certain limits. The slit lamp assisted in determining location, extent, and depth of corneal, iridial, and lens damage, and also permitted observation of changes in the anterior and posterior chambers of the eye. The use of the slit lamp has been advocated by others (Marzulli, 1968; Baldwin et al., 1973; Marzulli and Ruggles, 1973). Weltman et al. (1965) also noted that histologic procedures could more fully ascertain and permanently record the structural damage done to tissues and cells of the eye.

Ballantyne and Swanston (1972) pointed out that ocular scores published in the literature were uninformative about responses of individual tissues and this was a major limitation of the Draize system (Draize et al., 1944). Identical mean Draize scores could result from two entirely different reactions. Investigators, they felt, must keep ocular scores separate for each ocular tissue, as indicated in the *Illustrated guide* (FDA, 1965). In contrast, Ashford and Lamble (1974) pointed out that their method of assigning numerical values to a number of suitable symptoms and totaling them to give an overall description of the syndrome is valid if it correctly arranges the eyes in order of clinical severity. Shuster and Kaufman (1974), however, noted that addition of the scores assigned to different tissues or responses was statistically improper since some lesions or signs are more important than others. For example, mild but persistent corneal lesions are more ominous than severe but transient conjunctival hyperemia.

Ocular irritation is now evaluated routinely for a wide variety of materials. Some aspects of potential importance have received relatively little attention. For example, Aronson et al. (1966) demonstrated that the prolonged topical ocular instillation of allergenic materials could result in ocular lesions. More studies are needed to determine whether an allergenic or sensitizing response can be observed by the topical instillation of materials.

Schuck et al. (1966) devised a procedure for evaluating the ocular irritation potential of atmospheric pollutants in human eyes. A dose-response study of the major pollutants was performed to determine the level at which an irritation response was observed.

MECHANISMS OF OCULAR RESPONSE
TO IRRITANTS

An understanding of the origin and significance of ocular lesions is central to their recognition and correct interpretation. A brief summary of the pathogenesis of topical ocular injury is presented below, together with a brief description of the normal histology of each tissue (Prince et al., 1960; Marzulli and Simon, 1971; Fine and Yanoff, 1972).

Conjunctiva

The conjunctiva is squamous, nonkeratinized epithelium that contains numerous mucus-secreting cells. The bulbar conjunctival epithelium has fewer goblet cells and is less glandular than the palpebral conjunctival epithelium. More polyhedral cells appear in the palpebral conjunctiva and the surface cells are more stratified, like those of corneal epithelium. The outermost cell surfaces are covered by numerous microvilli (Phister, 1975). Melanophores are frequently present in the conjunctiva, particularly the bulbar conjunctiva near the limbus. They are, of course, absent in albino rabbits.

Visible through the conjunctiva on the posterior surface of the lids are the Meibomian glands (specialized sebaceous glands), which are parallel rows of lobulated glands with ducts opening into the rims of the eyelids. Modified sweat glands (of Moll) are also present in the eyelid and they open near the cilia (eyelashes) somewhat anterior to the outlets of the Meibomian glands. Many of the ducts of the glands of Moll also empty into the ciliary follicles. In some species there are also rudimentary sebaceous glands (of Zeiss), which open into the ciliary follicles. Rabbits also have accessory lacrimal glands in the conjunctiva around the Meibomian glands.

The nictitating membrane or third eyelid is a prominent and important structure in many common animal species and is especially prominent in rabbits. It is attached in the medial canthus of the eye and moves laterally or diagonally across the eye behind the external lids. The membrana nictitans consists of a T-shaped skeleton of cartilage covered by a layer of squamous epithelium. There are small lymphoid follicles and a prominent secretory gland, which is similar in many ways to accessory lacrimal glands. In rabbits, the gland of the nictitating membrane and Harder's glands are very similar histologically. The nictitating gland may be continuous with Harder's gland, which lies adjacent to the globe at the depth of the medial canthus (Prince et al., 1960). Harder's gland is present in rabbits but not in humans and nonhuman primates. The lacrimal gland is very large in the rabbit. It nearly encloses the globe near the orbital rim. The lacrimal gland is serous, while the glans nicitans and Harder's glands of the rabbit secrete lipid materials. Each of these glandular structures can affect ocular irritation scores, either directly by contributing to exudates and discharges or indirectly by altering the properties or concentrations of materials applied to the eye. Despite the relatively large size of the ocular glands, tearing in the rabbit is much less vigorous than in humans (Buehler and Newmann, 1964).

Vessels of the conjunctiva are prominent. They generally run in two layers, a deep and a more superficial group. The deep vessels are direct branches of the anterior ciliary arteries, while the superficial vessels are derived from the branches of this artery that supply the fornix. The vascular supply is greatest on the bulbar conjunctiva and less on the conjunctiva of the lids. There are two systems of lymphatics. The one within the fibrous layer contains larger vessels, while the one adjacent to the more superficial capillary blood vessels contains smaller lymphatic channels.

The various secretory cells and glands of the lids and orbit contribute significantly to normal corneal function. In addition to the washing and sweeping actions alluded to earlier, secretions of serous, fatty, and mucinous materials contribute to the tear film (precorneal film). This thin layer of liquid covers the cornea under normal circumstances and plays a vital role in the wettability of corneal epithelium. In particular, glycoproteins from the conjunctiva contribute to the stability and effectiveness of the tear film (Holly and Lemp, 1971). Materials that interfere with the stability or sources of the components of the film can seriously affect the corneal epithelium and may eventually result in corneal ulcers (Dohlman, 1971).

There is frequently a rather rapid response following topical administration of irritants. The subject often blinks rapidly, tearing may occur, and a sudden increase in the apparent vascularity of the conjunctiva is seen. It is difficult to evaluate accurately the effect these responses play in diluting and changing the pH, ionic concentration, and so forth of ocular irritants.

If the irritant persists or if it elicits a more prolonged reaction, more dramatic changes occur. They include continued secretion from the various conjunctival and orbital glands and accumulation of these materials on lid margins, at the medial canthus, and even on the haired skin of the lower lid. Continued irritation results in continued dilation of the conjunctival vascular bed. This is recognized clinically as increased redness and vascular injection (congestion). Intravascular stasis and/or injury to endothelial cells of the microcirculation (directly by the irritant or indirectly by release of chemical mediators of inflammation) results in escape of intravascular fluids and their accumulation in the loose subjunctival connective tissues. This results in edema (chemosis) and is recognized by bulging of the conjunctiva, especially of the palpebral conjunctiva, which may eventually prevent normal lid closure (Hogan and Zimmerman, 1962).

Cornea

The cornea consists of five layers; from without inwards they are epithelium, Bowman's membrane, stroma, Descemet's membrane, and endothelium. The epithelial layer is made up of several layers of cells and is approximately 10% of the total corneal thickness in humans and most other mammals. The innermost layer of cells is a basal cell layer, which is columnar and closely packed. Middle layer cells are more flattened and become thinner and wider, until finally in the superficial layers the outermost cells are flat and squamoid. Cell membranes are markedly interdigitated and connected by desmosomes. Interdigitation become less tortuous and intercellular spaces widen between the desmosomes as the surface is approached (Phister, 1973). Cytoplasmic projections exist on the outer surfaces of the superficial epithelial cells. The density of these projections per unit surface area and their organization vary from area to area on the cornea. Shifts in the organization occur apparently as part of normal metabolic events. On the outermost surface there is an osmophilic layer of material, which constitutes the lipid film on the surface of the corneal epithelium.

Stroma makes up about nine-tenths of the thickness of the cornea in most mammals. It is divided into sheets of collagenous material, which lie parallel to the surface and have numerous cells (corneal keratocytes) scattered throughout them. Blood vessels and lymphatics are absent except at the extreme periphery. The lamellae are formed of fibrous bands of collagen that run uninterruptedly from limbus to limbus, with the possible exception of the most superficial layer of the stroma, which appears to be slightly inter-digitated. The most anterior portion of the stromal zone forms Bowman's membrane in humans and nonhuman primates. This is a sheet approximately 12 μm thick that is distinguishable under ordinary light microscopic conditions. In most other mammals this zone is very thin (in rabbits it is about 2μm thick) or suggested only as a condensation of the stromal surface.

In addition to the specialized organization in sheets or lamellae and the relatively smaller diameters of the collagen fibrils, the other unique feature of the corneal stroma which contributes to transparency is its relative degree of hydration in comparison to the sclera. The water content of the stroma is approximately 78% in most species, while, in comparison, the sclera is approximately 68% water (Maurice, 1969).

The endothelium is a single layer of cells, which completely covers the posterior surface of the cornea and forms a hexagonal matrix when viewed from the flat surface or via the slit lamp. The cells vary slightly in thickness from species to species, being approximately 4-5 μm thick in humans but somewhat thinner in other species. Nuclei are large, flat, and oval or round. There are intracellular spaces, although the passageways between the anterior chamber and basement membrane are very tortuous. On the apical surfaces the cells are attached by zonula occludentes.

Descemet's membrane is an elastic sheet, which is 5-10 μm thick in humans (7 or 8 μm in the rabbit) and bounds the inner surface of the stroma. It is the exaggerated basement membrane of the endothelium. While appearing structureless under light microscopy, in the electron microscope it has some organization, particularly in the anterior zone.

The transitional zone (limbus) is the region in which the cornea adjoins the sclera; it is important in the study of corneal injury because one of the sources of fluid and cells is the blood vessel meshwork lying in the limbus. As one approaches the limbus the number of cells in the epithelial layer of the cornea increases and their morphologic appearance varies to approach that of conjunctival epithelium. Descemet's layer splits and begins to merge with the trabeculae of the angle of the anterior chamber together with the endo-thelium. The collagen fibrils continue into the scleral stroma. In the limbus the diameter of the fibrils is greater than that in the cornea, and they begin to assume the appearance of twisted bundles of fibers. There is a rich vascular plexus and capillary loops enter a short distance into the stroma, particularly in the superficial layers. This is quite prominent in albino rabbits (Prince et al., 1960).

Animal corneas differ from those of humans in several ways. Those in the rabbit and other common infrahuman species are thinner than those of humans. Epithelial layers are usually somewhat thinner, although usually five or six layers can be seen in rabbits and seven to ten layers occur in humans. Major differences occur in the structure of Bowman's membrane, which is essentially unrecognizable in rabbits but is prominent in human and nonhuman primate eyes. Thicknesses are given as 8–12 μm (human) and 1.75–2.0 μm (rabbit) in histological sections (Carpenter and Smyth, 1946; Prince et al., 1960). The stromal thickness accounts for the bulk of the difference in corneal thickness among most mammals. The stromal lamellae are more loosely arranged in the rabbit than the human eye. Descemet's membrane and the endothelial layer are quite similar among various mammals.

The cornea maintains its normal state of transparency in part by maintaining the peculiar arrangement of lamellae of collagen fibers. Destruction of either of the limiting cell layers will result in swelling of the corneal stroma. The swelling is the result of imbibition of fluid through the damaged epithelial or endothelial cell layers. Fluid can also enter from the capillary plexus at the limbus, particularly in situations where inflammatory irritation of the vascular endothelium occurs. Swelling appears to take place first in the anterior, more irregular layers of the stroma. The expansion takes place within lamellae and may be the result of fluid imbibition into the mucopolysaccharide ground substance around the collagen fibers. In the grossly swollen cornea of the rabbit, stroma appears to be divided sharply into anterior and posterior zones. The posterior zones show lamination into alternate sheets of greater or lesser cloudiness, suggesting that the lamellae are separating.

The corneal epithelium is highly resistant to fat-insoluble substances. Since it is probable that many substances penetrate at the epithelium largely by way of intracellular spaces, the outer layers of cells may offer great resistance to the movement, because the flattened forms increase the path distance from one face to the other, while at the same time the total area into which ions may penetrate is very much reduced.

Examination of the cornea includes evaluation of stromal lesions and epithelial lesions. Corneal cloudiness is contributed to by edema of the stroma and infiltration of inflammatory cells into the cornea. Increases in intensity or severity of corneal cloudiness indicate increasingly severe stromal lesions. Epithelial lesions may occur independently of corneal opacity (cloudiness) provided the basal cell layer of the corneal epithelium is not destroyed. Careful examination is necessary to detect these changes, and fluorescein is frequently recommended as an aid in detecting small epithelial defects. Careful examination of the cornea with magnification and various light sources will also often reveal fine opacities associated with mild epithelial injury. Materials that cause denudation of epithelium and exposure of the stroma are of much greater consequence. Corneal epithelium can rapidly migrate across epithelial defects and cover even denuded but otherwise intact Bowman's membrane. Rabbit cornea seems to reepithelize much more slowly than human cornea (Carpenter and Smyth, 1946). Injuries that affect large areas of the corneal surface and penetrate to Bowman's membrane significantly interfere with this process. Even punctate lesions that penetrate into and damage Bowman's membrane are serious because of the vital role played by the superficial stromal layers in effecting epithelization.

It should be noted that ocular irritants can induce corneal stromal edema by their action on the prominent vessels at the limbus and that this can occur without substantial injury to corneal epithelium. Prolonged damage to the cornea, especially persistent corneal edema, results in endothelial proliferation from limbal vessels and the extension of vascular loops toward the center of the cornea (pannus). Vascularization of the cornea occurs readily in rabbits. Permanent corneal opacities may result from the more severe lesions of stroma and epithelium.

Iris

There are close anatomic relationships involving both nerves and blood vessels between the cornea and the iris. In addition, the posterior surfaces of the cornea and the iris communicate directly via the aqueous humor, which bathes them both. Therefore, ocular irritants applied topically may produce alterations in the iris.

The iris is an extremely vascular structure which is heavily pigmented (except in albinos). The bulk of the iris is made up of loose connective tissue stroma in which the vessels, muscles, and pigmented cells are included. Vascular patterns vary. In humans a major arterial circle is recognized at the root of the iris, from which vessels extend in a radial pattern toward the pupil. They join to form a lesser vascular circle at the collarette. Small vessels then continue to supply the thinner portion of the iris between the collarette and the pupillary margin.

The New Zealand albino rabbit usually employed in ocular irritation studies allows one to observe the iris vessels easily. Beginning from the 3:00 and 9:00 o'clock positions there are four vessels, two going to the upper part of the iris, while two others go to the lower part of the iris (Fig. 1; Figs. 1–12, reproduced in full color, are found between pages 568 and 569). These vessels are referred to as primary vessels. Branches coming off the primary vessels which are parallel to each other in a line in the direction of the pupillary border are referred to as secondary vessels. Branching off from the secondary vessels are very small branches (tertiary vessels).

The surface topography of the iris is characterized by a series of radiating furrows, which run from base to pupillary margin. The posterior surface is covered by a layer of cuboidal epithelial cells, which are heavily pigmented except in albinos.

Injury to the iris is detected by observing changes in the vessels of the iris, the thickness of the iridal stroma, and aqueous flare. As in the conjunctiva, the vessels of the iris become hyperemic following irritation. This change can be observed directly. Additional fluid may leak from the vessels and be imbibed by the iris stroma, causing swelling (edema) of the stroma. More severe injury may result in exudation of high molecular weight proteins and cells, resulting in more severe edema and aqueous flare.

The Tyndall phenomenon observed in the anterior chamber is known as aqueous flare. In the normal anterior chamber, there is the absence of an observable light beam as it passes through the aqueous humor. Release of proteinaceous material or cells contributes to changing the refractive index of light in the anterior chamber and gives rise to the Tyndall phenomenon. The presence of aqueous flare is presumptive evidence of breakdown of the blood-aqueous barrier. An interesting phenomenon of direct importance for eye irritation studies is known as "consensual breakdown" of the blood-aqueous barrier (Davson, 1969). It has been observed that a highly irritative substance applied topically to one eye potentiates the breakdown of the barrier by a less irritating substance in the opposite eye. This can be detected by observing an increase in the aqueous level of intravenously administered Evans blue. The importance of this phenomenon in conventional ocular irritation testing has not been determined. However, it seems possible that a highly irritative substance in one eye could give an artificially high reading in the iritis and flare scores of a less irritative substance in the opposite eye.

Although the term iritis is sometimes used to describe all changes in the iris, it should be recognized that iritis correctly refers to inflammation of the iris. Other, less severe changes such as injection of iridial vessels (hyperemia) and leakage of fluids into the iris stroma (edema) precede frank iritis.

Marzulli and Simon (1971) recently reviewed many of the factors that influence animal responses to ocular irritants. In addition to the anatomical features reviewed above, methods of application of irritants and the chemical nature of the material are important. The chemical structure will influence the rate of corneal penetration. Penetration is related to the lipoidal and hydrophilic properties of the material, since substances must first mix with the fatty precorneal film and then penetrate the hydropic corneal tissue. Penetration is achieved best by substances with maximum aqueous and lipid solubility (Havener, 1966). Osmolarity of the materials bathing the cornea and their ability to combine with corneal fluid and structural components also influence the action of these materials as irritants (Marzulli and Simon, 1971).

ANIMAL TESTS AS PREDICTORS OF HUMAN RESPONSES

One of the major issues in any test conducted to evaluate hazard to humans is how nearly the test animals actually predict the human response.

Probably the single most important factor is selection of a test animal. Ideally, the animal would be neither more nor less sensitive than the human, would predict human response accurately over a wide range of materials and their attendant effects, and would be readily available, inexpensive, and yield consistently reproducible data. In ocular irritation testing the albino rabbit has been used most frequently. However, other species, especially dogs and nonhuman primates (Rhesus monkey), have also been suggested as suitable animals in some circumstances (Beckley, 1965b).

The albino rabbit has obvious advantages for testing ocular irritants. The animal itself is readily available; it is docile, easily handled, relatively inexpensive, and easy to maintain. The eye is large and the corneal surface and bulbar conjunctival areas are both large and easily observed. The iris is unpigmented, allowing ready observation of the iridal vessels.

There are also deficiencies in the rabbit model. Some anatomic differences between rabbit and human eyes have already been mentioned. In addition, despite the general marked improvement in standardization of laboratory animals over the last few years, there are still significant variations among laboratory rabbits. Age, strain, and sex differences as well as variations in general health status can be expected to influence ocular irritation tests (Weltman et al., 1965).

Limited experience with Rhesus monkeys (Beckley et al., 1969) indicated that these animals more nearly reflected human responses than did rabbits. However, there are very real problems in using monkeys. They are very costly and are now very difficult to obtain. Restraint can be difficult, and they are even less uniform than rabbits. Their pigmented irises make observation of some irritation responses more difficult to evaluate, although Mann and Pullinger (1942) suggested that rabbits with pigmented irises are more appropriate than albinos for studying iris lesions.

Another important problem in selecting an animal model that will accurately predict the nature of the human response is lack of adequate information on how humans can be expected to react. Thus, it is not entirely clear what the animal model is expected to predict. McLaughlin (1946) did a retrospective study on industrial accidents in humans which resulted in ocular damage. A total of 602 cases of ocular injury were recorded among 3,566 patients referred to the dispensary of a manufacturing plant. Of these, 458 cases demonstrated mild, reversible (by 48 hr) ocular lesions, 37 cases required up to 10 days to heal, and 7 involved loss of vision. The majority of the offending agents were alkalis, but many details were not provided. Clinical studies of this type are needed, but information on the irritating substance, its concentration, and the exposure conditions would enhance their value.

A number of studies have been made in which the ocular irritative effects of various materials in humans and animals can be compared. The bulk of these studies were done in rabbits. Despite the relative lack of studies in which animal and human responses have been carefully compared under comparable, controlled conditions, there are a number of instances in which reactions in rabbits have generally predicted the observed effects in humans. Leopold (1945) observed that benzalkonium chloride concentrations of 0.03% or greater were irritating in rabbits. A similar reaction has been noted in humans, and several ophthalmic formulations that contain 0.02% benzalkonium chloride have not had any obvious effects. Our own experience is that 0.02% causes no conjunctival irritation in the rabbit, but 0.04% produces obvious ocular irritation (conjunctival congestion, swelling, discharge, and occasional corneal cloudiness).

Slight conjunctival hyperemia was observed after topical ocular instillation in rabbits of propylene glycol (Carpenter and Smyth, 1946). It is noninjurious for human eyes but does produce a transient stinging, blepharospasm, and lacrimation followed by mild conjunctiva hyperemia (Grant, 1974). A 70% concentration has been used as a treatment for corneal edema (Bietti and Giraldi, 1969).

Several liquid hydrocarbons of petroleum, including kerosene, Deo-Base, Stoddard solvent, and petroleum oil, were not harmful for the rabbit and human cornea after direct external contact (Carpenter and Smyth, 1946; Grant, 1974). Similar threshold concentrations (0.5%) for conjunctival irritation were noted for phenethyl alcohol in humans and rabbits (Nakano, 1958; Barkman et al., 1969). Comparable evidence of blepharospasm without ocular damage was noted for rabbit and human eyes after ocular exposure to a commercial preparation of dimercaprol (Grant, 1974).

Human and rabbit eyes reacted similarly to topical ocular oxalic acid (Suker, 1913; McLaughlin, 1946; Grant, 1974). It produced a corneal burn with loss of epithelium but recovery followed in a few days.

No ocular effects were noted in monkeys, humans, and rabbits when 0.1% cytarabine HCl was topically instilled six times a day for 6-10 days (Elliott and Schut, 1965). However, 0.5 and 1.0% solutions produced transient speckling, which resembled fine dust particles as seen on retroillumination of rabbit, monkey, and human corneas. McLaughlin (1946) and Grant (1974) reported that humans exhibited only slight corneal epithelial disturbances (clearing within 24-48 hr) after a splash of 5% sodium hypochlorite. There was transient corneal haze and conjunctival edema in rabbits, with a return to normal by a day or less (Grant, 1974). Carter and Griffith (1965) reported that monkey eyes healed faster than rabbit eyes after exposure to 5.5% sodium hypochlorite.

The threshold irritation concentration for tetraethoxysilane was 700 ppm for rabbit, guinea pig, and human eyes (Grant, 1974; Smyth and Seaton, 1940). Friemann and Overhoff (1956) and Grant (1974) noted that local application of a 1:5,000 (0.02%) solution of colchicine in humans produced very little ocular change, whereas serious reactions were noted with a 1% solution. The 1% solution caused clouding of the stroma with reduced vision, but the cornea cleared in a few weeks. In rabbit eyes, the same solution caused cellular infiltration in the cornea and vascularization which required several weeks before the eyes began to clear.

Full-strength polysorbate 80 (Tween 80) was nonirritating for rabbits. It was well tolerated and nonirritating at 20% concentration in several ophthalmic formulations and at a 9:1 ratio in castor oil for prolonged daily clinical use in humans (Hagiwara and Sugiwia, 1953; Treon, 1965). In our laboratories, we observed comparable minimal to moderate conjunctival congestion in rabbits and humans for 1% and 10% tetracycline ointments.

Podophyllum (Grant, 1974) in humans can produce discomfort, epiphora, and conjunctival hyperemia with slight exposure, but greater exposures may involve loss of the corneal epithelium, severe keratitis, and deposits on the back of the cornea associated with wrinkling of Descemet's membrane. Application of podophyllum as a dry powder to the rabbit eye caused an immediate pain reaction, blepharospasm, and a rapid progressive inflammatory reaction (Estable, 1948).

Grant and Kern (1956) evaluated the actions of various alkalis in the corneal stroma, since these are among the most common and the most devastating of chemical injuries to the eye. They noted that the severity of the injury to the corneal stroma by alkalis is governed by the pH rather than the nature of the base. However, they observed certain exceptions to this rule, including long-chain quaternary ammonia compounds, certain dyes, and beryllium. Regardless of the type of alkali used, as long as the pH was greater than 12.0 severe ocular damage was noted. Grant (1974) generally confirms that alkalis above this pH in humans can cause severe ocular damage that is usually irreversible. A comprehensive study of human ocular injury (McLaughlin, 1946) included reports on six or seven eyes lost in industrial accidents due to exposure to alkalis. Accidental ocular exposure of humans to pure thioglycolic acid produced ocular changes corresponding to that observed for rabbits (Grant, 1974; Butscher, 1953). The eyes progressively deteriorated with the presence of conjunctival edema, hyperemia and discharge, and diffuse corneal opacity requiring several weeks to months to clear.

Turpentine vapors were irritating to human eyes at 720–1,100 ppm and to cat eyes at 540–720 ppm (Flury and Zernik, 1931; Patty, 1949). Accidental splash caused comparable conjunctival hyperemia and slight transient injury of the corneal epithelium but no corneal stromal damage for humans and rabbits (Lewin and Guillery, 1913).

Ooka (1967) concluded from rabbit studies and data available for industry workers that Blasticidin-S induced similar ocular reactions for humans and rabbits. Experimental and clinical use of 0.4% chlorobutanol in a 1.4% sodium chloride solution produced comparable keratitis epithelialis for anesthetized (0.5% tetracaine) rabbit and human corneas (Grant, 1974).

Concentrated phenol produced comparable, instantaneous clouding of the cornea with subsequent conjunctival necrosis and scarring for humans and rabbits (D'Asaro Biondo, 1933; Carter, 1906). Polyethylene glycol ethers (2%)

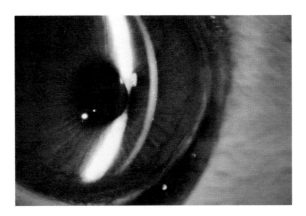

FIGURE 1 Normal albino rabbit eye.

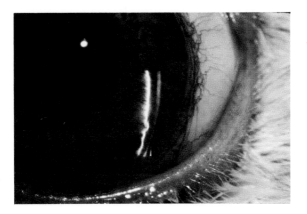

FIGURE 2 +2 Conjunctival congestion: bright red color with perilimbal injection.

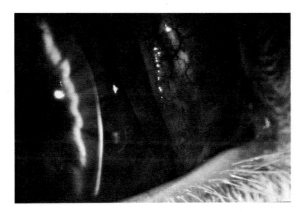

FIGURE 3 +3 Conjunctival congestion: dark, beefy red color, perilimbal injection, and petechia.

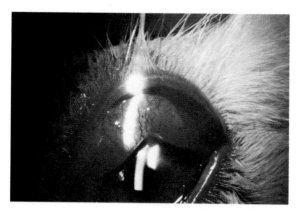

FIGURE 4 +2 Conjunctival swelling: partial eversion
of upper eyelid.

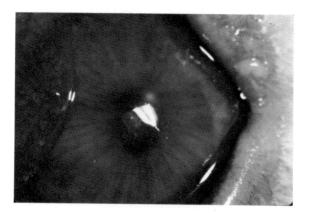

FIGURE 5 +2 Conjunctival discharge: grayish white
precipitate on lids.

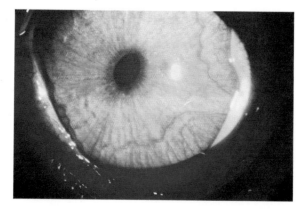

FIGURE 6 +2 Iris involvement: moderate injection of
secondary vessels and minimal injection of tertiary vessels.

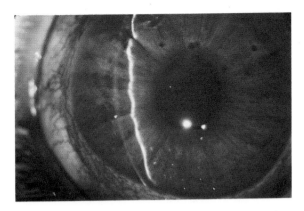

FIGURE 7 +4 Iritis: marked injection of vessels and marked swelling of iris muscle fibers.

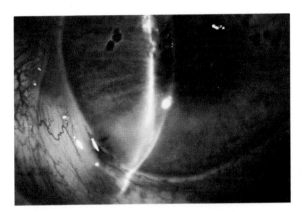

FIGURE 8 Corneal cloudiness (+1 intensity; +1 area): edema of anterior half of stroma; >25% area.

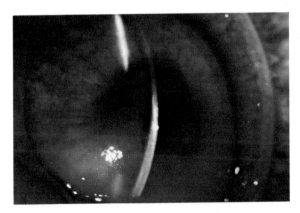

FIGURE 9 Corneal cloudiness (+2 intensity; +2 area): edema of entire stroma, 25–50% area.

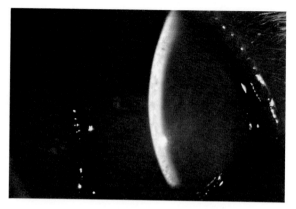

FIGURE 10 Corneal cloudiness (+4 intensity; +4 area): underlying structures obscured, 75–100% area.

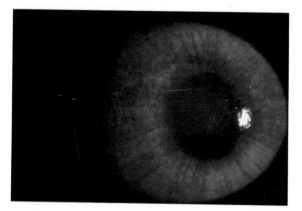

FIGURE 11 Fluorescein staining (+1 intensity; +1 area): diffuse and common in normal rabbit population, >25% area.

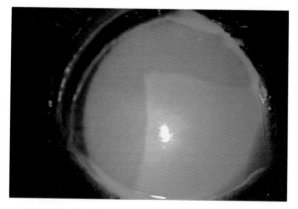

FIGURE 12 Fluorescein staining (+4 intensity; +3 area): obscures underlying structures, 75–100% area.

in an ointment caused corneal anesthesia, keratitis epithelialis, loss of epithelium, and corneal edema with wrinkling of Descemet's membrane in humans, while it caused conjunctivitis and long-lasting corneal ulceration and vascularization in rabbits (Popp, 1955).

In contrast to the results noted above, in which rabbits generally predicted the results in humans, there have been other studies in which results were disparate in the two species. Estable (1948) noted that a solution of 1:200 histamine biphosphate immediately produced a sensory reaction with slight but acute conjunctival vasodilatation that disappeared very soon in the rabbit eye. He noted that the slight conjunctival reaction with a highly concentrated solution in rabbits was in contrast to the potent vasodilatory effect produced in the human eye by 1:40,000 and 1:50,000 solutions (Gartner, 1944). Grant and Loeb (1948) noted that several antihistamine drugs that were noninjurious to the rabbit eye could not be employed in the treatment of human eyes because they produced considerable pain. The concentrations in the rabbit eye that were noninjurious had to be reduced by one-half to cause no pain or slight conjunctival congestion in human eyes.

McDonald et al. (1973b) demonstrated that concentrations of ethylene glycol as high as 80% only caused moderate conjunctivitis and mild swelling, discharge, flare, and iritis in the rabbit eye, even when instilled over a 6-hr period. Accidental exposure of 100% ethylene glycol in the eye of a man produced marked edema, considerable chemosis, substantial conjunctival congestion, considerable flare, diminished light reflex, and marked keratitis; it was 4 wk before the eye became clear (Skyowski, 1951). No ocular damage in rabbits was noted for topical ocular use of 0.5% selenium sulfide (Rosenthal and Adler, 1962) but an occasional irritation or transient keratitis was noted in human eyes (Bahn, 1954; Cohen, 1954). Ozone at 2-37 ppm caused irritation in human eyes but similar concentrations were not injurious to rabbits and dogs (Hine et al., 1960; Stokinger et al., 1957).

Conjunctival congestion and swelling with opacification and superficial vascularization of the cornea of man after a splash of 2.5% cresol was recorded (Lewin and Guillery, 1913). Only a mild epithelial defect was caused by topical ocular use of 2.5% cresol in rabbits, guinea pigs, and monkey eyes with a 10 to 12% solution caused marked conjunctival and corneal changes for rabbits (Lewin and Guillery, 1913).

Marsh and Maurice (1971) reported the influence of nonionic detergents and other surfactants on human corneal permeability. They used 1% concentrations of various nonionic detergents and noted that the most severe symptoms in humans were associated with 1% Brij 58, which caused discomfort, blurred vision, and halos with corneal epithelial bedewing, although these changes disappeared within 24 hr. Duponol (1%) caused severe and immediate pain. Grant (1974), on the other hand, has noted that these surfactants are generally nondamaging to the rabbit eye when administered at high concentrations. Marsh and Maurice (1971) also observed that Tween 20 caused no untoward effect in human eyes in concentrations up to 40%, while Brij 35 caused delayed irritation and punctate staining at concentrations above 3%. Hazelton (1952) considered both substances to be nonirritating to the rabbit eye when administered undiluted.

In another study, eye irritation evaluation was conducted on a male hairdressing formulation in rabbits prior to marketing (Van Abbe, 1973). The data indicated that the substance was nonirritating. When the product was marketed there were a high number of eye irritancy reports. The irritancy test in the laboratory for both monkey and rabbit had failed to indicate the likelihood of an adverse effect in humans. However, if the material was placed on the hair and then eluted, the concentrated aqueous eluant caused an immediate slight conjunctivitis and pitting of the corneal epithelium in the human eye but failed to do so in animal eyes.

Harris et al. (1975) demonstrated that some soaps and surfactants induce prolonged and profound corneal anesthesia in rabbits but not in humans. They indicated that studies of corneal anesthesia in rabbits may not be extrapolated to the human eye. Concentrations greater than those which produced corneal anesthesia in the rabbits were not tested in humans. It may be that the dose response for corneal anesthesia in humans is substantially larger than that in rabbits.

Test animals other than rabbits have also been used in eye irritation tests with variable results. Fairhall (1957) showed that piperonyl butoxide (undiluted) was nondamaging but irritating when tested on eyes of rabbits, cats, rats, and dogs. Phosphorus trichloride vapors were irritating to human eyes, while mild conjunctivitis was observed in cats at 2–4 ppm and corneal cloudiness at 23–90 ppm (von Oettingen, 1958; Flury and Zernik, 1931). A splash of liquid phosgene in the eyes of one human patient caused complete opacification of the cornea and subsequent loss of the eyes (D'Osvaldo, 1928) and high concentrations of the gas caused corneal opacification in cats (Laquer and Magnus, 1921).

One of the most comprehensive studies to compare the eye irritation potential of monkeys and rabbits was conducted by Buehler and Newmann (1964). They noted that materials that were moderately irritating to the monkey (primarily superficial changes such as edema and slight surface alterations) produced more severe ocular reactions in rabbits, including various degrees of corneal opacity, pannus formation, and conjunctivitis. They felt that the different degrees of irritation produced in monkey and rabbit eyes may be due in part to anatomical differences. Bowman's membrane is thin in the rabbit eye, and Buehler and Newmann postulated that this might have been the reason for the type of response noted in the monkey eye. However, Hood et al. (1971) compared the responses of rabbit eyes and monkey eyes with Bowman's membrane removed, and demonstrated that Bowman's membrane and the superficial stroma in the monkey eye had no protective or enhancing effect against the irritating effects of iodine.

Buehler and Newmann (1964) mentioned that the nictitating membrane might be a device for keeping irritating substances in close contact with the eye and might therefore provide a reservoir for an irritating substance. However, they could not demonstrate that surgical removal of the nictitating membrane affected the healing rates of damaged corneas. A study by Mann and Pullinger (1942) implicated the nictitating membrane to the extent that damage to it will result in prolongation of the ocular healing time.

Buehler and Newmann (1964) also postulated that the difference in tear flow volume from the rabbit and human eye could account for the differences noted in irritation potential of the various substances. However, no studies have been conducted to date to determine whether this mechanism plays a role. They also observed that the rabbit blinked much less frequently than the human. Our experience has been that the rabbit may blink on the order of 20 times in a 5-min period, which is less frequently than humans. However, it must be pointed out that when an irritant is applied to the rabbit's eye the animal quickly begins to lacrimate and to blink very frequently. To date, there have been no well-controlled studies to focus on whether the blink rate may effect a difference in irritation potential among rabbits, monkeys, and humans.

Pannus formation is very readily apparent in rabbits after a corneal injury (much more so than in humans). Usually it occurs some 4–7 days later, and if the corneal injury is substantial it will envelop the entire cornea within a 14-day period. Generally speaking, the pannus does not disappear and remains throughout the lifetime, although it may regress somewhat (Buehler and Newmann, 1964). Pannus response when seen in humans is usually associated with a chronic disease and is not an acute irritative effect. Pannus generally disappears in humans following healing of the cornea.

Rabbit eyes have a rich vascular plexus at the limbus which responds rapidly and vigorously to ocular injury. This, combined with the looser stromal lamellae of the cornea, may account for the fact that neovascularization and pannus are common responses in the rabbit but occur less readily in human and monkey eyes (Mann and Pullinger, 1942; Buehler and Newmann, 1964).

Other functional and anatomic differences that may contribute to differences in response include pH of the tears (7.1–7.3, human; 8.2, rabbit; 7.4, monkey); looser lids in the rabbit, which may allow irritants to remain in contact with the globe longer; and differences in tear secretion (Buehler and Newmann, 1964). Rabbits also require more time to repair corneal epithelial lesions than do humans and monkeys (Carpenter and Smyth, 1946; Buehler and Newmann, 1964).

Another factor that influences the response of the rabbit cornea to irritants is the effect of the conjunctival response. Buehler and Newmann (1964) noted that application of irritants to rabbit corneas by means of a cup which confined the material to the cornea resulted in less severe responses, which were more similar to those of humans and monkeys.

Beckley (1965b) conducted comparative eye irritation tests on humans, dogs, rabbits, and monkeys. In a limited number of animal trials (six rabbits, six dogs, and four monkeys) he observed that corneal effects caused by a liquid detergent were most severe in the dogs, while iridial and conjunctival responses were most pronounced in the rabbits. Monkeys were generally less responsive than the other species but exhibited more corneal lesions than humans. Test methods used in the human subjects did not duplicate those used in the animals. In the human subjects the detergent was applied in increasing concentrations and eyes were washed 12 min following exposure. Human subjects experienced burning, mild pain, and conjunctival erythema, and 8 (of 45) exhibited conjunctivitis. The study did not permit direct correlation between the results in animals and humans.

Battista and McSweeney (1965) reviewed the literature on comparative results for ocular irritants in rabbits, monkeys, and humans. They concluded that the rabbit should be considered a more sensitive species. In a later study, Beckley et al. (1969) compared the use of the Rhesus monkey for predicting human response to eye irritancy. In their study, the instillation of a 5% soap solution in rabbit eyes produced almost no effect on corneal epithelium. However, the same material caused corneal epithelial damage in both monkeys and humans. The lesions were not visible without slit-lamp examination. These studies indicated the potential usefulness of nonhuman primates in predicting human ocular responses to irritating substances. Harris et al. (1975) did not observe a similar relationship of epithelial defects for rabbits and humans for soap solutions.

Despite the many problems associated with using rabbits as model animals in which to predict human responses, they are a good test animal. In some instances, the more difficult and expensive tests in monkeys or other species may be justified.

REGULATORY GUIDELINES

Various governmental bodies have published guidelines for eye irritancy procedures. These guidelines are for ophthalmic containers, cosmetics, chemicals, ophthalmic formulations, and other materials that may accidentally or intentionally contact the eye during use.

Ophthalmic Plastic Containers

The *National formulary XIV* (National Formulary, 1975) sets forth a 72-hr ocular irritation test in rabbits for saline and cottonseed oil extracts of plastic containers used for packaging ophthalmic formulations. The plastic strips are cleansed and sterilized as per intended use before the extracts are made. After topical ocular instillation of the extracts and respective blanks, ocular changes are graded by macroscopic examination. A plastic is rated satisfactory if the ocular changes for the extract-treated eyes are equivalent to or less than those for the blank.

Eye Irritancy

Five federal agencies (Consumer Product Safety Commission, Occupational Safety and Health Administration, Food and Drug Administration, Environmental Protection Agency, and Food Safety and Quality Service of the Department of Agriculture) formed the Interagency Regulatory Liaison Group (IRLG) (*Fed. Regist.*, 1977, 1979). One task was the development of a testing standard including eye irritancy studies. The guidelines for eye irritation (*Fed. Regist.*, 1981) delineated test procedures for liquids, solids, aerosols, and liquids under pressure in order to place in perspective ocular irritancy to laboratory animals. For humane reasons, substances known to be corrosive may be assumed to be eye irritants and should not be tested in the eye. Substances shown to be severe irritants in dermal toxicity tests may be assumed to be eye irritants and need not be tested in the eye.

The guidelines are summarized below:

1. General Considerations
    a. Good laboratory practices. Studies should be conducted according to good laboratory practice regulations.
    b. Test substance. As far as is practical, composition of the test substance should be known and should include the names and quantities of all major components, known contaminants and impurities, and the percentages of unknown materials. The lot of the substance tested should be the same throughout the study and the substance should be stored under conditions that maintain its stability, strength, quality, and purity from the date of its production until the tests are complete.
    c. Animals. Healthy animals, without eye defects or irritation and not subjected to any previous experimental procedures, must be used. The test animal shall be characterized as to species, strain, sex, weight and/or age. Each animal must be assigned an appropriate identification number. Recommendations contained in DHEW publication (NIH) 74-23, entitled "Guide for the care and use of laboratory animals," should be followed for the care, maintenance, and housing of animals.
    d. Documentation. Color photographic documentation may be used to verify gross and microscopic findings.
2. Specific Considerations
    a. Test preparation. Testing should be performed on young, adult, albino rabbits (male or female) weighing about 2.0-3.0 kg. Other species may also be tested for comparative purposes. For a valid eye irritation test, at least six rabbits must survive the test for each test substance. A trial test on three rabbits is suggested. If the substance produces corrosion, severe irritation, or no irritation, no further testing is necessary. However, if equivocal

responses occur, testing in at least three additional animals should
be performed. If the test substance is intended for use in or
around the eye, testing on at least six animals should be performed.

b. Test procedure. Both eyes of each animal in the test groups must
be examined by appropriate means within 24 h before substance
administration. For most purposes, anesthetics should not be used;
however, if the test substance is likely to cause extreme pain,
local anesthetics may be used prior to instillation of the test
substance for humane reasons. In such cases, anesthetics should be
used only once, just prior to instillation of the test substance; the
eye used as the control in each rabbit should also be anesthetized.
The test substance is placed in one eye of each animal by gently
pulling the lower lid away from the eyeball (conjunctival cul-de-
sac) to form a cup into which the test substance is dropped. The
lids are then gently held together for 1 s and the animal is
released. The other eye, remaining untreated, serves as a control.
Vehicle controls are not included. If a vehicle is suspected of
causing irritation, additional studies should be conducted, using
the vehicle as the test substance. For testing liquids, 0.1 ml is
used. For solid, paste, or particulate substances (flake, granule,
powder, or other particulate form), the amount used must have a
volume of 0.1 ml weighing not more than 100 mg. For aerosol
products, the eye should be held open and the substance administered in a single, short burst for about 1 s at a distance of about
4 in directly in front of the eye. The dose should be approxi-
mated by weighing the aerosol can before and after each treatment for liquids. After the 24-h examination, the eyes may be
washed, if desired. Tap water or isotonic solution of sodium
chloride (USP or equivalent) should be used for all washings.

c. Observations. The eyes should be examined 24, 28, and 72 h after
treatment. At the option of the investigator, the eyes may also be
examined at 1 h and at 7, 14, and 21 d. In addition to the
required observations of the cornea, iris, and conjunctivae, serious
lesions such as pannus, phlyctena, and rupture of the globe should
be reported. The grades of ocular reaction (Table 1) must be
recorded at each examination. Evaluation of reactions can be
facilitated by using a binocular loupe, hand slit-lamp, or other
appropriate means. After the recording of observations at 24 h,
the eyes of any or all rabbits may be further examined after
applying fluorescein stain. An animal has exhibited a positive
reaction if the test substance has produced at any observation one
or more of the following signs:

  i. Ulceration of the cornea (other than a fine stippling).

TABLE 1 Grades for Ocular Lesions

Description	Grade
Cornea	
Opacity: degree of density (area most dense taken for reading)	
No ulceration or opacity	0
Scattered or diffuse areas of opacity (other than slight dulling of normal luster), details of iris clearly visible	1[a]
Easily discernible translucent areas, details of iris slightly obscured	2
Nacreous areas, no details of iris visible, size of pupil barely discernible	3
Opaque cornea, iris not discernible through opacity	4
Iris	
Normal	0
Markedly deepened rugae, congestion, swelling, moderate circumcorneal hyperemia, or injection, any of these or any combination thereof, iris still reacting to light (sluggish reaction is positive)	1[a]
No reaction to light, hemorrhage, gross destruction (any or all of these)	2
Conjunctivae	
Redness (refers to palpebral and bulbar conjunctivae excluding cornea and iris)	
Blood vessels normal	0
Same blood vessels definitely hyperemic (injected)	1
Diffuse, crimson color, individual vessels not easily discernible	2[a]
Diffuse beefy red	3
Chemosis: lids and/or nictitating membranes	
No swelling	0
Any swelling above normal (includes nictitating membranes)	1
Obvious swelling with partial eversion of lids	2[a]
Swelling with lids about half closed	3
Swelling with lids more than half closed	4

[a]Readings at these numerical values or greater indicate positive responses.

    ii. Opacity of the cornea (other than a slight dulling of the normal luster).

    iii. Inflammation of the iris (other than slight deepening of the rugae or light hyperemia of the circumcorneal blood vessels).

    iv. An obvious swelling in the conjunctivae (excluding the cornea and iris) with partial eversion of the eyelids or a diffuse crimson color with individual vessels not easily discernible.

  d. Evaluation. The test result is considered positive if four or more animals in either test group exhibit a positive reaction. If only one animal exhibits a positive reaction, the test result is regarded as negative. If two or three animals exhibit a positive reaction, the investigator may designate the substance an irritant. When two or three animals exhibit a positive reaction and the investigator does not designate the substance an irritant, the test shall be repeated with a different group of six animals. The second test result is considered positive if three or more of the animals exhibit a positive reaction. Opacity grades 2-4 and/or perforation of the cornea are considered to be corrosive effects when opacities persist to 21 d. If only one or two animals in the second test exhibit a positive reaction, the test should be repeated with a different group of six animals. When a third test is needed, the substance will be regarded as an irritant if any animal exhibits a positive response.

3. Data Reporting

a. Identification. Each test report should be signed by the persons responsible for the test, identify the laboratory where the test was performed by name and address, and give inclusive dates of the test.

b. Body of report. The test report must include all information necessary to provide a complete and accurate description and evaluation of the test procedures and results in the following sections:

i. Summary and conclusions.

ii. Materials, including the identification of the test substance, (chemical name, molecular structure, and a qualitative and quantitative determination of its chemical composition), manufacturer and lot number of the substance tested, and specific identification of diluents, suspending agents, emulsifiers, or other materials used in administering the test substance. Specific animal data are to be included in the report. This includes species and strain, source of supply of the animals, description of any pretest conditioning, and number, age, and condition of animals of each sex in each test group.

iii. Methods, such as deviation from guidelines, specifications of test methods, data on dosage administration, and data on observation methods.

iv. Results, such as tabulation of data and individual, must accompany each report in sufficient detail to permit independent evaluation of results, including summaries and tables that show relation of effects to time of dosing, etc.

Testing of Ophthalmic Therapeutic Formulations

The basic guideline for ocular irritancy evaluation of ophthalmic formulations was a 20-day test recommended by Draize (1959). Goldenthal (1968) set forth more complete general guidelines for toxicity evaluation of ophthalmic formulations (OTC or Rx). The guidelines are not for contact lenses or lens solutions. Goldenthal's guidelines are summarized in Table 2.

TABLE 2 Guidelines for Toxicity Evaluation of Ophthalmic
Formulations from Goldenthal (1968)

Category	Duration of human administration	Phase[a]	Subacute or chronic toxicity[b]
Ophthalmic	Single application	I	
	Multiple application	I, II, III	One species; 3 wk daily applications, as in clinical use
		NDA	One species; duration commensurate with period of drug administration

[a]Phases I, II, and III are defined in section 130.0 of the New Drug Regulations.
[b]Acute toxicity should be determined in three to four species; subacute or chronic studies should be by the route to be used clinically.

An ophthalmic safety test is conducted on each manufactured lot of an ophthalmic product. This test is designed to check on gross misformulation during manufacture. A single instillation in two eyes is followed by macroscopic examination at 15 min and 24 hr. Eyes with congestion (greater than 2+) or any other ocular change (chemosis, discharge, iris involvement, or corneal cloudiness) would warrant a retest. A rejection of the lot would follow if the above ocular changes are noted in the four retest eyes.

CONTACT LENS PRODUCTS

The FDA in 1979 provided new guidelines for testing new contact lenses (substances other than polymethyl methacrylate) and solutions used with new contact lenses. These guidelines were developed as a consequence of interest in soft contact lenses and the unique problems associated with good daily hygiene. The ophthalmic guidelines for testing new contact lenses and solutions are

1. A 3-wk ocular study in rabbits with normal and irritated eyes, employing various thicknesses of the lenses as they are to be used clinically, with and without sterilization procedures, and including solutions that may be used with the lens.
2. For the study of exaggerated effects, lenses should be worn continuously on normal and irritated eyes 24 hr/day for 21 days with interim observation. The cornea should be examined and cornea metabolism monitored. Gross and histopathologic evaluations are included.
3. Primary ocular irritation study in rabbits of extractives obtained from representative lots of the lenses, utilizing the National Formulary (1975) test described for opthalmic plastic containers.

4. Appropriate test with lenses to determine possible effects of inadvertent use of common OTC and prescription ophthalmic preparations.
5. National Formulary (1975) biological test for ophthalmic plastic containers to determine the suitability of a plastic for use as a container for the ophthalmic formulation(s) and lenses.

In the case of solutions, the FDA recommends the National Formulary (1975) plastic toxicity test for ophthalmic plastic containers to determine whether the container to be used for the solution is suitable. They also request a 3-wk ocular irritation study in rabbits, employing the final formulation as it is to be used clinically. Each formulation to be used for each proposed lens should be tested separately.

APPLIED OCULAR IRRITATION TESTING

In addition to directly applying the test protocols prescribed by various regulatory bodies, it is often necessary to interpret regulatory guidelines and devise additional protocols for a variety of circumstances. Here we present one approach for applied ophthalmic toxicology.

Ocular Examination and Slit-Lamp Scoring Procedure

The most critical feature of eye irritation tests in animals and humans is the ocular examination, since data produced by such examinations form the basis for subsequent evaluation, interpretation, and extrapolation.

In addition to scoring materials as irritants or nonirritants, it is often desirable to compare similar materials in various combinations in order to select a preparation with the least potential for producing human eye irritation. To assist in this endeavor, the Draize (1959) scoring system was modified to include routine slit-lamp examination. By regularly using a magnifying instrument that is also used with humans, we hope to correlate more precisely ocular irritation events in humans and animals. This method also assists in increasing the reproducibility of ocular irritation scores and permits inclusion of some changes in the anterior chamber for monitoring irritation.

McDonald et al. (1973a) discussed the techniques and types of illumination that can be utilized with the slit lamp (Vogt, 1931; Goldman, 1968) when studying the normal and irritated rabbit eye. Adjuncts to conventional slit-lamp microscopy include attachments to ascertain fluorescein staining, measure corneal thickness, determine anterior chamber depth, measure intraocular pressure, and take slit-image or anterior segment photographs.

Baldwin et al. (1973) briefly described an ocular scoring system for rabbits based on slit-lamp examination. The following scoring system is an updated version.

Conjunctiva. A normal rabbit eye is shown in Fig. 1. Conjunctival changes can be divided clinically (Draize et al., 1944) into congestion, swelling (chemosis), and discharge. Generally, the sequence of events for these changes is congestion, discharge, and swelling.

Conjunctival congestion.

0 = Normal. May appear blanched to reddish pink without perilimbal injection (except at 12:00 and 6:00 o'clock positions) with vessels of the palpebral and bulbar conjunctiva easily observed (Fig. 2).

+1 = A flushed, reddish color predominately confined to the palpebral conjunctival with some perilimbal injection but primarily confined to the lower and upper parts of the eye from the 4:00 and 7:00 and 11:00 to 1:00 o'clock positions.

+2 = Bright red color of the palpebral conjunctiva with accompanying perilimbal injection covering at least 75% of the circumference of the perilimbal region (Fig. 3).

+3 = Dark, beefy red color with congestion of both the bulbar and the palpebral conjunctiva along with pronounced perilimbal injection and the presence of petechia on the conjunctiva. The petechia generally predominate along the nictitating membrane and the upper palpebral conjunctiva (Fig. 4).

Conjunctival swelling. There are five divisions from 0 to +4.

0 = Normal or no swelling of the conjunctival tissue.

+1 = Swelling above normal without eversion of the lids (can be easily ascertained by noting that the upper and lower eyelids are positioned as in the normal eye); swelling generally starts in the lower cul-de-sac near the inner canthus, which needs slit-lamp examination.

+2 = Swelling with misalignment of the normal approximation of the lower and upper eyelids; primarily confined to the upper eyelid so that in the initial stages the misapproximation of the eyelids begins by partial eversion of the upper eyelid (Fig. 2). In this stage, swelling is confined generally to the upper eyelid, although it exists in the lower cul-de-sac (observed best with the slit lamp).

+3 = Swelling definite with partial eversion of the upper and lower eyelids essentially equivalent. This can be easily ascertained by looking at the animal head-on and noticing the positioning of the eyelids; if the eye margins do not meet, eversion has occurred.

+4 = Eversion of the upper eyelid is pronounced with less pronounced eversion of the lower eyelid. It is difficult to retract the lids and observe the perilimbal region.

Conjunctival discharge. Discharge is defined as a whitish; gray precipi-

tate, which should not be confused with the small amount of clear, inspissated, mucoid material that can be formed in the medial canthus of a substantial number of rabbit eyes. This material can be removed with a cotton swab before the animals are used.

  0 = Normal. No discharge.
+1 = Discharge above normal and present on the inner portion of the eye but not on the lids or hairs of the eyelids. One can ignore the small amount that is in the inner and outer canthus if it has not been removed prior to starting the study.
+2 = Discharge is abundant, easily observed, and has collected on the lids and around the hairs of the eyelids (Fig. 5).
+3 = Discharge has been flowing over the eyelids so as to wet the hairs substantially on the skin around the eye.

For reporting and tabulation, each numerical value for the conjunctiva is multiplied by 2, as proposed by Draize (1955).

Aqueous flare. The intensity of the Tyndall phenomenon is scored by comparing the normal Tyndall effect observed when the slit-lamp beam passes through the lens with that seen in the anterior chamber. The presence of aqueous flare is presumptive evidence of breakdown of the blood-aqueous barrier.

  0 = Absence of visible light beam light in the anterior chamber (no Tyndall effect).
+1 = The Tyndall effect is barely discernible. The intensity of the light beam in the anterior chamber is less than the intensity of the slit beam as it passes through the lens.
+2 = The Tyndall beam in the anterior chamber is easily discernible and is equal in intensity to the slit beam as it passes through the lens.
+3 = The Tyndall beam in the anterior chamber is easily discernible; its intensity is greater than the intensity of the slit beam as it passes through the lens.

Iris involvement. In the following definitions the primary, secondary, and tertiary vessels are utilized as an aid to determining a subjective ocular score for iris involvement. The assumption is made that the greater the hyperemia of the vessels and the more the secondary and tertiary vessels are involved, the greater the intensity of iris involvement. The scores range from 0 to +4.

  0 = Normal iris without any hyperemia of the iris vessels. Occasionally around the 12:00 to 1:00 o'clock position near the pupillary border and the 6:00 and 7:00 o'clock position near the pupillary

border there is a small area around 1-3 mm in diameter in which both the secondary and tertiary vessels are slightly hyperemic.

+1 = Minimal injection of secondary vessels but not tertiary. Generally, it is uniform, but may be of greater intensity at the 1:00 or 6:00 o'clock position. If it is confined to the 1:00 or 6:00 o'clock position, the tertiary vessels must be substantially hyperemic.

+2 = Minimal injection of tertiary vessels and minimal to moderate injection of the secondary vessels (Fig. 6).

+3 = Moderate injection of the secondary and tertiary vessels with slight swelling of the iris stroma (this gives the iris surface a slightly rugose appearance, which is usually most prominent near the 3:00 and 9:00 o'clock positions).

+4 = Marked injection of the secondary and tertiary vessels with marked swelling of the iris stroma. The iris appears rugose; may be accompanied by hemorrhage (hyphema) in the anterior chamber (Fig. 7).

Cornea. The scoring scheme measures the severity of corneal cloudiness and the area of the cornea involved. Severity of corneal cloudiness is graded as follows.

0 = Normal cornea. Appears with the slit lamp as having a bright gray line on the epithelial surface and a bright gray line on the endothelial surface with a marblelike gray appearance of the stroma.

+1 = Some loss of transparency. Only the anterior half of the stroma is involved as observed with an optical section of the slit lamp. The underlying structures are clearly visible with diffuse illumination, although some cloudiness can be readily apparent with diffuse illumination (Fig. 8).

+2 = Moderate loss of transparency. In addition to involving the anterior stroma, the cloudiness extends all the way to the endothelium. The stroma has lost its marblelike appearance and is homogeneously white. With diffuse illumination, underlying structures are clearly visible (Fig. 9).

+3 = Involvement of the entire thickness of the stroma. With optical section, the endothelial surface is still visible. However, with diffuse illumination the underlying structures are just barely visible (to the extent that the observer is still able to grade flare, iritis, observe for pupillary response, and note lenticular changes).

+4 = Involvement of the entire thickness of the stroma. With the optical section, cannot clearly visualize the endothelium. With diffuse illumination, the underlying structures cannot be seen. Cloudiness removes the capability for judging and grading aqueous flare, iritis, lenticular changes, and pupillary response (Fig. 10).

The surface area of the cornea relative to the area of cloudiness is divided into five grades from 0 to +4.

0 = Normal cornea with no area of cloudiness.
+1 = 1-25% area of stromal cloudiness (Fig. 8).
+2 = 26-50% area of stromal cloudiness (Fig. 9).
+3 = 51-75% area of stromal cloudiness.
+4 = 76-100% area of stromal cloudiness (Fig. 10).

Pannus is vascularization or the penetration of new blood vessels into the corneal stroma. The vessels are derived from the limbal vascular loops. Pannus is divided into three grades.

0 = No pannus.
+1 = Vascularization is present but vessels have not invaded the entire corneal circumference. Where localized vessel invasion has occurred, they have not penetrated beyond 2 mm.
+2 = Vessels have invaded 2 mm or more around the entire corneal circumference.

The use of fluorescein is a valuable aid in defining epithelial damage (Norn, 1971). For fluorescein staining, the area can be judged on a 0 to +4 scale using the same terminology as for corneal cloudiness. The intensity of fluorescein staining can be divided into a 0 to +4 scale.

0 = Absence of fluorescein staining.
+1 = Slight fluorescein staining confined to a small focus. With diffuse illumination the underlying structures are easily visible. (The outline of the pupillary margin is as if there were no fluorescein staining.) (Fig. 11).
+2 = Moderate fluorescein staining confined to a small focus. With diffuse illumination the underlying structures are clearly visible, although there is some loss of detail.
+3 = Marked fluorescein staining. Staining may involve a larger portion of the cornea. With diffuse illumination underlying structures are barely visible but are not completely obliterated.
+4 = Extreme fluorescein staining. With diffuse illumination the underlying structures cannot be observed (Fig. 12).

Interpretation is facilitated by rinsing the eye with an irrigating solution in order to remove excess and nonadsorbed fluorescein.

Slit lamps are equipped with cobalt blue filters, which can be placed in front of the light from the slit illuminator in order to excite fluorescence of the fluorescein. Photographs utilizing fluorescein staining require the use of this filter and fluorescence will be enhanced by a yellow filter placed in front of the objectives of the corneal microscope.

Fluorescein staining is an indication of corneal epithelial damage, which may precede underlying stromal damage. Kikkawa (1972) reported that 10-20% of rabbits examined exhibited focal, punctate fluorescein staining normally. There may be involvement of the whole cornea, or the foci may be limited to one area.

Reproducing Ocular Scores

Draize and Kelley (1952) noted variation of toxicity scores among different lots of the same surfactant and believed that this was due to investigator variability. Russell and Hoch (1962) reported variability of ocular scores for various shampoos submitted to several contract laboratories. Weil and Scala (1971), in a collaborative study, documented substantial variation in ocular scores within and among 24 laboratories (regulatory, contract, and industrial). They concluded that variability could be related to investigator training, rabbit strain differences, test procedures, and interpretation of ocular changes. Marzulli and Ruggles (1973) reported a similar collaborative study. They concluded that laboratory variability was reduced to insignificance if the laboratory was asked only to distinguish an irritant from a nonirritant and if all four criteria (cornea, iris, conjunctival congestion, and conjunctival swelling) were used. Weil and Scala (1971) and Marzulli and Ruggles (1973) recommended additional collaborative studies in order to identify and eliminate sources of variability in eye irritancy studies.

We attempted to address this problem by devising a statistically based experimental procedure to measure, monitor, and correct variability among investigators (analyst precision) and within the same investigator (analyst uniformity). We are collecting ocular irritation data for several substances that were evaluated on numerous occasions and have used only one source of rabbits. Later the data base will be expanded to include several rabbit sources. This approach is designed to isolate what many have thought are the two major causes (investigator and animal) of laboratory variability of eye irritancy studies. The first objective has been achieved and briefly reported (McDonald et al., 1975) while the second is still in progress.

The experimental design for the statistically based procedure is presented in Table 3. The previously described semiquantitative, slit-lamp ocular scoring system is used. The design provides a sufficient number of eyes for statistical evaluation of analyst precision (intervariability) and analyst uniformity (intravariability). Four treatment groups of 24 eyes per group are used. Each group receives a topical ocular treatment, providing groups with a range of changes from nonirritating to severe. Half of the eyes are tested in the morning and the other half in the afternoon. One hour is allowed for observation of each group of 24 rabbits (48 eyes) in order to minimize the effect of time on ocular reactions. Also, careful selection of test materials can

TABLE 3   Experimental Design for Reproducibility Test

Animals: 48 New Zealand albino rabbits

Test groups: 24 Eyes, not irritated
               24 Eyes, slight irritation
               24 Eyes, moderate irritation
               24 Eyes, severe irritation

Ocular scoring systems: Modifications of Draize (1955) and Baldwin et al. (1972) (0 to 3 or 4+)

Observations: (1) Each eye observed twice, (2) rabbits randomly selected, (3) ocular scores assigned under blind conditions, (4) scores maintained separately for each ocular parameter

Statistical evaluation:
  (1) Analyst uniformity (between investigators), method of correlation
  (2) Analyst precision (within the investigator), ratio of trial 1 to trial 2 matches for total possible matches (96); assumed 80% reproducibility

---

minimize this time influence. Other important features of the experimental design are: (1) each eye is observed twice without prior knowledge of treatment, (2) each eye is randomly selected for observation, and (3) scores are maintained and evaluated separately for each ocular parameter. This last feature permits one to determine weak areas of reproducibility for each investigator.

Frequency counts are made for each ocular parameter. An example of a frequency count for conjunctival swelling by three observers is shown in Table 4. The frequency counts compare trial 1 (first observation for an eye) to trial 2 (second observation for the same eye). On seven occasions investigator A gave a score of 3 in the first trial and a score of 2 in the second trial. This tabulation provides a basis for statistical evaluation.

An example of analyst uniformity is shown in Table 5. Here R values, (correlation coefficients) are used to evaluate uniformity. The maximum value is 1. Table 4 indicates that analyst uniformity for the three investigators is very good for swelling, light reflex, flare, iritis, and corneal cloudiness (intensity and area). Higher R values for congestion and discharge would be desirable.

Analyst precision is shown in Table 6. For conjunctival congestion, percentages ranged from 73-88% for the three analysts. This is, in our opinion, good reproducibility for a subjective scoring system. For discharge, percentages ranged from 57-79% for the three analysts, suggesting that the investigators need more training in evaluating this parameter in order to improve their precision. For swelling, light reflex, corneal intensity, iritis, and flare, reproducibility was generally 80% or better. This amount of precision for an investigator is considered good, since it demonstrates that an investigator can reproduce a score eight out of ten times.

During the time this system has been used in our laboratory (3 yr),

TABLE 4 Example of Tabulation of Ocular Scores (Frequency Counts) for Conjunctival Swelling

Trial 2	Trial 1				
	0	1	2	3	4
Investigator A					
0	48	1	0	0	0
1	2	7	3	0	0
2	0	5	12	7	0
3	0	0	3	8	0
4	0	0	0	0	0
Investigator B					
0	52	1	0	0	0
1	1	0	0	0	0
2	3	6	33	0	0
3	0	0	0	0	0
4	0	0	0	0	0
Investigator C					
0	48	0	0	0	0
1	2	14	3	0	0
2	0	9	11	6	0
3	0	1	1	1	0
4	0	0	0	0	0

reproducibility between and within investigators improved substantially. Demonstrated reproducibility within and between investigators increases the reliability of tests, even when the data have been collected several months apart or by separate investigators or laboratories. This test is used twice a year to monitor investigator reproducibility. It also provides a means of introducing

TABLE 5 Analyst Uniformity for Three Observers

Parameter	R values[a]		
	A vs. B	A vs. C	C vs. B
Congestion	0.63	0.59	0.61
Discharge	0.79	0.60	0.20
Swelling	0.82	0.95	0.81
Light reflex	0.94	0.95	0.99
Flare	0.82	0.94	0.86
Iritis	0.86	0.91	0.94
Corneal cloudiness (intensity)	0.90	0.97	0.92
Corneal cloudiness (area)	0.96	0.95	0.96

[a]R = correlation coefficient.

TABLE 6 Analyst Precision for Three Observers

| | Ratio of trial 1 — trial 2 matches to total possible matches (96) | | |
Parameter	A	B	C
Congestion	73	84	88
Swelling	78	86	77
Discharge	74	57	79
Flare	74	78	83
Iritis	70	79	83
Corneal cloudiness			
Intensity	82	80	87
Area	80	87	85

new investigators to the ocular scoring system, monitoring their progress, and permits corrective instruction.

Adaptation of Guidelines and Experimental Models

As noted before, the FHSA method or Draize test indicates the amount and mode of administration for solutions, pastes, powders, and aerosols. Materials whose application includes use with water are routinely diluted (one part of the formulation plus one part of water) prior to topical ocular instillation. In this manner, the investigator obtains an ocular irritation potential perspective for the effects of water on the formulation. The dilution is still near the concentrated form, so the data can be rationally extrapolated for the concentrate. Data to support this view are shown in Table 7. Too high

TABLE 7 Conjunctival Congestion, Swelling, Discharge, and Corneal Cloudiness for Rabbits 24 Hr after Single Topical Ocular Instillation of a Gel-Type Shampoo (Undiluted or Diluted 1 : 2)

Treatment		Conjunctiva			Corneal cloudiness	
		Congestion	Swelling	Discharge	Severity	Area
Undiluted shampoo	Mean[b]	6.0	4.0	5.3	4.0	3.7
	Incidence[c]	6/6	6/6	6/6	6/6	6/6
Diluted shampoo[a]	Mean	6.0	3.3	4.3	3.7	3.7
	Incidence	6/6	6/6	6/6	6/6	6/6
Untreated controls	Mean	0.3	0.0	0.0	0.0	0.0
	Incidence	1/6	0/6	0/6	0/6	0/6

[a]One part shampoo diluted with one part water.

[b]Maximum scores: congestion, 6; swelling, 8; discharge, 6; corneal cloudiness (severity and area), 4.

[c]Number of eyes with response/number of eyes in test group.

a dilution (1:10) may prevent the investigator from gaining a true perspective on the ocular damaging potential. Such products as hand lotions and sunscreens are evaluated undiluted since undiluted products are used.

We have combined and modified the FHSA method and the Draize test for evaluation of "dermatologic-type" products. The procedure is as follows:

1. Six eyes per test group.
2. Six eyes treated, washed at 20 sec.
3. Six eyes treated, washed at 5 min.
4. Six eyes treated, washed at 24 hr.
5. Wash with 200 ml tap water for 1 min.
6. Include marketed product control (use the three wash times as above).
7. Examine and grade eyes by slit-lamp scoring system at 1, 24, 48, and 72 hr and on days 7 and 14 (test may be terminated at any point if all treated eyes have returned to normal).
8. Use albino rabbits (about 2 kg).
9. Six sham control eyes washed on day 0.
10. Six sham control eyes washed at 24 hr.
11. Six untreated controls.

The control groups are important in ascertaining the incidence of normal fluorescein staining of the rabbit cornea, the incidence of normal conjunctival congestion, and the effect of washing on the eye. Both eyes of each rabbit are used. Control eyes but never treated eyes can be used again.

These wash times were selected because ocular changes for different types of products were different depending on the wash period. For about 80% of the 75 shampoos tested, the ocular reaction was more severe, of a higher incidence, and longer duration for the 5-min wash group compared to the 20-sec and 24-hr wash group. Examples of this are shown in Table 8. For some products, the earlier washing produced more marked ocular change (Table 9) while other products gave less severe ocular changes when the eyes were washed early.

TESTING OF OPHTHALMIC THERAPEUTIC FORMULATIONS

Guidelines by Goldenthal (1968) are used in designing the experimental protocol. Screening protocols have been developed and ophthalmic formulations have been evaluated according to the following scheme.

1. One-day acute (short-term) ocular irritation test. Use multiples of the active ingredients when possible and include a similar marketed product, if available, for comparison. This test is used prior to release of an ophthalmic formulation for ingredients that have been placed in category I by FDA ophthalmic panel(s).

TABLE 8 Conjunctival Congestion and Swelling in Rabbits after Single Topical Ocular Instillations of Shampoos

Test formulation	Wash time[a]		Congestion					Swelling				
			1 hr	24 hr	48 hr	72 hr	7 days	1 hr	24 hr	48 hr	72 hr	7 days
Nondandruff shampoo	20 sec	Intensity[b]	6.0	3.0	2.3	1.0	0.0	1.3	0.3	0.0	0.0	0.0
		Incidence[c]	6/6	5/6	4/6	1/6	0/4[d]	4/6	1/6	0/6	0/6	0/4[d]
	5 min	Intensity	6.0	5.3	4.7	0.7	0.0	3.3	1.0	0.0	0.0	0.0
		Incidence	6/6	6/6	5/6	2/6	0/6	6/6	3/6	0/6	0/6	0/6
	24 hr	Intensity	5.3	5.7	1.3	0.0	0.0	0.7	0.3	0.0	0.0	0.0
		Incidence	6/6	6/6	4/6	0/6	0/6	2/6	1/6	0/6	0/6	0/6
Mild shampoo	20 sec	Intensity	4.0	1.7	0.0	0.0	0.0	0.0	0.0	0.0	0.0	0.0
		Incidence	6/6	4/6	0/6	0/6	0/6	0/6	0/6	0/6	0/6	0/6
	5 min	Intensity	5.3	1.7	0.7	0.3	0.0	0.0	0.0	0.0	0.0	0.0
		Incidence	6/6	4/6	2/6	1/6	0/6	0/6	0/6	0/6	0/6	0/6
	24 hr	Intensity	4.3	1.7	0.3	0.7	0.0	0.0	0.0	0.0	0.0	0.0
		Incidence	6/6	3/6	1/6	2/6	0/6	0/6	0/6	0/6	0/6	0/6
Dandruff shampoo	20 sec	Intensity	5.3	4.7	2.7	1.0	1.3	2.7	0.0	0.0	0.0	0.0
		Incidence	6/6	6/6	4/6	3/6	4/6	5/6	0/6	0/6	0/6	0/6
	5 min	Intensity	6.0	6.0	4.7	4.0	1.7	4.0	1.7	1.3	0.0	0.0
		Incidence	6/6	6/6	6/6	6/6	5/6	6/6	5/6	4/6	0/6	0/6
	24 hr	Intensity	6.0	4.7	3.7	1.0	2.0	3.3	0.7	1.3	0.0	0.0
		Incidence	6/6	6/6	6/6	3/6	4/6	6/6	2/6	1/6	0/6	0/6

[a]Interval of time after dosing until eye was washed.
[b]Parameter scored by the method of Draize (1955). Maximum scores: congestion, 6; swelling, 8. Total score for the observation period(s). Mean score calculated by multiplying each individual score by 2, adding, and dividing by the number of observations.
[c]Number of eyes with response/number of eyes in test.
[d]Rabbit died in test.

588

TABLE 9 Conjunctival Congestion and Swelling after Single Topical Ocular Instillation of Acne Scrub Product

Test formulation	Wash time[a]		Congestion					Swelling				
			1 hr	24 hr	48 hr	72 hr	7 days	1 hr	24 hr	48 hr	72 hr	7 days
Acne scrub product	20 sec	Intensity[b]	5.7	6.0	6.0	6.0	1.3	2.0	2.0	1.3	0.7	0.3
		Incidence[c]	6/6	6/6	6/6	6/6	4/6	6/6	6/6	4/6	1/6	1/6
	5 min	Intensity	6.0	6.0	4.0	4.0	1.3	3.3	2.0	0.3	0.0	0.0
		Incidence	6/6	6/6	6/6	6/6	4/6	6/6	6/6	1/6	1/6	0/6
	24 hr	Intensity	5.3	5.3	3.3	2.0	0.0	2.7	1.0	0.0	0.0	0.0
		Incidence	6/6	6/6	6/6	5/6	0/6	6/6	2/6	0/6	0/6	0/6
Sham control[d]	0	Intensity	2.3	0.7	0.0	0.0	0.7	0.0	0.0	0.0	0.0	0.0
		Incidence	6/6	2/6	0/6	0/6	2/6	0/6	0/6	0/6	0/6	0/6
	24 hr	Intensity	2.0	0.0	0.7	0.2	0.0	0.0	0.0	0.0	0.0	0.0
		Incidence	4/6	0/6	2/6	1/6	0/6	0/6	0/6	0/6	0/6	0/6
Untreated control		Intensity	1.0	0.0	0.0	0.0	0.0	0.0	0.0	0.0	0.0	0.0
		Incidence	3/6	0/6	0/6	0/6	0/6	0/6	0/6	0/6	0/6	0/6

[a]Interval of time after dosing until eye was washed.

[b]Parameter scored by the method of Draize (1955). Maximum scores: congestion, 6; swelling, 8. Total score for the observation period(s). Mean score calculated by multiplying each individual score by 2, adding, and dividing by the number of observations.

[c]Number of eyes with response/number of eyes on test.

[d]Sham control; eyes were not treated but washed with water as per treated eyes.

589

2. Five-day ocular irritation test. When possible, use multiples of the active ingredients and include marketed products. The dosing regimen should be similar to the clinical regimen. This study is an extension of the 1-day test and may be in addition to or in lieu of the 1-day test for ingredients placed in category I by FDA ophthalmic panel(s).

3. Twenty-one-day topical ocular irritation test. Use of multiples of the active ingredients, when possible, is essential, as well as inclusion of a marketed product, when available. Dosing is according to the anticipated clinical regimen. This study is used for ingredients that have not been previously used by the topical ocular route. Hematology, clinical chemistry, urinalysis, and histopathology are not included if the ingredients have adequate published safety data or an FDA panel has placed them in a category I rating by some other route of administration.

4. Twenty-one-day topical ocular irritation test with systemic toxicologic studies. Multiples of the active ingredient are used, if possible, as well as a comparable marketed product, if available. The regimen should be similar to the clinical dosing regimen. Since the ingredients have not been investigated by any route and have no category rating by any FDA ophthalmic panel, or there are no published toxicology data, systemic toxicity is monitored by including hematology, clinical chemistry, urinalysis, and histopathology of tissues, including the eyes.

In the 1-day test, the test materials are instilled at 0.05 ml every 20 min for six consecutive hours, using at least six eyes (McDonald et al., 1973b). This is considered to be essentially continuous exposure for 6 hr. For tetracycline ointment, ethylene glycol, and ethylene chlorohydrin, the concentrations that were irritating in 1-day acute tests were less than or equal to the concentrations that were irritating in the 21-day test. A typical comparison of ocular changes produced by ethylene glycol is shown in Table 10. Histology confirmed these observations. The 1-day acute model does not reflect human usage, since most, if not all, OTC and prescription ophthalmic formulations are instilled three, four, or several times per day. The dosing frequency can be adjusted and the investigator must make a judgment on what is appropriate, keeping in mind the clinical dosing regimen and the concept that one wishes to enhance the chance of observing toxicity.

The 5-day test is an extension of the 1-day test and is used to confirm findings from the 1-day test. In the 5-day test, six eyes are used and the animals are dosed at a regimen similar to that to be used clinically. The eyes are evaluated every day for five consecutive days by slit-lamp observation. Examinations are usually done 1 hr after the last dose of the afternoon.

The 21-day test dosing regimen should be analogous to that used clinically. For instance, in studying an antifungal or antiviral product, the

TABLE 10 Comparison of Rabbit Ocular Scores Elicited after 6-Hr Acute Topical Ocular Instillation[a] and 21-Day Topical Ocular Instillation[b] of Ethylene Glycol

Ethylene glycol (%)	Parameter	Ocular scores[c]					
		6 hr[a]	Day 3[b]	Day 7[b]	Day 14[b]	Day 21[b]
80	Conjunctival congestion	3.0 (6/6)	1.3 (8/10)	2.0 (10/10)	1.7 (8/9)	2.0 (9/9)
	Conjunctival discharge	3.0 (6/6)	0.3 (3/10)	0.6 (6/10)	0.7 (6/9)	1.0 (9/9)
	Conjunctival swelling	3.0 (6/6)	0.1 (1/10)	0.4 (4/10)	0.2 (2/9)	0.2 (2/9)
	Iritis	2.2 (6/6)	0.0 (0/10)	0.0 (0/10)	0.0 (0/9)	0.0 (0/9)
	Flare	1.0 (4/6)	0.0 (0/10)	0.0 (0/10)	0.0 (0/9)	0.0 (0/9)
	Corneal cloudiness	2.5 (6/6)	0.0 (0/10)	0.0 (0/10)	0.0 (0/9)	0.1 (1/9)
20	Conjunctival congestion	2.8 (6/6)	0.8 (7/10)	1.5 (9/10)	0.9 (6/10)	0.8 (6/10)
	Conjunctival discharge	0.5 (6/6)	0.0 (0/10)	0.0 (0/10)	0.0 (0/10)	0.0 (0/10)
	Conjunctival swelling	0.3 (3/6)	0.0 (0/10)	0.0 (0/10)	0.0 (0/10)	0.0 (0/10)
	Iritis	1.0 (3/6)	0.0 (0/10)	0.0 (0/10)	0.0 (0/10)	0.0 (0/10)
	Flare	0.3 (2/6)	0.0 (0/10)	0.0 (0/10)	0.0 (0/10)	0.0 (0/10)
	Corneal cloudiness	0.2 (1/6)	0.0 (0/10)	0.0 (0/10)	0.0 (0/10)	0.0 (0/10)
5	Conjunctival congestion	0.8 (4/6)	0.4 (3/10)	0.4 (4/10)	0.3 (3/10)	0.5 (5/10)
	Conjunctival discharge	0.0 (0/6)	0.0 (0/10)	0.0 (0/10)	0.0 (0/10)	0.0 (0/10)
	Conjunctival swelling	0.0 (0/6)	0.0 (0/10)	0.0 (0/10)	0.0 (0/10)	0.0 (0/10)
	Iritis	0.0 (0/6)	0.0 (0/10)	0.0 (0/10)	0.0 (0/10)	0.0 (0/10)
	Flare	0.0 (0/6)	0.0 (0/10)	0.0 (0/10)	0.0 (0/10)	0.0 (0/10)
	Corneal cloudiness	0.0 (0/6)	0.0 (0/10)	0.0 (0/10)	0.0 (0/10)	0.0 (0/10)

[a]0.05 ml/dose at 20 min intervals for 6 hr, grade ocular reactions at 6 hr.
[b]0.1 ml/dose five times per day for 21 days, grade ocular reaction on days 3, 7, 14, and 21.
[c]Mean ocular score, incidence in parentheses; maximum scores: congestion, 3; swelling, 4; discharge, 3; flare, 3; iritis, 4; corneal cloudiness, 4.

formulations might be instilled quite frequently (generally at 1- or 2-hr intervals) in the first few days since this is the usual clinical regimen in humans. One might also decrease dosing frequency in a way that might be expected to be recommended clinically.

It seems reasonable to omit hematology, clinical chemistry, urinalysis, and histopathology if the substance has a published or known toxicity profile or has been given a safe, effective rating by the FDA (McDonald et al., 1970b). However, if the material is a novel drug these cannot be eliminated (McDonald et al., 1971, 1973c). Histopathology can be of value when it is needed to characterize the nature of reactions cytologically and is important for toxicity evaluation of vitreous chamber and retina. Histologic evaluation has not been shown to be more sensitive than careful, clinical examination in ocular irritation tests.

TESTING OF CONTACT LENSES AND SOLUTIONS

FDA guidelines for contact lenses and solutions were presented earlier.

Corneal physiology under contact lenses has been emphasized by Mishima (1972) and Morrison et al. (1972). The effects of a potential soft contact lens on corneal metabolism were measured by using histochemical methods for LDH and glycogen (de la Iglesia et al., 1974, 1976). Kikkawa (1975) suggested that only corneal thickness be included as a measurement for corneal effects of hydrogel (soft) contact lenses. Corneal thickness measurements (pachymetry) provide a rough measure of corneal metabolism. Corneal metabolism is disrupted if the lids are sutured to keep the lens on the eye (Kikkawa, 1975). Driefus and Wobmann (1975) observed that several bacteriostatic solutions intended for soft contact lenses, as well as water and saline, produced conjunctival edema, hyperemia, and corneal epithelial lesions (by electron microscopy) in rabbits, but the eyes for this study were sutured. Other investigators (Bailey and Carney, 1973; Davies, 1972; Uniacke et al., 1972) have used or proposed procedures for assessing the safety of soft contact lenses. Rucker et al. (1972) used corneal epithelial regeneration as an index for assessing the safety of hard contact lens wetting solutions. Some solutions inhibited epithelial regeneration while others did not.

Screening protocols for evaluating soft and hard contact lenses and support solutions have been briefly discussed (McDonald et al., 1973d). The protocol for the soft lens test follows.

1. Albino rabbits (3.5–4 kg).
2. Lens dimensions: diameter, 12–13 mm; base curve, 7.5–8.4; center thickness, no greater than 0.5 mm (Lindmark et al., 1972).
3. Treat lens with support solutions as per intended clinical use; as an option, the sterilizing solution may or may not be rinsed prior to insertion on the rabbit eye.

4. Six eyes per test group.
5. Lenses worn for 20 hr.
6. Remove lenses and grade ocular changes by slit-lamp scoring system.
7. Ocular changes can be graded at 24-hr intervals until the eyes are normal.
8. Corneal thickness measurements can be made.
9. Controls: eyes with lenses, without solutions; untreated eyes.

Three potential sterilizing solutions caused no ocular damage other than minimal conjunctival congestions when instilled topically without lenses (Table 11). When the solutions were tested with lenses, either rinsed or unrinsed, in the soft contact lens screening protocol a variety of ocular changes were noted. Moderate congestion, minimal swelling, discharge, flare, iritis, and corneal cloudiness were observed for solutions 1 and 2, while solution 3 produced only minimal conjunctival congestion (Table 12). The ocular reactions for solution 3 were similar to those for soft contact lenses sterilized by boiling in saline (without solutions).

The protocol for the hard contact lenses with solutions is below.

1. Albino rabbits (3.5–4 kg).
2. Lens dimensions: diameter, 12.3 mm; base curve, 7.8; center thickness, 0.2 mm.
3. Six eyes per test group.

TABLE 11 Ocular Changes of Rabbit Eyes during 6-Hr Acute Topical Ocular Instillation of Soft Contact Lens Sanitizing Solutions

Test formulation		Congestion	Swelling	Discharge	Flare	Iritis	Intensity	Area
		Conjunctiva					**Corneal cloudiness**	
Solution 1	$\bar{X}^a$	1.6	0.0	0.0	0.0	0.0	0.0	0.0
($n = 18$; 3 exp.)	Inc.[b]	83%	0%	0%	0%	0%	0%	0%
Solution 2	$\bar{X}$	1.4	0.0	0.0	0.0	0.0	0.0	0.0
($n = 18$; 3 exp.)	Inc.	78%	0%	0%	0%	0%	0%	0%
Solution 3	$\bar{X}$	1.4	0.0	0.0	0.0	0.0	0.0	0.0
($n = 12$; 2 exp.)	Inc.	75%	0%	0%	0%	0%	0%	0%
Untreated control eyes ($n = 42$; 8 exp.)	$\bar{X}$	0.3	0.0	0.0	0.0	0.0	0.0	0.0
	Inc.	17%	0%	0%	0%	0%	0%	0%

[a]Each individual score multiplied by 2; added; divided by number of observations for conjunctiva. For remaining each score added and divided by number of observations. Maximum score = 6 for congestion; 8 for swelling; 6 for discharge; and 4 for flare, iritis, and corneal opacity.
[b]Incidence = number of observations with response/number of observations.

TABLE 12 Ocular Changes of Rabbit Eyes Exposed to Soft Contact Lens Processed in Sanitizing Solutions

Formulation	Time (hr)	Congestion	Swelling	Discharge	Flare	Iritis	Corneal cloudiness	
							Intensity	Area
Solution 1 (n = 27; 9 exp.) (unrinsed)	20	3.8[a] (100%)[b]	0.5 (22%)	1.0 (33%)	0.2 (23%)	0.3 (27%)	1.0 (64%)	1.6 (64%)
	48	1.6 (48%)	0	0.2 (8%)	0	0	0.4 (41%)	0.7 (41%)
	96	0.3 (11%)					0.1 (4%)	0.1 (4%)
	144	0.2 (8%)					0.1 (4%)	0.1 (4%)
Solution 1 (n = 14; 5 exp.) (rinsed)	20	3.5 (100%)	0.1 (7%)	1.2 (50%)	0	0.1 (14%)	0.7 (57%)	1.6 (57%)
	48	1.6 (42%)	0	0.1 (7%)		0	0.1 (14%)	0.3 (14%)
	96	0		0			0	0
Solution 2 (n = 9; 3 exp.) (unrinsed)	20	4.7 (100%)	1.1 (44%)	3.1 (89%)	0.3 (33%)	0.4 (44%)	1.2 (56%)	1.8 (56%)
	48	3.1 (78%)	0	0.9 (22%)	0	0	0.8 (56%)	1.2 (56%)
	96	1.3 (67%)					0	0
	144	0.4 (11%)						
Solution 3 (n = 5; 2 exp.) (unrinsed)	20	2.7 (100%)	0	0	0	0	0	0
	48	0.7 (40%)						
	96	0.5 (20%)						
	144							
Soft lens control (n = 21; 7 exp.) (in saline)	20	1.5 (76%)	0	0	0	0	0	0
	48	0.4 (19%)						
	96	0						

[a]Mean score.
[b]Incidence.

594

4. Lenses are worn continuously for 3 days with a 2-hr removal (for lens cleaning and ocular examination) each 24 hr.
5. Ocular changes graded by slit-lamp scoring system at 24-hr intervals, up to 7 days.
6. During lens wearing, topically instill (0.1 ml/dose) test solutions at 4-hr intervals for 72 hr.
7. Corneal thickness measurements can be made.
8. Controls: untreated eyes; eyes with lenses, without solutions; eyes treated with solutions but without lenses.

An example of the ocular changes observed in this experimental model is shown in Table 13 for the same contact lens solutions evaluated in the 1-day acute study (Table 14). In the 1-day acute protocol, contact lens solution 1 produced congestion, swelling, discharge, iritis, and corneal cloudiness. These were enhanced and increased in intensity in the hard contact lens protocol. Contact lens solutions 2 and 3 produced minimal conjunctival congestion in the 1-day acute test. With the hard contact lens protocol, congestion, swelling, discharge, flare, iritis, and corneal cloudiness were associated with contact lens solution 2. These were generally of minimal intensity and at a high incidence. Contact lens solution 3 did not produce any swelling or flare, but there were rare instances of minimal iritis and discharge and a moderate incidence of minimal corneal cloudiness and conjunctival

TABLE 13 Ocular Changes of Rabbit Eyes during 6-Hr Acute Topical Ocular Instillation of Hard Contact Lens Wetting Solutions

Test formulation		Conjunctival Congestion	Conjunctival Swelling	Conjunctival Discharge	Flare	Iritis	Corneal cloudiness Intensity	Corneal cloudiness Area
CLS 1	$\bar{X}^a$	2.1	0.1	0.6	0.0	0.3	0.7	1.0
($n = 66$; 11 exp.)	Inc.[b]	100%	4%	30%	0%	21%	56%	56%
CLS 2	$\bar{X}$	0.9	0.0	0.0	0.0	0.0	0.0	0.0
($n = 18$; 3 exp.)	Inc.	61%	0%	0%	0%	0%	0%	0%
CLS 3	$\bar{X}$	1.7	0.0	0.0	0.0	0.0	0.0	0.0
($n = 42$; 7 exp.)	Inc.	83%	0%	0%	0%	0%	0%	0%
Untreated control	$\bar{X}$	0.3	0.0	0.0	0.0	0.0	0.0	0.0
eyes ($n = 42$; 8 exp.)	Inc.	17%	0%	0%	0%	0%	0%	0%

[a]Each score multiplied by 2; added; divided by number of observations for conjunctiva. For remaining each score added and divided by number of observations. Maximum score = 6 for congestion; 8 for swelling; 6 for discharge; and 4 for flare, iritis, and corneal opacity.

[b]Incidence = number of observations with response/number of observations.

TABLE 14 Ocular Changes of Rabbit Eyes Exposed to Hard Contact Lens and Topical Ocular Instillations of Contact Lens Wetting Solutions

Test formulation	Time (hr)	Conjunctiva					Corneal cloudiness	
		Congestion	Swelling	Discharge	Flare	Iritis	Intensity	Area
Test 1	24	3.3[a] (6/6)[b]	0.0 (0/6)	1.3 (2/6)	0.5 (3/6)	0.5 (3/6)	1.1 (6/6)	2.8 (6/6)
	→72[c]	5.0 (6/6)	1.3 (4/6)	3.0 (6/6)	0.3 (2/6)	0.7 (4/6)	2.3 (6/6)	3.5 (6/6)
	120	3.0 (5/6)	0.0 (0/6)	0.0 (0/6)	0.0 (0/6)	0.0 (0/6)	0.5 (3/6)	1.7 (3/6)
CLS 1								
Test 2	24	4.5 (6/6)	0.0 (0/0)	2.0 (4/6)	0.0 (0/6)	0.2 (1/6)	1.1 (6/6)	2.3 (6/6)
	→72	5.7 (6/6)	1.7 (4/6)	4.4 (6/6)	0.3 (2/6)	0.8 (4/6)	2.3 (6/6)	3.5 (6/6)
	120	3.0 (5/5)[d]	0.0 (0/5)	1.2 (2/5)	0.0 (0/5)	0.0 (0/5)	0.6 (2/6)	1.0 (2/5)
Test 1	24	3.0 (5/6)	0.3 (1/6)	1.3 (3/6)	0.2 (1/6)	0.3 (1/6)	0.7 (3/6)	0.8 (3/6)
	→72	4.7 (6/6)	0.0 (0/6)	2.3 (5/6)	0.0 (0/6)	0.2 (1/6)	1.7 (6/6)	2.5 (6/6)
	120	0.3 (1/6)	0.0 (0/6)	0.0 (0/6)	0.0 (0/6)	0.0 (0/6)	0.0 (0/6)	0.0 (0/6)
CLS 2								
Test 2	24	3.3 (6/6)	0.0 (0/6)	1.3 (3/6)	0.0 (0/0)	0.0 (0/6)	0.5 (3/6)	0.8 (3/6)
	→72	4.0 (6/6)	0.3 (1/6)	1.3 (2/6)	0.2 (1/6)	0.2 (1/6)	1.2 (5/6)	2.0 (5/6)
	120	0.4 (1/5)[d]	0.0 (0/5)	0.0 (0/5)	0.0 (0/5)	0.0 (0/5)	0.0 (0/5)	0.0 (0/5)
Test 1	24	2.0 (4/6)	0.0 (0/6)	0.0 (0/6)	0.0 (0/6)	0.0 (0/6)	0.3 (2/6)	0.3 (2/6)
	→72	3.7 (6/6)	0.0 (0/6)	0.0 (0/6)	0.0 (0/6)	0.2 (1/6)	0.3 (1/6)	0.3 (1/6)
	120	0.7 (2/6)	0.0 (0/6)	0.0 (0/6)	0.0 (0/6)	0.0 (0/6)	0.0 (0/6)	0.0 (0/6)
CLS 3								
Test 2	24	2.7 (6/6)	0.0 (0/6)	0.3 (1/6)	0.0 (0/6)	0.0 (0/6)	0.3 (2/6)	0.5 (2/6)
	→72	3.3 (6/6)	0.0 (0/6)	2.0 (4/6)	0.0 (0/6)	0.3 (2/6)	1.3 (4/6)	1.5 (4/6)
	120	1.0 (3/6)	0.0 (0/6)	0.0 (0/6)	0.0 (0/6)	0.0 (0/6)	0.0 (0/6)	0.0 (0/6)
Test 1	24	3.3 (6/6)	0.0 (0/6)	0.7 (2/6)	0.2 (1/6)	0.2 (1/6)	0.5 (2/6)	1.0 (2/6)
	→72	4.7 (6/6)	0.3 (1/6)	1.7 (5/6)	0.5 (3/6)	0.8 (5/6)	1.7 (6/6)	2.7 (6/6)
	120	2.0 (4/6)	0.0 (0/6)	0.0 (0/6)	0.0 (0/6)	0.0 (0/6)	0.0 (0/6)	0.0 (0/6)
Contact lens control								
Test 2	24	2.7 (6/6)	0.0 (0/6)	0.0 (0/6)	0.0 (0/6)	0.0 (0/6)	0.7 (2/6)	0.5 (2/6)
	→72	5.3 (6/6)	0.3 (1/6)	3.3 (4/6)	0.2 (1/6)	0.8 (4/6)	1.7 (5/6)	2.3 (5/6)
	120	2.0 (3/5)[c]	0.0 (0/5)	0.8 (2/5)	0.0 (0/5)	0.0 (0/5)	0.4 (2/5)	0.8 (2/5)

[a] Mean score.
[b] Incidence.
[c] Topical ocular instillation terminated.
[d] One rabbit died.

congestion. The ocular reactions for contact lens solution 3 were substantially less than for the contact lens control group. The ocular changes for the contact lens control group were substantial and comparable to those for contact lens wetting solution 1. Contact lens wetting solution 3 appeared to protect the rabbit eye from the harmful effects of a hard contact lens.

An example of the value of corneal thickness measurements is shown in Fig. 13. These represent the corneal thickness measurements for both experiments for the hard contact lens procedure. The test formulation with the highest ocular irritative change produced the greatest increase in corneal thickness, while the formulation with the minimal ocular change produced the least change in corneal thickness.

At present, there are no published guidelines for evaluating the ocular irritation potential of drug delivery ocular inserts. Perhaps the general guidelines for soft contact lenses can be used, with alteration of the protocols to fit the specific use condition of the insert.

CORNEAL WOUND HEALING

While not strictly ocular irritation, the effects of materials on corneal wound healing may be important since many ophthalmic formulations are used in injured eyes. Wounds may be induced, as by surgery or trauma, or may be the result of a disease, such as herpetic, fungal, or bacterial keratitis. Corneal wounds are stromal and/or epithelial in nature. Corneal epithelial

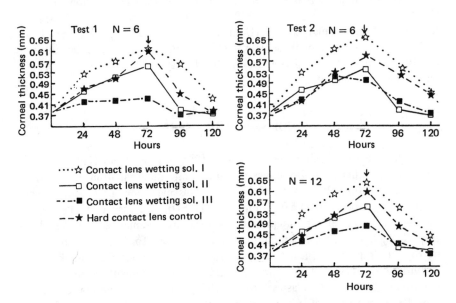

FIGURE 13 Change in corneal thickness of rabbit eyes exposed to hard contact lens and topical ocular instillation of contact lens wetting solutions. Two experiments: test 1 and test 2. Lower right graph represents combination of data for experiments 1 and 2.

wound healing has been discussed and reviewed by several authors (ARVO, 1975; Bellows, 1943; Hanna, 1966; Sigelman et al., 1954; McDonald et al., 1970a; McDonald, 1973). The kinetics of epithelial regeneration and an epithelial growth factor were recently discussed by Ho et al. (1974).

SPECULAR MICROSCOPY

The use of the *in vitro* specular microscope has enabled toxicity studies to be conducted on isolated cornea of rabbit, monkey, and human (Maurice, 1968; McCarey et al., 1973; Schimmelpfenning, 1979). Once the cornea has been isolated and the endothelium perfused with a physiological salt solution that is known to maintain the corneal endothelial structure and function for extended periods of time (Dickstein and Maurice, 1972; Edelhauser et al., 1975, 1976, 1978), a chemical or substance to be evaluated can be either added to the corneal endothelial perfusion medium or topically applied to the epithelial surface. During the perfusion the corneal thickness can be measured with an accuracy of 5 μm, the endothelial cells visualized, and at various times or at the end of a perfusion the cornea can be fixed for scanning and transmission electron microscopy. Corneal toxicity would be measured as a change in corneal thickness and/or ultrastructural damage to the component layers of the cornea that may ultimately lead to corneal opacity.

This technique has been used to evaluate intraocular irrigation solutions (Edelhauser et al., 1975, 1976, 1978), the establishment of pH and osmotic tolerance of intraocular tissues (Gonnering et al., 1979; Edelhauser et al., 1981), and the effect of preservatives (Van Horn et al., 1977; Edelhauser et al., 1979a) (Figs. 14 and 15) and drugs (Hull et al., 1975; Staatz et al., 1980) on corneal endothelium.

CORNEAL THICKNESS

The use of a pachometer (Mishima, 1968; Mishima and Hedbys, 1968) attached to a slit lamp also allows for an accurate determination of the effect of chemicals topically applied to the eye. This measurement is reproducible for a 2.2-kg rabbit 0.400 ± 0.02 mm (mean ± SD), and easy to make. Figure 16 illustrates the effect of epithelial removal by scraping and heptanol on corneal thickness. This technique has also been used to determine the effect of topical drugs on corneal thickness (Staatz et al., 1980; Edelhauser, et al., 1979b). The advantage of corneal thickness measurement is that it is a noninvasive procedure to assess the physiological state of the cornea, and it provides a measure of wound repair following a topical insult. Corneal thickness in conjunction with the Draize scoring method to determine eye irritation would allow a precise measurement of corneal toxicity and repair.

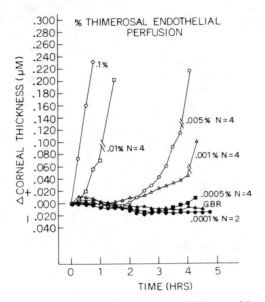

FIGURE 14 Changes in corneal thickness with time during perfusion of the endothelium of rabbit corneas with various concentrations of thimerosal in glutathione bicarbonate Ringer solution (GBR) (*N* = number of corneas).

CORNEAL PHOTOGRAPHY AND RE-EPITHELIALIZATION

Anterior segment photography with fluorescein staining provides a permanent record for eye irritation and complements the standard scoring method. It also provides uniformity between the various laboratories used to evaluate chemicals for irritation. Figure 17 illustrates corneal re-epithelialization following a 6-mm mechanical debridement of the epithelium. The degree of re-epithelialization can be assessed by fluorescein staining and measuring the healing rate [area (mm^2/h) or perimeter]. The rate of re-epithelialization following epithelial scraping and heptanol removal is shown in Fig. 18. Other investigators used this model to study the normal re-epithelialization of the

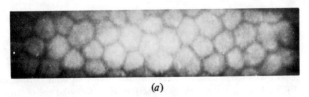

(a)

FIGURE 15 (*a*) Specular photomicrograph of rabbit cornea during 4 h of GBR perfusion, ×400.

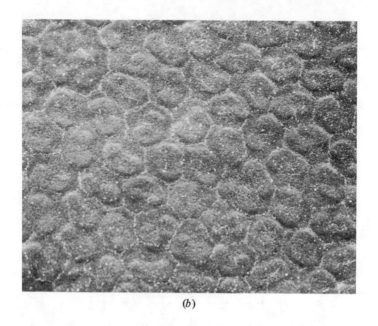

(b)

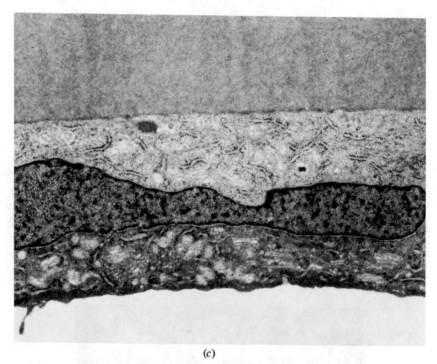

(c)

FIGURE 15 (*Continued*) (*b*) Scanning electron microscopy of same corneal endothelium after 4 h of GBR perfusion; normal mosaic pattern of endothelial cells is present and the posterior surface is smooth, ×800. (*c*) Transmission electron microscopy of same cornea; cell ultrastructure and subcellular organelles are normal, ×10, 300.

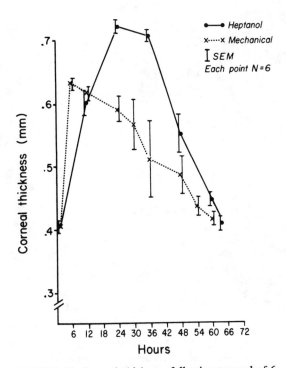

FIGURE 16 Corneal thickness following removal of 6 mm central corneal epithelium as measured with a pachometer. Note the initial swelling upon epithelial removal and the greater increase in corneal thickness in the heptanol group, indicating a degree of stromal damage. Corneal thickness does return to the initial thickness after 66 h.

cornea and the effect of growth factors (Ho et al., 1974; Friend and Thoft, 1978; Cintron et al., 1979; Moses et al., 1979; Jumblatt et al., 1980). This technique can be effectively used to evaluate the toxicity of chemicals and substances of the normal wound repair process of the cornea following chemical insult.

POTENTIALLY USEFUL TECHNIQUES

Electron microscopy has contributed to an understanding of corneal epithelial architecture (Harding et al., 1974; Sheldon, 1956; Hoffman, 1972; Rosen and Brown, 1974). The fingerprinting phenomenon of corneal epithelial surfaces has been detected by scanning electron microscopy (Rosen and Brown, 1974). Harding et al. (1974) observed a variety of corneal epithelial architectures for different animal species. Scanning and transmission electron

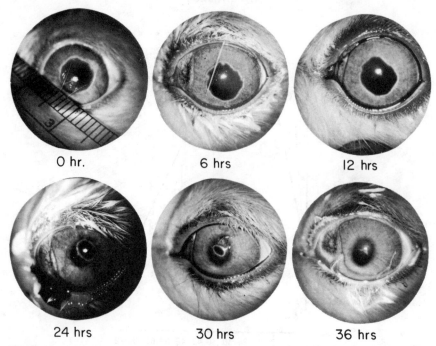

FIGURE 17 Fluorescein staining of the central corneal epithelium following 6-mm mechanical debridement. Note the progressive re-epithelialization throughout the 36-h period.

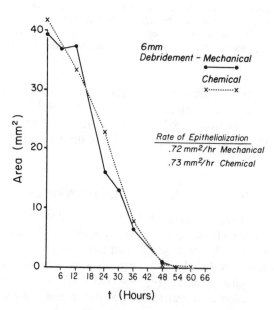

FIGURE 18 Rate of corneal re-epithelialization following mechanical and chemical epithelial debridement.

microscopy may prove useful for evaluating cellular toxicity of topically instilled products.

Maurice described the specular microscope in 1968. This in an *in vitro* instrument in which the cornea is isolated and perfused from the endothelial surface. The endothelial surface can be observed easily and corneal thickness measurements can be made accurately. McCarey et al. (1973) have included the specular microscope in a study using transmission and scanning electron microscopy. *In vitro* specular microscopy can also be used to evaluate epithelial surfaces of isolated rabbit corneas (Maurice, 1974).

A natural extension of the *in vitro* technique is *in vivo* specular microscopy (Laing et al., 1974). The specular microscope is mounted in the place of the slit lamp and its optics. The illumination is designed so that the observer can easily note the endothelial architecture. This instrument has not been applied or used in any ophthalmic toxicology study, but it represents a new area and technological advancement for ophthalmic toxicology. It may be possible to use *in vivo* specular microscopy to examine the epithelial surface as well.

Gasset et al. (1974) combined the techniques of enzyme histochemistry ($NADH_2$-oxidoreductase), electron microscopy, conventional histology, and *in vitro* specular microscopy to compare the effects of three ophthalmic preservatives on rabbit eyes. They showed that benzalkonium chloride (0.05 and 0.1%) was significantly more cytotoxic to corneal endothelial cells than 2% chlorobutanol or 2% thimerosal.

Ashford and Lamble (1974) noted that increased ocular inflammatory changes were correlated with increased ocular temperatures. Measurement of changes in ocular temperatures with an infrared thermometer may prove valuable in ophthalmic toxicology (Shuster and Kaufman, 1974).

Other quantitative techniques that can be used include corneal thickness measurements to quantitate corneal edema, and determination of corneal edema and amount of vascular leakage in the conjunctiva and aqueous humor by dye diffusion after intravenous injection of Evans blue (Laillier et al., 1975; Conquet et al., 1975).

SUMMARY

A large number of materials are subjected to ocular irritation tests. Significant advances have been made over the past 30 yr and several useful methods now exist for evaluating the ocular irritancy of materials in animals and predicting their effects in humans. However, several problems still exist. They include selection of appropriate test animals, accuracy and reproducibility of observations made in animals, and identifying test animals and protocols that more precisely predict human reactions.

In this chapter we have briefly reviewed the major papers that have influenced the direction of ocular irritation testing. The anatomical similarities and differences among the commonly used test animals have been described, with emphasis on the comparison of albino rabbits and humans. Despite significant anatomical dissimilarities, the rabbit eye appears to be the most useful system for most purposes, although use of other animals (e.g., monkeys) may be justified in special circumstances.

The predictive value for humans of irritation tests in animals (usually rabbits) has been discussed. The rabbit eye is often equally sensitive or more sensitive to a particular irritant than the human eye. However, there are also several examples of cases in which rabbit tests have failed to alert investigators to problems that appeared later in humans. Thus, as in most toxicologic studies, continued evaluation and improved methods are needed in eye irritation testing.

Because various test guidelines must often be adapted and applied to specific situations, some examples of specific protocols, with results obtained during tests of several materials, have been presented. A 1-day acute test, a 5-day test, and two types of 21-day tests have been discussed. The 1-day test is useful for rapid screening of the ocular irritation potential of numerous materials. The 5-day and 21-day tests allow longer application of the materials and evaluation of lesions that evolve more slowly. Modifications of these tests for contact lenses have also been discussed.

A few new techniques, such as specular microscopy, measurement of ocular temperature with an infrared thermometer, and measurement of vascular damage by leakage of dyes, have been briefly mentioned.

REFERENCES

Alexander, P. 1965. Evaluation of the irritation potential of shampoos and conditioning rinses. *Specialities* 9:33–37.

Aronson, S. B., Martenet, A. C. Yamamoto, E. A. and Bedford, M. J. 1966. Mechanisms of the host response in the eye. II. Variations in ocular diseases produced by several different antigens. *Arch. Ophthalmol.* 76:266–273.

ARVO (Association for Research in Vision and Ophthalmology). 1975. *Smelser symposium on corneal wound healing*, Sarasota, Fla., April 28 to May 2.

Ashford, J. J. and Lamble, J. W. 1974. A detailed assessment procedure of anti-inflammatory effects of drugs on experimental immunogenic uveitis in rabbits. *Invest. Ophthalmol.* 13:414–421.

Bahn, G. C. 1954. The treatment of seborrheic blepharitis. *South. Med. J.* 47:749–753.

Bailey, I. L. and Carney, L. G. 1973. Corneal changes from hydrophilic contact lenses. *Am. J. Optom.* 50:299–304.

Baldwin, H. A., McDonald, T. O. and Beasley, C. H. 1973. Slit examination of experimental animal eyes. II. Grading scales and photographic evaluation of induced pathological conditions. *J. Soc. Cosmet. Chem.* 24:181–195.

Ballantyne, B. and Swanston, D. W. 1972. Ocular irritation tests. *Br. J. Pharmacol.* 46:577–578.

Barkman, R., Germanis, M., Karpe, G. and Malmborg, A. S. 1969. Preservatives in drops. *Acta Ophthalmol.* 47:461–475.

Battista, S. P. and McSweeney, E. S., Jr. 1965. Approaches to a quantitative method of testing eye irritation. *J. Soc. Cosmet. Chem.* 16:119–131.

Bayard, S. and Hehir, R. 1976. Evaluation of proposed changes in the modified Draize rabbit eye irritation test. *Soc. Toxicol. 15th Meet.* Atlanta, Ga., March, paper 225.

Beckley, J. H. 1965a. Critique of the Draize eye test. *Am. Perfum. Cosmet.* 80:51–54.

Beckley, J. H. 1965b. Comparative eye testing: Man vs. animal. *Toxicol. Appl. Pharmacol.* 7:93–101.

Beckley, J. H., Russell, T. J. and Rubin, L. F. 1969. Use of Rhesus monkey for predicting human response to eye irritants. *Toxicol. Appl. Pharmacol.* 15:1–9.

Bellows, J. G. 1943. Local toxic effects of sulfanilamide and some of its derivatives. *Arch. Ophthalmol.* 36:65–69.

Bietti, G. B. and Giraldi, J. P. 1969. Topical osmotherapy of corneal edema. *Ann. Ophthalmol.* 1:40–49.

Bonfield, C. T. and Scala, R. A. 1965. The paradox in testing for eye irritation, a report on thirteen shampoos. *Proc. Sci. Sect. Toilet Goods Assoc.* 43:34–43.

Buehler, E. V. and Newmann, E. A. 1964. A comparison of eye irritation in monkeys and rabbits. *Toxicol. Appl. Pharmacol.* 6:701–710.

Butscher, P. 1953. Beitrag zur Therapie von Augenschadigunen durch Thioglykolsaur bei der Herstellung der sogenannten Kaltwelle. *Klin. Monatsbl. Augenheilkd.* 122:349–350.

Carpenter, C. P. and Smyth, H. F. 1946. Chemical burns of the rabbit cornea. *Am. J. Ophthalmol.* 29:1363–1372.

Carter, J. C. 1906. Instillation of pure carbolic acid into the eye. *J. Am. Med. Assoc.* 47:37–39.

Carter, L. M., Duncan, G. and Rennie, G. K. 1973. Effects of detergents on the ionic balance and permeability of isolated bovine cornea. *Exp. Eye Res.* 17:490–496.

Carter, R. O. and Griffith, J. G. 1965. Assessment of eye hazard. *Toxicol. Appl. Pharmacol.* 7(Suppl. 2):60–73.

Cintron, C., Hassinger, L., Kablin, C. L., and Friend, J. 1979. A simple method for the removal of rabbit corneal epithelium utilizing n-Heptanol. *Ophthalmic Res.* 11:90.

Cohen, L. B. 1954. Use of selsun in blepharitis marginalis. *Am. J. Ophthalmol.* 38:560–562.

Conquet, P., Durand, G., Laillier, J. and Plazonnet, B. 1975. Evaluation of ocular irritation in the rabbit. II. Objective versus subjective assessment. *17th Meet. Eur. Soc. Toxicol.*, Montpellier, France, June 16 to 18.

D'Asaro Biondo, M. 1933. Lesioni dell'occhio da catrame di carbon fossile e soui derivati. *Rass. Ital. Ottalmol.* 2:259–335.

Davies, M. 1972. Evaluating the toxicity of soft lens material. *Ophthalmic Optician* 12:939–947.

Davson, H. 1969. The intraocular fluids. In *The eye*, ed. H. Davson, vol. 1, p. 217–218. New York: Academic Press.

de la Iglesia, F. A., Mitchell, L. and Schwartz, E. 1974. Soft contact lens studies in rabbit eyes. *13th Meet. Soc. Toxicol.*, March 10 to 14.

de la Iglesia, F. A., Mitchell, L., Kayal, M. and Schwartz, E. 1976. Evaluation of hydrophilic contact lens effects on rabbit eyes. *Contacto* 20:18–24.

Dickstein, S. and Maurice, D. M. 1972. The metabolic basis to the fluid pump in the cornea. *J. Physiol.* 221:29.

Dohlman, C. H. 1971. The function of the corneal epithelium in health and disease. *Invest. Ophthalmol.* 10:376–407.

D'Osvaldo, 1928. Contributo clinico all'azione dei gas di guerra (fosgene). *Ann. Ottalmol.* 56:154.

Draize, J. H. 1955. Dermal toxicity. *Food Drug Cosmet. Law J.* 10:722–732.

Draize, J. H. 1959. *Appraisal of the safety of chemicals in foods, drugs, and cosmetics*, pp. 49–51. Austin, Texas: Association of Food and Drug Officials of the United States.

Draize, J. H. and Kelley, E. A. 1952. Toxicity to eye mucosa of certain cosmetic preparations containing surface-active agents. *Proc. Sci. Sect. Toilet Goods Assoc.* 17:1–4.

Draize, J. H., Woodard, G. and Calvery, H. O. 1944. Methods for the study of irritation and toxicity of substances applied topically to the skin and mucous membranes. *J. Pharmacol. Exp. Ther.* 82:377–390.

Driefus, M. and Wobmann, P. 1975. Influence of soft contact lens solutions on rabbit corneae. *Ophthalmic Res.* 7:140–151.

Edelhauser, H. F., Van Horn, D. L., Hyndiuk, R. A., and Schultz, R. O. 1975. Intraocular irrigating solutions: Their effect on the corneal endothelium. *Arch. Ophthalmol.* 93:648.

Edelhauser, H. F., Van Horn, D. L., Schultz, R. O., and Hyndiuk, R. A. 1976. Comparative toxicity of intraocular irrigating solutions on the corneal endothelium. *Am. J. Ophthalmol.* 81:473.

Edelhauser, H. F., Gonnering, R., and Van Horn, D. L. 1978. Intraocular irrigating solutions: A comparative study of BSS plus and lactated Ringer's solution. *Arch. Opthalmol.* 96:516.

Edelhauser, H. F., Van Horn, D. L., and Miller, P. M. 1979a. Modification of sulfhydryl groups in the corneal endothelium with organic mercurials. *Docum. Ophthalmol. Proc. Ser.* 18:271.

Edelhauser, H. F., Hine, J. E., Pederson, H. J., Van Horn, D. L., and Schultz, R. O. 1979b. The effect of phenylephrine on the cornea. *Arch. Ophthalmol.* 97:937.

Edelhauser, H. F., Hanneken, A. M., Pederson, H. J., and Van Horn, D. L. 1981. Osmotic tolerance of rabbit and human corneal endothelium. *Arch. Ophthalmol.* 99:1281.

Elliott, G. A. and Schut, A. L. 1965. Studies with cytarabine HCl (CA) in normal eyes of man, monkey and rabbit. *Am. J. Ophthalmol.* 60:1074–1082.

Estable, J. L. 1948. The ocular effect of several irritant drugs applied directly to the conjunctiva. *Am. J. Ophthalmol.* 31:837–844.

Fairhall, L. T. 1957. *Industrial toxicology*, 2d ed. Baltimore: Williams & Wilkins.

FDA (Food and Drug Administration). 1965. *Illustrated guide for grading eye irritation by hazardous substances*. Washington, D. C.: Government Printing Office.

Fed. Regist. 1972. 37(83):8534–8535.

Fed. Regist. 1977. 42:54856.

Fed. Regist. 1977. 42:59106.

Fed. Regist. 1979. 43:49015.

Fed. Regist. 1981. 46:7075.

Fine, B. S. and Yanoff, M. 1972. *Ocular histology. A text and atlas.* New York: Harper & Row.

Flury, F. and Zernik, F. 1931. *Schadliche Gase.* Springer, Berlin.

Food Drug Cosmet. Law Rep. 476:8310; 233:8311–8312; 440:8313.

Friedenwald, J. S., Hughes, W. F. and Herrmann, H. 1944. *Arch. Ophthalmol.* 31:379–383.

Friemann, W. and Overhoff, W. 1956. Keratitis als Berufserkrankung in der Ölheringsficherei. *Klin. Monatsbl. Augenheilkd.* 128:425–438.

Friend, J. and Thoft, R. A. 1978. Functional competence of regenerating ocular surface epithelium. *Invest. Ophthalmol.* 17:134.

Gartner, S. 1944. Blood vessels of the conjunctiva. *Arch. Ophthalmol.* 36:464–471.

Gasset, A. R., Ishii, Y., Kaufman, E. and Miller, T. 1974. Cytotoxicity of ophthalmic preservatives. *Am. J. Ophthalmol.* 78:98–105.

Gaunt, I. F. and Harper, K. H. 1964. The potential irritancy to the rabbit eye mucosa of certain commercially available shampoos. *J. Soc. Cosmet. Chem.* 15:290–230.

Goldman, H. 1968. Biomicroscopy of the eye. *Am. J. Ophthalmol.* 66:789–812.

Goldenthal, E. I. 1968. Current views on safety evaluation of drugs. *FDA Pap.* 2:13–18.

Gonnering, R., Edelhauser, H. F., Van Horn, D. L., and Durant, W. 1979. The pH tolerance of rabbit and human corneal endothelium. *Invest. Ophthalmol. Vis. Sci.* 18:373.

Grant, M. W. 1974. *Toxicology of the eye,* 2d ed. Springfield, Ill.: Thomas.

Grant, W. M. and Kern, H. L. 1956. Action of alkalies on the corneal stroma. *Arch. Ophthalmol.* 54:931–939.

Grant, W. M. and Loeb, D. R. 1948. Effect of locally applied antihistamine drugs on normal eyes. *Arch. Ophthalmol.* 39:553–554.

Hagiwara, H. and Sugiwia, S. 1953. The use of caster-oil and Tween 80 as an ophthalmic base. *Acta Soc. Ophthalmol. Jap.* 57:1–5.

Hanna, C. 1966. Proliferation and migration of epithelial cells during corneal wound repair in the rabbit and the rat. *Am. J. Ophthalmol.* 61:55–63.

Harding, C. V., Bagchi, M., Weinsieder, A. and Peters, V. 1974. A comparative study of corneal epithelial cell surfaces utilizing the scanning electron microscope. *Invest. Ophthalmol.* 13:906–912.

Harris, L. S., Kahanowica, Y. and Shimmyo, M. 1975. Corneal anesthesia induced by soaps and surfactants, lack of correlation in rabbits and humans. *Ophthalmologica* 170:320–325.

Havener, W. H. 1966. *Ocular pharmacology.* Saint Louis, Mo.: Mosley.

Hayes, W. 1971. *Toxicol. Pharmacol.* 20(Nov.):i–ii.

Hazelton, L. W. 1952. Relation of surface active properties to irritation of the rabbit eye. *Proc. Sci. Sect. Toilet Goods Assoc.* 17:5–9.

Hehir, R. M. 1973. Eye irritation and the consumer products. Eye Irritancy Workshop, 12th Meeting of the Society of Toxicology, New York, March 18 to 22.

Hine, C. H., Hogan, M. J. and McEwen, W. K. 1960. Eye irritation from air pollution. *J. Air Pollut. Control Assoc.* 10:17–20.

Ho, P. C., Davis, W. H., Elliott, J. H. and Cohen, S. 1974. Kinetics of corneal epithelial regeneration and epidermal growth factor. *Invest. Ophthalmol.* 13:804–809.

Hoffman, F. 1972. The surface of epithelial cells of the cornea under the scanning electron microscope. *Ophthalmol. Res.* 3:207–213.

Hogan, M. J. and Zimmerman, L. E. 1962. *Ophthalmic pathology: An atlas and textbook.* 2d ed. Philadelphia: Saunders.

Holly, F. J. and Lemp, M. A. 1971. Wettability and wetting of corneal epithelium. *Exp. Eye Res.* 11:239–250.

Hood, C. I., Gasset, A. R., Ellison, E. D. and Kaufman, H. E. 1971. The corneal reaction to selected chemical agents in the rabbit and squirrel monkey. *Am. J. Ophthalmol.* 71:1009–1017.

Hull, D. S., Chemotti, T., Edelhauser, H. F., Van Horn, D. L., and Hyndiuk, R. A. 1975. Effect of epinephrine on the corneal endothelium. *Am. J. Ophthalmol.* 79:245.

Jampol, L. M., Neufeld, A. H. and Sears, M. L. 1975. Pathway for the response of the eye to injury. *Invest. Ophthalmol.* 14:184–189.

Jumblatt, M. M., Fogle, J. A., and Neufeld, A. H. 1980. Cholera toxin stimulates adenosine 3′,5′-monophosphate synthesis and epithelial wound closure in the rabbit cornea. *Invest. Ophthalmol. Vis. Sci.* 19:1321.

Kay, J. H. and Calandra, J. C. 1962. Interpretation of eye irritation tests. *J. Soc. Cosmet. Chem.* 13:281–289.

Kikkawa, Y. 1972. Normal corneal staining with fluorescein. *Exp. Eye Res.* 14:13–20.

Kikkawa, Y. 1975. A procedure for evaluating corneal side-effects of the hydrogel contact lens. *Contacto* 19:5–11.

Laillier, J., Plazonnet, B. and LeDouarec, J. C. 1975. Evaluation of ocular irritation in the rabit. I. Development of an objective methodology to study eye irritation. *17th Meet. Eur. Soc. Toxicol.*, Montpellier, France, June 16 to 18.

Laing, R. A., Sandstrom, M. M. and Leibowitz, H. M. 1974. In-vivo corneal endothelial photomicrography. *Assoc. Res. Vision Ophthalmol.*, April 25 to 29.

Lang, K. 1969. Behandlung von Phenolveratzungen der Augen mit "Polyaethylenglykol 400". *Z. Aerztl. Fortbild. (Jena)* 63:705–708.

Laquer, E. and Magnus, R. 1921. Über Kampfagasvergiftung. V. Experimentelle und Theoretische Grundlagen zur Therapie der Phosgenerkrankung. *Z. Gesamte Exp. Med.* 13:200–205.

Leopold, I. H. 1945. Local toxic effect of detergents on ocular structures. *Arch. Ophthalmol.* 34:99–102.

Lewin, L. and Guillery, H. 1913. *Die Wirkungen von Arzneimitteln und Giften auf das Auge*, 2d ed. Berlin: Hirschwald.

Lindmark, R., Edelhauser, H. F. and McCarey, B. E. 1972. Design and fitting of rabbit hydrophilic contact lenses. *Contact Lens Soc. Am. J.* 6:21–28.

Mann, I. and Pullinger, B. D. 1942. A study of mustard gas lesions of the eyes of rabbits and men. *Proc. R. Soc. Med.* 35:229–244.

Markland, W. R. 1975. Eye irritation testing a difficult problem to bring into focus. *Norda Briefs No. 470.*

Marsh, R. J. and Maurice, D. M. 1971. The influence of non-ionic detergents and other surfactants on human corneal permeability. *Exp. Eye Res.* 11:43–48.

Marzulli, F. 1968. Ocular side effects of drugs. *Food Cosmet. Toxicol.* 6:221–224.

Marzulli, F. N. and Ruggles, D. I. 1973. Rabbit eye irritation test: Collaborative study. *J. Am. Assoc. Anal. Chem.* 56:905–914.

Marzulli, F. N. and Simon, M. E. 1971. Eye irritation from topically applied drugs and cosmetics: Preclinical studies. *Am. J. Optom.* 48:61–79.

Maurice, D. M. 1968. Cellular membrane activity in the corneal endothelium of the intact eye. *Experientia* 24:1094–1095.

Maurice D. M. 1969. The cornea and sclera. In *The eye*, ed. H. Davson, vol. 1, pp. 489–600. New York: Academic Press.

Maurice, D. M. 1974. A scanning slit optical microscope. *Invest. Ophthalmol.* 13:1033–1037.

McCarey, B. E., Edelhauser, H. F. and Van Horn, D. 1973. Functional and structural changes in the corneal endothelium during in-vitro perfusion. *Invest. Ophthalmol.* 12:410–417.

McDonald, T. O. 1973. Experimental ocular studies with polyinosinic acid:polycytidlylic acid. *Eye Ear Nose Throat Mon.* 52:27–34.

McDonald, T. O., Borgmann, A. R., Roberts, M. D. and Fox, L. G. 1970a. Corneal wound healing I. Inhibition of stromal healing by three dexamethasone derivatives. *Invest. Ophthalmol.* 9:703–709.

McDonald, T. O., Roberts, M. D. and Borgmann, A. R. 1970b. Intraocular safety of carbamylcholine chloride (carbachol) in rabbit eyes. *Ann. Ophthalmol.* 2:878–883.

McDonald, T. O., Fox, L. G., Timberlake, G., Belluscio, P. R. and Borgmann, A. R. 1971. Polyinosinic acid-polycylidylic acid in ophthalmology. I. Ocular irritation studies in rabbits. *Ann. Ophthalmol.* 3:371–376.

McDonald, T. O., Baldwin, H. A. and Beasley, C. H. 1973a. Slit-lamp examination of experimental animal eyes. I. Techniques of illumination and the normal animal eye. *J. Soc. Cosmet. Chem.* 24:163–180.

McDonald, T. O., Kasten, K., Hervey, R., Gregg, S., Borgmann, A. R. and Murchison, T. 1973b. Acute ocular toxicity of ethylene oxide, ethylene glycol, and ethylene chlorohydrin. *Bull. Parenter. Drug Assoc.* 27:153–164.

McDonald, T. O., Kasten, K., Hervey, R., Gregg, S., Smith, D. and Robb, C. A. 1973c. Comparative toxicity of dexamethasone and its tertiary butyl acetate ester after topical ocular instillation in rabbits. *Am. J. Ophthalmol.* 76:117–125.

McDonald, T. O., Kasten, K., Hervey, R., Gregg, S., Kellogg, M., Borgmann, A. R. and Hecht, G. 1973d. An animal model for toxicity evaluation of contact lens solutions. *Assoc. Res. Vision Ophthalmol.*, Sarasota, Fla., May 1 to 5, abstract.

McDonald, T. O., Britton, B., Kasten, K., Hervey, R. and McCallum, P. 1975. Reproducibility of ocular scores in the experimental animals. *Assoc. Res. Vision Ophthalmol.*, Sarasota, Fla., April 28 to May 2.

McLaughlin, R. S. 1946. Chemical burns of the human cornea. *Am. J. Ophthalmol.* 29:1355–1362.

Mishima, S. 1968. Corneal thickness. *Survey Ophthalmology* 13:57.

Mishima, S. 1972. Corneal physiology under contact lenses. In *Soft contact lenses,* eds. A. R. Gasset and H. E. Kaufman, pp. 19–36. St. Louis, Mo.: Mosby.

Mishima S. and Hedbys, B. O. 1968. Measurements of corneal thickness with the Haag-Streit pachometer. *Arch. Ophthalmol.* 80:710.

Morrison, D. R., Capella, J. A. and Schaefer, I. 1972. Dynamics of oxygen utilization under a soft contact lens. In *Soft contact lens,* eds. A. R. Gasset and H. Kaufman, pp. 44–58. St. Louis, Mo.: Mosby.

Moses, R. A., Parkinson, G., and Schuchardt, R. 1979. A standard large wound of the corneal epithelium in the rabbit. *Invest. Ophthalmol.* 18:103.

Nakano, M. 1958. Effect of various antifungal preparations on the conjunctiva and cornea of rabbits. *Yakuzaigaku* 18:94

National Formulary, Committee on the. 1975. *National formulary XIV,* pp. 884–887. Washington, D.C.: American Pharmaceutical Association.

Norn, M. S. 1971. Vital staining of cornea and conjunctiva. *Eye Ear Nose Throat Mon.* 50:294–299.

von Oettingen, W. F. 1958. *Poisoning,* 2d ed. Philadelphia: Saunders.

Ooka, R. 1967. Agricultural chemicals, blasticidin and the eyes. *Ophthalmology (Tokyo)* 9:166–175.

Patty, E. A. 1949. *Industrial hygiene and toxicology.* New York: Interscience.

Phister, R. R. 1973. The normal surface of corneal epithelium: A scanning electron microscopic study. *Invest. Ophthalmol.* 12:654–668.

Phister, R. R. 1975. The normal surface of conjunctiva epithelium. A scanning electron microscopic study. *Invest. Ophthalmol.* 14:267–279.

Popp, C. 1955. Kornaerosionen durch Polyäthyleneglykole. *Klin. Monatsbl. Augenheilkd.* 126:76-77.

Prince, J. H., Diesem, C. D., Eglitis, I. and Ruskell, G. L. 1960. *Anatomy and histology of the eye and orbit in domestic animals.* Springfield, Ill.: Thomas.

Rosen, J. and Brown, S. 1974. Scanning microscopy of healing corneal epithelium. *Assoc. Res. Vision Ophthalmol.*, Sarasota, Fla., April 25 to 29.

Rosenthal, J. W. and Adler, H. 1962. Effect of selenium disulfide on rabbit eyes. *South. Med. J.* 55:318-320.

Rucker, I., Kettrey, R., Bach, F. and Zeleznick, L. 1972. A safety test for contact lens wetting solutions. *Ann. Ophthalmol.* 4:1000-1006.

Russell, K. L. and Hoch, S. G. 1962. Product development and rabbit eye irritation. *Proc. Sci. Sect. Toilet Goods Assoc.* 37:27-32.

Schimmelpfenning, B. H. 1979. Long-term perfusion of human corneas. *Invest. Ophthalmol. Vis. Sci.* 18:107.

Schuck, E. A., Stephens, E. R. and Middleton, J. T. 1966. Eye irritation response at low concentrations of irritants. *Arch. Environ. Health* 13:570-575.

Seabaugh, V., Osterberg, R., Hoheisel, C. H., Murphy, J. and Bierbower, G. 1976. A comparative study of rabbit ocular reactions to various exposure times to chemicals. *Soc. Toxicol. 15th Annu. Meet.*, Atlanta, Ga., March, paper 227.

Sheldon, H. 1956. An electron microscope study of the epithelium in the normal mature and immature mouse cornea. *J. Biophys. Biochem. Cytol.* 2:253-260.

Shuster, J. and Kaufman, H. E. 1974. *Invest. Ophthalmol.* 13:892-893 (letter).

Sigelman, S., Dohlman, C. H. and Friedenwald, J. S. 1954. Miotic and wound healing activities in the rat corneal epithelium. *Arch. Ophthalmol.* 52:751-757.

Skyowski, P. 1951. Ethylene glycol toxicity. *Am. J. Ophthalmol.* 34:1599-1600.

Smyth, H. F. and Seaton, J. 1940. Acute response of guinea pigs and rats to inhalation of vapors of tetraethyl orthosilicate (ethyl silicate). *J. Ind. Hyg.* 22:288-296.

Staatz, W. D., Edelhauser, H. F., Lehner, R., and Van Horn, D. L. 1980. Cytotoxicity of pivalylphenylephrine and pivalic acid to the corneal endothelium. *Arch. Ophthalmol.* 98:1279.

Stokinger, H. E., Wagner, W. D. and Dobrogoski, O. J. 1957. Ozone toxicity studies. *Arch. Ind. Health* 16:514-522.

Suker, G. F. 1913. Injury to cornea from oxalic acid. *Ophthalmol. Rec.* 23:40-47.

Treon, J. F. 1965. Physiological properties of selected non-ionic surfactants. *Soap Perfum. Cosmet.* 38:47-54.

Uniacke, C. A., Hill, R. M., Greenberg, M. and Seward, S. 1972. Physiological tests for new contact lens material. I. Quantitative effects of selected oxygen atmospheres on glycogen storage, LDH concentration and thickness of the corneal epithelium. *Am. J. Optom.* 49:329-335.

Van Abbe, N. Y. 1973. Eye irritation: Studies relating to responses in man and laboratory animals. *J. Soc. Cosmet. Chem.* 24:685-692.

Van Horn, D. L., Edelhauser, H. F., Prodanovich, G., Eiferman, R. and Pederson, H. J. 1977. Effect of the ophthalmic preservative thimerosal on rabbit and human corneal endothelium. *Invest. Ophthalmol. Vis. Sci.* 16:273.

Vogt, A. 1931. *Lehrbuch und Atlas der Spaltlampenmikroskopie*, vol. 3, p. 227. Berlin: Springer.

Weil, C. S. and Scala, R. A. 1971. Study of intra- and interlaboratory variability in the results of rabbit eye and skin irritation tests. *Toxicol. Appl. Pharmacol.* 19:276-360.

Weltman, A. S., Sparber, S. B. and Jurtshuk, T. 1965. Comparative evaluation and the influence of various factors on eye-irritation scores. *Toxicol. Appl. Pharmacol.* 7:308-319.

29

skin as a route of entry for neurotoxic substances

Peter S. Spencer ▪ Monica C. Bischoff

INTRODUCTION

Skin as a major portal of entry for substances that induce degeneration of the nervous system is not a familiar concept. Most neurotoxic substances are assumed to enter the systemic circulation by a respiratory or gastro-intestinal route. Nevertheless, evidence amassed in recent years indicates that several widely used substances have the potential to traverse intact skin in sufficient quantities to precipitate neurologic disease.

Examples of neurotoxic substances that penetrate skin are found in both domestic and industrial settings. Neurotoxic chemicals used in the home have included (1) the antimicrobial agent hexachlorophene [HCP; 2,2'-methylenebis(3,4,6-trichlorophenol)], (2) the fragrance compounds musk tetralin or AETT (acetyl ethyl tetramethyl tetralin) and musk ambrette (2,4-dinitro-3-methyl-6-*tert*-butylanisole), and (3) the antiseborrheic drug zinc pyridinethione [ZPT; bis(*N*-oxopyridine-2-thionato)zinc II]. Of these four substances, only HCP is documented as a cause of neurotoxic disease in humans, the other three having been identified in experimentally treated animals. Use of HCP in over-the-counter drugs and AETT in fragrance formulations was discontinued after the recognition of percutaneous neuro-toxicity. Musk ambrette and ZPT are unregulated. The scabicide lindone or

Work discussed in this chapter was supported in part by the National Institute of Occupational Safety and Health (OH 00851), the National Institute of Environmental Sciences (ES 02168), and corporate donations.

Kwell (gamma-benzyl hydrochloride) is an example of a freely available drug with the potential to penetrate human skin in sufficient quantities to induce neurologic disease (delerium, choreoathetoid movements, diminished vision with optic atrophy, seizures, spasticity, and cerebellar dysfunction) (Orkin and Maibach, 1978).

Percutaneous absorption of neurotoxic agents is a major but widely unacknowledged route of intoxication in the occupational setting. Several commercially important chemicals have induced neurologic disease in workers ignorant of the hazards of skin exposure to such substances and unprotected by suitable clothing. Examples include the solvents *n*-hexane and methyl *n*-butyl ketone (M*n*BK), the monomer acrylamide, several organophosphorus compounds (pesticides and chemical warfare agents), and the foaming agent Lucel-7 (2-*tert*-butylazo-2-hydroxy-5-methyl hexane). Other industrial and commercial neurotoxic agents that penetrate skin include epichlorohydrin, lead tetraethyl, and biphenyl.

TYPES OF NEUROPATHOLOGY

There are no qualitative differences between the neuropathologic response to toxic agents absorbed through skin and that induced by toxins entering in other ways. Degree of structural damage to nervous tissue is usually dose-dependent and two types of cellular interruption are common. One involves distal degeneration of long and large-diameter axons; this picture underlies the symmetric sensorimotor neuropathies encountered with acrylamide, *n*-hexane, M*n*BK, Lucel-7, and organophosphorus insecticides. The second is a disease of myelin (or myelinating cells) and is associated with percutaneous intoxication with HCP and AETT. Distal axonopathies and myelinopathies usually involve the central and peripheral nervous systems (CNS and PNS) concurrently, the exact pattern and distribution of pathological change varying with each agent. Figures 1 and 2 illustrate commonly involved pathways in spinal cord and peripheral nerves only.

NEUROTOXIC SUBSTANCES
IN THE DOMESTIC ENVIRONMENT

Hexachlorophene

For over 20 yr, HCP was commonly used as an antimicrobial agent in soaps and liquid detergents and as a preservative in cosmetics. HCP is absorbed through the skin and mucous membranes of humans and experimental animals. While the mechanism of percutaneous entry is unknown, the degree of absorption depends on the concentration, the diluent, and the condition of the exposed epithelium (Carroll et al., 1967). Most cases of HCP intoxication in humans resulted from either dermal application or ingestion of liquid

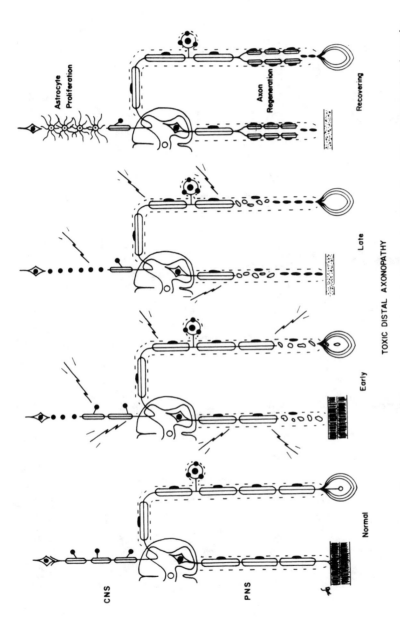

FIGURE 1 Diagram of the cardinal pathological features of a toxic distal axonopathy. Jagged lines indicate that the toxin is acting at multiple sites along motor and sensory axons in the PNS and CNS. Axon degeneration has moved proximally (dying-back) by the late stage. Recovery in the CNS is impeded by astroglial proliferation (Schaumburg et al., in press).

613

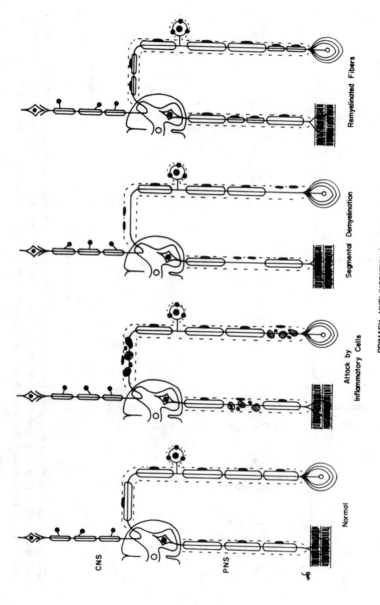

PRIMARY MYELINOPATHY (e.g. Inflammatory)

FIGURE 2 Diagram of the cardinal pathological features of an inflammatory PNS myelinopathy. Axons are spared as is CNS myelin. Following the attack, remaining Schwann cells divide. The denuded segments of axons are remyelinated, leaving them with shortened internodes (Schaumburg et al., in press).

detergents containing high concentrations of the agent. Occasionally, vaginal packing soaked with HCP was the source of exposure. Affected individuals presented with convulsions, focal or generalized motor weakness, behavioral changes, or CNS depression sometimes leading to coma and death. Premature infants were particularly susceptible to bathing in solutions containing HCP. Newborn babies bathed 1-3 times a day in 3.5-7.5 ml 3% HCP solution exhibited mean HCP blood levels of 0.1-0.5 μg/ml. Postmortem studies revealed extensive vacuolation of myelin in the brains of infants who died as a result of HCP encephalopathy (Powell et al., 1973; Shuman et al., 1975).

HCP is also absorbed by the shaved or abraded skin of experimental animals. Daily doses greater than 12 mg/kg applied to skin of adult rats induce lesions comparable to those seen in humans with HCP encephalopathy (Gaines et al., 1973). Rats 6-22 d old are more susceptible to daily dermal application than older animals. Histological studies demonstrate that HCP intoxication precipitates the formation of edematous spaces within the myelin sheaths of central and peripheral nerve fibers (Towfighi et al., 1974). Nerve roots are especially affected. Severe intoxication may precipitate additional damage to CNS axons, but not to those in peripheral nerves. Extensive pathological changes are seen in the retina: photoreceptors and ganglion cells are both disrupted, the latter resulting in degeneration of optic nerve fibers (Towfighi et al., 1975).

Acetyl Ethyl Tetramethyl Tetralin

AETT is a tetralin musk introduced into fragrance preparations in 1955. The compound was widely used as a significant ingredient of colognes, creams, after-shave lotions, and perfumes, and was often used to mask product odor in so-called unscented preparations. Behavioral abnormalities in treated rats were discovered during a routine safety evaluation of a new perfume oil containing AETT. This compound was found to be the responsible ingredient and studies were initiated to evaluate its safety. Repeated application of AETT in ethanol to the skin of experimental animals produced an extraordinary blue discoloration of all internal organs and pigmentation and vacuolar degeneration of the brain, spinal cord, and peripheral nerves (Spencer et al., 1980c). This evidence persuaded the fragrance industry in 1977 to discontinue use of AETT in all fragrance formulations.

The percutaneous LD50 of AETT in ethanol (10% w/v) proved to be 584 mg/kg for female rats. However, animals repetitively treated with only 18-36 mg/kg·d AETT in ethanol failed to gain weight normally and gradually developed behavioral and functional abnormalities characterized by hyper-irritability and hindlimb weakness. Treated rats startled easily upon auditory and tactile stimuli and exhibited excessive spontaneous motor activity. A peculiar, intermittent back-arching syndrome developed by 3-4 wk. As treatment continued, gait abnormalities developed, and ataxia, limb weakness, footdrop, and eversion of hindfeet were apparent by 9 wk. This clinical picture was unchanged throughout the remaining treatment period.

Onset of behavioral abnormalities was associated with a widespread blue discoloration of skin, eyes, and internal organs, including the nervous system. Structural damage to the nervous system developed concurrently with the first observations of behavioral changes and blue discoloration. The earliest pathological abnormality consisted of a granular lipopigmentation of neurons in brain, spinal cord, and spinal ganglia. This pigmentation increased with time, and, with continued exposure, massive intracellular inclusion bodies appeared in cortex and brainstem nuclei. Scattered pyramidal neurons underwent degeneration. Neuronal abnormalities were accompanied by a symmetrical pattern of vacuolar demyelination (similar to that seen with HCP) of nerve fibers in brain, spinal cord, and peripheral nerves. Hematogenous phagocytes stripped the edematous myelin sheaths, leaving denuded, shrunken axons. Demyelinated axons later underwent remyelination during AETT treatment (Spencer et al., 1979a, 1979b).

These data showed AETT to be a cumulative neurotoxin in the rat, capable of inducing a complex pattern of behavioral and neuropathologic changes after repeated skin application. Unlike the neurotoxic disease induced by HCP, where initial pathological changes were reversible and largely restricted to myelin, AETT not only precipitated widespread demyelination, but also caused irreversible degeneration of critical CNS neurons. The capacity of AETT to induce these neuropathologic changes may be related to its chromogenic properties, since methyl substitution of the ethyl residue on the benzene ring results in a compound that is nonchromogenic and free of neurotoxicity. This observation is of major significance for the petrochemical industry, since many widely used aromatic hydrocarbons (Table 1) exhibit the same chromogenic property (Spencer et al., 1980b), and some, such as biphenyl, are neurotoxins in humans (Seppalainen and Hakkinen, 1975). Most of the compounds listed probably penetrate human skin, and because of their widespread use they should all be tested for possible chronic neurotoxic properties.

TABLE 1   List of Aromatic Hydrocarbons Causing Production of Colored Urine[a]

Monocyclic	Dicyclic
Benzene	Indane
o-Xylene	Indene
o-Ethyltoluene	Tetrahydronaphthalene (Tetralin)[b]
o-Diethylbenzene	Diphenyl
m-Diethylbenzene	Diphenylmethane
o-Diisopropylbenzene	1-Methylnaphthalene[b]
Triethylbenzene (mixture)	2-Methylnaphthalene[b]
Diethyldiisopropylbenzene	1-Ethylnaphthalene[b]
	2-Ethylnaphthalene[b]

[a]Rats, single sc dose, ~5 ml/kg.
[b]Humans may also excrete colored (green) urine following exposure to Tetralin or naphthalene.

Musk Ambrette

Musk ambrette has been widely used as a nitro musk since the 1920s. Use in fragrances in the United States amounted to approximately 100,000 lb in 1979, with concentrations in fragrance formulations ranging between 0.03 and 2% (Opdyke, 1979). The Council of Europe included musk ambrette at a level of 1 ppm in the list of artificial flavoring substances that may be added to foodstuffs without hazard to public health, and the Flavoring Extract Manufacturer's Association has given the chemical GRAS (generally recognized as safe) status. These decisions were reached after publication of the results of a study that demonstrated marked loss in weight, progressive hindquarter weakness leading to paralysis, and other toxic effects in rats fed 1500–4000 ppm for 20–50 wk (Davis et al., 1967). Musk ambrette also penetrates skin when dissolved in a suitable medium and, in sufficient doses, causes structural breakdown of cellular elements in brain, spinal cord, and peripheral nerves (P. S. Spencer et al., unpublished data).

Zinc Pyridinethione

The toxic effects of ZPT, the water-insoluble salt of 1-hydroxy-2($1H$)-pyridinethione, have been studied since the late 1950s. ZPT is a broad-spectrum antibacterial and antifungal agent currently used in shampoos for its antiseborrheic properties. Its toxic effects on the nervous system established from animal studies represent the basis for concern over its widespread use in antidandruff shampoos and hairdressing creams (Sahenk and Mendell, 1980). The 1–2% level of ZPT now used in these marketed formulations has been stated to represent an adequate margin of safety (Snyder et al., 1965).

Studies to determine skin retention of radiolabeled pyridinethiones have been conducted by several investigators; in humans, more is absorbed from the forehead and scalp than from the forearm (Wedig et al., 1977). Repeated application, especially to abraded skin, or pretreatment of the skin with surfactants significantly increases ZPT absorption. Percutaneously treated rats fail to gain weight normally and display signs of hindlimb weakness 2–3 wk after commencement of daily applications. Footdrop progresses to hindlimb paralysis and muscle atrophy (especially at the site of application). Animals allowed to recover after repeated exposure to ZPT gradually regain hindlimb function (Sahenk and Mendell, 1980).

ZPT induces a characteristic pattern of nervous system degeneration in which long and large nerve fibers in spinal cord and peripheral nerves undergo distal axonal degeneration. Although ZPT has not been associated with neurologic damage in humans, CNS-PNS distal axonopathy is a pathological hallmark of many toxic/metabolic diseases (n-hexane, MnBK, organophosphorus compounds) in which the clinical expression is distal, symmetrical polyneuropathy. Animals with subclinical ZPT neuropathy display pathological axon terminals in gastrocnemius, lumbrical, and intrinsic foot muscles. With continued exposure, abnormal axons are observed in more proximal regions, while distal axons display overt breakdown. Concurrently, similar pathological changes are observed in vulnerable nerve fiber tracts in the spinal cord and cerebellar vermis.

NEUROTOXIC CHEMICALS
IN THE INDUSTRIAL SETTING

Aliphatic Hexacarbon Compounds

n-*Hexane and methyl* n-*butyl ketone.* Hexacarbon neuropathy was first discovered in industrially exposed humans. The solvent *n*-hexane was responsible for an outbreak of sensorimotor polyneuropathy in workers continually exposed to hexanes in a laminating factory in Japan in the early 1960s; subsequently, similar reports appeared from many parts of Europe and from the United States (Spencer et al., 1980c). M*n*BK, an oxidized derivative of *n*-hexane, was implicated as the neurotoxic agent in an outbreak of peripheral neuropathy in a fabric plant in Ohio in 1973 (Allen et al., 1975). These outbreaks were the impetus for a large number of experimental studies, which confirmed the neurotoxic properties of these agents. Although their neurotoxic potencies differ, *n*-hexane and M*n*BK induce identical patterns of neurologic disease and are therefore considered together.

The most common initial complaint is of an insidious onset of numbness symmetrically involving the hands and feet (stocking-and-glove sensory neuropathy). Moderate loss of touch, pin, vibration, and thermal sensation is usually prominent and may be accompanied by loss of the Achilles reflex. As the neuropathy becomes more severe, distal weakness and muscle atrophy dominate the clinical picture. Weakness most commonly involves intrinsic muscles of the hands and long extensors and flexors of the digits. A common complaint in these cases is difficulty with pinching movements, grasping objects, and stepping over curbs. Cessation of intoxication is associated with a continual progression of disability for at least several weeks before recovery supervenes. The degree of recovery in most cases is directly correlated with the intensity of the neurologic deficit, those with mild or moderate sensorimotor neuropathy usually recovering completely within 10 mo after exposure is terminated.

Individuals with hexacarbon neuropathy sustained predominantly respiratory and skin exposure to solvent mixtures containing *n*-hexane or M*n*BK. Human respiratory retention of *n*-hexane is much lower ($< 10\%$) than that of M*n*BK (60–90%) (Spencer et al., 1980c). Cutaneous absorption of *n*-hexane has yet to be measured, although it was suggested as a major route of entry in humans and claimed to be responsible for one outbreak of neuropathy (Nomiyama et al., 1973; Nomiyama and Nomiyama, 1974). Skin absorption of M*n*BK was examined in humans and found to be a significant route of body entry (DiVincenzo et al., 1978). The shaved skin of dogs absorbed 77 mg in 1 h, and human skin absorbed 16-27 mg in the same period. Subclinical neuropathy was reported in chickens exposed percutaneously to a solvent mixture containing 35.2% n-hexane, but attempts to induce experimental neuropathy by repeated application of MnBK to guinea pig skin have not been successful.

Subchronic exposure of experimental animals to n-hexane or MnBK by respiratory, subcutaneous, or intraperitoneal routes induced a characteristic pattern of CNS-PNS distal axonopathy (Spencer and Schaumburg, 1977). Both solvents have a common proximal neurotoxic metabolite, 2,5-hexanedione (a gamma diketone) (DiVincenzo et al., 1976), which also induces an identical pattern of nervous system damage in orally exposed animals. Intoxicated animals fail to gain weight normally and insidiously develop hindlimb foot-drop, which eventuates in atrophy and paralysis. Exposed rats also develop an orange-brown discoloration of the skin and hair. Paralyzed animals allowed to recover after the intoxication period gradually regain limb function.

Neuropathologic examination of animals with subclinical neuropathy reveals multifocal axonal swellings and associated focal demyelination in affected distal regions of long and large-diameter CNS and PNS nerve fibers (Spencer and Schaumburg, 1975). With time, swellings are observed in more proximal regions of affected pathways, while distal axons undergo complete degeneration, resulting in denervation atrophy of affected muscles. Regeneration of affected PNS axons occurs during and after the intoxication period, and functional recovery presumably corresponds to reinnervation of denervated muscles. In the spinal cord, long ascending and descending tracts are first affected: degeneration appears in the rostral part of the gracile tract and the caudal portion of lateral, ventrolateral, and ventromedial pathways. As the disease advances, degenerative changes spread retrogradely along affected tracts. Axonal degeneration also affects the spinocerebellar pathway in the cerebellar vermis, the distal optic tract, and the mammillary bodies. Spastic gait and impaired vision and memory, respectively, are believed to represent the human correlates of these experimental neuropathologic changes, but these appear only in individuals with severe neuropathy (Schaumburg and Spencer, 1979).

Lucel-7. In 1979 a new foaming agent, Lucel-7, was introduced in the manufacture of reinforced bath fixtures in a plant in Lancaster, Texas. Within 1 mo, four cases of neuropathy were reported to the National Institute of Occupational Safety and Health (Anon., 1980). Use of protective equipment while working with Lucel-7 reportedly had been variable. The four affected workers experienced weight loss, dizziness, loss of peripheral vision, motor and sensory neuropathy, memory impairment, and decreased attention span. Electrodiagnostic findings consistent with nerve damage persisted for up to 5 mo after their last exposure to the chemical. Although it could not be determined unequivocally that Lucel-7 was responsible, the association of the neuropathy outbreak with the introduction of the foaming agent strongly suggested a causal effect. Moreover, the physical properties of Lucel-7, which spontaneously dissociates to nonneurotoxic components at room temperature, suggested that skin exposure to the agent was most likely the route of intoxication.

Theoretical considerations suggest that Lucel-7 (a methyl hexane derivative) is unlikely to induce neuropathy by the same mechanism as n-hexane because the 5-methyl group presumably would prevent metabolism to a gamma diketone. If the t-butylazo group on the second carbon were cleaved, the oxidation product would be the 5-methyl derivative of MnBK, methyl isoamyl ketone, a solvent that penetrates skin but does not induce nervous system degeneration in orally treated experimental animals or in organotypic culture models of neuromuscular tissue exposed directly to this compound (O'Donoghue and Krasavage, 1979; J. Zagoren and P. S. Spencer, unpublished data).

Experimental rodent studies confirmed that percutaneous intoxication with Lucel-7 induces widespread nervous system degeneration, and the pattern and distribution of pathological changes differ from those seen with n-hexane or MnBK (P. S. Spencer et al., unpublished data). Groups of young adult male and female rats received 250–500 mg/kg·d Lucel-7 dissolved in ethanol, 5 d/wk, for up to 5 wk. The first signs of abnormality, observed after 10 d in female animals receiving large doses of Lucel-7, were weight loss and hindlimb dysfunction. Males treated with high concentrations of Lucel-7 and females treated with lower doses exhibited similar signs after 2 wk. Functional abnormalities increased with time and included weakness of all four limbs, corneal opacity, nasal discharge, and incontinence. Some animals died during intoxication.

Neuropathologic examination of affected animals revealed axonal degeneration in multiple sites of the CNS and PNS. Wallerian-like anonal degeneration was concurrent with the onset of functional abnormality. Degeneration first appeared in the brain and spinal cord, where dorsal columns (gracile tract) displayed a severe loss of fibers. Optic nerves also showed extensive breakdown of nerve fibers. Peripheral nerves and spinal roots supplying the hindlimbs were markedly affected, although sensory and motor neurons remained intact. A predominantly distal, retrograde pattern of degeneration was evident, at least in sensory nerve fibers coursing in dorsal roots and dorsal columns. These pathological features suggest that Lucel-7 induces another example of a central-peripheral distal axonopathy with involvement of optic nerves and mammillary bodies, the likely anatomic substrate for the human clinical manifestations of sensorimotor neuropathy, visual abnormalities, and memory loss. While this is the same overall type of neurologic disease induced by n-hexane and MnBK, the rapid progression and severity of impairment, coupled with the type and distribution of pathological changes, suggest that Lucel-7 induces nervous system degeneration by a molecular mechanism different from that affected by n-hexane or MnBK.

Organophosphorus Compounds

The commonly encountered organophosphorus compounds are mostly highly lipid-soluble liquids. The less volatile compounds employed as agricultural insecticides (e.g., parathion and malathion) are generally dispersed as aerosols or dusts consisting of the organophosphorus compound adsorbed to an inert, finely particulate material. Consequently, the compounds are rapidly and effectively absorbed by practically all routes, including the skin and mucous membranes (Taylor, 1980). Studies with human volunteers percutaneously exposed to radioactive malathion or parathion demonstrated wide regional differences in the ability of these compounds to penetrate skin; for example, scrotal skin is almost no barrier to labeled parathion, allowing 10 times greater penetration than skin of the forearm or the palm (Maibach et al., 1971). The retroauricular area and scrotum also present no barrier to tri-*n*-butyl phosphate, but plantar skin is less permeable to this compound than skin on the forearm (Marzulli, 1968).

The two best known neurotoxic effects of organophosphorus compounds are the cholinergic crisis and delayed neuropathy. Both effects can be reproduced in some species (humans and hens) by a single dose or repeated doses of a suitable organophosphorus compound. The cholinergic crisis results from widespread inhibition of acetylcholinesterase, the enzyme that hydrolyzes the neurotransmitter acetyl choline. Irreversible inhibitors of cholinesterase activity such as paraoxon, parathion, and the chemical warfare agents tabun, soman, and sarin, as well as reversible inhibitors such as physostigmine and neostigmine, cause excessive accumulation of acetyl choline at nerve terminals. Clinical effects may be localized (sweating, muscular fasciculation) or generalized; muscarinic effects result from excessive parasympathetic activity and include miosis, conjunctival congestion, nasal discharge, bronchial secretion and constriction, nausea, abdominal cramps, vomiting, and diarrhea. Severe intoxication is manifest by excessive salivation, involuntary defecation and urination, sweating, lacrimation, bradycardia, and hypotension. Confusion, ataxia, slurred speech, loss of reflexes, convulsions, coma, and central respiratory paralysis may supervene in severe poisoning. Nicotinic actions of organophosphorus anticholinesterases at the neuromuscular junctions include fatigability and generalized weakness, scattered fasciculation, and paralysis of respiratory muscles (Taylor, 1980).

Peripheral neuropathy is readily induced in hens by percutaneous exposure to compounds such as tri-*o*-cresyl phosphate (TOCP) or leptophos in acetone (Glees and White, 1961; Abou-Donia and Graham, 1978). Although these agents are effective cholinesterase inhibitors, this property is unrelated to their ability to induce neuropathy. Instead, neuropathy is closely correlated with their capacity to inhibit irreversibly "neurotoxic esterase" (NTE), an enzyme of unknown function resident in nervous and some other tissues. Organophosphorus compounds (phosphates, phosphoroamidates, and phosphonates) that irreversibly inhibit hen NTE approximately 75% within 1–40 h after a single exposure, or 45–65% after repetitive exposure, will induce neuropathy. Other compounds (sulfonates, phosphinates, and carbamates) that react covalently (reversibly) with the neurotoxic phosphorylation site fail to induce nervous system degeneration and protect against subsequent doses of organophosphorus esters that would otherwise cause neuropathy (Johnson, 1975).

Human organophosphorus neuropathy has most often resulted from oral intoxication via contaminated food, cooking oil, or beverages. Several thousand cases appeared in the southern states in 1930 when alcoholic extracts of Jamaica ginger, widely consumed during Prohibition, were adulterated with 2% TOCP (Airing, 1942). Cooking oil contaminated with lubricating oil containing cresyl phosphates was responsible for several outbreaks of organophosphorus neuropathy, including a major epidemic in Morocco in which more than 10,000 people were affected (Smith and Spaulding, 1959). Approximately 2 wk after ingestion, during which gastrointestinal disturbances may be manifest, victims experience pain, aches, and paresthesia in feet and calves, followed within days by progressive weakening of leg and foot muscles leading to paralysis. The thighs and then the hands and arms may become weak during succeeding days. Weakness is always more severe in the legs than in the arms, symmetrical, and greatest in distal muscles. During the progressive phase of the illness, which lasts 1–2 wk, depending on the dose, weakness spreads steadily but usually stops short of complete quadriplegia. Examination reveals hyperactive knee jerks, a positive Babinski response, and hypoactive ankle jerks, a spectrum of neurologic signs indicative of motor system damage in spinal cord and degeneration of peripheral nerves. Footdrop is pronounced and victims adopt a high-stepping gait, Muscle denervation is evident from electromyography, and atrophy in lower legs and hands may become severe. Mildly affected individuals gradually improve, but the more severely affected who recover some muscle strength may display permanent ataxia and spasticity. The latter clinical features were especially prominent in 12 factory workers who developed neurologic disease at a plant manufacturing and packaging leptophos in Bayport, Texas: some sustained a high level of dermal exposure to molten leptophos as it splashed from shallow trays; others were exposed to airborne particles during the process of splitting and breaking cakes of hardened leptophos before it was fed into a pulverizer (Xintaras and Burg, 1980).

Many types of experimental animals are vulnerable to the neurotoxic effects of organophosphorus compounds, although neurotoxic doses vary markedly from one species to another. Rodents are relatively resistant and fowl are very susceptible; the hen is widely used to assay acetylcholinesterase compounds for their ability to induce paralysis. In all sensitive species, onset of neurologic signs is preceded by a delay period during which weight loss and nerve fiber degeneration ensue. Long after the cessation of acute cholinergic signs, hens given TOCP develop a steadily increasing flaccid paresis of the hindlimbs, with an ataxic, broad-based gait. Weakness spreads over several days and, in severely intoxicated animals, may eventuate in death.

Tissue examination demonstrates that the pathological substrate of these clinical phenomena is central-peripheral distal axonopathy, with prominent and symmetrical involvement of long ascending (gracile and spinocerebellar) and descending (corticospinal) spinal cord tracts. Like other agents that induce distal axonopathy, organophosphorus esters precipitate neuropathologic changes multifocally in distal regions of affected pathways and structural and functional disconnection of motor terminals. Axonal degeneration progresses toward but stops short of neuronal perikarya (Cavanagh, 1964). Myelin debris is removed from affected regions of peripheral nerves and spinal cord, a feature of the disease erroneously described as *demyelination*. Clinical reversibility in mild cases is associated with the ability of damaged peripheral nerves to regenerate and restore structural and functional connection with end organs. Damaged central nerve fibers lack the capacity for functional regeneration, so that individuals who have recovered from severe neuropathy may display signs of ataxia and spasticity attributable to permanent damage of appropriate spinal cord tracts.

SIGNIFICANCE

Neurotoxic chemicals commonly used in agriculture, industry, and the home have the potential to penetrate skin and precipitate degeneration of brain, spinal cord, and peripheral nerves. In some cases, such as with the neurotoxic fragrance compounds AETT and musk ambrette, use of the agents in nonessential skin preparations continued for years before experimental animal studies revealed their potential to penetrate skin in sufficient quantities to induce degeneration of nervous tissue. With other agents, the failure to test compounds for neurotoxic properties has led to major outbreaks of neurologic disease among infants and adults. It can be concluded that experimental studies to determine the effects of topically applied compounds on the nervous system are imperative for public health and environmental control.

Nowhere is this statement more applicable than in the evaluation of workers exposed to solvents. It is generally supposed that the system of threshold limit values for regulating the concentration of volatile substances in workroom air provides adequate protection for individuals occupationally exposed to solvents, and that nonvolatile solvents represent a small health hazard. This opinion must be questioned, since it ignores the potential of these agents to penetrate skin in significant quantities. Calculations based on experimental studies of respiratory and skin absorption of MnBK showed that a dose of 314 mg would be absorbed during a 1-h period by an individual breathing 25 ppm and working with hands immersed in the solvent. Only 30% of this would be derived from respiratory absorption; 70% would be absorbed percutaneously (DiVincenzo et al., 1978).

Another important point emerging from this brief survey of percutaneous neurotoxicity concerns the number and range of neurotoxic agents discovered in fragrance formulations and cosmetic preparations. In some cases, as with AETT, the fragrance industry moved rapidly and responsibly once definitive evidence of neurotoxicity was obtained from animal studies. Other widely used compounds, such as zinc pyridinethione and musk ambrette, have been unregulated for many years even though experimental evidence demonstrates neurotoxic properties. Such decisions are based in part on the neurotoxic dose in animals versus the use level in humans. However, this type of reasoning fails to consider several points: (1) differences in response among species, (2) variability in susceptibility with age, (3) presence of neurotoxic drugs and chemicals in the human environment that might have an additive effect, and (4) possible special vulnerability of individuals with metabolic conditions (diabetes mellitus, alcoholism) associated with neurologic disease. Moreover, methods for the evaluation of no-effect levels have often been based on insensitive techniques such as evaluation of clinical behavior or on outdated neuropathologic methods. These considerations indicate that it will be necessary to increase the range and depth of studies to evaluate fragrance chemicals for neurotoxic effects. Experience shows that a major part of this assessment is the evaluation of nervous tissue with state-of-the-art morphological techniques that allow detection of subclinical pathology and estimation of reversibility (Spencer et al., 1980a).

REFERENCES

Abou-Donia, M. B. and Graham, D. G. 1978. Delayed neurotoxicity from long-term low-level topical administration of leptophos to the comb of hens. *Toxicol. Appl. Pharmacol.* 46:199.

Airing, C. D. 1942. The systemic nervous affinity of tri-*ortho*-cresyl phosphate. *Brain* 65:34.

Allen, N., Mendell, J. R., Billmaier, D. J., Fontaine, R. E., and O'Neill, J. 1975. Toxic polyneuropathy due to methyl *n*-butyl ketone. An industrial outbreak. *Arch. Neurol.* 32:209.

Anonymous. 1980. Toxic occupational neuropathy—Texas. *Morbid. Mortal. Weekly Rep.* 29:529.

Carroll, F. E., Jr., Salak, W. W., Howard, J. M., and Pairent, F. W. 1967. Absorption of antimicrobial agents across experimental wounds. *Surg. Gynecol. Obstet.* 125:974.

Cavanagh, J. B. 1964. The significance of the "dying-back" process in experimental and human neurological disease. *Int. Rev. Exp. Pathol.* 3:129.

Davis, D. A., Taylor, J. M., Jones, W. I., and Brouwer, J. B. 1967. Toxicity of musk ambrette. *Toxicol. Appl. Pharmacol.* 10:405.

Di Vincenzo, G. D., Kaplan, C. J., and Dedinas, J. 1976. Characterization of the metabolites of methyl *n*-butyl ketone, methyl *iso*-butyl ketone, and methyl ethyl ketone in guinea pig serum and their clearance. *Toxicol. Appl. Pharmacol.* 36:511.

Di Vincenzo, G. D., Hamilton, M. L., Kaplan, C. J., Krasavage, W. J., and

O'Donoghue, J. L. 1978. Studies on the respiratory uptake and excretion and skin absorption of MnBK in humans and dogs. *Toxicol. Appl. Pharmacol.* 44:593.

Gaines, T. B., Kimbrough, R. D., and Linder, R. E. 1973. The oral and dermal toxicity of hexachlorophene in rats. *Toxicol. Appl. Pharmacol.* 25:332.

Glees, P. and White, W. G. 1961. The absorption of tri-*ortho*-cresyl phosphate through the skin of hens and its neurotoxic effects. *J. Neurol. Neurosurg. Psychiat.* 24:271.

Johnson, M. K. 1975. Organophosphorus esters causing delayed neurotoxic effects. *Arch. Toxicol.* 34:259.

Maibach, H. I., Feldmann, R. J., Milby, T. H., and Serat, W. F. 1971. Regional variation in percutaneous penetration in man. *Arch. Environ. Health* 23:208.

Marzulli, F. 1968. Barriers to skin penetration. *J. Invest. Dermatol.* 39:334.

Nomiyama, K. and Nomiyama, H. 1974. Respiratory retention, uptake and excretion of organic solvents in man. Benzene, toluene, *n*-hexane, trichloroethylene, acetone, ethyl acetate and ethyl alcohol. *Int. Arch. Arbeitsmed.* 32:75.

Nomiyama, K., Yoshida, T., and Yanagisawa, H. 1973. Percutaneous absorption of *n*-hexane caused severe polyneuropathy. *Proc. 46th Annu. Meet. Jpn. Assoc. Ind. Health*, p. 420.

O'Donoghue, J. L. and Krasavage, W. J. 1979. The structure-activity relationships of aliphatic diketones and their potential neurotoxicity. *Toxicol. Appl. Pharmacol.* 48:A55.

Opdyke, D. L. J. 1979. *Monographs on Fragrance Raw Materials*. New York: Pergamon.

Orkin, M. and Maibach, M. I. 1978. Scabies in children. *Pediatr. Clin. North Am.* 25:371.

Powell, H., Swarner, O., Gluck, L., and Lampert, P. 1973. Hexachlorophene myelinopathy in premature infants. *J. Pediatr.* 82:976.

Sahenk, Z. and Mendell, J. R. 1980. Zinc pyridinethione. In *Experimental and Clinical Neurotoxicology*, eds. P. S. Spencer and H. H. Schaumburg, pp. 578–592. Baltimore, Md.: Williams & Wilkins.

Schaumburg, H. H. and Spencer, P. S. 1979. Clinical and experimental studies of distal axonopathy—a frequent form of nerve damage produced by environmental chemical hazards. *Ann. N.Y. Acad. Sci.* 329:14.

Schaumburg, H. H., Spencer, P. S., and Thomas, P. K. 1982. *Introduction to Peripheral Neuropathy*. Philadelphia, Pa.: Davis. In press.

Seppalainen, A. M. and Hakkinen, I. 1975. Electrophysiological findings in diphenyl poisoning. *J. Neurol. Neurosurg. Psychiat.* 38:248.

Shuman, R. M., Leech, R. W., and Alvord, E. C., Jr. 1975. Neurotoxicity of hexachlorophene in humans. II. A clinicopathologic study of 46 premature infants. *Arch. Neurol.* 32:320.

Smith, H. B. and Spaulding, J. M. K. 1959. Outbreak of paralysis in Morocco due to *ortho*-cresyl phosphate poisoning. *Lancet* ii:1019.

Snyder, F. H., Buehler, E. R., and Winek, C. L. 1965. Safety evaluation of zinc 2-pyridinethiol-1-oxide in a shampoo formulation. *Toxicol. Appl. Pharmacol.* 7:425.

Spencer, P. S. and Schaumburg, H. H. 1975. Experimental neuropathy produced by 2,5-hexanedione, a major metabolite of the neurotoxic industrial solvent methyl *n*-butyl ketone. *J. Neurol. Neurosurg. Psychiat.* 38:771.

Spencer, P. S. and Schaumburg, H. H. 1977. Ultrastructural studies of the dying-back process. IV. Differential vulnerability of PNS and CNS fibers in experimental central-peripheral distal axonopathies. *J. Neuropathol. Exp. Neurol.* 36:300.

Spencer, P. S., Sterman, A. S., Houroupian, D., Bischoff, M., and Foster, G.: 1979a. Neurotoxic changes in rats exposed to the fragrance compound acetyl ethyl tetramethyl tetralin. *Neurotoxicology* 1:221.

Spencer, P. S., Sterman, A. B., Horoupian, D. S., and Foulds, M. M. 1979b. Neurotoxic fragrance produces ceroid and myelin disease. *Science* 204:663.

Spencer, P. S., Bischoff, M. C., and Schaumburg, H. H. 1980a. Neuropathological methods for the detection of neurotoxic disease. In *Experimental and Clinical Neurotoxicology*, eds. P. S. Spencer and H. H. Schaumburg, pp. 743–757. Baltimore, Md.: Williams & Wilkins.

Spencer, P. S., Foster, G. V., Sterman, A. B., and Horoupian, D. 1980b. Acetyl ethyl tetramethyl tetralin. In *Experimental and Clinical Neurotoxicology*, eds. P. S. Spencer and H. H. Schaumburg, pp. 296–308. Baltimore, Md.: Williams & Wilkins.

Spencer, P. S., Schaumburg, H. H., Sabri, M. I., and Veronesi, B. 1980c. The enlarging view of hexacarbon neurotoxicity. *Crit. Rev. Toxicol.* 7:4.

Taylor, P. 1980. Acetylcholinesterase agents. In *The Pharmacological Basis of Therapeutics*, eds. A. Goodman Gilman, L. S. Goodman, and A. Gilman, 6th ed., pp. 100–119. New York: Macmillan.

Towfighi, J., Gonotas, N. K., and McGree, L. 1974. Hexachlorophene-induced changes in central and peripheral myelinated axons of developed and adult rats. *Lab. Invest.* 31:712.

Towfighi, J., Gonatas, N. K., and McGree, L. 1975. Hexachlorophene retinopathy in rats. *Lab. Invest.* 32:330.

Wedig, J. H., Feldmann, R. J., and Maibach, H. I. 1977. Percutaneous penetration of the magnesium sulfate adduct of dipyrithione in man. *Toxicol. Appl. Pharmacol.* 41:1.

Xintaras, C. and Burg, J. E. 1980. Screening and prevention of human neurotoxic outbreaks: Issues and problems. In *Experimental and Clinical Neurotoxicology*, eds. P. S. Spencer and H. H. Schaumburg, pp. 663–674. Baltimore, Md.: Williams & Wilkins.

30

identification of contact pustulogens

Jan E. Wahlberg ■ Howard I. Maibach

INTRODUCTION

Pustular patch test reactions in humans have been observed with metal compounds (e.g., nickel, chromium, mercury, arsenic) and halogens (e.g., iodide, fluoride) (Becker and O'Brien, 1959; Bjornberg, 1968; Eberhartinger et al., 1969; Fisher et al., 1959; Plewig and Kligman, 1972; Stone and Johnson, 1967; Sulzberger, 1940; Uehara et al., 1975; Wahlberg and Skog, 1971). Such reactions are more common in patients with atopic dermatitis (Sulzberger, 1940) and seem distinct, clinically and histopathologically, from allergic and irritant reactions (Fisher, 1973). When performing serial dilution tests in nickel-allergic patients, pustular reactions were observed in 3 of 53 (Wahlberg and Skog, 1971). Pustules were seen only at the highest concentrations and the vehicle (petrolatum, water) seemed to play a role. Pustulation seems concentration- and vehicle-dependent (Wahlberg, 1976). Our aim was to develop an animal model to define chemicals that are pustulogens on topical application and to analyze factors that contribute to pustulation. A pustulogen can be defined as a chemical that causes sterile pustulation on topical application.

Reprinted with permission from the *Journal of Investigative Dermatology*, vol. 76, pp. 381–383 (1981).

MATERIALS AND METHODS

Experimental Animals

New Zealand white rabbits weighing 2.5-4 kg were used. The hair on the back was clipped with an Oster animal electric clipper, blade sizes 10, ANG-RA, and 40. Skin that was visibly damaged was not tested.

Chemicals

Ammonium fluoride (NH_4F) was obtained from Baker & Adamsson, Morristown, N. J.; benzalkonium chloride, UC Hospital Pharmacy, San Francisco, Calif.; croton oil, Robinson Laboratories, San Francisco; mercuric chloride ($HgCl_2$), J. T. Baker, Phillipsburg, N.J.; nickel sulfate ($NiSO_4 \cdot 6 H_2O$), J. T. Baker; potassium iodide (KI), Mallinckrodt, St. Louis, Mo.; sodium arsenate ($Na_2HAsO_4 \cdot 7 H_2O$), Matheson, Coleman & Bell, Los Angeles, Calif.; sodium lauryl sulfate (SLS), Matheson, Coleman & Bell.

Vehicles

White petrolatum USP (w/w), nonionic base UC-hydrous (w/w), hydrophilic ointment USP (w/w), distilled water (w/v). Liquid petrolatum USP was used for control oil (v/v). A vehicle control was applied in each experiment.

Concentrations

Concentrations of 0.01-50% were used. The first concentration chosen was based on results obtained from patch testing in humans (see above); this was gradually increased. The lower concentrations (0.01-1%) were mainly used in series with damaged skin to find a threshold for pustulation.

Test Patches, Tapes, Wrapping

Al-test (diameter, 10 mm), Big Finn chamber (diameter, 12 mm) (V. Pirila, personal communication, 1979), Finn chamber (diameter, 8 mm), and Webril (1 cm^2). Scanpore (Norgeplaster A/S, Norway) and Scotch transparent tape (No. 600, 3M) were used to attach and to secure the patches.

Wrapping was Elastoplast (Beiersdorf Inc., Norwalk, Conn.) was used to obtain optimal occlusion. Exposure time was 24 h.

Physical Damage

For some chemicals it was necessary to damage the skin to obtain pustules. Premarked sites were treated with a sterile knife; scraping or scratching in the shape of an X (Stone and Willis, 1969) with needle stabbings (sterile 20 or 22 gauge) (Uehara et al., 1975) or with a Berkley scarifier (Phillips et al., 1972).

Reading

Erythema, papules, vesicles, pustules, induration, necrosis, scaling, and scarring were recorded by visual examination. In the text and tables, however, mainly the presence or absence of pustules is presented. Reactions were assessed daily for 4–5 d.

Sterility

To exclude a bacterial cause or contamination of the pustules, culture and/or Gram staining of their contents were performed.

RESULTS

Macroscopic Picture

Solitary, yellow pustules, 1–2 mm in diameter, were obtained from application of SLS and $HgCl_2$ on normal skin. The few pustules obtained from 40% $NiSO_4$ and Na_2HAsO_4 had the same appearance. Erythema around the pustules was usually slight. The yellow pustules from NH_4F were 2–4 mm in diameter. Croton oil caused erythema and edema; the dark yellow pustules were sometimes difficult to detect.

Time Course

Pustules were present at 24 h and persisted for 1–3 d. A delayed appearance, at the 48 h reading, was not observed.

Sterility

If culture and/or Gram staining of pustule content was positive, the experiment was discarded. This occurred mainly in the damaged skin experiments (see below). In the damaged skin experiments, approximately 5% of pustules revealed Gram-positive cocci that were, on culture, identified as *Staphylococcus pyogenes* variety *aureus*.

Comparison of Test Patches

In each of 12 rabbits, 4 types of patches were applied simultaneously. Experiments were performed with three concentrations of $HgCl_2$ (5, 10, 20%), four of NH_4F (10, 15, 20, and 30%), and 5% SLS in petrolatum. Pustules were obtained in all 12 experiments with Big Finn chambers, in 8 with Al patches and in 6 with small Finn chambers and Webril, respectively. Pustule absence was not related to the test substance used.

Based on these results, Big Finn chambers were used in subsequent experiments.

Vehicle Comparison

In each of 11 rabbits, the same concentration of the test substance was applied in petrolatum and in water. With 5% $HgCl_2$, pustules were observed only with petrolatum; with NH_4F and SLS similar numbers of pustules were obtained with both vehicles. In an experiment with 40% $NiSO_4$ in petrolatum,

1 pustule was obtained, while the remaining 5 with petrolatum and water were negative. In 4 experiments with 40% NiSO$_4$ in 2 other vehicles (nonionic base and hydrophilic ointment) no pustules were obtained. Based on these findings, petrolatum was selected for further studies because this vehicle seemed to be more reliable. If no pustules were obtained with petrolatum, the other vehicles were tried.

Effect of Clipping

In each of 4 rabbits, the left side of the dorsal skin was clipped 3 times (48 h, 24 h, and immediately before exposure), while the right side was clipped only once, 48 h before exposure. Three sites on each side were exposed to the same concentration of the test substances (HgCl$_2$ and SLS). In one of the 12 sites where clipping had been performed 3 times, 2 pustules were obtained. Pustulation was not seen in any of the 12 sites where clipping was performed 48 h before exposure.

Based on these preliminary findings, clipping was performed once, 24 h before exposure.

Variability in Pustulation (Table 1)

Identical patches were applied on 5 sites in each of 10 rabbits. Pustulation was independent of which anatomic site (anterior-posterior, left-right) was exposed.

Effect of Concentration: Croton Oil, HgCl$_2$, SLS, NH$_4$F

Five to seven concentrations were applied in each rabbit. Clear dose response relations (Fig. 1) were obtained for croton oil (10 rabbits), HgCl$_2$ (6 rabbits, Table 2), and SLS (8 rabbits). For NH$_4$F (16 rabbits) the response was less certain; even when the concentration was raised to 20–30%, no more than 70% of the sites showed pustules.

NiSO$_4$

Nine concentrations (0.1–50% in petrolatum) were studied (minimum of 10 sites for each concentration). In 3 of 19 sites exposed to 40%, pustules were obtained, while all other experiments were negative, including 50% NiSO$_4$ in water, nonionic base, and hydrophilic ointment.

KI

Thirteen sites exposed to 50% in petrolatum and in water were negative.

Na$_2$HAsO$_4$

Exposure to 40% in petrolatum gave one pustule in 1 of 12 sites.

TABLE 1 Regional Variation in Pustulation; the Same Concentration in Petrolatum Was Applied to 5 Sites in the Same Rabbit[a]

Rabbit	Test substance and concentration (%)	Site[b] (no. of pustules)					6 (petrolatum control)
		1	2	3	4	5	
1	HgCl$_2$, 5	1	2	4	2	4	0
2	HgCl$_2$, 10	15	10	ct[c]	8	12	0
3	NH$_4$F, 15	0	0	1	1	0	0
4	NH$_4$F, 20	2	0	1	2	1	0
5	NH$_4$F, 30	0	2	1	1	1	0
6	NH$_4$F, 30	5	2	2	1	2	0
7	SLS, 1	2	1	0	1	2	0
8	SLS, 1	1	2	0	0	1	0
9	SLS, 5	ct	ct	ct	ct	ct	0
10	NiSO$_4$, 40	5	5	0	0	0	0
Total no. of positive sites		8	8	7	8	8	0

[a] Big Finn Chambers, 24 h exposure.

[b] Site 1, anterior left; 2, midleft; 3, posterior left; 4, anterior right; 5, midright; and 6, posterior right.

[c] Confluent.

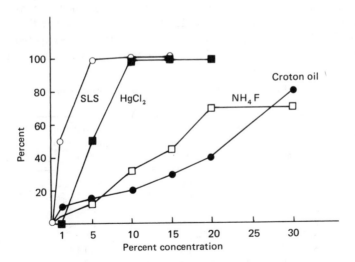

FIGURE 1 Dose-response curves. The y-axis shows the percent of exposed sites with pustules.

TABLE 2   Pustulation at Various Concentrations
of HgCl$_2$ in Petrolatum

| Rabbit | No. of pustules at site[a] | | | | | |
	1	2	3	4	5	6 (petrolatum control)
11	0	0	4	6	ct	0
12	0	0	1	10	ct	0
13	0	3	3	10	ct	0
14	0	0	10	3	10	0
15	0	2	7	10	ct	0
16	0	2	ct	ct	ct	0

[a]Concentration at site 1, 1%; site 2, 5%; site 3, 10%; site 4, 15%; and site 5, 20%.

Benzalkonium Chloride

At 0.1, 1.5, and 10% in water, benzalkonium chloride gave a light-yellow staining and a severe induration of the test sites (5 rabbits). No solitary pustules were observed.

Physical Damage

Of the methods tried, stabbings with a needle gave the most reproducible results: At the corners of an equilateral triangle (side, 5 mm) the skin was stabbed with a sterile needle, which then was rotated a few times. Six to eight sites and corresponding numbers of control sites were exposed to each concentration (0.01, 0.1, 1, and 10%) of the test compounds. At the reading,

TABLE 3   Threshold Concentrations for Pustulations
in Normal and Damaged Skin[a]

Agent	Normal skin concentration (%)	After stabbing concentration (%)
Croton oil	1.0	0.1
NH$_4$F	1.0	0.1
SLS	1.0	Not tested
HgCl$_2$	5.0	Not tested
Na$_2$HAsO$_4$	40.0	1.0
NiSO$_4$	40.0	0.1
KI	>50.0	10.0

[a]Benzalkonium chloride: induration, necrosis, but no pustules. Note the $\geq$10-fold difference in concentration between normal and stabbed skin sites.

the holes in the skin were surrounded by an inner yellow ring (1–3 mm) and an outer erythema. With this maneuver, pustulation was easily obtained with KI, Na_2HAsO_4, and $NiSO_4$ (Table 3) and the number of positive responses was related to concentration.

To study the effect of tissue damage (Stone and Willis, 1968) the following experiments were performed. After penetrating the epidermis outside a premarked area, 10 mm of the needle was inserted through the dermis parallel to the skin surface, rotated and redrawn. No injection was performed. The same number of pustules was obtained at 3 sites with preexisting trauma and at 3 control sites in an experiment with 5% $HgCl_2$. In the experiments with 1% SLS (2 rabbits) and 40% $NiSO_4$ (1 rabbit) no pustules were obtained at either pretreated or control sites. The tissue damage caused by the needle did not lower the concentration for obtaining pustules.

DISCUSSION

Sterile pustules occur in several skin diseases, including pustular psoriasis, pustulosis palmoplantaris, subcorneal pustulosis [for a review, see Wilkinson (1969)]; the final steps in the evolution of the pustules from internal or external factors might be similar. By disclosing the external factors, which are easier to study and define, we hope to gain insight into the mechanism for the pustulation seen in some dermatoses and triggered by mainly internal factors. A possible mechanism for the pustule formation has been proposed by Tagami and Ofuju (1978).

Of the 8 chemicals studied, SLS and $HgCl_2$ gave reproducible pustulation and clear dose-response curves (Figs. 1 and 2a,b). The findings support the idea that this pustulation is an expression of irritancy.

The pustules from the application of NH_4F were not always reproducible. Raising the concentration to 30% gave a positive response in only 70% of the exposures (Fig. 1). The reason is not known, but possibly implies another mechanism for pustulation than for SLS and $HgCl_2$. Pustules were obtained from Webril, so this is not ascribed to interaction with the Al in the other patches.

For KI, Na_2HAsO_4, and $NiSO_4$ reproducible pustulation was obtained when the skin barriers had been damaged (Table 3). Similar findings were described for $NiSO_4$ by Stone and Willis (1968) and Uehara et al. (1975).

Biopsies were taken to verify the histological picture of pustules described by others (Becker and O'Brien, 1959; Eberhartinger et al., 1969; Fisher et al., 1959; Plewig and Kligman, 1972; Stone and Willis, 1969; Uehara et al., 1975). Our findings were identical to those of Stone and Willis (1968, 1969). Pustular reactions in patch testing have engendered considerable discussion (Becker and O'Brien, 1959; Bjornberg, 1968; Eberhartinger et al., 1969; Fisher et al., 1959; Plewig and Kligman, 1972; Stone and Johnson, 1967; Sulzberger, 1940; Uehara et al., 1975; Wahlberg and Skog, 1971). We

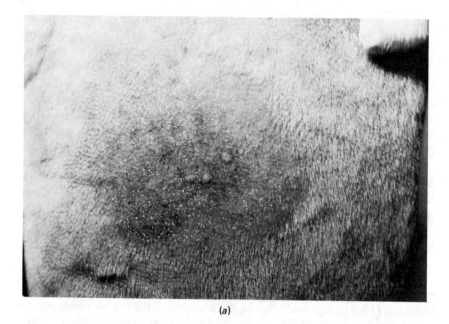

(a)

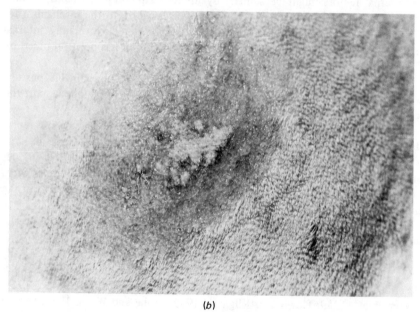

(b)

FIGURE 2 Solitary pustules (*a*) and more confluent reactions (*b*) 24 h after application of 5% HgCl$_2$ in petrolatum (rabbits).

note that they are often not reproducible. We wonder whether these patches were, in fact, unwittingly placed on microscopically damaged skin, similar to that produced by stabbing in these experiments?

These experiments show that certain chemicals (SLS and $HgCl_2$) readily produce pustules in this model, whereas others (Na_2HAsO_4, $NiSO_4$, and KI) require prior skin damage. We noted sparse sterile pustules in occupational irritant dermatitis in humans but have not made a systematic survey of their frequency. Clearly, this is required to ascertain how this predictive type of testing relates to pustulogens in humans.

REFERENCES

Becker, S. W. and O'Brien, M. P. 1959. Value of patch tests in dermatology. *Arch. Dermatol.* 79:569.

Bjornberg, A. 1968. *Skin Reactions to Primary Irritants in Patient with Hand Eczema.* Göteborg, Sweden: Isacsons.

Eberhartinger, C., Ebner, H., and Klotz, L. 1969. Zur Kenntnis under interpretation follikulärer, papulo-pustuloser Reaktionen im Epikutantest. *Berufs Dermatosen* 17:241.

Fisher, A. A. 1973. *Contact Dermatitis,* pp. 30–31. Philadelphia, Pa.: Lea & Febiger.

Fisher, A. A., Chargin, L., Fleischmajer, R., and Hyman, A. 1959. Pustular patch test reactions. *Arch. Dermatol.* 80:742.

Phillips, L., Steinberg, M., Maibach, H. I., and Akers, W. A. 1972. A comparison of rabbit and human skin response to certain irritants. *Toxicol. Appl. Pharmacol.* 21:369.

Plewig, G. and Kligman, A. M. 1972. Follikuläre Pusteln im Kaliumjodid-Epicutantest. *Arch. Dermatol. Forsch.* 242:137.

Stone, O. J. and Willis, C. J. 1968. Sterile cutaneous pustular reaction. *J. Invest. Dermatol.* 50:280.

Stone, O. J. and Johnson, D. A. 1967. Pustular patch test-experimentally induced. *Arch. Dermatol.* 95:618.

Stone, O. J. and Willis, C. J. 1969. Enhancement of inflammation by fluorides. *Tex. Rep. Biol. Med.* 25:601.

Sulzberger, M. B. 1940. *Dermatologic Allergy,* p. 175. Springfield, Ill.: Thomas.

Tagami, H. and Ofuju, S. 1978. A leukotactic factor in the stratum corneum of pustulosis palmaris et plantaris: A possible mechanism for the formation of intra-epidermal sterile pustules. *Acta Derm. Venereol. (Stockh.)* 58:401.

Uehara, M., Takahashi, C., and Ofuji, S. 1975. Pustular patch test reactions in atopic dermatitis. *Arch. Dermatol.* 111:1154.

Wahlberg, J. E. and Skog, E. 1971. Nickel allergy and atopy. Threshold of nickel sensitivity and immunoglobulin E determinations. *Br. J. Dermatol.* 85:97.

Wahlberg, J. E. 1976. Immunoglobulin E., atopy, and nickel allergy. *Cutis* 18:715.

Wilkinson, D. S. 1969. Pustular dermatoses. *Br. J. Dermatol.* 8 (Suppl.)3:38.

appendixes

Appendixes

oecd guidelines
for testing of chemicals[1]

PREFACE

General

1. This publication contains the official OECD[2] Guidelines for Testing of Chemicals as adopted by the OECD Council.

2. The Test Guidelines have been developed initially under the OECD Chemicals Testing Programme (see paragraphs 10-16 below), and subsequently, since 1981, as provided by the council under the OECD Updating Programme for Test Guidelines.

3. Whenever testing of chemicals is contemplated, the OECD Test Guidelines should be consulted. Since the Test Guidelines have been endorsed by the OECD Member countries, their use in the generation of data provides a common basis for the acceptance of data internationally, together with the opportunity to reduce direct and indirect costs to governments and industry associated with testing and assessment of chemicals.

4. Other methods and guidelines not included in this publication may be judged to be appropriate in testing chemicals in certain scientific, legal, and administrative contexts.

5. The OECD Council Decision on Mutual Acceptance of Data [12th May, 1981; C(81)30] affirms that data generated in one country in

---

[1] The following portions of the *OECD Guidelines for Testing of Chemicals* are reprinted with permission.

[2] Organization for Economic Cooperation and Development.

accordance with the OECD Test Guidelines—and additionally in accordance with the OECD Principles of Good Laboratory Practice—should be accepted in OECD countries for purposes of assessment and other uses relating to protection of man and the environment. The full text of this Decision and the OECD Principles of Good Laboratory Practice may be found in the Appendix to the OECD Guidelines for Testing of Chemicals.

6. The OECD Test Guidelines contain generally formulated procedures for the laboratory testing of a property or effect deemed important for the evaluation of health and environmental hazards of a chemical. The Guidelines vary somewhat in respect of detail, but include all the essential elements which, assuming good laboratory practice, should enable an operator to carry out the required test.

7. OECD Test Guidelines are not designed to serve as rigid test protocols. They are instead designed to allow flexibility for expert judgment and adjustment to new developments.

8. It is intended that the OECD Test Guidelines be used by experienced laboratory staff familiar with the type(s) of testing involved. Proper conduct of testing and associated interpretation of results can only be achieved by appropriately trained personnel with access to adequately equipped laboratory facilities.

9. The loose-leaf system chosen for the Guidelines allows for additions and changes to be made when necessary. Information will be circulated when such changes occur resulting from work under the Updating Programme.

OECD Chemicals Testing Programme

10. The OECD Chemicals Testing Programme was launched by the Chemicals Group in November, 1977. It comprised six Expert Groups under the leadership of individual Member countries. One of these Groups, the Step Systems Group, worked on phased approaches to testing and assessment of chemicals (see paragraphs 30–32 below).

11. Five of the groups reviewed the state-of-the-art of methods and produced draft Test Guidelines. The following areas were covered:

    i. Physical-chemical properties (Lead country—Germany).
    ii. Effects on biotic systems other than man (Lead country—the Netherlands).
    iii. Degradation/accumulation (Lead countries—Japan/Germany).
    iv. Long term health effects (Lead country—The United States).
    v. Short term health effects (Lead country—The United Kingdom).

12. Some 300 experts, drawn from academia, government, industry, international organisations, and other sectors, took part in the Programme. In all, some 50 meetings were held during 1978-1979 under the auspices of the OECD Chemicals Testing Programme.

13. In order to improve the international validation of tests, several methods were subjected to laboratory intercomparison exercises in the Chemicals Testing Programme. This work is being continued under the OECD Updating Programme.

14. In December, 1979, the five Expert Groups working on test methods submitted their reports to the OECD. The two Groups on health effects submitted a combined report. The reports contained draft Test Guidelines and an analysis of approaches to testing within the respective areas.

15. During 1980, the draft Test Guidelines were subjected to an extensive commentary and review process. Member countries were invited to submit comments to the OECD which were subsequently taken into account by a Review Panel, established to finalise the product for adoption and printing. The Panel worked in close collaboration with the Chairman of the Expert Groups.

16. The review process was concluded by the Chemicals Group and the Environment Committee of the Organisation, which endorsed these Test Guidelines prior to their formal submission to the OECD Council.

17. The subject areas covered by the Expert Groups under the Chemicals Testing Programme have largely been kept separate in this publication. Thus, OECD Test Guidelines are presented under four different sections:

- physical-chemical properties
- effects on biotic systems other than man
- degradation/accumulation
- health effects

18. Each section is preceded by a summary of considerations raised in the individual expert group reports. These summaries reflect some of the major observations and explanations made at the scientific level during the preparatory process. Further, major portions of the expert group reports have been absorbed into the on-going activities of OECD on chemicals.

OECD Updating Programme for Test Guidelines

19. In 1981, the OECD Updating Programme for Test Guidelines was established by Member countries in consultation with the Commission of the European Communities. The aim was to ensure that OECD Test Guidelines will not become outdated as a result of major changes in the state-of-the-art or scientific advances.

20. The Updating Programme is considering:

a. Proposals for new or modified tests which offer conspicuous advantages over those already adopted.
b. New guidelines which are being developed in areas not yet covered.

    c. Incorporation of results from the Chemicals Testing Programme into OECD Test Guidelines.

    d. Those matters which need further investigation and research.

OECD Principles for Testing and Assessment of Chemicals

21. The OECD Test Guidelines are but one component in an OECD strategy to make testing of chemicals more systematic, relevant, and cost effective within an international framework which could lead to increased exchange and acceptance of test data between countries. This strategy has been developed with vigour in the Organisation during the 1970s leaving several important questions yet to be resolved.

22. While the OECD Test Guidelines can properly be used in establishing one effect or property, the Guidelines were developed under programmes directed towards an integrated and comprehensive approach to testing and assessment. Thus, the OECD Council, in 1974 and 1977, developed recommendations which deal respectively with "The Assessment of the Potential Environmental Effects of Chemicals" [C(74)215] and "Guidelines in Respect to Procedures and Requirements for Anticipating the Effects of Chemicals on Man and in the Environment" [C(77)97(Final)].

23. In 1974, the OECD Council recommended that prior to marketing of chemicals their potential effects on man and his environment should be assessed.

24. This concern, that assessments should encompass both man and his environment, was reflected in the subject areas chosen for the OECD Chemicals Testing Programme, and is also reflected in the disposition of the Test Guidelines into sections.

25. Some outstanding features with respect to testing and assessment which derive from the 1977 OECD Council Recommendation can be summarised as follows:

    i. Chemical substances—with special emphasis on new substances—should be subjected to systematic assessment for potential effects, in relation to both human and environmental hazard.

    ii. It is possible to determine no more than the likelihood of adverse effects from chemicals, and this can only be done through the application of expert judgment based on methods that are technically practicable, as well as economically acceptable.

    iii. Responsibility for generating and assessing the data necessary to determine the potential effects of chemicals must be part of the overall function and liability of industry.

    iv. A phased approach should be applied in data gathering and assessments.

26. These four principles also provided guidance to the Expert Groups in their work in the Chemicals Testing Programme.

27. The need for expert judgment in testing and assessment has been emphasised throughout the work on chemicals in OECD. The Expert Groups under the OECD Chemicals Testing Programme reaffirmed this need when they selected methods that were regarded as technically practicable and economically acceptable for inclusion into OECD Test Guidelines.

28. The question of a phased approach to testing and assessment is an important concept which is under continuing active consideration in OECD within the Chemicals Testing Programme. All the expert groups have contributed to the framework of an overall scheme for testing and assessment of chemicals.

29. In their work the five Expert Groups on test methods identified steps in which testing and assessment might proceed. The early steps were usually simple in character with the objective of establishing a first indication of hazard. Further steps brought the testing and assessment into a sophisticated and time-consuming range of tests, characterised by increased confidence in the assessments.

30. The Step Systems Group, the sixth Expert Group established under the Chemicals Testing Programme, draws upon the work of the other Expert Groups and is currently developing an integrated stepwise approach to testing and assessment of chemical hazard to man and his environment.

31. An important outcome of the work of the Step Systems Group is the OECD Minimum Pre-marketing set of Data (MPD).

32. MPD lists some thirty-five individual data components that normally would be sufficient to perform a meaningful first assessment of the potential hazard of a chemical.

33. Finally, it should be recognised that elaboration of principles for testing and assessment of chemicals is a continuing process within OECD. This process has been, and remains, possible only through the generous provision of time, knowledge, and enthusiasm from the participating experts, and the active support of Member countries.

ACUTE DERMAL TOXICITY
(GUIDELINE #402)[1]

1. Introductory Information

Prerequisites

- Solid or liquid test substance
- Chemical identification of test substance
- Purity (impurities) of test substance
- Solubility characteristics
- Melting point/boiling point
- pH (where appropriate)

Standard Documents

There are no relevant international standards.

2. Method

A. Introduction, Purpose, Scope, Relevance, Application and Limits of Test

In the assessment and evaluation of the toxic characteristics of a substance, determination of acute dermal toxicity is useful where exposure by the dermal route is likely. It provides information on health hazards likely to arise from a short term exposure by the dermal route. Data from an acute dermal toxicity study may serve as a basis for classification and labelling. It is an initial step in establishing a dosage regimen in subchronic and other studies and may provide information on dermal absorption and the mode of toxic action of a substance by this route.

Definitions

Acute dermal toxicity is the adverse effects occurring within a short time of dermal application of a single dose of a test substance.

Dose is the amount of test substance applied. Dose is expressed as weight (g, mg) or as weight of test substance per unit weight of test animal (e.g., mg/kg).

[1] Adopted May 12, 1981. Users of this Test Guideline should consult the Preface, in particular paragraphs 3, 4, 7, and 8.

The LD50 (median lethal dose), dermal, is a statistically derived single dose of a substance that can be expected to cause death in 50 per cent of treated animals when applied to the skin. The LD50 value is expressed in terms of weight of test substance per unit weight of test animal (mg/kg).

Dosage is a general term comprising the dose, its frequency and the duration of dosing.

Dose-response is the relationship between the dose and the proportion of a population sample showing a defined effect.

Dose-effect is the relationship between the dose and the magnitude of a defined biological effect either in an individual or in a population sample.

Principles of the Test Method

The test substance is applied to the skin in graduated doses to several groups of experimental animals, one dose being used per group. Subsequently, observations of effects and deaths are made. Animals which die during the test are necropsied, and at the conclusion of the test the surviving animals are sacrificed and necropsied as necessary.

Description of the Test Procedure

Preparations

Healthy young adult animals are acclimatised to the laboratory conditions for at least 5 days prior to the test. Before the test, animals are randomised and assigned to the treatment groups. Approximately 24 hours before the test, fur should be removed from the dorsal area of the trunk of the test animals by clipping or shaving. Care must be taken to avoid abrading the skin which could alter its permeability.

Not less than 10 per cent of the body surface area should be clear for the application of the test substance. The weight of the animal should be taken into account when deciding on the area to be cleared and on the dimensions of the covering.

When testing solids, which may be pulverised if appropriate, the test substance should be moistened sufficiently with water or, where necessary, a suitable vehicle to ensure good contact with the skin. When a vehicle is used, the influence of the vehicle on penetration of skin by the test substance should be taken into account. Liquid test substances are generally used undiluted.

Experimental Animals

Selection of species. The adult rat, rabbit or guinea pig may be used. Other species may be used but their use would require justification. The following weight ranges are suggested to provide animals of a size which facilitates the conduct of the test: rats, 200 to 300 g; rabbits, 2.0 to 3.0 kg; guinea pigs, 350 to 450 g.

Number and sex. Equal numbers of animals of each sex with healthy intact skin are required for each dose level. At least 10 animals (5 female and 5 male) should be used at each dose level. The females should be nulliparous and non-pregnant. A smaller number of animals may sometimes be used, especially in the case of the rabbit, but this may prevent the determination of an acceptable LD50.

Housing and feeding conditions. Animals should be caged individually. The temperature of the experimental animal room should be 22°C (±3°) for rodents, 20°C (±3°) for rabbits, and the relative humidity 30–70 per cent. Where the lighting is artificial, the sequence should be 12 hours light, 12 hours dark. For feeding, conventional laboratory diets may be used with an unlimited supply of drinking water.

Test Conditions

Dose levels. These should be sufficient in number, at least three, and spaced appropriately to produce test groups with a range of toxic effects and mortality rates. The data should be sufficient to produce a dose-response curve and, where possible, permit an acceptable determination of the LD50.

Limit test. If a test at one dose level of at least 2000 mg/kg body weight, using the procedures described for this study, produces no compound-related mortality, then a full study using three dose levels may not be necessary.

Observation period. The observation period should be at least 14 days. However, the duration of observation should not be fixed rigidly. It should be determined by the toxic reactions, rate of onset and length of recovery period, and may thus be extended when considered necessary. The time at which signs of toxicity appear and disappear, their duration and the time of death are important, especially if there is a tendency for deaths to be delayed.

Procedure

The test substance should be applied uniformly over an area which is approximately 10 per cent of the total body surface area. With highly toxic substances the surface area covered may be less, but as much of the area should be covered with as thin and uniform a film as possible.

Test substances should be held in contact with the skin with a porous gauze dressing and non-irritating tape throughout a 24-hour exposure period. The test site should be further covered in a suitable manner to retain the gauze dressing and test substance and ensure that the animals cannot ingest the test substance. Restrainers may be used to prevent the ingestion of the test substance, but complete immobilisation is not a recommended method.

At the end of the exposure period, residual test substance should be removed, where practicable using water or an appropriate solvent.

Clinical Examinations

Observations should be recorded systematically as they are made. Individual records should be maintained for each animal. Following application of the test substance, the animals should be observed frequently during the first day and then a careful clinical examination should be made at least once each day. Additional observations should be made daily with appropriate actions taken to minimise loss of animals to the study, e.g. necropsy or refrigeration of those animals found dead and isolation or sacrifice of weak or moribund animals. Cageside observations should include changes in fur, eyes, and mucous membranes, and also respiratory, circulatory, autonomic and central nervous system, and somatomotor activity and behaviour pattern. Particular attention should be directed to observations of tremors, convulsions, salivation, diarrhoea, lethargy, sleep, and coma. The time of death must be recorded as precisely as possible.

Individual weights of animals should be determined shortly before the test substance is applied, weekly thereafter, and at death; changes in weight should be calculated and recorded when survival exceeds one day. At the end of the test surviving animals are weighed and then sacrificed.

Pathology

Consideration should be given to gross necropsy of all animals where indicated by the nature of the toxic effects observed. All gross pathological changes should be recorded. Microscopic examination of organs showing evidence of gross pathology in animals surviving 24 or more hours should also be considered because it may yield useful information.

Data and Reporting

Treatment of Results

Data may be summarised in tabular form, showing for each test group the number of animals at the start of the test, time of death of individual animals at different dose levels, number of animals displaying other signs of toxicity, description of toxic effects, and necropsy findings.

The LD50 may be determined by any accepted method, e.g., Bliss (4), Litchfield and Wilcoxon (3), Finney (5), Weil (6), Thompson (7), Miller and Tainter (8).

Evaluation of Results

The dermal LD50 value should always be considered in conjunction with the observed toxic effects and the necropsy findings. The LD50 value is a relatively coarse measurement, useful only as a reference value for classification and labelling purposes, and an expression of the lethal potential of the test substance following dermal exposure.

Reference should always be made to the experimental animal species in which the LD50 value was obtained. An evaluation should include an evaluation of relationships, if any, between the animals' exposure to the test substance and the incidence and severity of all abnormalities, including behavioural and clinical abnormalities, gross lesions, body weight changes, effect on mortality, and any other toxic effects.

Test Report

The test report should include the following information:

- Species/strain used
- Tabulation of response data by sex and dose level (i.e., number of animals dying, number of animals showing signs of toxicity, number of animals exposed)
- Time of death after dosing
- LD50 value for each sex (intact skin) determined at 14 days with the method of determination specified
- 95 per cent confidence interval for the LD50 (where this can be provided)
- Dose-mortality curve and slope (where permitted by the method of determination)
- Pathology findings

Interpretation of the Results

A study of acute toxicity by the dermal (percutaneous) route and determination of a dermal LD50 provides an estimate of the relative toxicity of a substance by the dermal route of exposure.

Extrapolation of the results of acute dermal toxicity studies and dermal LD50 values in animals to man is valid only to a limited degree. The results of an acute dermal toxicity study should be considered in conjunction with data from acute toxicity studies by other routes.

Literature

(1) WHO Publication: Environmental Health Criteria 6, *Principles and Methods for Evaluating the Toxicity of Chemicals*. Part I, Geneva, 1978.

(2) National Academy of Sciences, Committee for the Revision of NAS Publication 1138, *Principles and Procedures for Evaluating the Toxicity of Household Substances,* Washington, 1977.

(3) Litchfield, J. T. and Wilcoxon, F., *J. Pharmacol., Exp. Ther.,* 96, 99-113, 1949.

(4) Bliss, C. I., *Quart. J. Pharm. Pharmacol.,* 11, 192-216, 1938.

(5) Finney, D. G., *Probit Analysis* (3rd Ed.), London, Cambridge University Press, 1971.

(6) Weil, C. S., *Biometrics,* 8, 249-263, 1952.

(7) Thompson, W., *Bact. Rev.,* 11, 115-141, 1947.

(8) Miller, L. C. and Tainter, M. L., *Proc. Soc. Exp. Biol. Med. NY,* 57, 261-264, 1944.

ACUTE DERMAL IRRITATION/CORROSION
(GUIDELINE #404)[1]

Introductory Information

Prerequisites

- Solid or liquid test substance
- Chemical identification of test substance
- Purity (impurities) of test substance
- Solubility characteristics
- pH (where appropriate)
- Melting point/boiling point

Standard Documents

There are no relevant international standards.

Method

Introduction, Purpose, Scope, Relevance, Application and Limits of Test

In the assessment and evaluation of the toxic characteristics of a substance, determination of the irritant or corrosive effects on skin of mammals is an important initial step. Information derived from this test serves to indicate the existence of possible hazards likely to arise from exposure to the skin.

Definitions

Dermal irritation is the production of reversible inflammatory changes in the skin following the application of a test substance.

Dermal corrosion is the production of irreversible tissue damage in the skin following the application of a test substance.

Principle of the Test Method

The substance to be tested is applied in a single dose to the skin of several experimental animals, each animal serving as its own control. The

[1] Adopted May 12, 1981. Users of this Test Guideline should consult the Preface, in particular paragraphs 3, 4, 7, and 8.

647

degree of irritation is read and scored at specified intervals and is further described to provide complete evaluation of the effects. The duration of the study should be sufficient to evaluate fully the reversibility or irreversibility of the effects observed.

Description of the Test Procedure

Preparations

Approximately 24 hours before the test, fur should be removed by clipping or shaving from the dorsal area of the trunk of the animals. Care should be taken to avoid abrading the skin. Only animals with healthy intact skin should be used.

When testing solids (which may be pulverised if considered necessary) the test substance should be moistened sufficiently with water or, where necessary, a suitable vehicle, to ensure good contact with the skin. When vehicles are used, the influence of the vehicle on irritation of skin by the test substance should be taken into account. Liquid test substances are generally used undiluted.

Strongly acidic or alkaline substances, for example with a demonstrated pH of 2 or less or 11.5 or greater, need not be tested for primary dermal irritation, owing to their predictable corrosive properties. The testing of materials which have been shown to be highly toxic by the dermal route is unnecessary.

Experimental Animals

Selection of species. Although several mammalian species may be used, the albino rabbit is recommended as the preferred species.

Number of animals. At least 3 healthy adult animals should be used. Additional animals may be required to clarify equivocal responses.

Housing and feeding conditions. Animals should be individually housed. The temperature of the experimental animal room should be 22°C (±3°) for rodents, 20°C (±3°) for rabbits, and the relative humidity 30 to 70 per cent. Where the lighting is artificial, the sequence should be 12 hours light, 12 hours dark. Conventional laboratory diets are suitable for feeding and an unrestricted supply of drinking water should be available.

Test Conditions

Dose level. A dose of 0.5 ml of liquid or 0.5 g of solid or semisolid is applied to the test site. Separate animals are not required for an untreated control group. Adjacent areas of untreated skin of each animal serve as control for the test.

Observation period. The duration of the observation period should not be fixed rigidly but should be sufficient to evaluate fully the reversibility or irreversibility of the effects observed. It need not normally exceed 14 days after application.

Procedure

The test substance should be applied to a small area (approximately 6 cm^2) of skin and covered with a gauze patch; which is held in place with nonirritating tape. In the case of liquids or some pastes it may be necessary to apply the test substance to the gauze patch and then apply that to the skin. The patch should be loosely held in contact with the skin by means of a suitable semi-occlusive dressing for the duration of the exposure period. However, the use of occlusive dressing may be considered appropriate in some cases. Access by the animal to the patch and resultant ingestion/inhalation of the test substance should be prevented.

Exposure duration is four hours. Longer exposures may be indicated under certain conditions, e.g., expected pattern of human use and exposure. At the end of the exposure period, residual test substance should be removed, where practicable, using water or an appropriate solvent, without altering the existing response or the integrity of the epidermis.

Clinical Observations and Scoring

Animals should be examined for signs of erythema and oedema and the responses scored at 30–60 minutes, and then at 24, 48, and 72 hours after patch removal.

Dermal irritation is scored and recorded according to the grades in Table 1. Further observations may be needed, as necessary, to establish reversibility. In addition to the observation of irritation, any serious lesions and other toxic effects should be fully described.

Data and Reporting

Treatment of Results

Data may be summarised in tabular form, showing for each individual animal the irritation scores for erythema and oedema at 30–60 minutes, 24, 48, and 72 hours after patch removal, any serious lesions, a description of the degree and nature of irritation, corrosion or reversibility, and any other toxic effects observed.

Evaluation of Results

The dermal irritation scores should be evaluated in conjunction with the nature and reversibility or otherwise of the responses observed. The individual scores do not represent an absolute standard for the irritant properties of a material, and they should be viewed as reference values which are only meaningful when supported by a full description and evaluation of the observation(s). The use of an occlusive dressing is a severe test and the results are relevant to very few likely human exposure conditions.

TABLE 1 Evaluation of Skin Reaction

Reaction	Value
Erythema and eschar formation	
No erythema	0
Very slight erythema (barely perceptible)	1
Well-defined erythema	2
Moderate to severe erythema	3
Severe erythema (beet redness) to slight eschar formation	
(injuries in depth)	4
Maximum possible	4
Oedema formation	
No oedema	0
Very slight oedema (barely perceptible)	1
Slight oedema (edges of area well defined by definite raising)	2
Moderate oedema (raised approximately 1 millimetre)	3
Severe oedema (raised more than 1 millimetre and extending	
beyond area of exposure)	4
Maximum possible	4

Test Report

The test report must include the following information:

- Species/strain used
- Physical nature and, where appropriate, concentration and pH value for the test substance
- Tabulation of irritation response data for each individual animal for each observation time period (e.g., 30-60 minutes, 24, 48, and 72 hours after patch removal)
- Description of any serious lesions observed
- Narrative description of the degree and nature of irritation observed
- Description of any toxic effects other than dermal irritation

Interpretation of the Results

Extrapolation of the results of dermal irritancy/corrosivity studies in animals to man is valid only to a limited degree. The albino rabbit is more sensitive than man to irritant substances in most cases. The finding of similar results in tests on other animal species may give more weight to extrapolation from animal studies to man.

Literature

(1) WHO Publication: Environmental Health Criteria 6, *Principles and Methods for Evaluating the Toxicity of Chemicals.* Part II, (in preparation).

(2) United States National Academy of Sciences, Committee for the

Review of NAS Publication 1138, *Principles and Procedures for Evaluating the Toxicity of Household Substances,* Washington, 1977.

(3) Draize, J. H., Woodward, G. and Calvery, H. O., *J. Pharmacol. Exp. Ther.,* 83, 377-390, 1944.

(4) Draize, J. H. *The Appraisal of Chemicals in Foods, Drugs, and Cosmetics,* pp. 46-48. Association of Food and Drug Officials of the United States, Austin, Texas, 1959.

(5) *Advances in Modern Toxicology,* Vol. 4, Dermato-Toxicology and Pharmacology, (Eds. Marzulli, F. N. and Maibach, H. I.), Hemisphere Publ. Co., Washington-London, 1977.

(6) Draize, J. H. *Appraisal of the Safety of Chemicals in Foods, Drugs and Cosmetics:* pp. 46-59. Assoc. of Food and Drug Officials of the United States, Topeka, Kansas, 1965.

ACUTE EYE IRRITATION/CORROSION
(GUIDELINE #405)[1]

Introductory Information

Prerequisites

- Solid or liquid test substance
- Chemical identification of test substance
- Purity (impurities) of test substance
- Solubility characteristics
- pH (where appropriate)
- Melting point/boiling point

Standard Documents

There are no relevant international standards.

Method

Introduction, Purpose, Scope, Relevance, Application and Limits of Test

In the assessment and evaluation of the toxic characteristics of a substance, determination of the irritant and/or corrosive effects on eyes of mammals is an important initial step. Information derived from this test serves to indicate the existence of possible hazards likely to arise from exposure of the eyes and associated mucous membranes to the test substance.

Definitions

Eye irritation is the production of reversible changes in the eye following the application of a test substance to the anterior surface of the eye.

Eye corrosion is the production of irreversible tissue damage in the eye following application of a test substance to the anterior surface of the eye.

Principle of the Test Method

The substance to be tested is applied in a single dose to one of the eyes in each of several experimental animals; the untreated eye is used to provide

[1] Adopted May 12, 1981. Users of this Test Guideline should consult the Preface, in particular paragraphs 3, 4, 7, and 8.

control information. The degree of irritation/corrosion is evaluated and scored at specific intervals and is further described to provide a complete evaluation of the effects. The duration of the study should be sufficient to evaluate fully the reversibility or irreversibility of the effects observed.

Description of the Test Procedure

Preparations

Both eyes of each experimental animal provisionally selected for testing should be examined within 24 hours before testing starts. Animals showing eye irritation, ocular defects or pre-existing corneal injury should not be used.

Strongly acidic or alkaline substances, for example with a demonstrated pH of 2 or less or 11.5 or greater, need not be tested owing to their probable corrosive properties.

Materials which have demonstrated definite corrosion or severe irritation in a dermal study need not be further tested for eye irritation. It may be presumed such substances will produce similarly severe effects in the eyes.

Experimental Animals

Selection of species. A variety of experimental animals have been used, but it is recommended that testing should be performed using healthy adult albino rabbits.

Number of animals. At least 3 animals should be used. Additional animals may be required to clarify equivocal responses.

Housing and feeding conditions. Animals should be individually housed. The temperature of the experimental animal room should be 22°C (±3°) for rodents, 20°C (±3°) for rabbits, and the relative humidity 30 to 70 per cent. Where the lighting is artificial, the sequence should be 12 hours light, 12 hours dark. Conventional laboratory diets are suitable for feeding and an unrestricted supply of drinking water should be available.

Test Conditions

Dose level. For testing liquids, a dose of 0.1 ml is used. In testing solids, pastes, and particulate substances, the amount used should have a volume of 0.1 ml, or a weight of not more than 100 mg (the weight must always be recorded). If the test material is solid or granular it should be ground to a fine dust. The volume of particulates should be measured after gently compacting them, e.g., by tapping the measuring container. To test a substance contained in a pressurised aerosol container the eye should be held open and the test substance administered in a single burst of about one second from a distance of 10 cm directly in front of the eye. The dose may be estimated by weighing the container before and after use. Care should be taken not to damage the eye. Pump sprays should not be used but instead the liquid should be expelled and 0.1 ml collected and instilled into the eye as described for liquids.

Observation period. The duration of the observation period should not be fixed rigidly but should be sufficient to evaluate fully the reversibility or irreversibility of the effects observed. It normally need not exceed 21 days after instillation.

Procedure

The test substance should be placed in the conjunctival sac of one eye of each animal after gently pulling the lower lid away from the eyeball. The lids are then gently held together for about one second in order to prevent loss of the material. The other eye, which remains untreated, serves as a control. If it is thought that the substance could cause extreme pain, a local anaesthetic may be used prior to instillation of the test substance. The type and concentration of the local anaesthetic should be carefully selected to ensure that no significant differences in reaction to the test substance will result from its use. The control eye should be similarly anaesthetised.

The eyes of the test animals should not be washed out for 24 hours following instillation of the test substance. At 24 hours a washout may be used if considered appropriate.

For some substances shown to be irritating by this test, additional tests using rabbits with eyes washed soon after instillation of the substance may be indicated. In these cases it is recommended that 6 rabbits be used. Four seconds after instillation of the test substance, the eyes of 3 rabbits are washed, and 30 seconds after instillation the eyes of the other 3 rabbits are washed. For both groups, the eyes are washed for 5 minutes using a volume and velocity of flow which will not cause injury.

Clinical Observations and Scoring

The eyes should be examined at 1, 24, 48, and 72 hours. If there is no evidence of irritation' at 72 hours the study may be ended. Extended observation may be necessary if there is persistent corneal involvement or other ocular irritation in order to determine the progress of the lesions and their reversibility or irreversibility. In addition to the observations of the cornea, iris and conjunctivae, any other lesions which are noted should be recorded and reported. The grades of ocular reaction (Table 1) should be recorded at each examination.

Examination of reactions can be facilitated by use of a binocular loupe, hand slit-lamp, biomicroscope, or other suitable devices. After recording the observations at 24 hours, the eyes of any or all rabbits may be further examined with the aid of fluoroscein.

The grading of ocular responses is subject to various interpretations. To promote harmonization and to assist testing laboratories and those involved in making and interpreting the observations an illustrated guide in grading eye irritation should be used. (Such an illustrated guide is in use in the United

TABLE 1   Grades for Ocular Lesions

Lesions	Grade
Cornea	
Opacity: degree of density (area most dense taken for reading).	
No ulceration or opacity	0
Scattered or diffuse areas of opacity (other than slight dulling of normal lustre), details of iris clearly visible	1^a
Easily discernible translucent area, details of iris slightly obscured	2^a
Nacrous area, no details of iris visible, size of pupil barely discernible	3^a
Opaque cornea, iris not discernible through the opacity	4^a
Conjunctivae	
Redness (refers to palpebral and bulbar conjunctivae, cornea, and iris).	
Blood vessels normal	0
Some blood vessels definitely hyperaemic (injected)	1
Diffuse, crimson colour, individual vessels not easily discernible	2^a
Diffuse beefy red	3^a
Chemosis: lids and/or nictating membranes	
No swelling	0
Any swelling above normal (includes nictating membranes)	1
Obvious swelling with partial eversion of lids	2^a
Swelling with lids about half closed	3^a
Swelling with lids more than half closed	4^a
Iris	
Normal	0
Markedly deepened rugae, congestion, swelling, moderate circumcorneal hyperaemia, or injection, any of these or combination of any thereof, iris still reacting to light (sluggish reaction is positive)	1^a
No reaction to light, haemorrhage, gross destruction (any or all of these)	2^a

^{a}Indicates positive effect.

States and can be obtained from the Consumer Product Safety Commission, Washington, D.C.)

Data and Reporting

Treatment of Results

Data may be summarised in tabular form, showing for each individual animal the irritation scores at the designated observation time; a description of the degree and nature of irritation; the presence of serious lesions and any effects other than ocular which were observed.

Evaluation of the Results

The ocular irritation scores should be evaluated in conjunction with the nature and reversibility or otherwise of the responses observed. The individual scores do not represent an absolute standard for the irritant properties of a material. They should be viewed as reference values and are only meaningful when supported by a full description and evaluation of the observations.

Test Report

The test report should include the following information:

- Species/strain used
- Physical nature and, where applicable, concentration and pH value for the test substance
- Tabulation of irritant/corrosive response data for each individual animal at each observation time (e.g., 1, 24, 48 and 72 hours)
- Description of any serious lesions observed
- Narrative description of the degree and nature of irritation or corrosion observed
- Description of the method used to score the irritation at 1, 24, 48 and 72 hours (e.g., hand slit-lamp, biomicroscope, fluorescein)
- Description of any non-ocular topical effects noted

Interpretation of the Results

Extrapolation of the results of eye irritation studies in animals to man is valid only to a limited degree. The albino rabbit is more sensitive than man to ocular irritants or corrosives in most cases. Similar results in tests on other animal species can give more weight to extrapolation from animal studies to man.

Care should be taken in the interpretation of data to exclude irritation resulting from secondary infection.

Literature

(1) WHO Publication: Environmental Health Criteria 6, *Principles and Methods for Evaluating the Toxicity of Chemicals.* Part II, (in preparation).

(2) United States National Academy of Sciences, Committee for the Revision of NAS Publication 1138, *Principles and Procedures for Evaluating the Toxicity of Household Substances,* Washington, 1977.

(3) Draize, J. H., Woodward, G. and Calvery, H. O., *J. Pharmacol. Exp. Ther.,* 83, 377-390, 1944.

(4) Draize, J. H. *Appraisal of the Safety of Chemicals in Foods, Drugs, and Cosmetics–Dermal Toxicity,* pp. 49-52. Assoc. of Food and Drug Officials of the United States, Topeka, Kansas, 1965.

(5) Draize, J. H. *The Appraisal of Chemicals in Foods, Drugs and Cosmetics,* pp. 36-45. Association of Food and Drug Officials of the United States, Austin, Texas, 1965.

(6) United States Federal Hazardous Substances Act Regulations. Title 16, Code of Federal Regulations, 38 FR 27012, Sept. 27, 1973; 38 FR 30105, Nov. 1, 1973.

(7) Loomis, T. A. *Essentials of Toxicology,* 2d ed., pp. 207-213. Lea & Febiger, Philadelphia, 1974.

SKIN SENSITISATION
(GUIDELINE #406)[1]

Introductory Information

Prerequisites

- Solid or liquid test substance
- Chemical identification of test substance
- Purity (impurities) of test substance
- Solubility characteristics
- pH (where appropriate)
- Melting point/boiling point

Standard Documents

There are no relevant international standards.

Method

Introduction, Purpose, Scope, Relevance, Application and Limits of Test

In the assessment and evaluation of the toxic characteristics of a substance, determination of its potential to provoke skin sensitisation reactions is important. Information derived from tests for the skin sensitisation serves to identify the possible hazard to a population repeatedly exposed to the substance.

While the desirability of this type of safety evaluation is recognised, there are some real differences of opinion about the best method of testing for skin sensitising properties of a new substance. The test selected should be a reliable screening procedure which should not fail to identify substances with significant allergenic potential, while at the same time avoiding false negative results.

Definitions

Skin sensitisation (allergic contact dermatitis) is an immunologically mediated cutaneous reaction to a substance. In the human, the responses may

---

[1] Adopted May 12, 1981. Users of this Test Guideline should consult the Preface, in particular paragraphs 3, 4, 7, and 8.

be characterised by pruritis, erythema, oedema, papules, vesicles, bullae or a combination of these. In other species the reactions may differ and only erythema and oedema may be seen.

Induction period. A period of at least one week following a sensitisation exposure during which a hypersensitive state is developed.

Induction exposure. An experimental exposure of a subject to a test substance with the intention of inducing a hypersensitive state.

Challenge exposure. An experimental exposure of a previously treated subject to a test substance following an induction period, to determine if the subject will react in a hypersensitive manner.

Principle of the Test Method

Following initial exposure(s) to a test substance, the animals are subsequently subjected, after a period of not less than one week, to a challenge exposure with the test substance to establish whether a hypersensitive state has been induced. Sensitisation is determined by examining the reaction to the challenge exposure.

Description of the Test Procedure

Any of the following seven methods is considered to be acceptable. However, it is realised that the methods differ in their probability and degree of reaction to sensitising substances. Periodic use of a positive control substance with an acceptable level of response in test animals is recommended to assess the reliability of a test system.

- Draise Test
- Freund's Complete Adjuvant Test
- Guinea Pig Maximisation Test
- Split Adjuvant Technique
- Buehler Test
- Open Epicutaneous Test
- Mauer Optimisation Test

An additional method which has not, however, been widely used is described in the Annex.

Preparations

Healthy young adult animals are acclimatised to the laboratory conditions for at least 5 days prior to the test. Before the test, animals are randomised and assigned to the treatment groups. Removal of hair is by clipping, shaving or possibly by chemical depilation, depending on the test method used.

Experimental Animals

Selection of species. The guinea pig is the generally recommended species. If other species are used this should be justified.

Number and sex. The number and sex of animals used will depend on the method employed. If females are used, they should be nulliparous and non-pregnant. Animals may act as their own controls or groups if induced animals can be compared to groups which have received only a challenge exposure.

Housing and feeding conditions. The temperature of the experimental animal room should be 22°C (±3°) and the relative humidity 30-70 per cent. Where the lighting is artificial, the sequence should be 12 hours light, 12 hours dark. For feeding, conventional laboratory diets may be used with an unlimited supply of drinking water. It is essential that guinea pigs receive an adequate amount of ascorbic acid.

Test Conditions

Dose levels. Depending on the method, the concentration used should produce skin reaction following the induction exposure and should be non-irritating following the challenge exposure. These concentrations can be determined by a small scale (2 or 3 animals) pilot study. The use of a control group is recommended.

Observation period. Skin reactions should be recorded 24 hours and 48 hours after the pertinent exposures. These exposures will vary depending on the method used.

Procedures

The principle features of the seven methods mentioned above are given in Table 1.

Data and Reporting

Treatment of Results

Data may be summarised in tabular form, showing for each individual animal the skin reaction results of the induction exposure(s) at 1 and 24 hours, and the challenge exposure(s) at 24 and 48 hours after exposure. As a minimum, the erythema and oedema should be graded. Any unusual finding should be recorded.

Evaluation of the Results

Evaluation of the results will provide information on the proportion of each group that became sensitised and the extent (slight, moderate, severe) of the sensitisation reaction in each individual animal.

Test Report

The test report should contain the following information:

- A description of the method used (and commonly accepted name)
- Species/strain used

TABLE 1 Principal Features of Test Methods

	Draize	Freund's complete adjuvant (FCA)	Mauer optimisation	Buehler	Open epicutaneous test	Maximisation	Split adjuvant
Species	Guinea pig	Guinea pig	Guinea pig	Guinea pig	Guinea pig	Guinea pig	Guinea pig
Route	id[a]	id	id	ec[b]	ec	id and ec	id and ec
Number in test group	20	8–10	10–10	10–20	6–8	20–25	10–20
Number of test group	1	1	1	1	up to 6	1	1
Number in control group	20	8–10	10–10	10–20	6–8	20–25	10–20
Induction exposure route	id	id	id	dermal	dermal	id and dermal	id and dermal
Number of exposures	10	5	9	3	20 or 21	1 id, 1 dermal	4
Exposure period	—	—	24 hr	6 hr each	continuous	48 hr	48 hr each
Patch type	—	—	—	closed	open	closed	closed
Test group(s)	TS	TS in FCA	TS in FCA	TS	TS	TS, TS + FCA, FCA	TS
Control group	—	FCA only	—	—	vehicle (v) only	FCA, FCA + V, V	—
Site	L. flank	R. flank	Back	L. flank	R. flank	shoulder	shoulder
Frequency	every 2nd day	every 2nd day	every other day	every 7 days	daily	0 (id), 7d (dermal)	0, 2, 4, 7d
Duration	0–18d	0–8d	0–21d	0–14d	0–20d	0–7d	0–7d
Concentration	2–10 times that of first	same throughout	0.1 ml of 0.1%	same throughout	same per group different between groups	—	same throughout
Challenge exposure route	id	dermal	id	dermal	dermal	dermal	dermal
Number of exposure		2	2	1	2	1	1
Day(s)	35	22 & 35	14 & 28	28	21 & 35	21	20
Exposure period	—	—	24 hr	6 hr	—	24 hr	24 hr
Patch type	—	open	—	closed	open	closed	closed
Test group(s)	TS	TS	TS	TS	TS	TS	TS
Control group	TS	TS	TS	TS	TS	TS	TS
Site	R. flank	L. flank	back, new site	R. flank	L. flank	L. flank TS R. flank vehicle	shoulder
Concentration	same as first	4 different	0.1 ml of 0.1%	same as induction	4 different	same as 2nd induction	half induction
Evaluation (hr after challenge)	24, 48	24, 48, 72	24 hr	24, 48	24, 48 and/ or 72	24, 48	24, 48
Reference	(2)	(3)	(7)	(4)	(3)	(5)	(6)

[a] Intradermal.
[b] Epicutaneous.

- The number and sex of the animals
- Individual weights of the animals at the start of the test
- Individual weights of the animals at the conclusion of the test
- A brief description of the grading system
- Each reading made on each individual animal

Interpretation of the Results

The test results should provide an estimate of the overall sensitisation potential of the test substance, i.e., essentially a non-sensitiser, a weak sensitiser, a moderate sensitiser, or a potent sensitiser.

A skin sensitisation study thus provides an assessment of whether or not a test substance could be a likely sensitiser. Extrapolation of these results to man is valid only to a very limited degree. The only generalisation that can be made is that substances which are strong sensitisers in guinea pigs also cause a substantial number of sensitisation reactions in man, whereas weak sensitisers in guinea pigs may or may not cause reactions in man.

Literature

(1) Klecak, G., Chapter 9 in *Advances in Modern Toxicology,* Vol. 4, *Dermatology and Pharmacology* (eds. Marzulli, F. N. and Maibach, H.), publ.: Hemisphere Publishing Corporation, Washington and London, 1977.

(2) Draize, J. H., Food Drug Cosmets. Law J., 10, 722, 1955.

(3) Klecak, G. et al., *J. Soc. Cosm. Chem.,* 28, 53, 1977.

(4) Buehler, E. V., *Toxicol. Appl. Pharmacol.* 6, 341, 1964, also *Arch. Dermatol.* 91, 171, 1965.

(5) Magnusson, B. and Kligman, A. M., *J. Invest. Dermatol.,* 52, 268, 1969; also *Allergic Contact Dermatitis in the Guinea Pig,* publ. Thomas, Springfield, Illinois, 1970.

(6) Maguire, A. C., Immunol. Commun., 1973, 1, 239, *J. Soc. Cosm. Chem.* 24, 151, 1973; also *Animal Models in Dermatology,* (ed. Maibach), publ. Churchill Livingstone, Edinburgh, 1975.

(7) Mauer, T. et al., *Agents and Actions,* 5, 174–179, 1975; also *Int. Cong. Series Excerpts Medica* No. 376.203, 1975.

Annex to Skin Sensitisation Test

Introductory Information

Prerequisites

- Solid or liquid test substance
- Chemical identification of test substance
- Purity (impurities) of test substance
- Solubility characteristics
- pH (where appropriate)
- Melting point/boiling point

Standard Documents

There are no relevant international standards.

Method

Skin sensitisation (allergic contact dermatitis) is a condition occurring in man and some other animals in which skin reactions are exacerbated after two or more exposures to sensitising materials.

Footpad Technique for Evaluating
Sensitisation Potential in Guinea Pigs

A 1.0 per cent mixture (w/v) of the test material is prepared in Freund's Complete Adjuvant (FCA) and stirred gently at room temperature for three hours.

After being allowed to settle for a few minutes, 0.05 ml of the mixture is injected into the front footpad of ten white guinea pigs which have not previously been exposed to test materials by any route.

One week later the test material is dissolved at a concentration of 1.0 per cent in a solvent system of guinea pig fat[2]:dioxane:acetone, 1:2:7. Each previously injected animal is challenged by dropping 0.3 ml on the clipped (not depilated) skin of the lower back. (If a 1.0 per cent solution produces moderate irritation, an 0.1 per cent solution is used.)

An equal number of control guinea pigs which have not been previously exposed to test material, but were injected with FCA, are challenged in an identical manner.

Twenty-four hours after the "drop on" exposure, the stubble of the exposed area is removed with a suitable depilatory[3] followed by a wash with warm (approximately 37°C) tap water.

[2] Method of Preparing Guinea Pig Fat: Any method that produces clean guinea pig fat should be suitable. The following method has consistently provided an adequate product.
1. Strip fat from large, preferably obese, guinea pigs.
2. Freeze.
3. Grind frozen fat with a kitchen-style meat grinder.
4. Add acetone to ground fat (approximately 10:1, acetone:fat). Stir well and heat by placing flask in a hot water bath.
5. Filter (Whatman No. 4 paper or similar, through a Buchner funnel).
6. Add and stir with Norite—warmed.
7. Filter through Whatman No. 4 and Super Cel, pour into beaker.
8. Freeze, fat will solidify on bottom of beaker.
9. Decant acetone and discard.
10. Gently warm fat and vacuum distill off acetone.
11. Pour warmed fat into vials of a size which allow use of one vial per group of sensitisations.
12. Freeze all vials and use as needed. Frozen fat will remain acceptable for at least one year.

[3] Depilatory: Any depilatory can, if misused, cause serious skin burns and death and therefore should be handled and used correctly. The following depilatory is preferred

Approximately three hours after depilation, the challenged skin site is scored under uniform fluorescent lighting for irritation (erythema and oedema) compared to untreated skin areas.

The grading of redness is as follows: 0 = normal; 1 = slight, just detectable; 2 = moderate, easily seen; 3 = definite deep red, usually hot, not haemorrhagic; 4 = dark red, may show haemorrhagic areas, usually accompanied by marked swelling and increase in temperature of the skin.

The degree of swelling of the skin is determined by picking up a fold of skin about 1 cm in length, feeling it between thumb and forefinger, and grading as follows: 0 = normal; 1 = slight, just detectable; 2 = moderate, easily felt; 3 = marked, difficult to pick up a fold of skin, often visible without feeling the skin.

The total irritation score for each animal equals the sum of redness and swelling and ranges from zero for no irritation to seven for severe irritation.

The exposed skin sites are again graded 24 hours later (48 hours after the "drop on").

The difference between the control guinea pigs (primary irritation) and the injected guinea pigs (sensitisation response) is considered to be a measure of the degree of skin sensitisation.

---

because of easy handling and excellent results: 6 parts soluble starch, 6 parts talc, 6 parts barium sulphide, 2.7 parts of a granular nonirritant anionic surfactant.

Add the parts in the order listed and mix well. Add cold water to make a viscous paste. Apply to the clipped skin of guinea pigs and allow to remain for about four minutes. Rinse off all traces of depilatory.

REPEATED DOSE DERMAL TOXICITY: 21/28-DAY STUDY (GUIDELINE #410)[1]

Introductory Information

Prerequisites

- Solid or liquid test substance
- Chemical identification of test substance
- Purity (impurities) of test substance
- Solubility characteristics
- pH (where appropriate)
- Stability, including stability in vehicle when so applied
- Melting point/boiling point

Standard Documents

There are no relevant international standards.

Method

Introduction, Purpose, Scope, Relevance, Application and Limits of Test

In the assessment and evaluation of the toxic characteristics of a chemical the determination of subchronic dermal toxicity may be carried out after initial information on toxicity has been obtained by acute testing. It provides information on possible health hazards likely to arise from repeated exposures by the dermal route over a limited period of time.

There is sufficient similarity between the considerations involved in the conduct of a 21-day or 28-day repeated dose dermal study to allow one Guideline to cover both test durations. The main difference lies in the time over which dosing takes place (indicated in the text).

Definitions

Dose in a dermal test is the amount of test substance applied to the skin. Dose is expressed as weight (g, mg) or as weight of test substance per unit weight of test animal (e.g., mg/kg).

[1] Adopted May 12, 1981. Users of this Test Guideline should consult the Preface, in particular paragraphs 3, 4, 7, and 8.

No-effect level/No-toxic-effect level/No-adverse-effect level is the maximum dose used in a test which produces no adverse effects. A no-effect level is expressed in terms of the weight of a substance given daily per unit weight of test animal (mg/kg).

Cumulative toxicity is the adverse effects of repeated doses occurring as a result of prolonged action on, or increased concentration of the administered substance or its metabolites in, susceptible tissues.

Principle of the Test Method

The test substance is applied daily to the skin in graduated doses to several groups of experimental animals, one dose per group, for a period of 21/28 days. During the period of application the animals are observed daily to detect signs of toxicity. Animals which die during the test are necropsied, and at the conclusion of the test the surviving animals are sacrificed and necropsied.

Description of the Test Procedure

Preparations

Healthy young adult animals are acclimatised to the laboratory conditions for at least 5 days prior to the test. Before the test, animals are randomised and assigned to the treatment and control groups. Shortly before testing fur is clipped from the dorsal area of the trunk of the test animals. Shaving may be employed but it should be carried out approximately 24 hours before the test. Repeat clipping or shaving is usually needed at approximately weekly intervals. When clipping or shaving the fur care must be taken to avoid abrading the skin, which could alter its permeability, unless a requirement for abraded skin is part of the test design. Not less than 10 per cent of the body surface area should be clear for the application of the test substance. The weight of the animal should be taken into account when deciding on the area to be cleared and on the dimensions of the covering. When testing solids, which may be pulverised if appropriate, the test substance should be moistened sufficiently with water or, where necessary, a suitable vehicle to ensure good contact with the skin. When a vehicle is used, the influence of the vehicle on penetration of skin by the test substance should be taken into account. Liquid test substances are generally used undiluted.

Experimental Animals

Selection of species. The adult rat, rabbit, or guinea pig may be used. Other species may be used but their use would require justification.

The following weight ranges at the start of the test are suggested in order to provide animals of a size which facilitates the conduct of the test: rats, 200 to 300 g; rabbits, 2.0 to 3.0 kg; guinea pigs, 350 to 450 g.

Where a repeated dose dermal study is conducted as a preliminary to a long term study, the same species and strain should be used in both studies.

Number and sex. At least 10 animals (5 female and 5 male) with healthy skin should be used at each dose level. The females should be nulliparous and non-pregnant. If interim sacrifices are planned the number should be increased by the number of animals scheduled to be sacrificed before the completion of the study. In addition, a satellite group of 10 animals (5 animals per sex) may be treated with the high dose level for 21/28 days and observed for reversibility, persistence, or delayed occurrence of toxic effects for 14 days post-treatment.

Housing and feeding conditions. Animals should be caged individually. The temperature in the experimental animal room should be 22°C (±3°) for rodents or 20°C (±3°) for rabbits and the relative humidity 30–70 per cent. When the lighting is artificial, the sequence should be 12 hours light, 12 hours dark. For feeding, conventional laboratory diets may be used with an unlimited supply of drinking water.

Test Conditions

Dose levels. At least three dose levels, with a control and, where appropriate, a vehicle control, should be used. Except for treatment with the test substances, animals in the control group should be handled in an identical manner to the test group subjects. The highest dose level should result in toxic effects but not produce an incidence of fatalities which would prevent a meaningful evaluation. The lowest dose level should not produce any evidence of toxicity. Where there is a usable estimation of human exposure the lowest level should exceed this. Ideally, the intermediate dose level(s) should produce minimal observable toxic effects. If more than one intermediate dose is used the dose levels should be spaced to produce a gradation of toxic effects. In the low and intermediate groups and in the controls the incidence of fatalities should be low, in order to permit a meaningful evaluation of the results.

If application of the test substance produces severe skin irritation, the concentration may be reduced although this may result in a reduction in, or absence of, other toxic effects at the high dose level. However, if the skin has been badly damaged early in the study it may be necessary to terminate the study and undertake a new study at lower concentrations.

Limit test. If a test at one dose level of at least 1000 mg/kg body weight (but expected human exposure may indicate the need for a higher dose level), using the procedures described for this study, produces no observable toxic effects and if toxicity would not be expected based upon data from structurally related compounds, then a full study using three dose levels may not be considered necessary.

Observations. A careful clinical examination should be made at least once each day. Additional observations should be made daily with appropriate actions taken to minimise loss of animals to the study, e.g., necropsy or refrigeration of those animals found dead and isolation or sacrifice of weak or moribund animals.

Procedure

The animals are treated with the test substance, ideally for at least 6 hours per day on a 7-day per week basis, for a period of 21/28 days. However, based primarily on practical considerations, application on a 5-day per week basis is considered to be acceptable. Animals in a satellite group scheduled for follow-up observations should be kept for a further 14 days without treatment to detect recovery from, or persistence of, toxic effects.

The test substance should be applied uniformly over an area which is approximately 10 per cent of the total body surface area. With highly toxic substances the surface area covered may be less but as much of the area should be covered with as thin and uniform a film as possible.

Between applications the test substance is held in contact with the skin with a porous gauze dressing and non-irritating tape. The test site should be further covered in a suitable manner to retain the gauze dressing and test substance and ensure that the animals cannot ingest the test substance. Restrainers may be used to prevent ingestion of the test substance but complete immobilisation is not a recommended method.

Signs of toxicity should be recorded as they are observed including the time of onset, the degree and duration. Cage-side observations should include, but not be limited to, changes in skin and fur, eyes and mucous membranes and also respiratory, circulatory, autonomic and central nervous system, somatomotor activity and behaviour pattern. Measurements should be made of food consumption weekly and the animals weighed weekly. Regular observation of the animals is necessary to ensure that animals are not lost from the study due to causes such as cannibalism, autolysis of tissues or misplacement. At the end of the study period all survivors in the non-satellite treatment groups are sacrificed. Moribund animals should be removed and sacrificed when noticed.

Clinical Examinations

The following examinations should be made on all animals:

a. Haematology, including haematocrit, haemoglobin concentration, erythrocyte count, total and differential leucocyte count, and a measure of clotting potential such as clotting time, prothrombin time, thromboplastin time, or platelet count should be investigated at the end of the test period.

b. Clinical biochemistry determination on blood should be carried out at the end of the test period. Blood parameters of liver and kidney function are appropriate. The selection of specific tests will be influenced by observations on the mode of action of the substance. Suggested determinations are: calcium, phosphorus, chloride, sodium, potassium, fasting glucose (with period of fasting appropriate to the species), serum glutamic-pyruvic transaminase,[2] serum glutamic-oxaloacetic transaminase,[3] ornithine decarboxylase, gamma glutamyl transpeptidase, urea nitrogen, albumen, blood creatinine, total bilirubin and total serum protein measurements. Other determinations which may be necessary for an adequate toxicological evaluation include analyses of lipids, hormones, acid/base balance, methaemoglobin, and cholinesterase activity. Additional clinical biochemistry may be employed, where necessary, to extend the investigation of observed effects.

c. Urinalysis is not required on a routine basis, but only when there is an indication based on expected or observed toxicity.

If historical baseline data are inadequate, consideration should be given to determination of haematological and clinical biochemistry parameters before dosing commences.

Pathology

Gross necropsy. All animals in the study should be subjected to a full gross necropsy which includes examination of the external surface of the body, all orifices, and the cranial, thoracic and abdominal cavities and their contents. The liver, kidneys, adrenals and testes must be weighed wet as soon as possible after dissection to avoid drying. The following organs and tissues should be preserved in a suitable medium for possible future histopathological examination: normal and treated skin, liver, kidney and target organs, that is, those organs showing gross lesions or changes in size.

Histopathology. Histological examination should be performed on the preserved organs and tissues of the high dose group and the control group. These examinations may be extended to animals of other dosage groups, if considered necessary to investigate the changes observed in the high dose group. Animals in the satellite group should be examined histologically with particular emphasis on those organs and tissues identified as showing effects in the other treated groups.

Data and Reporting

Treatment of Results

Data may be summarised in tabular form, showing for each test group the number of animals at the start of the test, the number of animals showing lesions, the type of lesions and the percentage of animals displaying each type of lesion.

All observed results, quantitative and incidental, should be evaluated by

---

[2] Now known as serum alanine aminotransferase.
[3] Now known as serum aspartate aminotransferase.

an appropriate statistical method. Any generally accepted statistical method may be used; the statistical methods should be selected during the design of the study.

Evaluation of the Results

The findings of a repeated dose dermal toxicity study should be considered in terms of the observed toxic effects and the necropsy and histopathological findings. The evaluation will include the relationship between the dose of the test substance and the presence or absence, the incidence and severity, of abnormalities, including behavioural and clinical abnormalities, gross lesions, identified target organs, body weight changes, effects on mortality and any other general or specific toxic effects. A properly conducted 21/28-day study will provide information on the effects of repeated dermal application of a substance and can indicate the need for further longer term studies. It can also provide information on the selection of dose levels for longer term studies.

Test Report

The test report must include the following information:

- Species/strain used
- Toxic response data by sex and dose
- Time of death during the study or whether animals survived to termination
- Toxic or other effects
- The time of observation of each abnormal sign and its subsequent course
- Food and body weight data
- Haematological tests employed and results with relevant baseline data
- Clinical biochemistry tests employed and results with relevant baseline data
- Necropsy findings
- A detailed description of all histopathological findings
- Statistical treatment of results where appropriate

Interpretation of the Results

A repeated dose dermal study will provide information on the effects of repeated dermal exposure to a substance. Extrapolation from the results of the study to man is valid to a limited degree, but it can provide useful information on the degree of percutaneous absorption of a substance.

Literature

(1) WHO Publication: Environmental Health Criteria. No. 6, *Principles and Methods for Evaluating the Toxicity of Chemicals.* Part I. Geneva, 1978.

(2) United States National Academy of Sciences, Committee for the Revision of NAS Publication 1138. *Principles and Procedures for Evaluating the Toxicity of Household Substances.* Washington, 1977.

(3) Draize, J. H. *The Appraisal of Chemicals in Food, Drugs and Cosmetics,* 26–30. Association of Food and Drug Officials of the United States, Austin, Texas, 1959.

(4) Hagan, E. G., *Appraisal of the Safety of Chemicals. Appraisal of Chemicals in Foods, Drugs and Cosmetics,* 17–25. Association of Food and Drug Officials of the United States, Topeka, Kansas, 1965.

SUBCHRONIC DERMAL TOXICITY:
90–DAY STUDY
(GUIDELINE #411)[1]

Introductory Information

Prerequisites

- Solid or liquid test substance
- Chemical identification of test substance
- Purity (impurities) of test substance
- Solubility characteristics
- pH (where appropriate)
- Stability, including stability in vehicle when so applied
- Melting point/boiling point

Standard Documents

There are no relevant international standards.

Method

Introduction, Purpose, Scope,
Relevance, Application and Limits of Test

In the assessment and evaluation of the toxic characteristics of a chemical the determination of subchronic dermal toxicity may be carried out after initial information on toxicity has been obtained by acute testing. It provides information on possible health hazards likely to arise from repeated exposure by the dermal route over a limited period of time.

Definitions

Subchronic dermal toxicity is the adverse effects occurring as a result of the repeated daily dermal application of a chemical to experimental animals for part (not exceeding 10 per cent) of a life span.

Dose in a dermal test is the amount of test substance applied to the skin (applied daily in subchronic tests). Dose is expressed as weight (g, mg) or as weight of the test substance per unit weight of test animal (e.g., mg/kg).

[1] Adopted May 12, 1981. Users of this Test Guideline should consult the Preface, in particular paragraphs 3, 4, 7, and 8.

672

No-effect level/No-toxic-effect level/No-adverse-effect level is the maximum dose used in a test which produces no adverse effects. A no-effect level is expressed in terms of the weight of a substance given daily per unit weight of test animal (mg/kg).

Cumulative toxicity is the adverse effects of repeated doses occurring as a result of prolonged action on, or increased concentration of the administered substance or its metabolites in, susceptible tissue.

Principle of the Test Method

The test substance is applied daily to the skin in graduated doses to several groups of experimental animals, one dose per group, for a period of 90 days. During the period of application the animals are observed daily to detect signs of toxicity. Animals which die during the test are necropsied, and at the conclusion of the test the surviving animals are sacrificed and necropsied.

Description of the Test Procedure

Preparations

Healthy young adult animals are acclimatised to the laboratory conditions for at least 5 days prior to the test. Before the test, animals are randomised and assigned to the treatment and control groups. Shortly before testing fur is clipped from the dorsal area of the trunk of the test animals. Shaving may be employed, but it should be carried out approximately 24 hours before the test. Repeat clipping or shaving is usually needed at approximately weekly intervals. When clipping or shaving the fur care must be taken to avoid abrading the skin, which could alter its permeability. Not less than 10 per cent of the body surface area should be clear for the application of the test substance. The weight of the animal should be taken into account when deciding on the area to be cleared and on the dimensions of the covering. When testing solids, which may be pulverised if appropriate, the test substance should be moistened sufficiently with water or, where necessary, a suitable vehicle to ensure good contact with the skin. When a vehicle is used, the influence of the vehicle on penetration of skin by the test substance should be taken into account. Liquid test substances are generally used undiluted.

Experimental Animals

Selection of species. The adult rat, rabbit or guinea pig may be used. Other species may be used, but their use would require justification.

The following weight ranges at the start of the test are suggested in order to provide animals of a size which facilitates the conduct of the test: rats, 200 to 300 g; rabbits, 2.0 to 3.0 kg; guinea pigs, 350 to 450 g.

Where a subchronic dermal study is conducted as a preliminary to a long term study, the same species and strain should be used in both studies.

Number and sex. At least 20 animals (10 female and 10 male) with healthy skin should be used at each dose level. The females should be nulliparous and non-pregnant. If interim sacrifices are planned the number should be increased by the number of animals scheduled to be sacrificed before the completion of the study. A satellite group of 20 animals (10 animals per sex) may be treated with the high dose level for 90 days and observed for reversibility, persistence, or delayed occurrence, of toxic effects for a post-treatment period of appropriate length, normally not less than 28 days.

Housing and feeding conditions. Animals should be caged individually. The temperature in the experimental animal room should be 22°C (±3°) for rodents or 20°C (±3°) for rabbits and the relative humidity 30–70 per cent. When the lighting is artificial, the sequence should be 12 hours light, 12 hours dark. For feeding, conventional laboratory diets may be used with an unlimited supply of drinking water.

Test Conditions

Dose levels. At least three dose levels with a control and (where appropriate) a vehicle control should be used. Except for treatment with test substances, animals in the control group should be handled in an identical manner to the test group subjects. The highest dose level should result in toxic effects but not produce an incidence of fatalities which would prevent a meaningful evaluation. The lowest dose level should not produce any evidence of toxicity. Where there is a usable estimation of human exposure the lowest level should exceed this. Ideally, the intermediate dose level(s) should produce minimal observable toxic effects. If more than one intermediate dose is used the dose levels should be spaced to produce a gradation of toxic effects. In the low and intermediate groups and in the controls the incidence of fatalities should be low, in order to permit a meaningful evaluation of the results.

If application of the test substance produces severe skin irritation the concentration should be reduced, although this may result in a reduction in, or absence of, other toxic effects at the high dose level. However, if the skin has been badly damaged early in the study, it may be necessary to terminate the study and undertake a new study at lower concentrations.

Limit test. If a test at one dose level of at least 1000 mg/kg body weight (but expected human exposure may indicate the need for a high dose level), using the procedures described for this study, produces no observable toxic effects and if toxicity would not be expected based upon data from structurally related compounds, then a full study using three dose levels may not be considered necessary.

Observations. A careful clinical examination should be made at least once each day. Additional observations should be made daily with appropriate actions taken to minimise loss of animals to the study, e.g., necropsy or refrigeration of those animals found dead and isolation or sacrifice of weak or moribund animals.

Procedure

The animals are treated with the test substance, ideally for at least 6 hours per day on a 7-day per week basis, for a period of 90 days. However, based primarily on practical considerations, application on a 5-day per week basis is considered to be acceptable. Animals in a satellite group scheduled for follow-up observations should be kept for at least a further 28 days without treatment to detect recovery from, or persistence of, toxic effects.

The test substance should be applied uniformly over an area which is approximately 10 per cent of the total body surface area. With highly toxic substances the surface area covered may be less, but as much of the area should be covered with as thin and uniform a film as possible.

Between applications the test substance is held in contact with the skin with a porous gauze dressing and non-irritating tape. The test site should be further covered in a suitable manner to retain the gauze dressing and test substance and ensure that the animals cannot ingest the test substance. Restrainers may be used to prevent ingestion of the test substance, but complete immobilisation is not a recommended method.

Signs of toxicity should be recorded as they are observed, including the time of onset, the degree and duration. Cage-side observations should include, but not be limited to, changes in skin and fur, eyes and mucous membranes, as well as respiratory, circulatory, autonomic and central nervous system, somatomotor activity and behaviour pattern. Measurements should be made of food consumption weekly and the animals weighed weekly. Regular observation of the animals is necessary to ensure that animals are not lost from the study due to causes such as cannibalism, autolysis of tissues or misplacement. At the end of the study period all survivors in the non-satellite treatment groups are sacrificed. Moribund animals should be removed and sacrificed when noticed.

Clinical Examinations

The following examinations should be made:

a. Ophthalmological examination, using an ophthalmoscope or equivalent suitable equipment, should be made prior to exposure to the test substance and at the termination of the study, preferably in all animals but at least in the high dose and control groups. If changes in the eyes are detected all animals should be examined.

b. Haematology, including haematocrit, haemoglobin concentration, erythrocyte count, total and differential leucocyte count, and a measure of clotting potential, such as clotting time, prothrombin time, thromboplastin time, or platelet count, should be investigated at the end of the test period.

c. Clinical biochemistry determinations on blood should be carried out at the end of the test period. Test areas which are considered appropriate to all studies are electrolyte balance, carbohydrate metabolism, liver and and kidney function. The selection of specific tests will be influenced by observations on the mode of action of the substance. Suggested determinations are calcium, phosphorus, chloride, sodium, potassium, fasting glucose (with the period of fasting appropriate to the species), serum glutamicpyruvic trans-aminase,[2] serum glutamic oxaloacetic transaminase,[3] ornithine decarboxylase, gamma glutamyl transpeptidase, urea nitrogen, albumen, blood creatinine, total bilirubin and total serum protein measurements. Other determinations which may be necessary for an adequate toxicological evaluation include analyses of lipids, hor-mones, acid/base balance, methaemoglobin, cholinesterase activity. Additional clinical biochemistry may be employed, where necessary, to extend the investigation of observed effects.

d. Urinalysis is not required on a routine basis, but only when there is an indication based on expected or observed toxicity.

If historical baseline data are inadequate, consideration should be given to determination of haematological and clinical biochemistry parameters before dosing commences.

Pathology

  Gross necropsy. All animals should be subjected to a full gross necropsy which includes examination of the external surface of the body, all orifices, and the cranial, thoracic and abdominal cavities and their contents. The liver, kidneys, adrenals and testes must be weighed wet as soon as possible after dissection to avoid drying. The following organs and tissues should be preserved in a suitable medium for possible future histopathological examina-tion: all gross lesions, brain—including sections of medulla/pons, cerebellar cortex and cerebral cortex, pituitary, thyroid/parathyroid, thymus, (trachea), lungs, heart, aorta, salivary glands, liver, spleen, kidneys, adrenals, pancreas, gonads, accessory genital organs, gall bladder (if present), oesophagus, stomach, duodenum, jejunum, ileum, caecum, colon, rectum, urinary bladder, representative lymph node, (female mammary gland), (thigh musculature), peripheral nerve, (eyes), (sternum with bone marrow), (femur—including articular surface), (spinal cord at three levels—cervical, midthoracic and lumbar), and (exorbital lachrymal glands). (The tissues mentioned in paren-theses need only be examined if indicated by signs of toxicity or target organ involvement.)

  Histopathology. (a) Full histopathology should be carried out on normal and treated skin and on organs and tissues of all animals in the control and

---

[2] Now known as serum alanine aminotransferase.
[3] Now known as serum aspartate aminotransferase.

high dose groups. (b) All gross lesions should be examined. (c) Target organs in other dose groups should be examined. (d) Where rats are used lungs of animals in the low and intermediate dose groups should be subjected to histopathological examination for evidence of infection, since this provides a convenient assessment of the state of health of the animals. Further histopathological examination may not be required routinely on the animals in these groups but must always be carried out in organs which showed evidence of lesions in the high dose group. (e) When a satellite group is used histopathology should be performed on tissues and organs identified as showing effects in other treated groups.

Data and Reporting

Treatment of Results

Data may be summarised in tabular form, showing for each test group the number of animals at the start of the test, the number of animals showing lesions, the types of lesions and the percentage of animals displaying each type of lesion.

All observed results, quantitative and incidental, should be evaluated by an appropriate statistical method. Any generally accepted statistical method may be used; the statistical methods should be selected during the design of the study.

Evaluation of Results

The findings of a subchronic dermal toxicity study should be evaluated in conjunction with the findings of preceding studies and considered in terms of the observed toxic effects and the necropsy and histopathological findings. The evaluation will include the relationship between the dose of the test substance and the presence or absence, the incidence and severity, of abnormalities, including behavioural and clinical abnormalities, gross lesions, identified target organs, body weight changes, effects on mortality and any other general or specific toxic effects. A properly conducted subchronic test should provide a satisfactory estimation of a no-effect level.

Test Report

The test report must include the following information:

- Species/strain used
- Toxic response data by sex and dose
- Time of death during the study or whether animals survived to termination
- Toxic or other effects
- The time of observation of each abnormal sign and its subsequent course

- Food and body weight data
- Haematological tests employed and results with relevant baseline data
- Clinical biochemistry tests employed and results with relevant baseline data
- Necropsy findings
- A detailed description of all histopathological findings
- Statistical treatment of results where appropriate

Interpretation of the Results

A subchronic dermal study will provide information on the effects of repeated dermal exposure to a substance. Extrapolation from the results of the study to man is valid to a limited degree, but it can provide useful information on the degree of percutaneous absorption of a substance, no-effect levels and permissible human exposure.

Literature

(1) WHO Publication: Environmental Health Criteria No. 6, *Principles and Methods for Evaluating the Toxicity of Chemicals.* Part I. Geneva, 1978.

(2) United States National Academy of Sciences, Committee for the Revision of NAS Publication 1138, *Principles and Procedures for Evaluating the Toxicity of Household Substance,* Washington, 1977.

(3) Draize, J. H., *The Appraisal of Chemicals in Food, Drugs and Cosmetics,* 26–30. Association of Food and Drug Officials of the United States, Austin, Texas, 1959.

(4) Hagan, E. G., *Appraisal of the Safety of Chemicals. Appraisal of Chemicals in Foods, Drugs and Cosmetics,* 17–25. Association of Food and Drug Officials of the United States, Topeka, Kansas, 1965.

recommended guideline for acute dermal toxicity test[1]

■ **INTERAGENCY REGULATORY LIAISON GROUP** ■
(Testing Standards and Guidelines Work Group[2])

GENERAL CONSIDERATIONS

Good Laboratory Practices

Studies should be conducted according to good laboratory practice regulations (e.g., "Nonclinical Laboratory Studies, Good Laboratory Practice Regulations," 43 FR 59986, 22 December 1978).

Test Substance

1. The specific substance or mixture of substances to be tested should be determined in consultation with the responsible agency. As far as is practical, composition of the test substance should be known. Information should include the name and quantities of all major components, known contaminants and impurities, and the percentage of unidentifiable materials, if any, to account for 100% of the test sample.

2. Ideally, the lot of the substance tested should be the same throughout the study. The test sample should be stored under conditions that maintain its stability, strength, quality, and purity from the date of its production until the tests are complete.

[1] January 1981.
[2] U.S. Consumer Product Safety Commission, U.S. Environmental Protection Agency, Food and Drug Administration (U.S. Dept. of HHS), Food Safety and Quality Service (U.S. Dept. of Agriculture), Occupational Safety and Health Administration (U.S. Dept. of Labor).

Animals

1. Healthy animals, not subjected to any previous experimental procedures, must be used.
2. The test animal shall be characterized as to species, strain, sex, weight and/or age. Each animal must be assigned an appropriate identification number.
3. Recommendations contained in DHEW pub. no. (NIH) 74-23, entitled *Guide for the Care and Use of Laboratory Animals*, should be followed for the care, maintenance, and housing of animals.
4. Animals should be caged individually for this test.
5. Animals must be assigned to groups in such a manner as to minimize bias and assure comparability of pertinent variables (for example, weight variation in animals used in a test should not exceed ±20% of the mean weight).

Dead Animals, Necropsy, and Histopathology

Animals should be observed as necessary to insure that there is minimal loss due to cannibalism or management problems. Where possible, necropsy must be performed soon after an animal is sacrificed or found dead to minimize loss of tissues due to autolysis. When necropsy cannot be performed immediately, the animal must be refrigerated at temperatures low enough to minimize autolysis. If histopathological examination is to be conducted, tissue specimens should be placed in appropriate fixative when they are taken from the animal.

SPECIFIC CONSIDERATIONS

Test Preparation

Animals

The rat, rabbit or guinea pig may be used; however, the young, adult, albino rabbit weighing 2.0 to 3.0 kg is the preferred species because of its size, ease of handling and restraint, and skin permeability. If rats or guinea pigs are used, rats weighing 200 to 300 g or guinea pigs weighing 350 to 450 g are suggested. Selection of other species may be acceptable but must be justified.

Preparation of Skin

Approximately twenty-four hours before testing, fur from the back of animals should be clipped so that no less than 10% (about 240 cm²) of the total body surface area is available for application of material.

Limit Test

A trial test on abraded skin is recommended. The abraded area may be prepared by making four epidermal incisions with a clean needle through the stratum cornum (not deep enough to disturb the derma or produce bleeding), but other acceptable methods may be used. If a test at a dose of 2 g/kg body weight (or 2 ml/kg) or more, using the procedures described for this study, produces no compound related mortality, then a full study using 3 dose levels may not be necessary.

Number and Sex

Equal numbers of animals of each sex with intact skin are required for each dose level. The number of animals per dose depends on the level of statistical confidence desired. Five animals per sex per dose are recommended in most cases. Females should be nulliparous and non-pregnant.

Dose Levels

If mortality occurs in the limit test, an additional test should be conducted using rabbits with intact skin. At least three dose levels spaced appropriately to produce test groups with a range of toxic effects and mortality rates should be used.

Test Procedure

Test Substance

Liquids should be tested directly, but solid test substances should be moistened sufficiently with normal saline or tap water to make a paste that will insure good contact with the skin. For some applications, it may be appropriate or necessary to use other vehicles. If a carrier or diluent is used, it should be nonirritating and of known low toxicity. When such vehicles are used, consideration should be given to the effects of those vehicles on absorption of the test substance.

Dosage

When technically feasible, the maximum quantity of substance plus vehicle to be applied is 2 g/kg body weight. The test substance should be applied uniformly over the dorsal surface area.

Administration (Application)

The test substance must remain in contact with the skin throughout the exposure period of 24 hours. Liquid or solid substances should be held in contact with the skin with a porous gauze dressing and nonirritating tape. The test site should be covered with an impermeable material such as plastic film or rubberized cloth in a semi-occlusive fashion, allowing air to pass between the skin and the covering. Occlusive skin dressings may enhance penetration of the test substance and should be used only when testing for effects that may occur under similar conditions in humans.

During exposure, animals should be prevented from ingesting or inhaling

TABLE 1   Evaluation of Skin Reaction

	Value
Erythema and eschar formation	
No erythema	0
Very slight erythema (barely perceptible)	1
Well-defined erythema	2
Moderate to severe erythema	3
Severe erythema (deep redness to slight eschar formation, injuries in depth)	4
Oedema formation	
No oedema	0
Very slight oedema (barely perceptible)	1
Slight oedema (edges of area well-defined by definite raising)	2
Moderate oedema (raised approximately 1 mm)	3
Severe oedema (raised more than 1 mm and extending beyond area of exposure	4
Severe eschar and/or corrosion	Note occurrence

the test substance. Restrainers, such as Elizabethan collars, that permit animals to move about their cages should be used for this purpose. Immobilization is not recommended.

At the end of the exposure period, all residual material should be removed by washing, using an appropriate solvent. About one half hour later, and once again at 72 hours, the exposed area should be examined, and all lesions noted and graded (Table 1).

Observation Period

The observation period must be at least 14 days. Although a 14-day observation period is sufficient for most compounds, animals demonstrating visible signs of toxicity at 14 days may be held together.

Clinical Observations

A careful clinical observation of each animal should be made at least once a day. Additional observations should be made daily with appropriate actions taken to minimize loss of animals to the study, e.g., necropsy or refrigeration of those animals found dead and isolation or sacrifice of weak or moribund animals. All toxicological and pharmacological signs should be recorded including time of onset, intensity, and duration. The time of death should also be noted. Individual records should be maintained for each animal.

Weight Change

Animals must be weighed individually on the day the test substance is administered, weekly thereafter, and at death or sacrifice.

Necropsy

A complete gross necropsy should be performed on all animals that die during the course of the test. Consideration should be given to gross necropsy of the animals sacrificed at termination of the test. Microscopic examination of gross lesions should also be considered. If the substance will not be subjected to additional acute or multiple dose testing that includes gross necropsy, or if the results of this test are to be used for labelling purposes. complete gross necropsy should be performed on all remaining animals at termination of the test.

DATA REPORTING

Identification

Each test report should be signed by the persons responsible for the test and identify:

1. The laboratory where the test was performed by name and address;
2. The inclusive dates of the test; and
3. Each person primarily responsible for separate components of the test including (a) the conduct of the test, (b) pathology, (c) analysis of the data, (d) the writing of the report, and (e) any written or other matter contained in the report.

Body of Report

The test report must include all information necessary to provide a complete and accurate description and evaluation of the test procedures and results, in the following sections:

1. Summary and conclusions: This section of the test report should contain a brief description of the methods, a summary of the data, an analysis of the data, and a statement of the conclusions drawn. The summary must highlight all positive data or observations and any deviations from control data which may be indicative of toxic effects.
2. Materials: This section of the test report should include, but not be limited to, the following information:

   a. Identification of the test substance, so far as practical, including:

      i. chemical name, molecular structure, and a qualitative and quantitative determination of its chemical composition, including names and quantities of known contaminants and impurities and listing the percentage of unidentifiable materials to account for 100% of the test sample.

    ii. manufacturer and lot number of the substance tested, and such information as physical state, pH, stability, and purity; and

    iii. specific identification of diluents, suspending agents, emulsifiers, or other materials used in administering the test substance.

  b. Animal data, including:

    i. species and strain used and rationale for selection of the strain if other than a common laboratory strain;

    ii. source of supply of the animals;

    iii. description of any pre-test conditioning;

    iv. description of the method used in randomization of animals to test or control groups; and

    v. numbers, age, and condition of animals of each sex in each test and control group.

  c. Data on husbandry should include description of the caging conditions including number of animals per cage, diet, bedding material, ambient temperature, humidity, and lighting conditions.

3. Methods:

  a. Deviation from guidelines—This section shall indicate all ways in which the test procedure deviates from these guidelines and shall state the rationale for such deviation.

  b. Specification of test methods—This section shall include a full description of the experimental design and procedure, the length of the study, and the dates on which the study began and ended.

  c. Statistical analysis—All statistical methods used should be fully described or identified by reference.

  d. Data on dosage administration, including:

    i. all dose levels administered, expressed as mg/kg of body weight;

    ii. method and frequency of administration; and

    iii. total volume of substance (i.e., test substance plus vehicle) contained in individual dosages.

  e. Data on observation methods, including:

    i. duration; and

    ii. method and frequency of observation of the animals.

4. Results:

The tabulation of data and individual results must accompany each report in sufficient detail to permit independent evaluation of results, including summaries and tables that show, as appropriate, the relationship of effects to time of dosing, sex, etc.

SUGGESTED READING

(1) Draize, J. H. 1959. Dermal toxicity. In *Appraisal of the Safety of Chemicals in Foods, Drugs, and Cosmetics,* Austin, Texas. Association of Food and Drug Officials of the U.S. pp. 46-59.

(2) National Academy of Sciences—National Research Council, 1977. Dermal and eye toxicity tests. In *Principles and Procedures for Evaluating the Toxicity of Household Substances,* Report No. 1138, prepared for the Consumer Product Safety Commission, pp. 23-28.

(3) McCreesh, A. H. and M. Steinberg, 1977. Dermato—Toxicology and Pharmacology, Hemisphere Publishing Corp., Washington, D.C.

(4) Maibach, H. I. and F. N. Marzulli. 1975. Animal Models in Dermatology. Churchill and Livingstone, Edinburgh.

index